Radiology: Techniques and Applications

Radiology: Techniques and Applications

Editor: Samuel Price

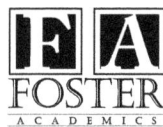

FA FOSTER
ACADEMICS

www.fosteracademics.com

www.fosteracademics.com

FA FOSTER
ACADEMICS

Cataloging-in-Publication Data

Radiology : techniques and applications / edited by Samuel Price.
    p. cm.
Includes bibliographical references and index.
ISBN 978-1-63242-911-7
1. Medical radiology. 2. Radiology. 3. Diagnostic imaging. 4. Imaging systems in medicine. I. Price, Samuel.
R895 .R33 2020
616.075 7--dc23

Foster Academics,
118-35 Queens Blvd., Suite 400,
Forest Hills, NY 11375, USA

ISBN 978-1-63242-911-7 (Hardback)

Contents

Preface

Radiology is a field concerned with the diagnosis and treatment of diseases, using medical imaging. Radiological imaging techniques include ultrasonography, X-ray radiography, nuclear medicine, computed tomography, magnetic resonance imaging, etc. Advanced imaging techniques allow the meaningful acquisition of images of the interior of the body with a high degree of accuracy. Such techniques are of immense use in neuroradiology, musculoskeletal imaging, abdomen imaging, pediatric radiology, interventional radiology, breast imaging, etc. Perfusion MRI techniques are useful for the characterization of tumors and assessment of the hemodynamic state of brain tissue. MR elastography allows examination of the viscoelastic properties of the liver. Digital subtraction angiography is the best method for the evaluation of cerebral aneurysms. This book aims to shed light on some of the unexplored aspects of radiology and the recent researches in this domain. The various studies that are constantly contributing towards advancing techniques, applications and evolution of this field are examined in detail. Scientists and students actively engaged in this field will find this book full of crucial and unexplored concepts.

Significant researches are present in this book. Intensive efforts have been employed by authors to make this book an outstanding discourse. This book contains the enlightening chapters which have been written on the basis of significant researches done by the experts.

Finally, I would also like to thank all the members involved in this book for being a team and meeting all the deadlines for the submission of their respective works. I would also like to thank my friends and family for being supportive in my efforts.

Editor

Assessment of Condylar Changes in Patients with Temporomandibular Joint Pain using Digital Volumetric Tomography

Ujwala Shivarama Shetty,[1] Krishna N. Burde,[2] Venkatesh G. Naikmasur,[2] and Atul P. Sattur[2]

[1] A J Institute of Dental Science and Hospital, Mangalore, Karnataka, India
[2] SDM College of Dental Science and Hospital, Dharwad, Karnataka, India

Correspondence should be addressed to Ujwala Shivarama Shetty; ujwalashetty@gmail.com

Academic Editor: Hans-Joachim Mentzel

Objective. To evaluate the efficiency of DVT in comparison with OPG in the assessment of bony condylar changes in patients of TMJ pain. *Methods*. 100 temporomandibular joints of 62 patients with the complaint of temporomandibular joint pain were included in the study. DVT and OPG radiographs were taken for all the 100 joints. Three observers interpreted the DVT and OPG radiograph for the bony changes separately for two times with an interval of one week. The bony changes seen in the condyle were given coding from 0 to 6. (0: Normal, 1: Erosion, 2: Flattening, 3: Osteophyte, 4: Sclerosis, 5: Resorption, and 6: other changes). Interobserver and intraobserver variability was assessed with one-way ANOVA statistics. Z test was used to see the significant difference between OPG and DVT. *Results*. In the present study the interexaminer reliability for OPG and DVT was 0.903 and 0.978, respectively. Intraexaminer reliability for OPG and DVT was 0.908 and 0.980, respectively. The most common condylar bony change seen in OPG and DVT was erosion followed by flattening and osteophyte. There was significant difference between OPG and DVT in detecting erosion and osteophytes. The other changes observed in our study were Ely's cyst, pointed condyle, and bifid condyle. All the bony changes are more commonly seen in females than males. *Conclusion*. DVT provides more valid and accurate information on condylar bony changes. The DVT has an added advantage of lesser radiation exposure to the patient and cost effectiveness and could be easily accessible in a dental hospital.

1. Introduction

Temporomandibular joint is one of the most fascinating and complex synovial systems in the body. It is the area in which the mandible articulates with the cranium [1]. The masticatory system is extremely complex, which comprises primarily of bones, muscles, ligaments, and teeth, all of which are responsible for activities like mastication, speech, and deglutition. All these movements are regulated by an intricate neurological controlling mechanism, which is important for the system to function normally and efficiently [1]. Lack of such harmony may lead to disruptive muscle behavior or structural damage to any of the components. The function of the TMJ is unique, in that the condyle both rotates within the fossa and translates anteriorly along the articular eminence. Because of the ability of the condyle to translate, the mandible can have a much higher maximal incisal opening than would be possible with rotation alone. Because of all these features, the TMJ is referred to as "ginglymodiarthrodial," which means a combination of the terms ginglymoid (rotation) and arthrodial (translation) [2].

In UK orofacial pain accounts for approximately 10% of pain in the adult population [3]. The prevalence rates of orofacial pain in the Indian population are not available. Temporomandibular disorders (TMD) is a term given to a heterogeneous group of pathologies affecting the temporomandibular joints, the masticatory muscles, or both. It is the most commonly occurring jaw disorder, with a prevalence rate of 28% to 86% of adults and adolescents showing one or more clinical signs or symptoms [4]. The etiology of the TMD is unknown. Occlusal disharmony and psychological distress are the two hypotheses which have dominated the literature. The psychological hypothesis proposes that the disorder evolves as a consequence of psychological distress that is usually due to the individual's stressful environment. The psychological distress in turn leads to parafunctional habits (tooth clenching and grinding) that result in muscle pain [5]. There are various signs and symptoms of TMJ dysfunction. It may include one or more of the following: pain in the TMJ or ear or both, headache, muscle tenderness, joint stiffness, clicking or other joint noises, reduced range of motion, locking, and subluxation [4]. TMJ imaging may be necessary to supplement information obtained from the clinical examination. It is useful particularly when an osseous abnormality or infection is suspected; conservative treatment has failed or symptoms are worsening. Screening projection used for TMJ is panoramic projection. It provides an overall view of the teeth and jaws. It also helps in identifying odontogenic diseases and other disorders that may be the source of TMJ symptoms. Specific TMJ programs are available in some of the panoramic machines. They have the disadvantage of thick image layers and the oblique, distorted view of the joint, which severely limits image quality. Hence there is a need for advanced radiographic imaging for TMJ. The main aim for TMJ imaging includes evaluation of the integrity of the structures when disease is suspected, determination of the extent of disease and its progression, and finally evaluation of the effects of treatment [6]. Recent imaging technology for TMJ is digital volumetric tomography (DVT). It was developed for angiography in 1982 and subsequently applied to maxillofacial imaging. It uses a divergent or "cone"-shaped source of ionizing radiation and a two dimensional area detector fixed on a rotating gantry to acquire multiple sequential projection images in one complete scan around the area of interest. It is only since late 1990s that it has become possible to produce clinical systems that are both inexpensive and small enough to be used in the dental office [7]. This technology has been given several names including dental volumetric tomography, cone beam volumetric tomography, cone beam computed tomography, dental computed tomography, cone beam imaging [5], and CB3D [8]. DVT provides high definition three-dimensional digital data on precise anatomical information of all oral and maxillofacial structures at reduced cost and less radiation to patient, in comparison to traditional imaging systems, which are limited by distortion, magnification changes, restricted clarity, lack of accuracy in measurements, and not allowing for 3D reconstruction. TMJ imaging poses a challenge because the bony components are small and superimpositions from the base of the skull often result in a lack of clear delineation of the joint. Different imaging modalities have been used for TMJ but they have disadvantages such as superimpositions, high radiation dose, and long scanning time present severe limitation. These disadvantages have led to an increase in popularity of the use of DVT for TMJ imaging [9].

2. Materials and Methods

62 patients who visited the Department of Oral Medicine and Radiology, SDM College of Dental Sciences and Hospital,

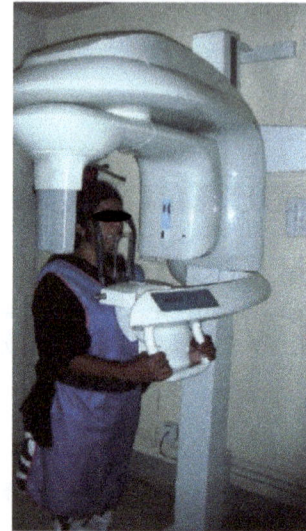

FIGURE 1: Patient positioned for DVT in Kodak 9000C 3D Extra oral imaging system.

Dharwad, with chief complaint of temporomandibular joint pain were selected for the study. Their age ranged from 15 to 72 years. A total of 100 joints were assessed in these patients. Approval from the ethical board has been obtained for this study.

Inclusion criteria are as follows:

(1) patients willing to participate in the study;

(2) patients with a complaint of chronic temporomandibular joint pain.

Exclusion criteria are as follows:

(1) systemic, rheumatic, neurologic/neuropathic, endocrine, and immune/autoimmune disease of widespread pain;

(2) TMJ pain associated with another joint pain;

(3) previous history of radiation treatment to the head and neck;

(4) previous history of TMJ surgery;

(5) previous history of trauma to jaw;

(6) pregnancy.

All the patients were subjected to conventional (OPG) and digital imaging (DVT) evaluation. KODAK 9000C 3D Extra oral imaging system (Care stream Health, Inc., 150 Verona Street, Rochester, NY 14 608) was used for obtaining both OPG and DVT images (Figures 1 and 2).

Technical specification of the machine is shown in Table 1.

2.1. Exposure Parameters

(i) Panoramic radiography is as follows: 70–74 Kv, 14.3–15.1 mAs with scan time of 13.9–15.1 seconds.

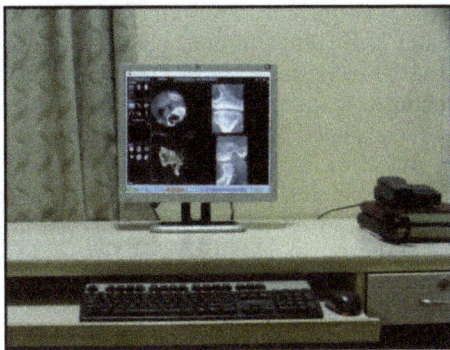

FIGURE 2: HP L1910 19-inch LCD Monitor used for interpretation of DVT and OPG images.

TABLE 1

X-ray generator	
Tube voltage	60–90 kv (max), pulsed mode for 3D modality
Tube current	2–15 mA (max)
Frequency	140 kHz (max)
Tube focal spot	0.5 mm
Total filtration	>2.5 mm eq.Al
Panoramic modality	
Technology	Digital volumetric tomography (DVT)
Sensor technology	(i) CCD
	(ii) Optical fibre sensor with Csi coating
Sensor matrix	61 × 1244 pixels
Image field	6.3 × 129.4 mm
Gray scale	16384—14 bits
Magnification	1.27
3D modality	
Technology	Digital volumetric tomography (DVT)
Sensor technology	(i) CMOS
	(ii) Optical fibre sensor with Csi coating
Gray scale	16384—14 bits
Volume size	50 × 37 mm
Voxel size	76.5 × 76.5 × 76.5 μm

(ii) Digital volumetric tomography is as follows: 70–80 kv, 10 × 10.8 mAs with a scan time of 24 seconds.

The temporomandibular joint was assessed by both panoramic and digital volumetric tomography images. In the DVT images and 200 μm tomographic sections were taken in sagittal, axial, and coronal planes. Tomographic sections were taken in the curved planar reformation (panorex), a series of multiplanar reconstructions (cross-sections) and oblique planar reformation.

2.2. Radiation Exposure to the Patient. Radiation exposure to the patient is as follows:

OPG—0.01 mSv (70–85 mGy cm^2)

DVT—1.02 mSv to 1.05 mSv (220–235 mGy cm^2)

The radiographic exposure for patients in both groups was well below the maximum permissible dose of 2.4 mSv as per the NCRP guidelines. Radiation safety precautions such as thyroid collar and lead apron were used before subjecting the patients for imaging evaluation.

The temporomandibular joints were assessed as follows:

0: normal;

1: erosion;

2: flattening;

3: osteophytes;

4: sclerosis;

5: resorption;

6: other changes.

2.3. Interpretation of Radiographs. The assessment of both OPG and DVT images was done by three observers blinded to each other. OPG and DVT images were assessed separately. All three observers assessed these images twice with an interval of one week. All the three observers were asked to interpret the images to see the bony changes in the condyle and gave the code ranging from 0 to 6. All three observers interpreted the OPG and DVT images on HP L1910 19-inch square LCD Monitor with 1280 × 1024 screen resolution.

2.4. Statistical Analysis. SPSS 10 software is used for statistical analysis. One-way ANOVA test was done to evaluate interobserver and intraobserver variation. The two imaging modalities were compared and subjected to statistical analysis with the help of Z test.

3. Results

A total of 100 TMJ in 62 patients with a complaint of TMJ pain were assessed for the different condylar changes as mentioned in the methodology. All the 100 TMJ was assessed by two radiological methods, one being OPG and the other being DVT. Three observers assessed the diagnostic information for each of the imaging modalities. The three observers assessed the diagnostic information for each of the imaging modalities twice with an interval of one week. Distribution of gender and age in the present study is shown in Table 2. Interpretation of OPG and DVT images done by all the three observers is shown in Tables 3 and 4, respectively. There was good agreement between all the observers suggestive of no inter- and intraobserver variation (Table 5). Statistically significant difference was observed between two imaging modalities in assessing erosion and osteophytes ($P < 0.05$) which is shown in Table 6.

4. Discussion

Imaging is considered as an important diagnostic adjunct to the clinical assessment [10]. Several radiographic methods

TABLE 2: Distribution of gender and age in this study.

Gender	Number	Age (average)	Range
Male	20	25.8 years	(15–49)
Female	42	30.5 years	(16–72)
Total	62	28.15 years	(15–72)

are used to assess bony changes that affect the TMJ. It is important to obtain a clear and precise image of the region. Superimposition of adjacent structures, different angulations of the condyle, limitation of mouth opening in some patients, presence of artifacts, and mandibular movements during the examination make the TMJ image difficult to obtain [11]. There are many radiographic techniques for TMJ examination. The most recent one is DVT or CBCT.

A recent "effective dose" survey showed that CBCT units delivered a broad range of doses (dependent on machine, field size, resolution, etc.) of between 13 Sv (minimum dose, small volume) and 82 Sv (maximum dose, large volume) which compared favorably with radiation dose inflicted by multislice CT (MSCT) of between 474 Sv and 1,160 Sv for mandibular and full head scans, respectively. To put these measurements into perspective, panoramic doses have recently been found to range between 3 and 24 Sv.

In the present study, we evaluated different bony changes of condyle seen in patient with TMJ pain using DVT and OPG. The diagnostic reliability of OPG and DVT radiographic techniques to see the condylar bony changes were assessed and compared with each other.

In our study, we used KODAK 9000C 3D Extra oral imaging system to obtain both OPG and DVT images. Using of this system can be justified by a study done by Alqerban et al. in which authors compared six different CBCT systems to assess the root resorption [12].

Different bony changes assessed in our study are as follows:

(i) erosion;
(ii) flattening;
(iii) osteophytes;
(iv) sclerosis;
(v) resorption;
(vi) other changes;

Erosion is defined as an area of decreased density of the cortical bone and the adjacent subcortical bone. Flattening is defined as a flat bony contour deviating from the convex form. Osteophyte is defined as marginal bony outgrowths on the condyle. Sclerosis is defined as an area of increased density of cortical bone extending into the bone marrow. Resorption is defined as a partial loss of the condylar head [11]. All the observers interpreted the images and gave the coding from 0 to 6, where 0 stands for normal (Figure 3), 1 for erosion (Figure 4), 2 for flattening (Figure 5), 3 for osteophytes (Figure 6), 4 for sclerosis (Figure 7), 5 for resorption (Figure 8), and 6 for other changes.

In our study, we included 100 TMJ of 62 patients who had complained of TMJ pain. Out of 62 patients, 44 were female (67.75%) and 20 were male (32.25%) (Table 2). All the 100 joints were subjected for OPG and DVT examination and the images were interpreted by the three observers separately.

In our study, we had three observers to interpret the images who were blinded to each other, so that interobserver variations can be assessed. All the three observers interpreted the DVT and OPG images twice with an interval of one week to assess intraobserver's variations.

Different bony changes as seen by the three observers in DVT and OPG are shown in Tables 3 and 4.

In our study, one-way ANOVA test was done to see interobserver and intraobserver variation (Table 5). According to this test there was no interobserver and intraobserver variation in any of the imaging modality. This presumes that the observers were experienced and well calibrated in interpreting the images. Also, the image quality of OPG and DVT was par adequate not to mislead the observers.

According to available literature bony changes of TMJ are more common in female than male. In our study out of 100 joints 64% were of female and 36% were of male. Results of the present study show that more common bony changes seen like erosion, flattening, osteophytes, and sclerosis are seen more commonly in female than male (Table 7). This is in accordance with the study done by Pontual et al. (2012) [13] in which 78% were female and 22% were male. Another study done by LeResche (1997) found that pain in the temporomandibular joint is twice as common in females as in males [14]. The greater occurrence in women may be explained by the hormonal influences of estrogen and prolactin, which may exacerbate degradation of cartilage and articular bone in addition to stimulating a series of immunological responses in the TMJ [14].

In our study most common bony change seen by all the three observers was erosion followed by flattening and osteophytes. The results of our study are consistent with other studies done by Alexiou et al. (2009) [15] and Martínez Blanco et al. (2004) [16]. Objective of the present was to evaluate the efficiency of DVT in comparison with OPG in the assessment of bony condylar changes in patients of TMJ pain. Comparison of both imaging modalities was done using the Z test. Results of the Z test are shown in Table 6.

Most common bony change seen in our study is erosion. According to the results of our study there was a significant difference between DVT and OPG in assessing erosion of the condyle ($P < 0.05$). Erosion is the initial stage of degenerative changes, indicating that the TMJ is unstable and changes in bone surfaces will occur, probably resulting in changes in occlusion [11]. In our study, 61% of erosion could be identified in DVT whereas OPG was able to detect only 21%. Hence DVT has proved to be more superior than OPG in detecting early bony changes like erosion. This can be explained by the fact that DVT is a three-dimensional imaging technique in which the images can be viewed in all the three sections, that is, axial, coronal, and sagittal. The thickness section is 200 μm. Hence minor changes can be well appreciated by this technique. Our results are in accordance with a study done by Lee et al. who compared the panoramic radiograph and

TABLE 3: Bony changes seen by three observers in OPG.

Condylar changes	Observer 1		Observer 2		Observer 3	
	Day 1	Day 7	Day 1	Day 7	Day 1	Day 7
Normal	56	55	55	54	58	59
Erosion	21	20	21	21	21	20
Flattening	29	29	30	28	26	25
Osteophytes	7	7	6	6	7	7
Sclerosis	5	5	5	5	6	6
Resorption	1	1	1	1	1	1
Others changes	4	4	4	4	4	4

TABLE 4: Bony changes seen by three observers in DVT.

Condylar changes	Observer 1		Observer 2		Observer 3	
	Day 1	Day 7	Day 1	Day 7	Day 1	Day 7
Normal	56	55	55	54	58	59
Erosion	21	20	21	21	21	20
Flattening	29	29	30	28	26	25
Osteophytes	7	7	6	6	7	7
Sclerosis	5	5	5	5	6	6
Resorption	1	1	1	1	1	1
Others changes	4	4	4	4	4	4

TABLE 5: One-way ANOVA test to see interobserver variation in DVT and OPG.

	N	Mean	Std. deviation	Std. error	F	P value
DVT						
Observer 1	100	1.4900	0.797	$7.977E-02$		
Observer 2	100	1.5400	0.845	$8.459E-02$	0.102	0.903
Observer 3	100	1.5300	0.846	$8.463E-02$		
Total	**300**	**1.5200**	**0.827**	**$4.779E-02$**		
OPG						
Observer 1	100	1.1300	0.393	$3.933E-02$		
Observer 2	100	1.1300	0.393	$3.933E-02$	0.22	0.978
Observer 3	100	1.1200	0.383	$3.835E-02$		
Total	**300**	**1.1267**	**0.388**	**$2.244E-02$**		

TABLE 6: Comparison of DVT and OPG groups.

Comparison of DVT and OPG groups	Z Test		P value
Condylar changes	OPG	DVT	
Normal	56	22	0.000*
Erosion	21	61	0.000*
Flattening	29	35	0.449
Osteophytes	4	20	0.001*
Sclerosis	5	10	0.283
Resorption	1	4	0.369
Others changes	3	5	1.000

*Statistically significant difference was observed between two imaging modality in assessing erosion and osteophytes as P value is less than 0.05.

cone beam computed tomographic images in detecting bony changes in patients with temporomandibular joint disorder and they found that CBCT was able to detect more percentage of erosion compared with OPG [17].

Second most common change observed in our study is flattening. Flattening is considered a degenerative alteration resulting from overload on the TMJ and it may be related to the involvement of the masseter and temporal muscles [11]. In our study, though DVT could detect more number of flattening than OPG, there was no statistically significant difference between two modalities in detecting this bony change. This can be explained by the fact that flattening is a gross change which can be easily detected by two-dimensional imaging like OPG. In a study done by Lee et al., they also found that OPG was able to detect more percentage of flattening [17].

Next common bony change detected in the present study was the presence of osteophytes.

Osteophytes occur in an advanced stage of degenerative change when the body adapts itself to repair the joint. The

TABLE 7: Most common bony changes in male and female in OPG and DVT.

Condylar changes	OPG			DVT		
	Male	Female	Total	Male	Female	Total
Erosion	8	13	21	21	40	61
Flattening	11	18	29	15	20	35
Osteophytes	3	4	7	9	11	20
Sclerosis	2	3	5	3	7	10

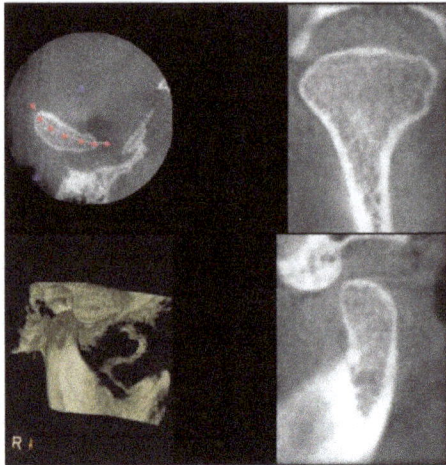

FIGURE 3: Normal condyle as seen in DVT.

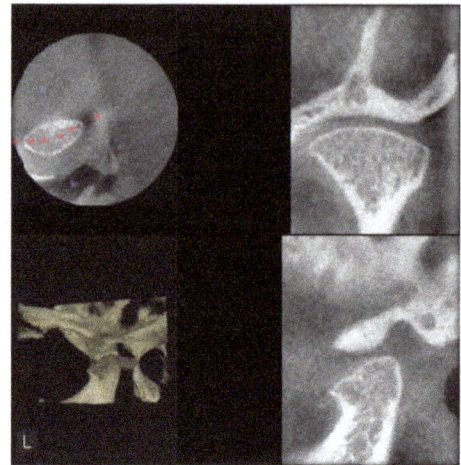

FIGURE 5: Flattening of condyle as seen in DVT.

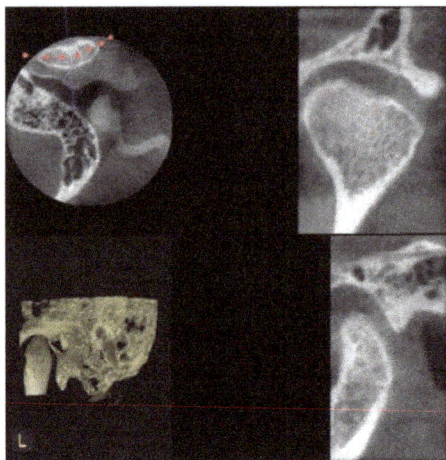

FIGURE 4: Erosion of condyle as seen in DVT.

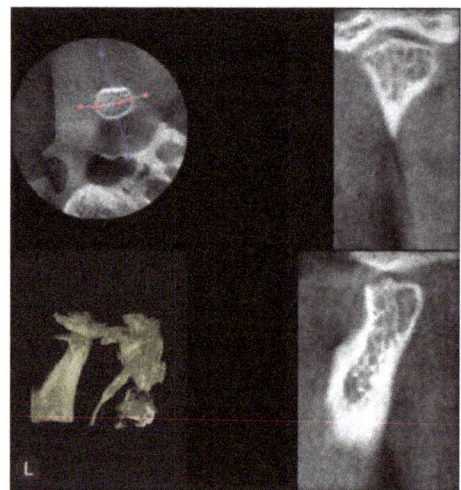

FIGURE 6: Osteophyte of condyle as seen in DVT.

osteophytes appear to stabilize and widen the surface in an attempt to improve the overload resulting from occlusal forces, representing areas of neoformed cartilage [11]. There was statistically significant difference between DVT and OPG in detecting osteophytes. These results are similar to a study by Lee et al. in which out of 212 joints CBCT was able to detect 2.1% of osteophytes whereas OPG detected only 0.9% and hence proving that CBCT is superior to OPG [17].

Sclerosis and resorption are the other two bony changes seen in our study. DVT was able to detect more number of sclerosis and resorption compared to OPG. But there

was no statistically significant results between the two imaging modality. Reason for no significant difference can be attributed to the small percentage of these changes observed in our study.

In our study, we also found other changes like Ely's cyst of the mandibular condyle (Figure 9), pointed shape of condylar head (Figure 10) and bifid condyle (Figure 11). Ely's cysts are also called subcortical cysts. These are rounded radiolucent areas that may be just below the cortical plate or deep in trabecular bone. There was no significant difference between

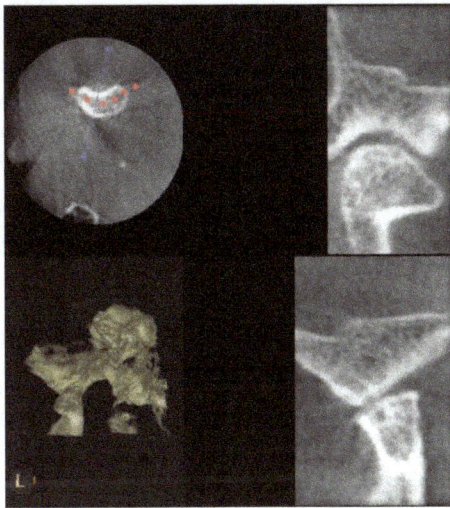

FIGURE 7: Sclerosis of condyle as seen in DVT.

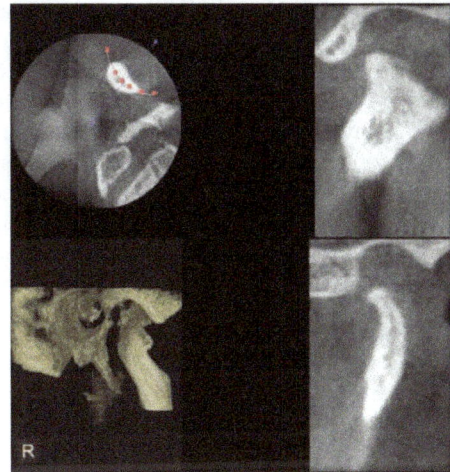

FIGURE 10: Pointed shape of condyle as seen in DVT.

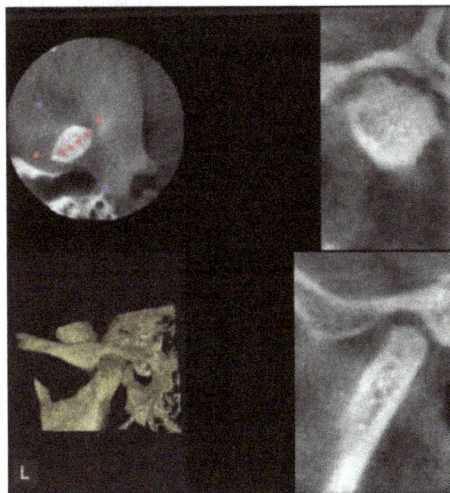

FIGURE 8: Resorption of condyle as seen in DVT.

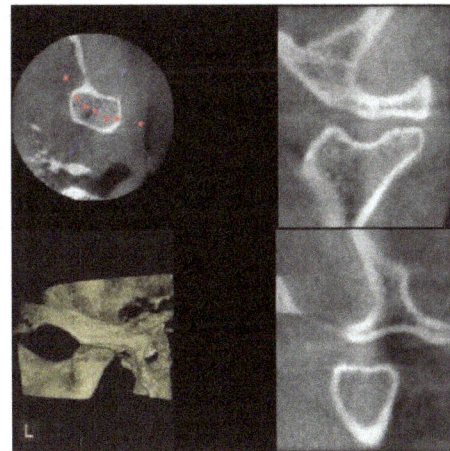

FIGURE 11: Bifid condyle as seen in DVT.

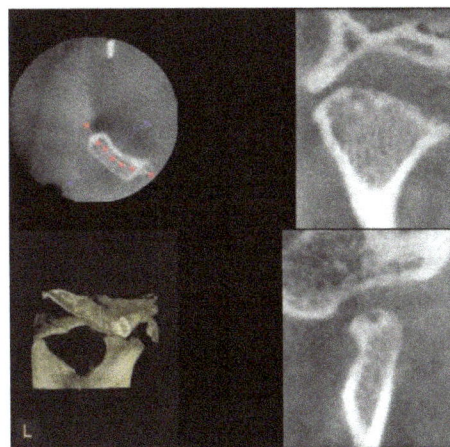

FIGURE 9: Ely's cyst of condyle as seen in DVT.

DVT and OPG to detect Ely's cysts. Out of 100 joints we found 2 joints having Ely's cysts. In a cross-sectional study done by Mathew et al. to see condylar changes and its association with age, TMD, and dentition status, they found 5 Ely's cysts out of 75 subjects [18].

In our study there were 2 joints with a pointed condylar head which was seen in both DVT and OPG. In a study done by Christiano Oliveira et al. 22.9% (129 condyles out of 566 condyles) of condyle had pointed condylar head [19]. A smaller amount of occurrence of pointed condylar head in our study may be due to a smaller number of sample sizes.

Bifid condyle is a rare anatomic variation of mandibular condyle. It can be symptomatic or diagnosed incidentally on routine radiographic examination. They appear to be more common on the left side in unilateral cases [20]. In a study done by Caǧlayan and Tozoǧlu in the year 2012 they found 2 bifid condyles out of 45 subjects [21]. In our study, we found one bifid mandibular condyle in left TMJ which was detected on DVT and not in OPG. This difference may have been due to the superiority of DVT for analyzing the TMJ region because of the absence of superimposition of anatomical structures.

To conclude, OPG alone can be used to detect gross bony changes of condyle like flattening and pointed condyle and DVT is helpful in detecting changes of condyle like erosion and osteophytes and Common bony changes seen in our study are erosion followed by flattening and osteophytes both in OPG and DVT. All the bony changes are seen more commonly in female than male. Other bony changes observed in our study are Ely's cyst, pointed condyle, and bifid condyle.

Conflict of Interests

The authors declare that there is no conflict of interests regarding the publication of this paper.

References

[1] J. P. Okeson, *Management of Temporomandibular Disorders and Occlusion*, Mosby, St. Louis, Mo, USA, 5th edition, 2003.

[2] K. Herb, S. Cho, and M. A. Stiles, "Temporomandibular joint pain and dysfunction," *Current Pain and Headache Reports*, vol. 10, no. 6, pp. 408–414, 2006.

[3] J. P. Okeson, *Bell's Orofacial Pain's the Clinical Management of Orofacial Pain*, Chicago Quintessence, Chicago, Ill, USA, 2005.

[4] S. P. Springer, S. M. Greenberg, and M. Glick, "Temporomandibular disorders," in *Burket's Oral Medicine Diagnosis and Treatment*, S. M. Greenberg and M. Glick, Eds., pp. 230–232, BC Decker, Ontario, Canada, 9th edition, 2003.

[5] W. C. Scarfe and A. G. Farman, "Diagnostic imaging of the temporomandibular joint," in *Oral Radiology, Principles and Interpretation*, S. C. White and M. J. Pharoah, Eds., pp. 473–478, Elsevier, Noida, India, 6th edition, 2010.

[6] E. L. Lewis, M. F. Dolwick, S. Abramowicz, and S. L. Reeder, "Contemporary imaging of the temporomandibular joint," *Dental Clinics of North America*, vol. 52, no. 4, pp. 875–890, 2008.

[7] W. C. Scarfe and A. G. Farman, "Cone beam computed tomography," in *Oral Radiology, Principles and Interpretation*, S. C. White and M. J. Pharoah, Eds., pp. 225–243, Elsevier, Noida, India, 6th edition, 2010.

[8] R. Molteni, "The so-called cone beam computed tomography technology (or CB3D, rather!)," *Dento Maxillo Facial Radiology*, vol. 37, no. 8, pp. 477–478, 2008.

[9] J. B. Ludlow, K. L. Davies, and D. A. Tyndall, "Temporomandibular joint imaging: a comparative study of diagnostic accuracy for the detection of bone change with biplanar multidirectional tomography and panoramic images," *Oral Surgery, Oral Medicine, Oral Pathology, Oral Radiology, and Endodontics*, vol. 80, no. 6, pp. 735–743, 1995.

[10] W. C. Scarfe and A. G. Farman, "What is cone-Beam CT and how does it work?" *Dental Clinics of North America*, vol. 52, no. 4, pp. 707–730, 2008.

[11] M. L. Dos Anjos Pontual, J. S. L. Freire, J. M. N. Barbosa, M. A. G. Frazão, and A. Dos Anjos Pontual, "Evaluation of bone changes in the temporomandibular joint using cone beam CT," *Dentomaxillofacial Radiology*, vol. 41, no. 1, pp. 24–29, 2012.

[12] A. Alqerban, R. Jacobs, S. Fieuws, O. Nackaerts, and G. Willems, "Comparison of 6 cone-beam computed tomography systems for image quality and detection of simulated canine impaction-induced external root resorption in maxillary lateral incisors," *The American Journal of Orthodontics and Dentofacial Orthopedics*, vol. 140, no. 3, pp. e129–e139, 2011.

[13] M. L. Pontual, J. S. L. Freire, J. M. N. Barbosa, M. A. G. Frazão, and A. Pontual, "Evaluation of bone changes in the temporomandibular joint using cone beam CT," *Dentomaxillofacial Radiology*, vol. 41, no. 1, pp. 24–29, 2012.

[14] L. LeResche, "Epidemiology of temporomandibular disorders: implications for the investigation of etiologic factors," *Critical Reviews in Oral Biology and Medicine*, vol. 8, no. 3, pp. 291–305, 1997.

[15] K. E. Alexiou, H. C. Stamatakis, and K. Tsiklakis, "Evaluation of the severity of temporomandibular joint osteoarthritic changes related to age using cone beam computed tomography," *Dentomaxillofacial Radiology*, vol. 38, no. 3, pp. 141–147, 2009.

[16] M. Martínez Blanco, J. V. Bagán, A. Fons, and R. Poveda Roda, "Osteoarthrosis of the temporomandibular joint. A clinical and radiological study of 16 patients," *Medicina Oral*, vol. 9, no. 2, pp. 106–115, 2004.

[17] D.-Y. Lee, Y.-J. Kim, Y.-H. Song et al., "Comparison of bony changes between panoramic radiograph and cone beam computed tomographic images in patients with temporomandibular joint disorders," *Korean Journal of Orthodontics*, vol. 40, no. 6, pp. 364–372, 2010.

[18] A. L. Mathew, A. A. Sholapurkar, and K. M. Pai, "Condylar changes and its association with age, TMD, and dentition status: a cross-sectional study," *International Journal of Dentistry*, vol. 2011, Article ID 413639, 7 pages, 2011.

[19] C. Christiano Oliveira, R. T. Bernardo, and A. Capelozza, "Mandibular condyle morphology on panoramic radiographs of asymptomatic temporomandibular joints," *International Journal of Dentistry*, vol. 8, no. 3, pp. 114–118, 2009.

[20] A. Faizal, I. Ali, U. S. Pai, and K. Bannerjee, "Bifid mandibular condyle-report of two cases of varied aetiology," *National Journal of Maxillofacial Surgery*, vol. 1, no. 1, pp. 78–80, 2010.

[21] F. Cağlayan and U. Tozoğlu, "Incidental findings in the maxillofacial region detected by cone beam CT," *Diagnostic and Interventional Radiology*, vol. 18, pp. 159–163, 2012.

Fat Necrosis of the Breast: A Pictorial Review of the Mammographic, Ultrasound, CT, and MRI Findings with Histopathologic Correlation

William D. Kerridge,[1] Oleksandr N. Kryvenko,[2] Afua Thompson,[3] and Biren A. Shah[4]

[1]*Department of Radiology and Imaging Sciences, Indiana University School of Medicine, Indianapolis, IN 46202, USA*
[2]*Departments of Pathology and Urology, University of Miami Miller School of Medicine, Miami, FL 33136, USA*
[3]*Department of Radiology, Meharry Medical College, Nashville, TN 37208, USA*
[4]*Department of Radiology, Henry Ford Hospital, Detroit, MI 48202, USA*

Correspondence should be addressed to Biren A. Shah; birens@rad.hfh.edu

Academic Editor: Henrique M. Lederman

Fat necrosis of the breast is a challenging diagnosis due to the various appearances on mammography, ultrasound, CT, PET-CT, and MRI. Although mammography is more specific, ultrasound is a very important tool in making the diagnosis of fat necrosis. MRI has a wide spectrum of findings for fat necrosis and the appearance is the result of the amount of the inflammatory reaction, the amount of liquefied fat, and the degree of fibrosis. While CT and PET-CT are not first line imaging examinations for the diagnosis of breast cancer or fat necrosis, they are frequently performed in the surveillance and staging of disease. Knowledge of how fat necrosis presents on these additional imaging techniques is important to prevent misinterpretation of the imaging findings. Gross and microscopic appearances of fat necrosis depend on the age of the lesion; the histologic examination of fat necrosis is usually straightforward. Knowledge of the variable appearances of fat necrosis on a vast array of imaging modalities will enhance a radiologist's accuracy in the analysis and interpretation of fat necrosis versus other diagnoses.

1. Introduction

Fat necrosis is a benign nonsuppurative inflammatory process of adipose tissue. It is important to diagnose fat necrosis because it can often mimic carcinoma of the breast. Fat necrosis in the breast is a common pathologic condition with a wide variety of presentations on mammography, ultrasound, and MRI.

The incidence of fat necrosis of the breast is estimated to be 0.6% in the breast, representing 2.75% of all breast lesions. Fat necrosis is found to be 0.8% of breast tumors and 1% in breast reduction mammoplasty cases. The average age of patients is 50 years [1].

Fat necrosis is most commonly the result of trauma to the breast (21–70%), radiotherapy, anticoagulation (warfarin), cyst aspiration, biopsy, lumpectomy, reduction mammoplasty, implant removal, breast reconstruction with tissue transfer, duct ectasia, and breast infection. Other rare causes for fat necrosis include polyarteritis nodosa, Weber-Christian disease, and granulomatous angiopanniculitis. In some patients, the cause for fat necrosis is unknown [1].

The typical clinical presentation of fat necrosis can range from an incidental benign finding to a lump. However, in around half of the cases patients do not report any injury to the breast and are clinically occult. Following injury to breast tissue, hemorrhage in the fat leads to induration and firmness, which demarcates and may result in a cavity caused by cystic degeneration. The clinical features of fat necrosis vary from indolent single or multiple smooth round nodules to clinically worrisome fixed, irregular masses with overlying skin retraction [2–6]. Other clinical features associated with fat necrosis include ecchymosis, erythema, inflammation, pain, skin retraction or thickening, nipple retraction, and occasionally lymphadenopathy [1, 2]. There is little difference

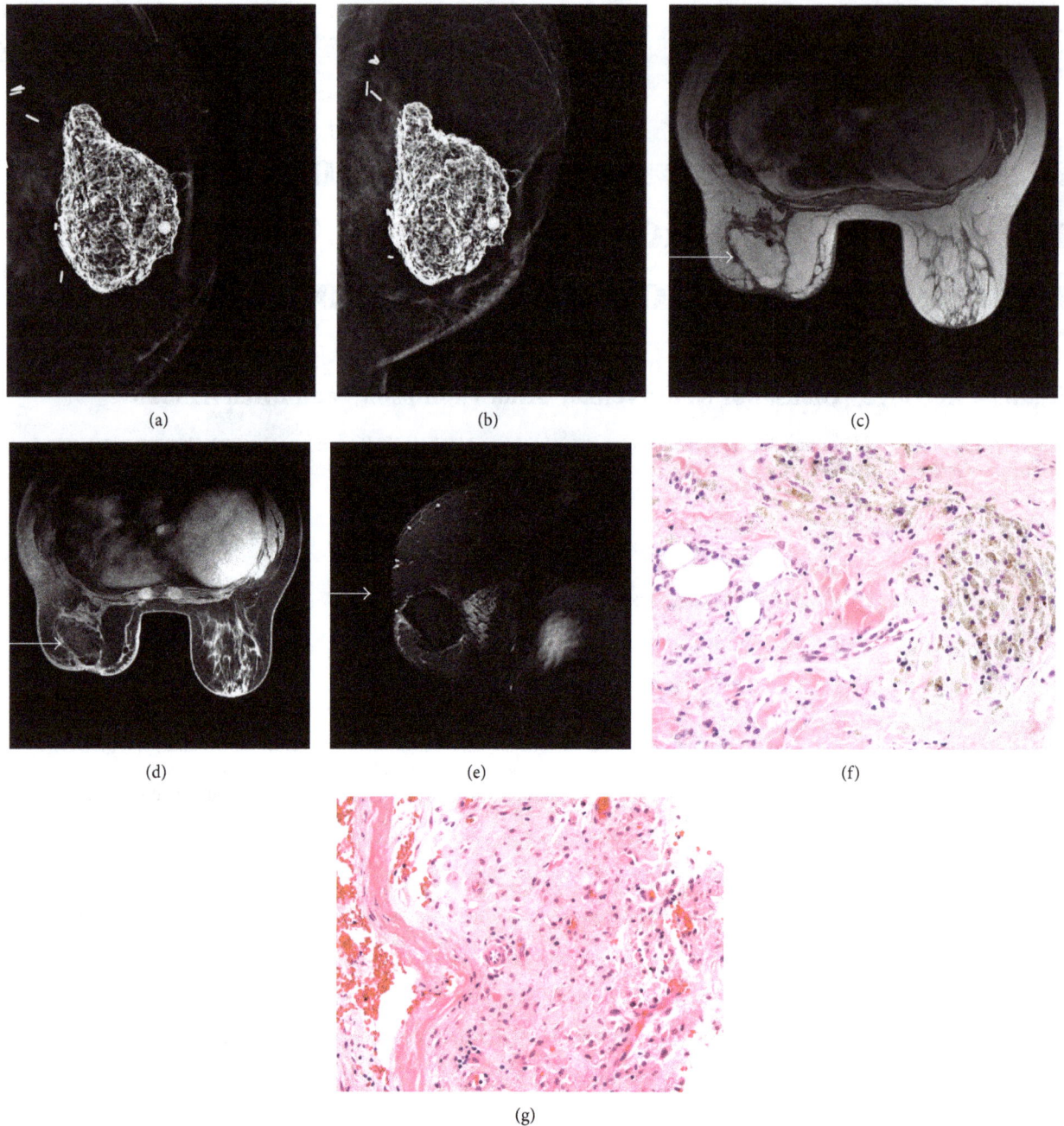

FIGURE 1: 49-year-old female with history of left modified radical mastectomy with transverse rectus abdominis myocutaneous (TRAM) flap reconstruction. Left TRAM flap reconstruction craniocaudal and mediolateral oblique projections ((a) and (b)) demonstrate a large mass of dystrophic calcification and fat. MRI breast T1-weighted nonfat saturation (c), T1-weighted fat saturation after gadolinium (d), and T2-weighted fat saturation images (e) demonstrate a mass in the central left TRAM which follows fat signal on all pulse sequences with a thin rim of enhancement (arrow). The biopsy ((f); H&E, 400x) demonstrating dense fibrotic tissue with foamy histiocytes (left) and hemosiderin-laden macrophages (upper and right). Rebiopsy ((g); H&E, 400x) demonstrating fibrous paucicellular cyst wall (left) surrounded by massive accumulation of foamy histiocytes (center and right).

in the clinical presentations of fat necrosis regardless of whether they are related to trauma. In cases related to trauma, the majority of patients presented with a breast lump. The mean time of patients to present with a breast lump from time of trauma is 68.5 weeks. Fat necrosis is commonly seen in the superficial breast tissues and subareolar regions in obese women with pendulous breasts [1]. The aim of this paper is to review the histopathological and radiological features of fat necrosis of the breast which distinguishes it from a cancer.

2. Histopathologic Findings of Fat Necrosis

Gross and microscopic appearances of the fat necrosis depend on the age of the lesion. Macroscopically, early lesions

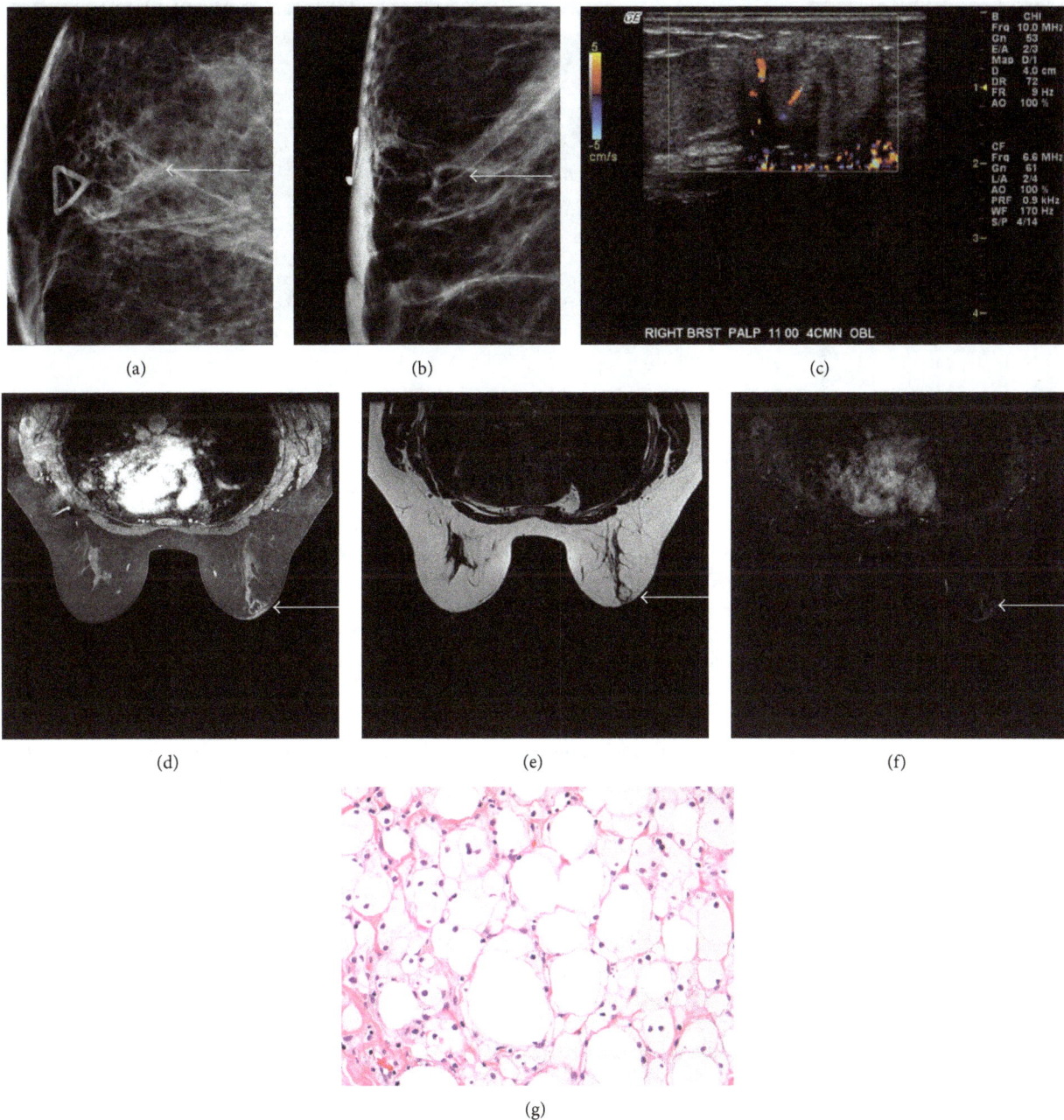

(a)

(b)

(c)

(d)

(e)

(f)

(g)

FIGURE 2: 51-year-old female with history of right lobular carcinoma in situ status after lumpectomy and radiation now with palpable lump. Right breast mediolateral oblique and craniocaudal projections ((a) and (b)) demonstrate a radiolucent lobular mass at site of palpable mass (arrow). Targeted ultrasound (c) at site of palpable mass shows a lobular heterogeneous hypoechoic mass with posterior acoustic shadowing. Axial T1-weighted fat saturation after gadolinium, T2-weighted nonfat saturation, and subtraction images ((d)–(f)) demonstrate a mass at 11 o'clock in the right breast anteriorly that follows fat signal on all sequences with thin rim enhancement (arrow). Histologically, tissue specimen ((g); H&E, 400x) demonstrating dead, anucleated adipocytes intermixed with foamy histiocytes.

appear as hemorrhagic foci or areas of indurated fat. In time, the lesion may become bright yellow (saponification), chalky white (calcification), or yellow-gray (fibrosis). Some lesions may develop a central cavity because of liquefactive necrosis (Figure 1). Poppiti Jr. et al. referred to such cystic lesions as membranous fat necrosis [7]. Microscopically, early lesions show hemorrhage, anucleated adipocytes, foamy (lipid-laden) histiocytes, and multinucleated giant cells (Figure 2).

Older lesions develop fibrosis with a few foamy histiocytes and multinucleated giant cells (Figures 3 and 4). However, the latter are usually seen even in older foci of fat necrosis which underwent subsequent transformation. Hemosiderin-laden macrophages may be seen as a morphologic evidence of remote hemorrhage (Figure 1). Dystrophic calcification may occur in older lesions. The morphologic examination of fat necrosis is usually straightforward. If needed,

(a)   (b)   (c)

(d)

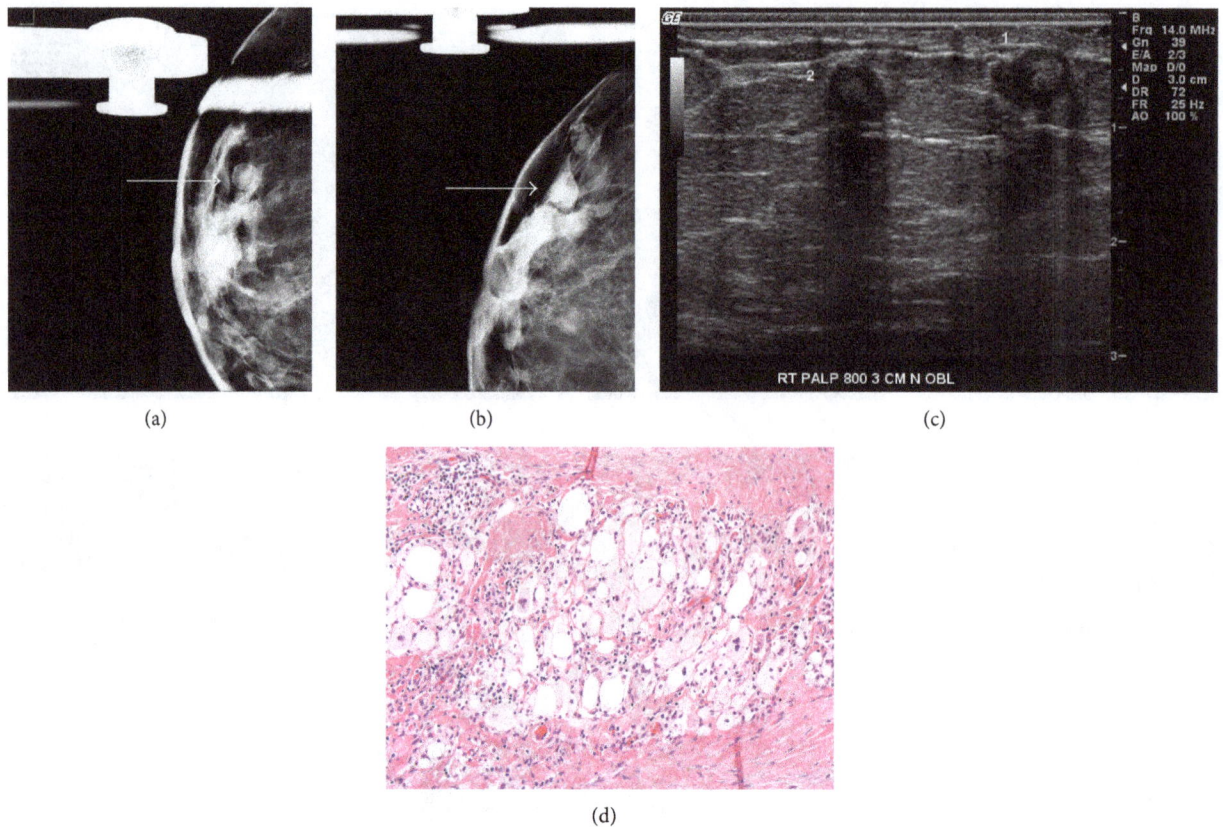

FIGURE 3: 78-year-old female with palpable right breast masses. Right breast mediolateral oblique and craniocaudal mammograms ((a) and (b)) demonstrate round masses with radiolucent centers at the site of palpable finding (arrow). Ultrasound of the right breast (c) at site of palpable finding demonstrate two hypoechoic round masses with central echogenicity with associated posterior acoustic shadowing. Hematoxylin and eosin (H&E, 200x) slide (d) shows fibrous areas around excision cavity with mixed chronic inflammatory cells, foamy histiocytes, and occasional giant cells.

the histogenesis of foamy histiocytes may be confirmed by positive CD68 and negative pan cytokeratin immunostains. However, older lesions with prominent fibrosis may warrant a more scrutinized examination of the specimen and pan cytokeratin immunostaining to rule out invasive lobular carcinoma in which discohesive single cells with small monomorphic nuclei infiltrate the stroma [8].

3. Imaging Findings of Fat Necrosis

On mammography, common findings of fat necrosis are oil cysts (Figure 5), coarse calcifications, focal asymmetries, microcalcifications, or spiculated masses. Lipid cysts are pathognomonic of benign fat necrosis, although the fibrous rim of the cyst may calcify or collapse and may produce an appearance that is mammographically indeterminate and requires biopsy to exclude malignancy (Figure 3). Calcifications may form in the cyst walls and are frequently seen on mammography, usually as smooth and round or curvilinear. Calcifications may be the only findings but may be of concern if they are branching, rod-like, or angular [9]. The clustered, pleomorphic microcalcifications may be indistinguishable from those of malignancy (Figure 4) [10, 11]. When fibrosis is present but the radiolucent fat is not completely replaced,

the oil cyst may have thickened, irregular, spiculated, or ill-defined walls. Fibrosis may lead to replacement of the radiolucent necrotic fat, resulting in the appearance of a focal asymmetric density, a focal dense mass, or an irregular spiculated mass on mammography [12]. Oil cysts with fat-fluid levels or serous-hemorrhagic contents, collapsed cysts, and cysts containing spherical densities are all atypical features of fat necrosis.

On sonography, the appearance of fat necrosis ranges from a solid hypoechoic mass with posterior acoustic shadowing to complex intracystic masses that evolve over time. These features depict the histological evolution of fat necrosis. Fat necrosis may appear as cystic or solid masses. Cystic lesions appear complex with mural nodules or internal echogenic bands. Solid masses have circumscribed or ill-defined margins and are often associated with distortion of the breast parenchyma [13]. In a retrospective study of the clinical, mammographic, and sonographic features of fat necrosis by Bilgen et al., 26.9% of lesions demonstrated increased echogenicity of the subcutaneous tissue with or without small cysts, 16.6% were anechoic masses with posterior acoustic enhancement, 14.2% were solid-appearing masses, 11.1% had cystic masses with internal echoes, and 3.9% had cystic masses with mural nodules [14].

(a)   (b)   (c)

(d)

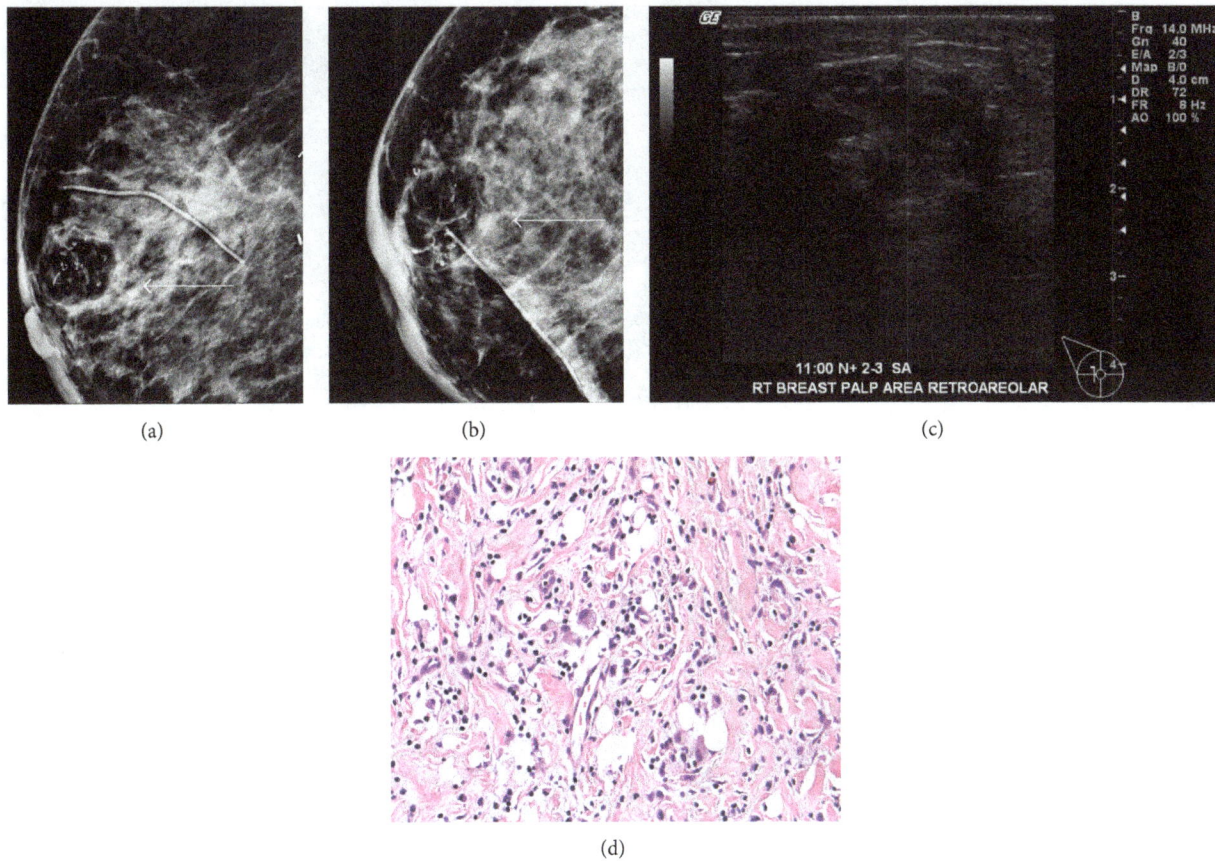

FIGURE 4: 85-year-old female with history of right breast mucinous carcinoma, lobular carcinoma in situ (LCIS), and ductal carcinoma in situ (DCIS) status after lumpectomy and radiation. Right breast mammogram ((a) and (b)) craniocaudal and mediolateral oblique views demonstrate a radiolucent round mass with dystrophic calcifications (arrow) (c). Targeted ultrasound demonstrates a heterogeneous hypoechoic mass with areas of posterior acoustic shadowing. The biopsy ((d); H&E, 400x) demonstrating dense fibrotic tissue with mixed chronic inflammatory infiltrate and scattered foamy histiocytes.

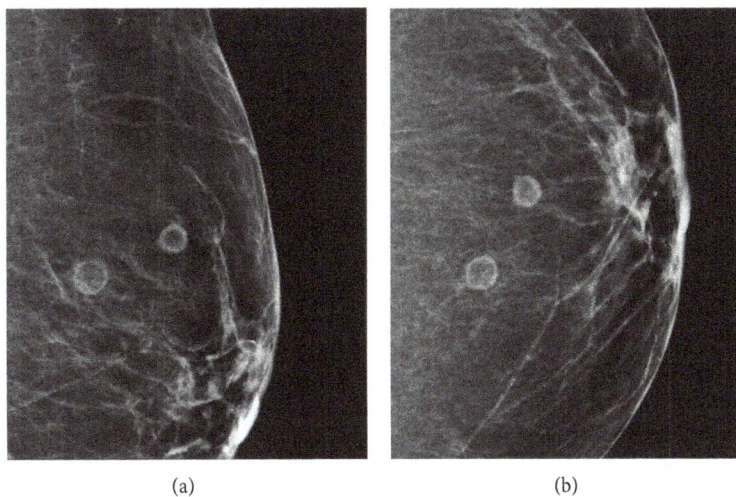

(a)   (b)

FIGURE 5: 69-year-old asymptomatic female with a stable screening mammogram for 18 years. Left breast mammogram craniocaudal and mediolateral oblique projections demonstrate two round masses with radiolucent centers at 12 o'clock position anteriorly.

(a)   (b)   (c)

(d)   (e)

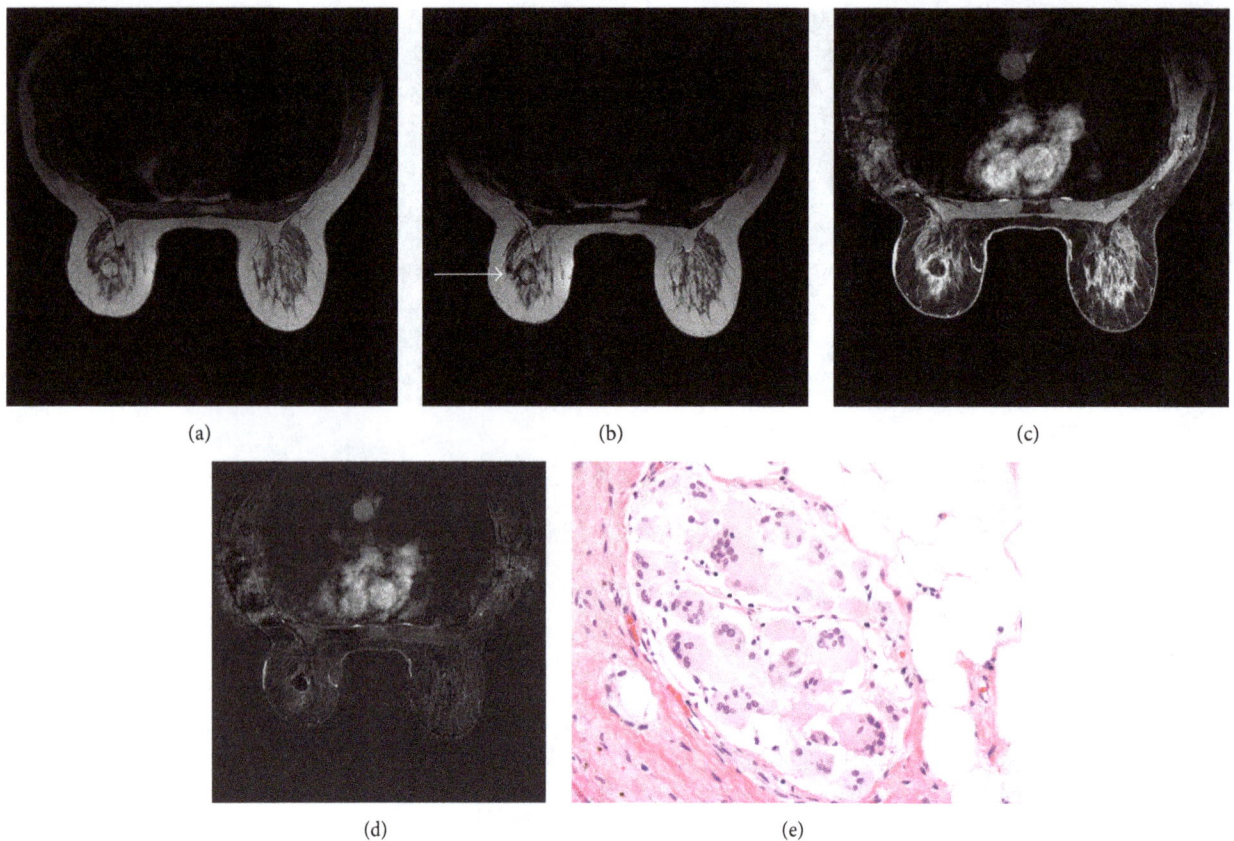

FIGURE 6: Axial T1-weighted nonfat saturation, T2-weighted nonfat saturation, and T1-weighted fat saturation after gadolinium and subtraction images ((a)–(d)) demonstrate a mass in the left breast which follows fat signal on all sequences (arrow). Histologically, excision ((e); H&E, 400x) shows collection of multinucleated cells in a fibrous area around excision cavity.

A specific sonographic indicator of fat necrosis is a mass with echogenic internal bands that shift in orientation with changes in patient position [15]. Hyperechoic masses very rarely represent malignancy; in fact, hyperechoic cancers are reported in less than 0.8% of tumors [16]. Although rare, malignant hyperechoic lesions include invasive ductal and lobular carcinoma, lymphoma, angiosarcoma, and liposarcoma [16]. The associated ultrasound characteristics (margin, shape, and hypervascularity) are important to consider when determining follow-up or when determining whether core needle biopsy is needed [16].

MRI also has a wide spectrum of findings for fat necrosis and the appearance is the result of the amount of the inflammatory reaction, the amount of liquefied fat, and the degree of fibrosis. The most common appearance of fat necrosis on MRI is a lipid cyst, round or oval mass with hypointense T1-weighted signal on fat saturation images [17]. Fat necrosis is usually isointense to fat elsewhere in the breast (Figure 2) and shows low signal intensity on T1-weighted MRI, which may be due to its hemorrhagic and inflammatory content [17]. Fat necrosis may show focal or diffuse and homogeneous or heterogeneous enhancement after the administration of IV paramagnetic contrast material. The amount of enhancement is correlated with the intensity of the inflammatory process [17]. As the high signal of fat interferes with the detection of

enhancing lesions on MRI, fat suppression is important for identifying enhancing breast cancers or enhancing regions of fat necrosis on MRI [15]. As mentioned before, fat necrosis is usually isointense to fat elsewhere in the breast, a key to diagnosis (Figure 6). In cases where fat necrosis is not isointense, the T1-weighted signal may be lower than fat elsewhere in the breast [12]. Another useful technique for ruling out necrotic tumors is using unenhanced non-fat-saturated T1-weighted images to evaluate the degree of lipid cyst formation, looking for a thin rim of enhancement [17]. Further, the "black hole" sign has been described as another characteristic on MRI to help diagnose fat necrosis, marked central hypointensity of the lesion on short tau inversion recovery (STIR) images when compared with surrounding fat [18]. Fat necrosis may mimic malignancy with varying appearances on MRI. Thin rim of enhancement (Figure 1) is common although it may also be thick, irregular, or spiculated, which are features of recurrent or residual cancer. Another confounding factor in the diagnosis is the different appearance that fat necrosis may have in the same patient. Kinetic analysis may be of little help because fat necrosis exhibits the full spectrum of benign and malignant enhancement patterns. Fat necrosis may also show FDG uptake on PET [19].

CT is not typically included in the imaging protocol for breast cancer detection; however, cancer patients may

TABLE 1: Common imaging features of fat necrosis.

Mammography	(i) Wide spectrum ranging from benign to indeterminate to malignant appearing masses or calcification
	(ii) Visualized masses may be as follows:
	  (a) radiolucent with a thin, well-defined capsule
	  (b) both radiolucent and dense with encapsulation
	  (c) dense and circumscribed mass
	  (d) mass with indistinct margins
	  (e) mass with spiculated margins

Ultrasound	(i) Sonographic spectrum with two most common appearances:
	  (a) mass (anechoic, hypoechoic, isoechoic, or hyperechoic with or without shadowing and enhancement)
	  (b) area of increased echogenicity of the subcutaneous tissue with or without small cysts and architectural distortion

CT	(i) Liquefied fat demonstrates low attenuation coefficients (ii) Fibrosis has attenuation similar to fibroglandular tissue or linear densities resembling fibrous bands (iii) Inflammation enhances after contrast injection
PET-CT	(i) Fat necrosis has increased FDG uptake secondary to presence of metabolically active inflammatory cells (ii) It may show intense activity in the setting of TRAM flap reconstruction
MRI	(i) Wide spectrum of appearance depending on amount of inflammatory reaction, liquefied fat, and degree of fibrosis (ii) It may demonstrate enhancement following administration of IV paramagnetic contrast material depending on the intensity of the inflammatory process (iii) Most common appearance are lipid cyst, round or oval mass with hypointense T1-weighted signal on fat saturation images (iv) It is usually isointense to fat elsewhere in the breast (v) "Black hole" sign, marked hypointensity on STIR images when compared with surrounding fat (vi) It may mimic malignancy with thin, thick, irregular or spiculated enhancement

undergo chest CT as part of staging and surveillance. CT can show areas of fat necrosis and knowledge of the CT appearance will help prevent misinterpretation of the imaging findings. The CT appearance is based on the main components found in fat necrosis: liquefied fat, fibrosis, and inflammation. Liquefied fat would present on CT as low attenuation coefficients, fibrosis would present as soft tissue coefficients similar to fibroglandular tissue or linear densities resembling fibrous bands, and inflammation would present with enhancement after contrast injection [12]. Calcifications typically are not evident until later in the evolution of fat necrosis when they become large in size.

Although F^{18}-FDG PET/CT is not recommended for the primary detection of breast cancer, it may play a role in the detection of local recurrence or distant metastases in the setting of locally advanced breast cancer when other imaging modalities are equivocal or confounding [20]. There are several entities within the breast that will show increased FDG-activity on PET/CT with F^{18}-FDG. These include acute and chronic inflammation, physiologic lactation, and benign focal breast masses including fat necrosis amongst others. Fat necrosis has increased FDG uptake secondary to the presence of metabolically active inflammatory cells in early stages of the process [19]. Fat necrosis of the breast is often hypermetabolic on PET/CT and may show intense FDG activity in the setting of transverse rectus abdominis myocutaneous (TRAM) flap reconstruction if the fat-rich tissue is damaged intraoperatively [21]. The presentation of a patient with a history of breast cancer status after mastectomy, palpable mass, and increased activity on PET/CT may be concerning, although this entity is more likely to be fat necrosis than recurrent tumor.

4. Conclusion

Fat necrosis of the breast may be a challenging diagnosis as it has a wide variety of presentations on mammography, ultrasound, CT, PET-CT, and MRI (Table 1). The extent of associated fibrosis, liquefied fat, and calcifications determine the imaging findings of fat necrosis. Mammography is more specific, although ultrasound is still a very important tool in making the diagnosis-increased echogenicity of subcutaneous tissue; in the event of recent trauma, it is the most common presentation and hyperechoic masses are almost always benign. MRI may be helpful in the diagnosis, for example, when internal signal characteristics are identical to those of the adjacent fat and no evidence of enhancement is seen after IV contrast.

Conflict of Interests

The authors declare that there is no conflict of interests regarding the publication of this paper.

References

[1] P. H. Tan, L. M. Lai, E. V. Carrington et al., "Fat necrosis of the breast—a review," *The Breast*, vol. 15, no. 3, pp. 313–318, 2006.

[2] C. D. Haagensen, "Diseases of the female breast," *Transactions of the New England Obstetrical and Gynecological Society*, vol. 10, pp. 141–156, 1956.

[3] J. P. Hogge, R. E. Robinson, C. M. Magnant, and R. A. Zuurbier, "The mammographic spectrum of fat necrosis of the breast," *RadioGraphics*, vol. 15, no. 6, pp. 1347–1356, 1995.

[4] B. J. Lee and J. T. Munzer, "Fat necrosis of the female breast and its differentiation from carcinoma," *Annals of Surgery*, vol. 37, pp. 188–195, 1920.

[5] A. M. Pullyblank, J. D. Davies, J. Basten, and Z. Rayter, "Fat necrosis of the female breast—Hadfield re-visited," *Breast*, vol. 10, no. 5, pp. 388–391, 2001.

[6] F. E. Adair and J. T. Munzer, "Fat necrosis of the female breast. Report of one hundred ten cases," *The American Journal of Surgery*, vol. 74, no. 2, pp. 117–128, 1947.

[7] R. J. Poppiti Jr., M. Margulies, B. Cabello, and A. M. Rywlin, "Membranous fat necrosis," *The American Journal of Surgical Pathology*, vol. 10, no. 1, pp. 62–69, 1986.

[8] V. Martinez and J. G. Azzopardi, "Invasive lobular carcinoma of the breast: incidence and variants," *Histopathology*, vol. 3, no. 6, pp. 467–488, 1979.

[9] G. Gatta, A. Pinto, S. Romano, A. Ancona, M. Scaglione, and L. Volterrani, "Clinical, mammographic and ultrasonographic features of blunt breast trauma," *European Journal of Radiology*, vol. 59, no. 3, pp. 327–330, 2006.

[10] C. E. Baber and H. I. Libshitz, "Bilateral fat necrosis of the breast following reduction mammoplasties," *The American Journal of Roentgenology*, vol. 128, no. 3, pp. 508–509, 1977.

[11] L. W. Bassett, R. H. Gold, and H. C. Cove, "Mammographic spectrum of traumatic fat necrosis: the fallibility of 'pathognomonic' signs of carcinoma," *American Journal of Roentgenology*, vol. 130, no. 1, pp. 119–122, 1978.

[12] L. Fernandes Chala, N. de Barros, P. de Camargo Moraes et al., "Fat necrosis of the breast: mammographic, sonographic, computed tomography, and magnetic resonance imaging findings," *Current Problems in Diagnostic Radiology*, vol. 33, no. 3, pp. 106–126, 2004.

[13] P. H. Tan, L. M. Lai, E. V. Carrington et al., "Fat necrosis of the breast—a review," *Breast*, vol. 15, no. 3, pp. 313–318, 2006.

[14] I. G. Bilgen, E. E. Ustun, and A. Memis, "Fat necrosis of the breast: clinical, mammographic and sonographic features," *European Journal of Radiology*, vol. 39, no. 2, pp. 92–99, 2001.

[15] J. L. Taboada, T. W. Stephens, S. Krishnamurthy, K. R. Brandt, and G. J. Whitman, "The many faces of fat necrosis in the breast," *The American Journal of Roentgenology*, vol. 192, no. 3, pp. 815–825, 2009.

[16] B. Adrada, Y. Wu, and W. Yang, "Hyperechoic lesions of the breast: radiologic-histopathologic correlation," *The American Journal of Roentgenology*, vol. 200, no. 5, pp. W518–W530, 2013.

[17] C. P. Daly, B. Jaeger, and D. S. Sill, "Pictorial essay: variable appearances of fat necrosis on breast MRI," *The American Journal of Roentgenology*, vol. 191, no. 5, pp. 1374–1380, 2008.

[18] R. M. Trimboli, L. A. Carbonaro, F. Cartia, G. Di Leo, and F. Sardanelli, "MRI of fat necrosis of the breast: the 'black hole' sign at short tau inversion recovery," *European Journal of Radiology*, vol. 81, no. 4, pp. e573–e579, 2012.

[19] M. Adejolu, L. Huo, E. Rohren, L. Santiago, and W. T. Yang, "False-positive lesions mimicking breast cancer on FDG PET and PET/CT," *American Journal of Roentgenology*, vol. 198, no. 3, pp. W304–W314, 2012.

[20] National Comprehensive Cancer Network (NCCN), *NCCN Clinical Practice Guidelines in Oncology. Breast Cancer*, BINV1–14; IBC1; M532, NCCN, 2011.

[21] N. B. Dobbs and H. R. Latifi, "Diffuse FDG uptake due to fat necrosis following transverse rectus abdominus myocutaneous (TRAM) flap reconstruction," *Clinical Nuclear Medicine*, vol. 38, no. 8, pp. 652–654, 2013.

3

Endovascular Embolisation of Visceral Artery Pseudoaneurysms

Yasir Jamil Khattak,[1] Tariq Alam,[2] Rana Hamid Shoaib,[1] Raza Sayani,[1] Tanveer-ul Haq,[1] and Muhammad Awais[1]

[1] Department of Radiology, Aga Khan University Hospital, Karachi, Pakistan
[2] Department of Radiology, French Medical Institute for Children, Aliabad, Kabul, Afghanistan

Correspondence should be addressed to Raza Sayani; raza.sayani@aku.edu

Academic Editor: Paul Sijens

Objective. To evaluate the technical success, safety, and outcome of endovascular embolization procedure in management of visceral artery pseudoaneurysms. *Materials and Methods.* 46 patients were treated for 53 visceral pseudoaneurysms at our institution. Preliminary diagnostic workup in all cases was performed by contrast enhanced abdominal CT scan and/or duplex ultrasound. In all patients, embolization was performed as per the standard departmental protocol. For data collection, medical records and radiology reports of all patients were retrospectively reviewed. Technical success, safety, and outcome of the procedure were analyzed. *Results.* Out of 46 patients, 13 were females and 33 were males. Mean patient age was 44.79 ± 13.9 years and mean pseudoaneurysm size was 35 ± 19.5 mm. Technical success rate for endovascular visceral pseudoaneurysm coiling was 93.47% ($n = 43$). Complication rate was 6.52% ($n = 3$). Followup was done for a mean duration of 21 ± 1.6 months (0.5–69 months). Complete resolution of symptoms or improvement in clinical condition was seen in 36 patients (80%) out of those 45 in whom procedure was technically successful. *Conclusion.* Results of embolization of visceral artery pseudoaneurysms with coils at our center showed high success rate and good short term outcome.

1. Introduction

Visceral arteries include arteries of the splanchnic circulation and the renal arteries [1]. The pseudoaneurysms of visceral arteries (VPAs) are uncommon and attributed to degeneration of the vessel wall mostly due to infections and adjacent inflammation, trauma, and iatrogenic causes [2]. Hemorrhage due to rupture of these pseudoaneurysms is a rare but often life threatening complication which manifests as intra-abdominal or retroperitoneal bleeding and requires emergency treatment [3, 4].

Using digital subtraction angiography the bleeding site can be evaluated followed by embolization of the bleeding vessel or pseudoaneurysm employing superselective catheterization technique [5, 6].

To the best of our knowledge there is no published data available from the developing world regarding clinical presentation, procedural results, and clinical outcome of endovascular management of visceral artery pseudoaneurysms. This study was hence carried out to present details of our initial experience with the procedure at a tertiary care hospital in a third world country.

2. Materials and Methods

This cross-sectional study was carried out at radiology department of a tertiary care hospital in third world country. The study was performed in accordance with the declaration of World Medical Association Declaration of Helsinki. The study was exempted from formal ethical approval as per the institution's policy on retrospective studies and the requirement of informed consent was waived. Data of patients was collected from July 2008 to December 2013. We included all patients who underwent endovascular coiling procedure for visceral artery pseudoaneurysms. A total of 46 patients were found to have visceral artery pseudoaneurysms during the study period.

The patients were referred for treatment to our interventional radiology section from clinical departments of our hospital and from other institutions after being diagnosed to

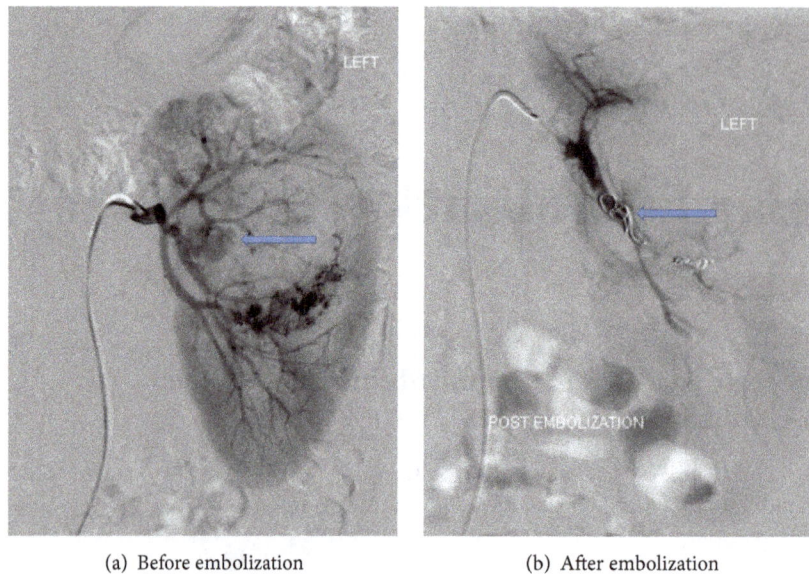

(a) Before embolization

(b) After embolization

FIGURE 1: Digital subtraction angiogram. (a) Arrow pointing to a large pseudoaneurysm arising from segmental branch of left renal artery supplying the interpolar region. (b) Arrow pointing to a platinum coil deployed in the segmental branch of left renal artery with successful exclusion of pseudoaneurysm.

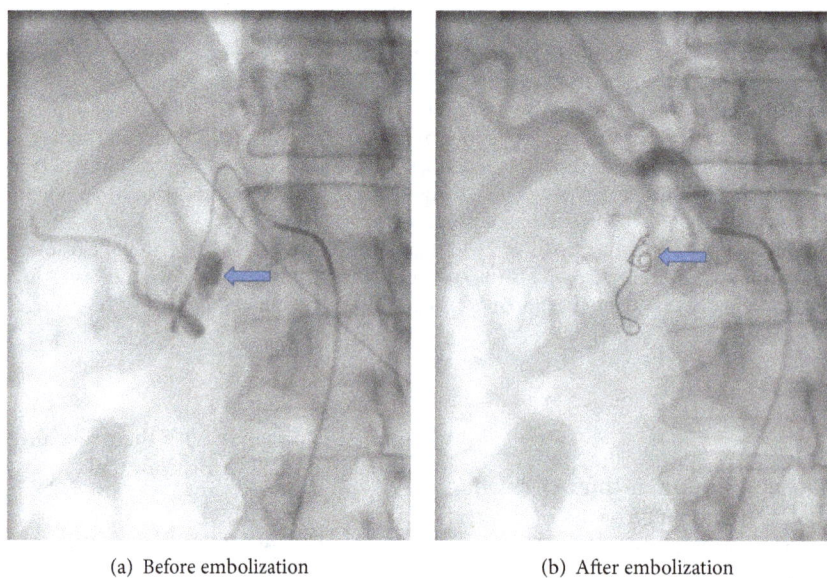

(a) Before embolization

(b) After embolization

FIGURE 2: (a) Arrow pointing to pseudoaneurysm arising from branch of gastroduodenal artery. (b) Arrow pointing to platinum coil placed in gastroduodenal artery with successful exclusion of pseudoaneurysm.

have pseudoaneurysm by contrast enhanced abdominal CT scan or duplex ultrasound examination.

Medical records and images were scrutinized to gather data regarding age, sex, clinical presentation including the symptoms, location, number, and size of aneurysms, technical success, complications, and outcome of the embolization procedures.

Informed consent for the embolization procedure was taken from all patients or their immediate attendants. Embolization was carried out by trained interventional radiologists in dedicated interventional radiology suite on a flat panel monoplane digital subtraction angiography machine (Axiom-Artis; Siemens Medical Systems, Erlangen, Germany). Majority of the cases (30 of 46) were performed under

local anesthesia. Femoral artery was punctured for vascular access and a 4 or 5Fr access sheath was placed. Either 4Fr or 5Fr renal double curve catheter (Cordis; Johnson & Johnson, Miami, FL), Sidewinder Simmons, Sim 1 (Cordis; Johnson & Johnsons, Miami, FL), or a Cobra, C1 angiographic catheter (Cook; Bloomington, IN), was advanced over a 0.035 inch guide wire. In cases where there was tortuosity of the vessels or superselective catheterization was required, a microcatheter (Progreat; Terumo, Tokyo, Japan) was used. It was coaxially taken as far as possible, proximal to the aneurysm. Platinum coils were deployed proximally to the aneurysm sac to block the inflow vessel to completely exclude the aneurysm in cases of end arteries (Figures 1 and 2). Outflow vessels were also coiled wherever required as in cases of collateral

TABLE 1: Number, size, and anatomical distribution of the aneurysms.

Artery of origin	Number of aneurysms	Size range
Total	53	
Renal	23	Range: 4.8–69 mm
Hepatic	14	Range: 7–44 mm
SMA	2	Range: 28–36 mm
Splenic	3	Range: 16–55 mm
IMA	1	Range: 15 mm
Cystic	1	Range: 19 mm
Celiac	2	Range: 43–45 mm
Gastroduodenal	3	Range: 11–13 mm
Pancreaticoduodenal	1	Range: 8 mm
Left colic	2	Range: 6–8.5 mm
Middle colic	1	Range: 4.5 mm

flow. Technical success was considered as total occlusion of the vascularity of lesion or aneurysmal sac and cessation of hemorrhage seen on postprocedural angiography. Patients were followed after procedure and if required reimaging was done via Doppler ultrasonography or contrast enhanced CT scan. Ultrasound diagnostic equipment (Xario; Toshiba Medical Systems, Tokyo, Japan) was used for performing Doppler examination using 3.6 Mhz convex probe (Xario PVT-674BT; Toshiba Medical Systems, Tokyo, Japan) and/or 7.5 Mhz linear probe (Xario PLT-704SBT; Toshiba Medical Systems, Tokyo, Japan). All CT scans were performed on 64- or 640-slice Multidetector CT (Aquilion; Toshiba Medical Systems, Tokyo, Japan).

3. Results

During the study period, 46 patients, 13 females and 33 males, were treated for 53 VPAs. Mean patient age was 44.79 ± 13.90 years (range: 10–77 years). Pseudoaneurysm size ranged from 2 to 69 mm (mean size: 32 ± 21.3 mm). Most common pseudoaneurysm site was renal artery, 23 out of 53 (43.39%), followed by hepatic artery, 14 out of 53 (26.41%). Anatomical distribution, number, and size of pseudoaneurysms are outlined in Table 1.

Four renal artery pseudoaneurysms were identified in a patient, which were filling from different subsegmental arteries; all were cannulated selectively and subsequently embolized. Twelve renal artery pseudoaneurysms were secondary to percutaneous nephrolithotomy (PCNL), two due to postpercutaneous nephrostomy (PCN) insertion and one as a complication of renal biopsy. In four patients renal artery pseudoaneurysms were associated with angiomyolipomas.

In one patient hepatic artery pseudoaneurysm was mycotic in nature due to adjacent liver abscess. Ten patients developed pseudoaneurysms secondary to liver lacerations following road traffic accidents (Figures 3(a), 3(b), and 3(c)). Another young patient who was a known case of embryonal sarcoma of liver developed multiple pseudoaneurysms within the liver mass.

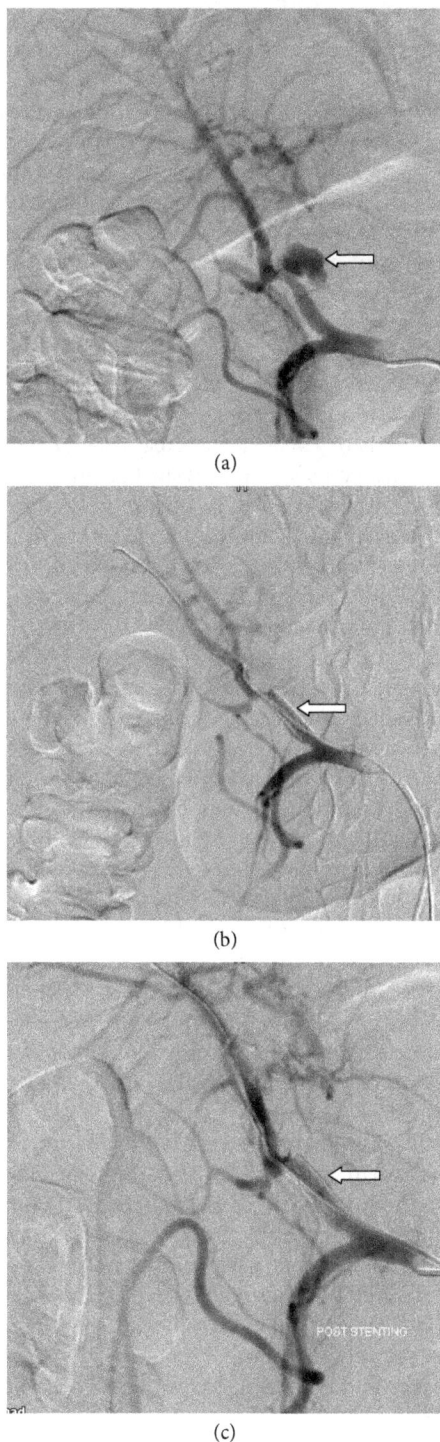

FIGURE 3: (a) Pseudoaneurysm arising from left hepatic artery (arrow in Figure 3(a)). (b) Covered stent placed across the site of pseudoaneurysm (arrow in Figure 3(b)). (c) Postcovered stent placement angiogram shows complete exclusion of pseudoaneurysm (arrow in Figure 3(c)).

There were three cases of visceral artery pseudoaneurysm secondary to hepatobiliary interventions, two following laparoscopic cholecystectomy (hepatic artery and cystic artery) and one patient developed pseudoaneurysm of hepatic artery secondary to biliary drain placement. This patient had history of anastomotic stricture following hepaticojejunostomy and underwent cholangioplasty on multiple occasions.

Of the 46 patients, technical success was achieved in 43 patients (93.47%) with preservation of native circulation. In two patients embolization was not successful and the reason of failure was difficult catheterization of the supplying artery, due to complex anatomy and vascular spasm. Both patients were subsequently managed by surgery. One patient had a large pseudoaneurysm of the celiac artery which ruptured during covered stent placement.

A common cause of visceral artery pseudoaneurysm in this series of patients was acute pancreatitis. There were three cases with gastroduodenal artery pseudoaneurysm amongst which two had history of acute pancreatitis. One patient with middle colic artery pseudoaneurysm had history of grade IV pancreatic transaction due to abdominal trauma during a road traffic accident. Another young patient with severe necrotizing pancreatitis developed pseudoaneurysm of left colic artery. Three patients had pseudoaneurysms arising from the splenic artery amongst which two patients had recent history pancreatitis. In one patient the cause was unknown. Two cases with SMA and one with pancreaticoduodenal artery pseudoaneurysms also had pancreatitis as the causative factor. There was one case of IMA (inferior mesenteric artery) pseudoaneurysm for which the cause could not be elucidated.

Complete resolution of symptoms or improvement in clinical condition was seen in 41 patients (91.11%) out of 45 in whom the procedure was technically successful. Six (13.04%) patients required second session of embolization or surgical intervention. Two of these had renal artery pseudoaneurysms associated with angiomyolipomas. One patient had hepatic artery pseudoaneurysm. One patient with embryonal sarcoma of liver had multiple pseudoaneurysms of hepatic artery and required a second session of embolization. One case of necrotizing pancreatitis developed small pseudoaneurysm in close proximity to the previously embolized branch of the middle colic artery. One patient with celiac artery pseudoaneurysm required second session of embolization followed by surgery due to intraprocedural complication.

Procedure related complication rate was 6.52% (3 patients out of 46). In one patient with splenic artery pseudoaneurysm, a small infarct was identified in spleen on followup CT examination. However, patient remained stable and was managed conservatively. In another patient with renal artery pseudoaneurysm, there was dislodgement of coil in the distal profunda femoris artery. However, no significant obstruction to flow was identified. One patient with a large celiac artery became tachycardiac and hypotensive {heart rate 170/min and blood pressure (BP): 60/40 mmHg} during the procedure just before placing the covered stent. Rupture of the aneurysm was suspected which was confirmed with angiogram. Rapid embolization was performed with covered stent. Angiogram showed exclusion of aneurysm; however, patient had low blood pressure and pulse with no spontaneous breathing. CPR was performed which went on for more than 40 minutes. Vitals reverted back and patient was shifted to OR. A second angiogram was performed in the OR as the pressures were still dropping to exclude a leaking pseudoaneurysm.

Endoleak was noted from the covered stent so a decision was made to perform laparotomy. During the surgery the patient went into DIC and could not be revived.

Followup was done for a mean duration of 21 ± 1.6 months (range: 0.5–69 months). Six patients were lost to follow up. None of the cases showed puncture site complications, large infarcts, postembolization syndrome, or renal abscess in the mean 21-month followup period. Three patients expired. Amongst these three one case was that of ruptured celiac artery pseudoaneurysm prior to deployment of covered stent. The second patient had necrotizing pancreatitis. There was active extravasation from the splenic artery with pseudoaneurysm formation which was successfully angioembolized with platinum coils; however, the patient had already gone into state of DIC by this time and developed profuse bleeding from multiple sites. Attempts made to resuscitate, however, were not successful. The third case was that of acute pancreatitis with pancreaticocolocutaneous fistula. During his hospital stay he developed multiple drug resistant organism infection. He was continuously kept on breathing support. The patient already had one session of successful angioembolization. In ICU he developed frank bleeding from the fistula in the epigastrium. Patient was taken to OR and attempts were made to control bleeding. Meanwhile the patient became asystolic. Attempts made to resuscitate the patient, however, could not be revived.

4. Discussion

In the past, surgery has been the method of treatment of both ruptured and unruptured aneurysms and pseudoaneurysms [7, 8]. With development of newer interventional techniques and increasing experience of interventional radiologists, traditional concepts of treatment have changed [9, 10].

Endovascular management is safe and effective with fewer complications, shorter hospital stay, and faster recovery [11–13]. The various methods for endovascular treatment include placement of coils, deployment of covered stents, injecting polyvinyl alcohol particles, gelfoam or glue, and endoluminal thrombin injection [9, 14–17]. In our series platinum coils of various lengths and diameters were used for endovascular treatment. Rare technical complications of coiling include parent artery occlusion, aneurysm perforation, coil migration, and aneurysm recurrence [18, 19].

Renal artery pseudoaneurysms were most common (43.39%) and most of these were related to iatrogenic vascular injury (22.64%, $n = 12$) especially due to percutaneous nephrolithotomy. Our technical success rate was 93.47% which is quite similar and comparable to that reported by Sethi et al., Piffaretti et al., and Zhu et al. [5, 20, 21].

Ruptured celiac artery pseudoaneurysm during covered stent placement was the only major complication in this series of patients. Minor procedural complications in our series were 6.6%. For both patients no active management was required and both were treated conservatively. Our complication rate is much better than the complication rate of 37.5 reported by Piffaretti et al. [20].

A total of 10 out of 46 patients (21.7%) received second session of endovascular embolization and/or surgical treatment as salvage procedure after the first procedure failed. In two out of these ten patients, first session of embolization was not technically successful due to complex vascular anatomy and vascular spasm. In four patients, reperfusion was the indication for subsequent session of endovascular or surgical treatment. One patient amongst these four had post-PCNL hematuria and pseudoaneurysm was successfully embolized in the first session but a repeat angiogram was later carried out because of persistent hematuria which showed contrast extravasation from a different subsegmental branch which was then superselectively catheterized and occluded successfully with a microcoil. Another patient had bilateral angiomyolipomas (AML); in this patient embolization was repeated three days later after the first session; however, hematuria persisted and nephrectomy had to be performed. Similarly in the other patient with AML, the small feeding vessel filling the pseudoaneurysm could not be successfully cannulated and therefore the segmental branch was embolized using PVA particles; however, hematuria could not be controlled and patient later underwent nephrectomy. One patient had a large pseudoaneurysm of the distal main hepatic artery which was compressing the main portal vein and common bile duct. The pseudoaneurysm was embolized; however, the patient presented three days later with recurrent hematemesis and melena and was managed by surgical ligation. On one occasion where an endoleak was suspected following covered stent placement angiography had to be performed just prior to laparotomy in the OR. One patient with history of pancreatic transaction underwent multiple angiograms to evaluate cause of dropping hemoglobin level. Mesenteric angiogram revealed active extravasation of contrast from branches of middle colic artery with pseudoaneurysm formation which was successfully embolized with platinum coils and PVA particles. The patient had multiple episodes of melena few days later, on account of which GI bleed was suspected and another angiogram was done which turned out to be negative. A CT was performed few days later which showed a large pancreataic pseudocyst. Since the hemoglobin levels were continuously dropping, a third angiogram was carried out. This time a small pseudoaneurysm was identified lying in close proximity to the previously embolized branch of the right colic artery.

The reintervention rate of 10.86% in our series is quite similar and comparable to that of Spiliopoulos et al. and Huang et al. [16, 22].

There was one procedure related mortality where a celiac artery pseudoaneurysm ruptured prior to deployment of a covered stent. One patient in our series had posttraumatic liver laceration and hepatic artery pseudoaneurysm on angiography which was successfully embolized but patient died due to disseminated intravascular coagulation and other multiorgan injuries. One patient with pancreaticocolocutaneous fistula developed multidrug resistant organism infection during his hospital stay. The patient already had one session of successful angioembolization of left colic artery. In ICU he developed frank bleeding from the fistula in the epigastrium. Patient was taken to OR and attempts were made to control bleeding. Meanwhile the patient became asystolic. Attempts made to resuscitate the patient, however, could not be revived.

We would like to mention a few limitations of our study. First, being a retrospective review, the study has inherent deficiencies, especially while recording the fine technical details of procedure and clinical examination of patients at presentation as well as at followups. Secondly since it is only our initial experience, the number of cases is also small. Lastly, the outcome measure was based on clinical criteria and followup angiograms were not performed if patient was clinically improving. Despite these limitations, this study is one of the first reported series of visceral artery aneurysm embolization from a third world country and in our opinion would serve as a baseline for monitoring further regional progress. Larger prospective studies are nevertheless recommended for even better evaluation and more detailed analysis of determinants of complications and outcome. The procedural success rates, safety, and eventually patient outcome are expected to improve further with increasing experience of interventional radiologists.

5. Conclusion

Results of endovascular pseudoaneurysm embolization with coils at our center showed high technical success rate and good short term clinical outcome.

Conflict of Interests

The authors declare that they have no conflict of interests regarding this study.

References

[1] M. Jana, S. Gamanagatti, A. Mukund, S. Paul, P. Gupta, and P. Garg, "Endovascular management in abdominal visceral arterial aneurysms: a pictorial essay," *World Journal of Radiology*, vol. 283, pp. 182–187, 2011.

[2] R. A. Jesinger, A. A. Thoreson, and R. Lamba, "Abdominal and pelvic aneurysms and pseudoaneurysms: imaging review with clinical, radiologic, and treatment correlation," *Radiographics*, vol. 33, no. 3, pp. E71–E96, 2013.

[3] D. Grotemeyer, M. Duran, E. Park et al., "Visceral artery aneurysms—follow-up of 23 patients with 31 aneurysms after surgical or interventional therapy," *Langenbeck's Archives of Surgery*, vol. 394, no. 6, pp. 1093–1100, 2009.

[4] H. G. Lee, J. S. Heo, S. H. Choi, and D. W. Choi, "Management of bleeding from pseudoaneurysms following pancreaticoduodenectomy," *World Journal of Gastroenterology*, vol. 16, no. 10, pp. 1239–1244, 2010.

[5] H. Sethi, P. Peddu, A. Prachalias et al., "Selective embolization for bleeding visceral artery pseudoaneurysms in patients with pancreatitis," *Hepatobiliary & Pancreatic Diseases International*, vol. 9, no. 6, pp. 634–638, 2010.

[6] O. Ikeda, Y. Tamura, Y. Nakasone, Y. Iryou, and Y. Yamashita, "Nonoperative management of unruptured visceral artery aneurysms: treatment by transcatheter coil embolization," *Journal of Vascular Surgery*, vol. 47, no. 6, pp. 1212–1219, 2008.

[7] R. Pulli, W. Dorigo, N. Troisi, G. Pratesi, A. A. Innocenti, and C. Pratesi, "Surgical treatment of visceral artery aneurysms: a 25-year experience," *Journal of Vascular Surgery*, vol. 48, no. 2, pp. 334–342, 2008.

[8] E. M. Marone, D. Mascia, A. Kahlberg, C. Brioschi, Y. Tshomba, and R. Chiesa, "Is open repair still the gold standard in visceral artery aneurysm management?" *Annals of Vascular Surgery*, vol. 25, no. 7, pp. 936–946, 2011.

[9] G. T. Fankhauser, W. M. Stone, S. G. Naidu et al., "The minimally invasive management of visceral artery aneurysms and pseudo-aneurysms," *Journal of Vascular Surgery*, vol. 53, no. 4, pp. 966–970, 2011.

[10] U. Sachdev, D. T. Baril, S. H. Ellozy et al., "Management of aneurysms involving branches of the celiac and superior mesenteric arteries: a comparison of surgical and endovascular therapy," *Journal of Vascular Surgery*, vol. 44, no. 4, pp. 718–724, 2006.

[11] A. M. Belli, G. Markose, and R. Morgan, "The role of interventional radiology in the management of abdominal visceral artery aneurysms," *CardioVascular and Interventional Radiology*, vol. 35, no. 2, pp. 234–243, 2012.

[12] X. Ding, J. Zhu, M. Zhu et al., "Therapeutic management of hemorrhage from visceral artery pseudoaneurysms after pancreatic surgery," *Journal of Gastrointestinal Surgery*, vol. 15, no. 8, pp. 1417–1425, 2011.

[13] M. Chadha and C. Ahuja, "Visceral artery aneurysms: diagnosis and percutaneous management," *Seminars in Interventional Radiology*, vol. 26, no. 3, pp. 196–206, 2009.

[14] O. Ikeda, Y. Nakasone, Y. Tamura, and Y. Yamashita, "Endovascular management of visceral artery pseudoaneurysms: transcatheter coil embolization using the isolation technique," *CardioVascular and Interventional Radiology*, vol. 33, no. 6, pp. 1128–1134, 2010.

[15] L. E. Francisco, L. C. Asunción, C. A. Antonio, R. C. Ricardo, R. P. Manuel, and M. H. Caridad, "Post-traumatic hepatic artery pseudoaneurysm treated with endovascular embolization and thrombin injection," *World Journal of Hepatology*, vol. 2, pp. 87–90, 2010.

[16] S. Spiliopoulos, T. Sabharwal, D. Karnabatidis et al., "Endovascular treatment of visceral aneurysms and pseudoaneurysms: long-term outcomes from a multicenter European study," *Cardiovascular and Interventional Radiology*, vol. 35, no. 6, pp. 1315–1325, 2012.

[17] K. Izaki, M. Yamaguchi, R. Kawasaki, T. Okada, K. Sugimura, and K. Sugimoto, "N-butyl cyanoacrylate embolization for pseudoaneurysms complicating pancreatitis or pancreatectomy," *Journal of Vascular and Interventional Radiology*, vol. 22, no. 3, pp. 302–308, 2011.

[18] J. R. A. Skipworth, C. Morkane, D. A. Raptis et al., "Coil migration—a rare complication of endovascular exclusion of visceral artery pseudoaneurysms and aneurysms," *Annals of the Royal College of Surgeons of England*, vol. 93, no. 4, pp. 19–23, 2011.

[19] F. Cochennec, C. V. Riga, E. Allaire et al., "Contemporary management of splanchnic and renal artery aneurysms: results of endovascular compared with open surgery from two European vascular centers," *European Journal of Vascular and Endovascular Surgery*, vol. 42, no. 3, pp. 340–346, 2011.

[20] G. Piffaretti, C. Lomazzi, G. Carrafiello, M. Tozzi, G. Mariscalco, and P. Castelli, "Visceral artery: management of 48 cases," *Journal of Cardiovascular Surgery*, vol. 52, no. 4, pp. 557–565, 2011.

[21] X. L. Zhu, C. F. Ni, Y. Z. Liu, Y. H. Jin, J. W. Zou, and L. Chen, "Treatment strategies and indications for interventional management of pseudoaneurysms," *Chinese Medical Journal*, vol. 124, no. 12, pp. 1784–1789, 2011.

[22] Y.-K. Huang, H.-C. Hsieh, F.-C. Tsai, S.-H. Chang, M.-S. Lu, and P.-J. Ko, "Visceral artery aneurysm: risk factor analysis and therapeutic opinion," *European Journal of Vascular and Endovascular Surgery*, vol. 33, no. 3, pp. 293–301, 2007.

4

Role of Barium Esophagography in Patients with Locally Advanced Esophageal Cancer: Evaluation of Response to Neoadjuvant Chemoradiotherapy

Daisuke Tsurumaru,[1] **Kiyohisa Hiraka,**[1] **Masahiro Komori,**[1] **Yoshiyuki Shioyama,**[2] **Masaru Morita,**[3] **and Hiroshi Honda**[1]

[1] *Department of Clinical Radiology, Graduate School of Medical Sciences, Kyushu University, 3-1-1 Maidashi, Higashi-ku, Fukuoka City 812-8582, Japan*
[2] *Department of Heavy Particle Therapy and Radiation Oncology, Graduate School of Medical Sciences, Kyushu University, 3-1-1 Maidashi, Higashi-ku, Fukuoka City 812-8582, Japan*
[3] *Department of Surgery and Sciences, Graduate School of Medical Sciences, Kyushu University, 3-1-1 Maidashi, Higashi-ku, Fukuoka City 812-8582, Japan*

Correspondence should be addressed to Daisuke Tsurumaru; tsuru-d@radiol.med.kyushu-u.ac.jp

Academic Editor: David Maintz

Purpose. This retrospective study examined the usefulness of barium esophagography, focusing on the luminal stenosis, in the response evaluation of neoadjuvant chemoradiotherapy (NACRT) in patients with esophageal cancer. *Materials and Methods.* Thirty-four patients with primary advanced esophageal cancer ($\geq$T2) who were treated with NACRT before surgical resection were analyzed. All patients underwent barium esophagography before and after NACRT. The tumor length, volume, and percent esophageal stenosis (PES) before and after NACRT were measured. These values and their changes were compared between histopathologic responders ($n = 22$) and nonresponders ($n = 12$). *Results.* Posttreatment tumor length and PES in responders (4.5 cm $\pm$ 1.1 and 33.0% $\pm$ 18.5) were significantly smaller than those in nonresponders (5.8 cm $\pm$ 1.9 and 48.0% $\pm$ 12.9) ($P = 0.018$). Regarding posttherapeutic changes, the decrease in PES in responders (31.5% $\pm$ 13.9) was significantly greater than that in nonresponders (14.4% $\pm$ 10.7) ($P < 0.001$). The best decrease in PES cutoff with which to differentiate between responders and nonresponders was 18.8%, which yielded a sensitivity of 91% and a specificity of 75%. *Conclusions.* Decrease in PES is a good parameter to differentiate responders from nonresponders for NACRT. Barium esophagography is useful in response evaluation to NACRT in patients with locally advanced esophageal cancer.

1. Introduction

In the treatment evaluation of chemoradiotherapy in patients with esophageal cancer, new guidelines published in 1999, known as the "Response Evaluation Criteria in Solid Tumors (RECIST)," have been commonly used [1]. RECIST gives specific size requirements for measurable lesions at baseline to distinguish target from nontarget lesions. It is difficult to measure accurately the primary site of esophageal cancer as distinct from the normal esophageal wall in one dimension, because a computed tomography (CT) scan detects a primary lesion of esophageal cancer according to wall thickness of the esophagus. Therefore, the primary site of esophageal cancer is often identified as a "nontarget lesion" [2]. Accordingly, in the case of patient who has no target lesion (i.e., nodal involvement), evaluation of response to chemoradiotherapy is not clinically available. The only way to verify the response is to pathologically evaluate the resected specimen after the treatment, neoadjuvant chemoradiotherapy (NACRT). NACRT is a treatment option for advanced esophageal cancer which main aim is downstaging before surgery to increase rates of curative resection [3, 4].

TABLE 1: Patient and tumor characteristics ($n = 34$).

Mean age (range), y	62 (47–82)
Male/female no.	30/4
Pathology no.	
Squamous cell carcinoma	34
Tumor stage no.	
T2	2
T3	23
T4	9
Tumor location no.	
Ce	3
Ut	7
Mt	15
Lt	8
Ae	1
Mean ± SD total radiation dose, Gy	41.3 ± 1.8
Chemotherapy regimen no.	
CDDP + 5-FU	34

Ce: cervical esophagus; Ut: upper thoracic esophagus; Mt: middle thoracic esophagus; Lt: lower thoracic esophagus; Ae: abdominal esophagus; SD: standard deviation; CDDP: cisplatin; FU: fluorouracil.

Barium esophagography has not generally been used in evaluating the response to chemoradiotherapy, because accurate measurement of esophageal tumor using barium esophagography was also considered to be difficult due to its diverse nature [5]. However, barium esophagography has a high potential of describing esophageal lesion and is useful for diagnosing depth of invasion of esophageal cancer [6].

The purpose of this study was to clarify whether evaluation of response to chemoradiotherapy is possible, by comparing the findings of double-contrast barium esophagography with histopathologic response in patients with esophageal cancer who underwent NACRT.

2. Methods and Materials

This study was performed with approval of the institutional review board of our institution.

2.1. Patients. We retrospectively analyzed 34 consecutive patients with primary advanced esophageal cancer (≥T2) who were treated with NACRT before surgical resection during the period from July 2006 to June 2011 at our institution. Stratification to initial T2-T4 category was based on the findings of EUS, CT, and FDG-PET. All patients included in this study had histologically diagnosed squamous cell carcinoma of the esophagus and underwent barium esophagography before and after NACRT. Patients were excluded if they had a previous or secondary malignancy, or had previously undergone radiation therapy, chemotherapy, endoscopic therapy, or had nonstenotic (polypoid) type tumor. Finally, the study group comprised 30 men and 4 women, with an age range of 47–82 years (mean age 62 years). The patients' profiles are shown in Table 1.

2.2. Treatment. Radiotherapy was performed using external photon beams delivered at a daily dose of 1.8 Gy, five times per week, at a dose of 38–41.4 Gy (mean 41.3 Gy). The concurrent chemotherapy consisted of cisplatin (CDDP) and 5-fluorouracil (5-FU) with a dose of 5–9 mg/m^2/d (mean 7.1 mg/m^2/d) and 250–500 mg/m^2/d (mean 413 mg/m^2/d), respectively. With an interval of 3–10 weeks after the completion of NACRT, patients underwent standard right thoracic esophagectomy with modified 3-field lymphatic dissection.

2.3. Esophagography. Both initial and second barium study were performed using double-contrast esophagography technique. To produce hypotonus of the esophagus, 20 mg of butyl scopolamine (Buscopan; Boehringer Ingelheim, Tokyo, Japan) was intramuscularly injected just before examination. The double-contrast esophagography images were obtained with a 170% w/v (weight/volume) suspension of barium (Baritogen HD; Fushimi Pharmaceutical Co., Ltd., Kagawa, Japan) and gas ingested via a 12 Fr nasogastric tube. In different positions (anterior-posterior, lateral, and right/left oblique) with multiple projections, the narrowest projection of the lesion and the most distended normal esophagus were chosen to prepare calibration. Tumor volume was determined, using conventional bidimensional measurement, by multiplying the maximal measured longitudinal length and perpendicular depth of the tumor [7, 8]. The percent esophageal stenosis (PES) was based on the diameter across the lesion at maximal narrowing and the average of the normal oral and anal side diameters by the following formula: PES = [(average of normal diameters − diameter of maximal narrowing)/average of normal diameters] × 100 (Figure 1) [6]. The second esophagography, for treatment evaluation, was performed 2 to 4 weeks after the completion of NACRT.

2.4. Histopathologic Analysis. Histopathologic responses were determined in the primary tumor site after operation according to the guidelines of the *Clinical and Pathologic Studies on Carcinoma of the Esophagus, the Japan Esophageal Society* [8]. The grading of histopathologic response was determined as follows: grade 0 indicates ineffective, grade 1 indicates slightly effective (viable cells occupied more than one-third of the entire tumor), grade 2 indicates moderately effective (viable cells occupied less than one-third of the entire tumor), and grade 3 indicates markedly effective (absence of residual tumor). All patients who demonstrated grade 0 or 1 regression were considered to be histopathologic nonresponders. All patients who showed grade 2 or 3 regression were considered to be responders.

2.5. Statistical Analysis. Pretreatment, posttreatment, and decrease in tumor length, volume (conventional volumetry), and PES were compared between responders and nonresponders using Student's t-test. P values less than 0.05 were considered to be statistically significant. To determine the best cutoff value with which to differentiate responders from nonresponders, we constructed a receiver operating characteristic curve (ROC). These statistical analyses were

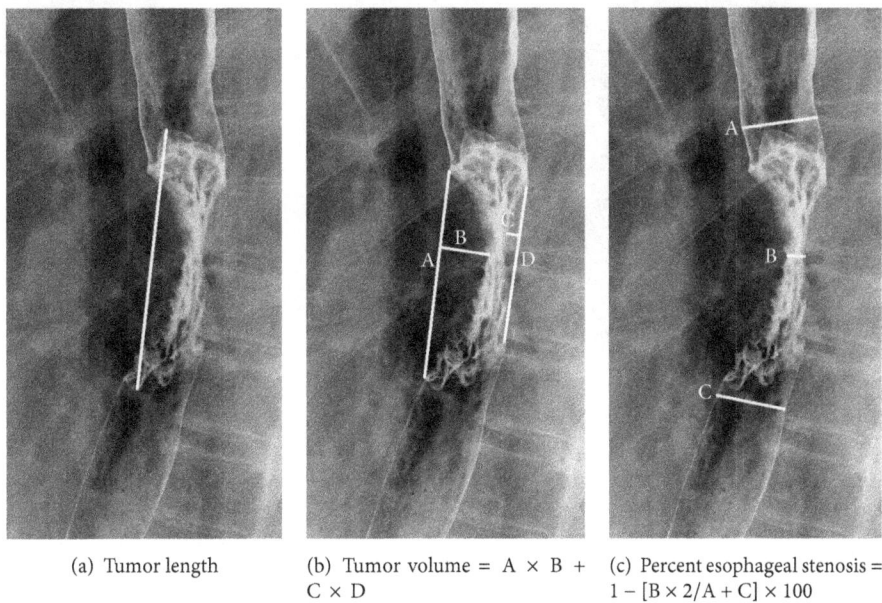

(a) Tumor length

(b) Tumor volume = A × B + C × D

(c) Percent esophageal stenosis = 1 − [B × 2/A + C] × 100

FIGURE 1: Measuring methods of esophageal stenosis.

TABLE 2: Tumor length, volume, and PES.

	Responders ($n = 22$)	Nonresponders ($n = 12$)	P value
Tumor length			
Pretreatment (cm)	5.5 ± 1.9	6.2 ± 2.3	0.336
Posttreatment (cm)	4.5 ± 1.1	5.8 ± 1.9	0.018
Decrease (%)	14.7 ± 16.1	8.9 ± 8.9	0.269
Tumor volume			
Pretreatment (cm^2)	10.3 ± 7.6	8.5 ± 3.3	0.439
Posttreatment (cm^2)	4.0 ± 2.8	4.7 ± 2.7	0.445
Decrease (%)	56.7 ± 24.9	44.8 ± 26.1	0.198
PES			
Pretreatment (%)	64.5 ± 12.9	62.4 ± 13.5	0.659
Posttreatment (%)	33.0 ± 18.5	48.0 ± 12.9	0.018
Decrease (%)	31.5 ± 13.9	14.4 ± 10.7	<0.001

Note: data are means ± standard deviations. PES: percent esophageal stenosis.

conducted with statistical software JMP (version 8.0; SAS Institute, Cary, NC).

3. Results and Discussion

Histopathologic specimens showed 22 responders (grade 2 or 3) and 12 nonresponders (grade 0 or 1). There was no significant difference in pretreatment tumor length, volume, and PES between responders and nonresponders. Posttreatment tumor length and PES in responders (4.5 cm ± 1.1 and 33.0% ± 18.5) were significantly smaller than those in nonresponders (5.8 cm ± 1.9 and 48.0% ± 12.9) ($P = 0.018$). However, there was no significant difference in posttreatment tumor volume between responders (4.0 cm^2 ± 2.8) and nonresponders (4.7 cm^2 ± 2.7) ($P = 0.445$). Regarding posttherapeutic changes, decrease in PES in responders (31.5% ± 13.9) was significantly greater than that in nonresponders (14.4% ± 10.7) ($P < 0.001$). However, there was no significant difference in decrease in tumor length and volume between responder (14.7% ± 16.1 and 56.7% ± 24.9) and nonresponder (8.9% ± 8.9 and 44.8% ± 26.1) ($P = 0.269$ and 0.198) (Table 2) (Figure 2). In the ROC analysis, area under the curve of decrease in PES was 0.84, and that of posttreatment tumor length and PES were 0.69 and 0.75. The best decrease in PES cutoff with which to differentiate between responders and nonresponders was 18.8%, which yielded a sensitivity of 91% and a specificity of 75% (Figure 3).

The results of this study indicated that posttreatment tumor length and PES in responders were significantly smaller than those in nonresponders, and that decrease in PES in responders was significantly greater than that in nonresponders. The change of PES of barium esophagography

(a)   (b)

(c)

(d)

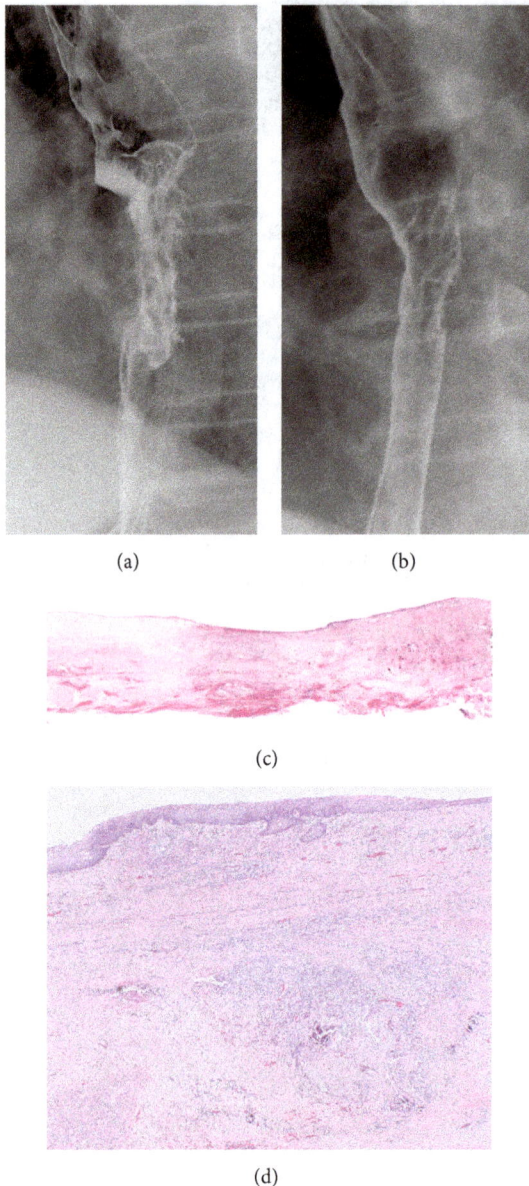

FIGURE 2: 76-year-old male with esophageal cancer who obtained a grade 3 pathologic response. (a) Before NACRT, esophagography shows irregular wall stenosis in the middle esophagus with the PES of 55.6%. (b) After NACRT, esophageal wall stenosis has improved result in the PES of 33.8%, which indicates the decrease in PES of 18.8%. (c), (d) Pathological specimen of the resected esophagus shows no carcinoma cells (grade 3). Many degenerative cells with keratinization and diffuse fibrosis are seen in the submucosa and muscularis propria.

FIGURE 3: ROC analysis. The best decrease in PES cutoff with which to differentiate between responders and nonresponders is 18.8%, which yields a sensitivity of 91% and a specificity of 75%.

might reflect the changes in tumor volume. Ito et al. reported that barium esophagography was useful diagnostic tool in the tumor staging of esophageal cancer and that the accuracy rate of the depth of invasion with barium esophagography was comparable to EUS [6]. The PES of barium esophagography increases according to the depth of tumor invasion, which is highly associated with tumor volume.

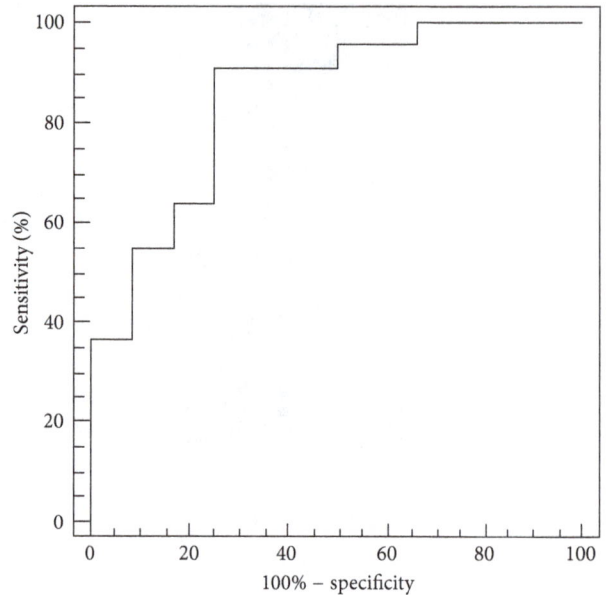

There was no significant difference in other parameters such as posttreatment tumor volume, decrease in tumor volume, and decrease in tumor length between responders and nonresponders. These results may support the inaccuracy of tumor volume measurement on 2 dimensional images such as esophagography. Regarding the posttreatment tumor length, it may not be suitable for the response evaluation, because it is very difficult to demarcate the ill-defined tumor from normal esophagus after chemoradiotherapy.

The results of this study indicated that a double-contrast barium esophagography using PES differentiated between responders and nonresponders with the sensitivity of 91% and specificity of 75%. Endoscopic ultrasound (EUS) or F-18 fluorodeoxyglucose positron emission tomography (FDG-PET) has been used for evaluation of therapeutic response in patients with esophageal cancer; the sensitivity and the specificity are 50% to 100% and 36% to 100% for EUS [9–12], and 50% to 100% and 55% to 100% for FDG-PET [10, 13–16]. Our result indicated that the diagnostic performance of barium esophagography could be comparable to EUS or FDG-PET.

In recent years, barium esophagography has not generally been used in evaluating the therapeutic response, because quantitative assessment of esophageal tumor using conventional volumetry was considered to be difficult due to its diverse nature [5]. Even pathologically markedly effective cases present esophageal wall thickening related to inflammatory change or fibrosis without residual cancer [17–19]. There were 10–11.9% mismatched cases shown to have a pathological complete response despite being diagnosed with residual tumors [20, 21]. Several studies investigated previously the use of endoscopic biopsy in predicting the pathological response to neoadjuvant therapy [22–24]. However, these studies suggested that endoscopic biopsy is not reliable for determining the presence of residual disease because of higher rates of false negative results.

In our study, most responders after NACRT had some degree of esophageal stenosis owing to inflammatory change or fibrosis. In clinical setting, it is more practical to differentiate responder from nonresponder rather than to diagnose no residual cancer, because it has been recently shown that patients responding to neoadjuvant therapy had a better survival than patients not responding to neoadjuvant therapy [25–28]. It is also useful if our results can be adapted to the response evaluation of definite chemoradiotherapy. Treatment response of definite chemoradiotherapy is generally determined by imaging examination or follow-up investigation several months later not by pathological findings. In the course of definitive chemoradiotherapy, a method that can be used to predict therapeutic response early after initiating chemoradiation is crucially important for avoiding chemoradiation-related side effects and unnecessary delay for surgery.

In the diagnosis or treatment evaluation of esophageal cancer, barium esophagography is the primary imaging technique, which is simple to perform, inexpensive, and noninvasive. Furthermore, double-contrast esophagography reveals the mucosal appearance and enables good reproduction of lesions. The value of barium esophagography should be reviewed because it can be useful for evaluation of treatment response to Chemoradiotherapy as well as staging of locally advanced esophageal cancer.

There are some limitations that need to be addressed regarding this study. First, the patients were examined between 2 and 4 weeks and operated between 3 and 10 weeks after completion of NACRT. There was great variability in the time interval between the examination and the operation among patients, which might have influence on our result. Secondly, association of nodal involvement or other prognostic factors were not discussed. They might be also important factors for evaluating the response of NACRT.

4. Conclusions

Decrease in PES after chemoradiotherapy is a good parameter to differentiate responders from nonresponders for NACRT. Barium esophagography, commonly or traditionally used modality, has still been a useful diagnostic tool which could determine the response to NACRT in patients with locally advanced esophageal cancer.

Conflict of Interests

The authors declare that there is no conflict of interests regarding the publication of this paper.

Acknowledgment

This work was supported by JSPS KAKENHI Grant no. 23591773.

References

[1] F. Duffaud and P. Therasse, "New guidelines to evaluate the response to treatment in solid tumors," *Bulletin du Cancer*, vol. 87, no. 12, pp. 881–886, 2000.

[2] M. Tahara, A. Ohtsu, S. Hironaka et al., "Clinical impact of criteria for complete response (CR) of primary site to treatment of esophageal cancer," *Japanese Journal of Clinical Oncology*, vol. 35, no. 6, pp. 316–323, 2005.

[3] J. R. Bessell, P. G. Devitt, P. G. Gill, S. Goyal, and G. G. Jamieson, "Prolonged survival follows resection of oesophageal SCC downstaged by prior chemoradiotherapy," *Australian and New Zealand Journal of Surgery*, vol. 66, no. 4, pp. 214–217, 1996.

[4] J. R. Hyngstrom and M. C. Posner, "Neoadjuvant strategies for the treatment of locally advanced esophageal cancer," *Journal of Surgical Oncology*, vol. 101, no. 4, pp. 299–304, 2010.

[5] S. J. Walker, S. M. Allen, A. Steel, M. H. Cullen, and H. R. Matthews, "Assessment of the response to chemotherapy in oesophageal cancer," *European Journal of Cardio-Thoracic Surgery*, vol. 5, no. 10, pp. 519–522, 1991.

[6] B. Ito, Y. Niwa, N. Ando et al., "Diagnosis of the depth of invasion of esophageal carcinoma using digital radiography," *European Journal of Radiology*, vol. 54, no. 3, pp. 377–382, 2005.

[7] F. P. Agha, M. A. Gennis, M. B. Orringer, and A. A. Forastiere, "Evaluation of response to preoperative chemotherapy in esophageal and gastric cardia cancer using biphasic esophagrams and surgical-pathologic correlation," *American Journal of Clinical Oncology*, vol. 9, no. 3, pp. 227–232, 1986.

[8] Japanese Society for Esophageal Diseases, *Guidelines for the Clinical and Pathologic Studies on Carcinoma of the Esophagus*, Kanehara, Tokyo, Japan, 9th edition, 1999.

[9] M. Giovannini, J. F. Seitz, P. Thomas et al., "Endoscopic ultrasonography for assessment of the response to combined radiation therapy and chemotherapy in patients with esophageal cancer," *Endoscopy*, vol. 29, no. 1, pp. 4–9, 1997.

[10] M. Westerterp, H. L. van Westreenen, J. B. Reitsma et al., "Esophageal cancer: CT, endoscopie US, and FDG PET for assessment of response to neoadjuvant therapy-systematic review," *Radiology*, vol. 236, no. 3, pp. 841–851, 2005.

[11] N. Hirata, K. Kawamoto, T. Ueyama, K. Masuda, T. Utsunomiya, and H. Kuwano, "Using endosonography to assess the effects of neoadjuvant therapy in patients with advanced esophageal cancer," *American Journal of Roentgenology*, vol. 169, no. 2, pp. 485–491, 1997.

[12] J. Willis, G. S. Cooper, G. Isenberg et al., "Correlation of EUS measurement with pathologic assessment of neoadjuvant therapy response in esophageal carcinoma," *Gastrointestinal Endoscopy*, vol. 55, no. 6, pp. 655–661, 2002.

[13] J. R. Kroep, C. J. van Groeningen, M. A. Cuesta et al., "Positron emission tomography using 2-deoxy-2-[18 F]-fluoro-D-glucose for response monitoring in locally advanced gastroesophageal cancer; a comparison of different analytical methods," *Molecular Imaging and Biology*, vol. 5, no. 5, pp. 337–346, 2003.

[14] B. L. D. M. Brucher, W. Weber, M. Bauer et al., "Neoadjuvant therapy of esophageal squamous cell carcinoma: response evaluation by positron emission tomography," *Annals of Surgery*, vol. 233, no. 3, pp. 300–309, 2001.

[15] W. A. Weber, K. Ott, K. Becker et al., "Prediction of response to preoperative chemotherapy in adenocarcinomas of the esophagogastric junction by metabolic imaging," *Journal of Clinical Oncology*, vol. 19, no. 12, pp. 3058–3065, 2001.

[16] P. Flamen, E. van Cutsem, A. Lerut et al., "Positron emission tomography for assessment of the response to induction radiochemotherapy in locally advanced oesophageal cancer," *Annals of Oncology*, vol. 13, no. 3, pp. 361–368, 2002.

[17] R. Earlam and J. R. Cunha-Melo, "Oesophageal squamous cell carcinoma. II: a critical review of radiotherapy," *British Journal of Surgery*, vol. 67, no. 7, pp. 457–461, 1980.

[18] J. M. Muller, H. Erasmi, M. Stelzner, U. Zieren, and H. Pichlmaier, "Surgical therapy of oesophageal carcinoma," *British Journal of Surgery*, vol. 77, no. 8, pp. 845–857, 1990.

[19] S. Y. K. Law, M. Fok, and J. Wong, "Pattern of recurrence after oesophageal resection for cancer: clinical implications," *British Journal of Surgery*, vol. 83, no. 1, pp. 107–111, 1996.

[20] Y. Okamoto, M. Murakami, Y. Kuroda et al., "Mismatched clinicopathological response after concurrent chemoradiotherapy for thoracic esophageal cancer," *Diseases of the Esophagus*, vol. 13, no. 1, pp. 80–86, 2000.

[21] K. Morita, I. Takagi, and M. Watanabe, "Relationship between the radiologic features of esophageal cancer and the local control by radiation therapy," *Cancer*, vol. 55, no. 11, pp. 2668–2676, 1985.

[22] I. S. Sarkaria, N. P. Rizk, M. S. Bains et al., "Post-treatment endoscopic biopsy is a poor-predictor of pathologic response in patients undergoing chemoradiation therapy for esophageal cancer," *Annals of Surgery*, vol. 249, no. 5, pp. 764–767, 2009.

[23] Q. Yang, K. R. Cleary, J. C. Yao et al., "Significance of post-chemoradiation biopsy in predicting residual esophageal carcinoma in the surgical specimen," *Diseases of the Esophagus*, vol. 17, no. 1, pp. 38–43, 2004.

[24] B. A. Bates, F. C. Detterbeck, S. A. Bernard, B. F. Qaqish, and J. E. Tepper, "Concurrent radiation therapy and chemotherapy followed by esophagectomy for localized esophageal carcinoma," *Journal of Clinical Oncology*, vol. 14, no. 1, pp. 156–163, 1996.

[25] M. A. Chidel, T. W. Rice, D. J. Adelstein, P. A. Kupelian, J. H. Suh, and M. Becker, "Resectable esophageal carcinoma: local control with neoadjuvant chemotherapy and radiation therapy," *Radiology*, vol. 213, no. 1, pp. 67–72, 1999.

[26] M. Morita, T. Masuda, S. Okada et al., "Preoperative chemodiotherapy for esophageal cancer: factors associated with clinical response and postoperative complications," *Anticancer Research*, vol. 29, no. 7, pp. 2555–2562, 2009.

[27] J. S. Donington, D. L. Miller, M. S. Allen, C. Deschamps, F. C. Nichols III, and P. C. Pairolero, "Tumor response to induction chemoradiation: influence on survival after esophagectomy," *European Journal of Cardio-Thoracic Surgery*, vol. 24, no. 4, pp. 631–637, 2003.

[28] A. A. Forastiere, M. B. Orringer, C. Perez-Tamayo, S. G. Urba, and M. Zahurak, "Preoperative chemoradiation followed by transhiatal esophagectomy for carcinoma of the esophagus: final report," *Journal of Clinical Oncology*, vol. 11, no. 6, pp. 1118–1123, 1993.

5

Treatment of Nonvariceal Gastrointestinal Hemorrhage by Transcatheter Embolization

Muhammad Ali, Tanveer Ul Haq, Basit Salam, Madiha Beg, Raza Sayani, and Muhammad Azeemuddin

Radiology Department, Aga Khan University Hospital, Stadium Road, P.O. Box 3500, Karachi 74800, Pakistan

Correspondence should be addressed to Raza Sayani; sayani_raza@yahoo.com

Academic Editor: Sotirios Bisdas

Purpose. To investigate the sensitivity of mesenteric angiography, technical success of hemostasis, clinical success rate, and complications of transcatheter embolization for the treatment of acute nonvariceal gastrointestinal hemorrhage. *Material and Methods.* A retrospective review of 200 consecutive patients who underwent mesenteric arteriography for acute nonvariceal gastrointestinal hemorrhage between February 2004 and February 2011 was done. *Results.* Of 200 angiographic studies, 114 correctly revealed the bleeding site with mesenteric angiography. 47 (41%) patients had upper gastrointestinal hemorrhage and 67 (59%) patients had lower gastrointestinal hemorrhage. Out of these 114, in 112 patients (98%) technical success was achieved with immediate cessation of bleeding. 81 patients could be followed for one month. Clinical success was achieved in 72 out of these 81 patients (89%). Seven patients rebled. 2 patients developed bowel ischemia. Four patients underwent surgery for bowel ischemia or rebleeding. *Conclusion.* The use of therapeutic transcatheter embolization for treatment of acute gastrointestinal hemorrhage is highly successful and relatively safe with 98% technical success and 2.4% postembolization ischemia in our series. In 89% of cases it was definitive without any further intervention.

1. Introduction

Acute gastrointestinal (GI) hemorrhage is a commonly presenting medical emergency having a hospital mortality of around 10% [1]. Presentation may vary from insidious blood loss to potentially life-threatening hemorrhage [2]. The bleeding site determination is challenging as it involves entire gastrointestinal tract [2]. Upper gastrointestinal hemorrhage patients present with hematemesis or melena and the bleeding point is proximal to the ligament of Treitz, whereas gastrointestinal lower haemorrhage patients present with melena or hematochezia and bleeding point is distal to the ligament of Treitz [3–5]. Bleeding ceases spontaneously in approximately 75% of cases and can recur in 25% of cases, resulting in significant morbidity and mortality [6].

Therapeutic options available for patients with acute GI hemorrhage include conservative medical management, endoscopic coagulation, vasopressin infusion, therapeutic transcatheter embolization, and surgery [7, 8]. Endoscopy is considered as a first-line diagnostic and therapeutic procedure; its sensitivity reaches 100% in upper gastrointestinal bleed but in case of lower gastrointestinal bleed only probable bleeding source can be found (60% of cases). In stable patients, radionuclide and CT imaging plays a great role. Tc-99m RBC scintigraphy is more than 90% sensitive and specific in detecting a bleeding site anywhere in gastrointestinal tract. However, its limited resolution does not allow precise gastrointestinal bleed localization.

Endoscopy can fail in approximately 32% of cases because of presence of stool, blood clots, and technical difficulties as time required for patient's preparation for colonoscopy [9]. In addition, bleeder source in small bowel is not accessible via colonoscope [10]. Significant morbidity and mortality are associated with emergency surgery [11]. Higher rates of complication and rebleeding were encountered in patients treated with vasopressin [12]. Nusbaum and Baum first described mesenteric angiography for acute GI hemorrhage in 1963 [13]. In 1972, Rösch et al. successfully controlled acute gastric hemorrhage by gastroepiploic artery embolization using autologous blood clot [14]. Due to significant technical improvements in the past 10 years selective therapeutic transcatheter embolization has become a safer procedure and is now widely used for acute GI hemorrhage management [15].

The purpose of our study was to investigate the sensitivity of mesenteric angiography, technical success of hemostasis, clinical success rate, and complications of therapeutic transcatheter embolization for the treatment of acute nonvariceal gastrointestinal hemorrhage.

2. Materials and Methods

2.1. Study Group. We performed a single-center (from February 2004 to February 2011) retrospective survey of all patients in whom therapeutic transcatheter embolization was attempted for control of acute gastrointestinal bleeding.

2.2. Patient Selection. All acute GI hemorrhage patients who underwent mesenteric angiograms during this period were enrolled. These patients had been referred to by abdominal surgeons, emergency room (ER) physicians, or gastroenterologists, and procedures were performed by experienced interventional radiologist.

2.3. Clinical Data. The clinical and laboratory data, imaging and endoscopic findings, and care provided as well as the outcome data were obtained from medical records of our hospital. The following parameters were collected for each patient: age, gender, presenting symptoms, severity of hemorrhage, site of bleeding, comorbid, number of units of blood or packed red blood cells transfused, history of coagulation disorder, and findings of prior endoscopy or scintigraphy. Angiographic characteristics include segmental localization of bleeding in the gastrointestinal tract, vascular territory which is corresponding, catheters used for embolization, technique of embolization whether selective (proximal) or superselective (distal), repeat angiographic procedures, and type of embolic agent(s) used. Complications were divided into intraoperative and postprocedural complications. Follow-up duration as well as conservative or surgical management of complications was also documented.

2.4. Angiography and Embolization. Celiac, superior mesenteric, and inferior mesenteric angiography was performed transfemorally using 4 Fr or 5 Fr Cobra or Simmons type catheters (Cordis). Selective SMA angiography was also done by advancing catheter in different branches to evaluate the jejunal, ileal, ileocolic, and colic branches. Once the bleeding site was determined, then superselective catheterization was usually performed using a 2.7 Fr microcatheter (Progreat-Terumo), which is inserted coaxially through the macrocatheter. Superselective embolization was attempted by positioning the catheter as close to the bleeding site as possible. The materials used for embolization included microcoils (Cook and Balt), gelfoam, and polyvinyl alcohol particles (Boston Scientific). Other than active bleeding or pseudoaneurysm indirect sign for abnormal site was described when there were arteriovenous fistula vascular tuft,

early filling vein, or a hyper vascular mass. In certain cases where there was endoscopic finding of active bleeding from duodenal region and a negative arteriography, a prophylactic embolization of the gastroduodenal artery was performed using Sandwich technique. In this the catheter is placed distal to the bleeding site followed by placement of coil, and then the catheter is withdrawn proximal to the bleeding site with deployment of another coil to sandwich the bleeding point in between. This technique ensures any retrograde filling of the targeted portion of the vessel embolized. In few cases with severe vasospasm intra-arterial nitroglycerine was also given.

All procedures were performed by vascular access at the level of the common femoral artery using 5 Fr vascular access sheath (Arrow, Medcomp). Postexamination, manual compression was maintained at puncture site with the patient lying in supine position for hemostasis.

2.5. Definition and Data Analysis. Successful embolization is termed when there is devascularization of a focal lesion or reduction or stoppage of flow to the vascular bed. We defined outcome criteria in accordance with the guidelines of the Society of Interventional Radiology (SIR) [16].

Technical success was described as immediate cessation of extravasation on postprocedure angiography [16].

Clinical success was described as nonoccurrence of bleed or hemodynamic instability within 30 days after embolization on follow-up evaluation. Monitoring was performed to evaluate signs and symptoms of intestinal infarction or ischemia [16].

Rebleeding was described as drop in hemoglobin >1 g/dL in the presence of overt GI hemorrhage within 30 days. An ischemic event was defined as bowel ischemia or infarction that required surgery [16].

Data was entered into SPSS statistical software version 19.0. Mean and standard deviations were computed for quantitative variables. Frequencies and descriptive analysis of the variables also measured.

3. Results

From February 2004 until February 2011, a total of 200 patients underwent mesenteric angiography for acute GI hemorrhage at our institution. 114 patients (57%) had contrast blush or abnormal vascularity in the GI tract and underwent therapeutic transcatheter embolization.

There were 134 (67%) male and 66 (33%) female patients with male-to-female ratio of 2 : 1. Median age was 57 years (range: 8–97 years).

28 patients present with hematemesis, 66 with melena, and 106 with per-rectal bleeding. Severity of the symptoms was also calculated which were mild ($n = 74$), moderate ($n = 96$), and severe ($n = 30$). These are summarized in Table 1.

We also evaluated the effect of associated comorbid conditions which predispose to GI hemorrhage. 44 patients had no comorbid disease, 28 had infectious disease, 24 had chronic liver disease, 22 had hypertension, 15 had diabetes mellitus, 20 had chronic renal disease, 21 had malignancy,

TABLE 1: Demographics and characteristics of 200 patients who had mesenteric angiogram for acute GI hemorrhage.

Characteristics	Results
Angiographic sensitivity	114 (57%)
Median age	55 years
Gender	
Male	134 (76%)
Female	66 (33%)
Presenting complaints	
Hematemesis	28 (14%)
Melena	66 (33%)
Perrectal bleeding	106 (53%)
Prior investigation	
Upper GI endoscopy	93
Positive	66 (71%)
Negative	27 (29%)
RBC-tagged scintigraphy	62
Positive	49 (79%)
Negative	13 (21%)
Prior blood transfusion	145 (72.5%)
Coagulation profile	
Normal	124 (62%)
Deranged	76 (38%)
Comorbid	
No comorbid	44 (22%)
Chronic liver disease	24 (12%)
Hypertension	22 (11%)
Diabetes mellitus	15 (7.5%)
Chronic renal failure	20 (10%)
Malignancy	21 (10.5%)
Trauma	10 (5.0%)
Infectious diseases	28 (14%)
Misc	16 (8.0%)

10 had trauma, and 16 patients had miscellaneous comorbid diseases.

Blood was transfused in 145 (72.5%) out of 200 patients. Coagulation profile was deranged in 76 (38%) patients; the rest presented with a normal coagulation profile.

Prior RBC-tagged scintigraphy was performed in 62 patients. In 49 (79%) it showed activity corresponding to bleeding site. Majority of these patients had lower GI haemorrhage. Endoscopy was also performed in 93 patients of which 66 (70.9%) were positive.

On mesenteric angiography 47 patients (41%) had upper gastrointestinal hemorrhage, whereas 67 (59%) had lower gastrointestinal hemorrhage.

Angiographically positive sites were stomach 10 (8.8%), duodenum 37 (32.5%), jejunum 9 (7.9%), ileum 10 (8.8%), caecum 29 (25.4%), ascending colon 8 (7.0%), transverse colon 1 (0.9%), descending colon 2 (1.8%), and rectosigmoid region 8 (7.0%).

Embolization was technically possible in 112 of 114 patients, reaching a technical success rate of 98.24%. In one

patient technical failure was due to inability to catheterize the supplying artery. This patient had blunt abdominal trauma and presented with a large pseudoaneurysm filling from the inferior pancreaticoduodenal artery. After selective catheterization of the superior mesenteric artery multiple collateral vessels was seen at the origin of inferior pancreaticoduodenal artery with retrograde filling of gastroduodenal artery. Despite multiple attempts the collaterals supplying the pseudoaneurysm could not be catheterized. The second patient was a young woman who presented with per-rectal bleeding. Angiogram demonstrated an abnormal lesion in the rectum filling in the venous phase. There were multiple phleboliths suggesting venous hemangioma. Findings were discussed with referring surgeon and it was decided not to embolize this lesion due to low vascularity and risk of bowel ischemia.

Arteries primarily embolized were the gastroduodenal artery ($n = 36$) Figure 1, ileocolic artery ($n = 28$) Figure 2, right colic artery ($n = 12$), jejunal branches of superior mesenteric artery ($n = 10$), left gastric artery ($n = 9$), superior rectal artery ($n = 7$), ileal braches of superior mesenteric artery ($n = 5$), left colic artery ($n = 4$), and middle colic artery ($n = 1$).

We also evaluated the catheters used for angiography. In 109 (54.5%) patients microcatheter was used, whereas in 91 (45.4%) angiography was performed with regular 4 Fr catheters. Cobra catheter was used in 174 patients while Simmons catheter was used in 26 patients.

The type of embolic material used was at the discretion of the interventional radiologist, and in few patients materials were used in combination. Microcoils were used in isolation in 69 patients (62%) and in combination with particles in 9 patients (8%). Particles were used in isolation in 33 patients (29%) and gel foam was used in 1 patient (0.9%).

Out of 114 patients 81 were followed up with for one month, 17 for 1 week, and 1 for 1 day while 15 patients were lost to followup. Hence clinical success was measured in only 81 patients.

Total clinical success in the 30-day followup (i.e., complete resolution of signs or symptoms that prompted the embolization procedure) was achieved in 72 of 81 patients (89%). Seven out of 81 patients (11.5%) experienced clinical signs of early rebleeding Table 2. Corresponding vessels were gastroduodenal artery ($n = 3$), Jejunal branches of SMA ($n = 2$), and a single case from right ileocolic and left gastric arteries each. In 6 of them repeat angiographies were done, but only one patient showed recurrent jejunal hemorrhage and underwent clinically successful repeat embolization.

The only major complication was early bowel ischemia experienced by 2 (2.4%) of the 81 patients. An elderly male was presented with perrectal bleeding. Arteriography showed abnormal vascularity in the territory of superior rectal artery which was partially embolized using PVA particles. He developed postembolization ischemia along with thrombosis of right common iliac vein. He underwent urgent rectosigmoid resection, while limb ischemia was successfully managed conservatively with oral anticoagulants. Second patient was an elderly male with bleeding duodenal ulcer on endoscopy.

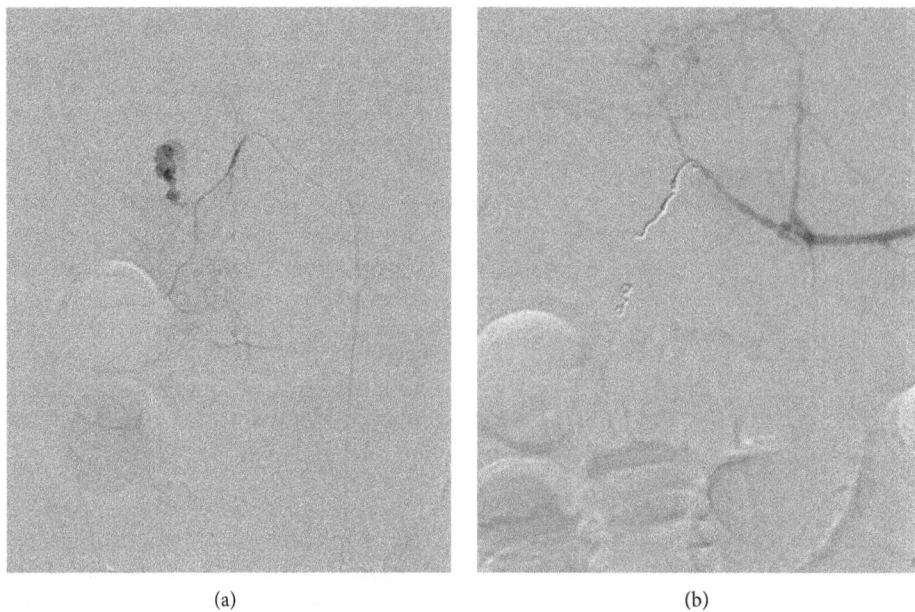

(a)   (b)

FIGURE 1: (a) Selective arteriogram of gastroduodenal artery demonstrates active bleeding from superior pancreaticoduodenal branch. (b) Postembolization arteriogram showed complete exclusion of the bleeding vessel by multiple platinum coils.

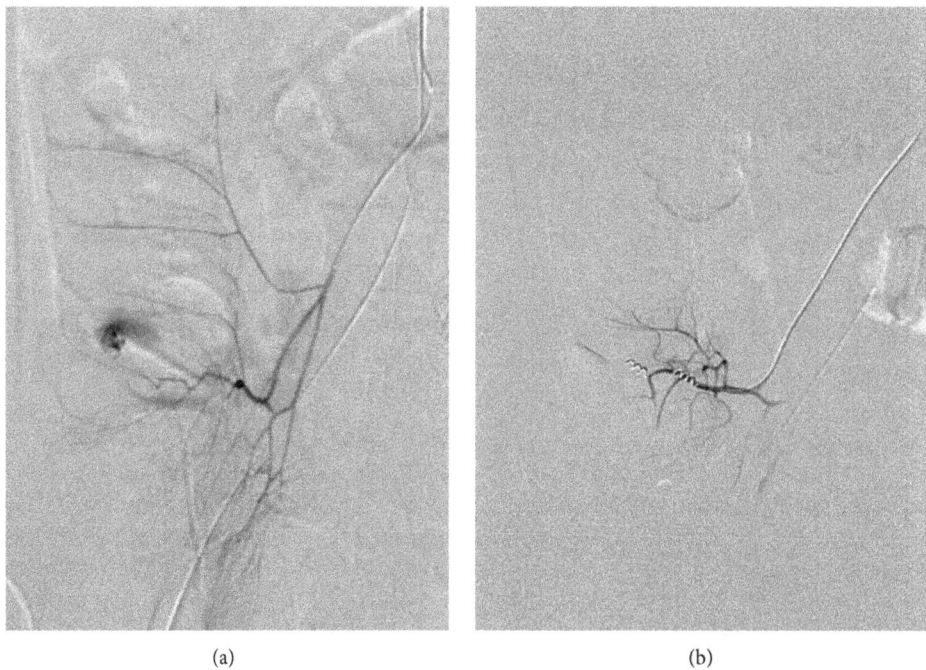

(a)   (b)

FIGURE 2: (a) Selective ileocolic artery angiogram demonstrates intraluminal extravasation of contrast in caecum. (b) Postembolization arteriogram after selective embolization shows total occlusion of feeding vessel and cessation of hemorrhaging.

His empiric embolization of gastroduodenal artery was done. He presented with symptoms of ischemia after three days and was managed conservatively (Table 3).

After embolization 4 patients underwent surgery 3 for recurrent bleeding and 1 for ischemia. No patient died as a consequence of complications caused by the procedure.

4. Discussion

Our data supports the present literature in demonstrating the efficiency of therapeutic transcatheter embolization in curing acute GI bleeding [5, 17]. In a recently published international consensus recommendation, arterial embolization

TABLE 2: Characteristics of 81 patients after one-month followup.

Characteristics	Results
Clinical success	72 (89%)
Complication (bowel ischemia)	02 (2.4%)
Rebleeding	07 (8.6%)
Repeat procedure	06 (7.4%)
Surgical management	04 (4.9%)

TABLE 3: Characteristics of 114 patients who revealed bleeding site and underwent therapeutic embolization.

Characteristics	Results
Technical success	112 (98%)
Site	
Upper GI hemorrhage	47 (41%)
Lower GI hemorrhage	67 (59%)
Embolization	
Proximal (selective)	21 (19%)
Distal (superselective)	91 (81%)
Arteries embolized	
Gastroduodenal artery	36 (32%)
Ileocolic artery	28 (25%)
Right colic artery	12 (11%)
Jejunal branches of SMA	10 (8.9%)
Left gastric artery	09 (8.0%)
Superior rectal artery	07 (6.2%)
Ileal branches of SMA	05 (4.4%)
Left colic artery	04 (3.6%)
Middle colic artery	01 (0.9%)
Embolization material	
Microcoils	69 (62%)
PVA particles	33 (29%)
PVA with microcoils	09 (8.0%)
Gel foam	01 (0.9%)

is considered as a surgical alternative in upper GI bleeding management in whom endoscopic haemostatic procedure has failed or who had recurrent bleeding [16]. Similarly arterial embolization is now considered a first-line therapy for patients with severe lower GI bleeding [18].

The first objective of arteriography is to identify the bleeding site which requires the patient to be actively bleeding [19, 20]. In few patients even a detailed workup may fail to identify an exact bleeding site, which resulted in the patients undergoing repeated blood transfusions and invasive investigations [20]. In our study 57% of the angiographies were positive. Charbonnet et al. [2] reported a positive rate of 37% while survey by Zuckerman and Prakash [9] found that the rate of positive angiograms can vary from 27% to 77%. Chevallier and colleagues [21] reported very high percentage (93.4%) of positive angiographies which can be explained by the increased frequency of superselective catheter placement in these patients. Nevertheless an angiography may give normal results despite superselective catheterization because even a massive hemorrhage can be intermittent [4]. In these

cases a blind or empirical embolization can be done, however, it is associated with an increased chance of rebleeding and ischemia [5, 7, 8]. To increase the positive rate prior to endoscopy, Tc 99 RBC-tagged scintigraphic evaluation or contrast enhanced CT scans could be helpful in identifying the bleeding vessel [6, 10, 20].

In our study prior Tc 99 RBC-tagged scintigraphy was performed in 62 patients with acute GI hemorrhage of which 49 (79%) were positive and helped in the identification of bleeding site. Similarly, endoscopy was performed in 93 patients of whom 66 (66%) were positive and guide towards the bleeding vessel.

Endoscopy for the management of gastrointestinal bleed still remains a feasible option whenever possible. Endoscopy can be diagnostic as well as therapeutic especially in upper GI bleed; however, in cases with massive GI bleed visualization becomes challenging and technically difficult. For lower GI bleed the technical success of endoscopy also depends on bowel preparation for optimal visualization. Evaluation of small bowel loops with endoscopy is not possible. For those patients in whom endoscopy was inconclusive or failed due to reasons described therapeutic transcatheter embolization is considered useful option. Surgery is rarely used for treatment of upper GI bleeds; however, it is still utilized for management of lower GI bleeds where endoscopic and transcatheter embolizations have failed or were not available. MDCT angio is considered as the initial radiological investigation as it is a very simple technique. It still requires active bleeding at the time of imaging but may be repeated in case of the first negative examination. A positive MDCT angio can select appropriate patients for rapid targeted embolization. The visualization of active extravasation of IV contrast in the GI tract requires careful attention to technique, including thin collimation, rapid IV contrast administration, and appropriate scan timing. The addition of multiplanar reconstructions (MPR) and 3D imaging is beneficial in identifying the exact source of the bleeding.

The present review, with a technical success rate of 98%, is concurrent with many other reports quoting technical success of more than 90% [4, 5, 8]. Defreyne and colleagues [22] reported technical success rate of 98%, while in a recent study Tan et al. [4] reported a technical success of 97%. In the literature only few technical failures have been reported, and they were mainly due to difficult vascular anatomy, vascular stenosis, and vascular spasms [15, 19]. In few cases intermittent contrast material extravasation can occur which reflects spontaneous bleeding arrests [22]. In such cases, the main arterial trunk should be vigorously studied to determine the point for safe embolization [3, 15, 22]. Because active extravasation was initially localized, we did not find indication for the use of anticoagulants or fibrinolytics, as recommended by some authors [22, 23].

There is a certain risk of complications with reported rates of major ischemic complications range from 0% to 16% [23, 24]. Very low rate (2.4%) of bowel ischemia in our study indicates that we delivered the right amount of embolic material in most of the cases. Luc Defreyne in 2001 observed absence of bowel ischemia in 40 patients [22]. Aina and colleagues [24] reviewed 75 consecutive patients who underwent arterial embolization for upper GI bleeding and reported a 99% technical success with a primary clinical success rate of 76%. Only three cases (4%) of ischemia were noted, two involving the duodenum and one the liver [24]. In our study rate of rebleeding was 8.6%. The reported rebleeding rate after therapeutic transcatheter embolization is approximately 33% (range: 9%–66%) [4]. Kwak et al. [5] found rebleeding in 21% of the patients while Wong and colleagues [11] reported high rate of rebleeding (34.4%). A possible explanation for the high rebleeding rate may be coiling the gastroduodenal artery from the celiac axis in these series as gastroduodenal artery can be later fed with collateral branches from the superior mesenteric artery [1, 11]. Our study also concurred with these results as 5 (38%) of the patients showed rebleeding from gastroduodenal artery. A sandwich technique can be used in these cases in which the gastroduodenal artery was coiled in a distal-to-proximal manner [1, 15]. Similarly inflammatory or ischemic reactions after embolization can trigger vasodilatation of the intramural collaterals and early rebleeding [12].

Our study had certain limitations, including the fact that it was a retrospective analysis, and the refinement and clinical validation of angiographic embolization require a prospective study. Secondly series of patients were enrolled from a single institution, and the cause of bleeding was not known in all cases.

In conclusion, therapeutic transcatheter embolization for the treatment of acute gastrointestinal hemorrhage is highly successful and relatively safe procedure with high technical and clinical success rates, and it should be reserved as a treatment option for patients who are high risk for surgery and failed endoscopic and medical management.

Conflict of Interests

The authors do not have any disclosures or conflict of interests that they would like to declare in relation to their paper.

References

[1] K. Palmer, "Acute upper gastrointestinal haemorrhage," British Medical Bulletin, vol. 83, no. 1, pp. 307–324, 2007.

[2] P. Charbonnet, J. Toman, L. Bühler et al., "Treatment of gastrointestinal hemorrhage," Abdominal Imaging, vol. 30, no. 6, pp. 719–726, 2005.

[3] B. J. D'Othée, P. Surapaneni, D. Rabkin, I. Nasser, and M. Clouse, "Microcoil embolization for acute lower gastrointestinal bleeding," CardioVascular and Interventional Radiology, vol. 29, no. 1, pp. 49–58, 2006.

[4] K.-K. Tan, D. Wong, and R. Sim, "Superselective embolization for lower gastrointestinal hemorrhage: an institutional review over 7 years," World Journal of Surgery, vol. 32, no. 12, pp. 2707–2715, 2008.

[5] H.-S. Kwak, Y.-M. Han, and S.-T. Lee, "The clinical outcomes of transcatheter microcoil embolization in patients with active lower gastrointestinal bleeding in the small bowel," Korean Journal of Radiology, vol. 10, no. 4, pp. 391–397, 2009.

[6] Y. Geffroy, M. H. Rodallec, I. Boulay-Coletta, M.-C. Jullès, C. Ridereau-Zins, and M. Zins, "Multidetector CT angiography in acute gastrointestinal bleeding: why, when, and how," Radiographics, vol. 31, no. 3, pp. E1–E12, 2011.

[7] M. P. Cherian, P. Mehta, T. M. Kalyanpur, S. S. Hedgire, and K. S. Narsinghpura, "Arterial interventions in gastrointestinal bleeding," Seminars in Interventional Radiology, vol. 26, no. 3, pp. 184–195, 2009.

[8] R. Sheth, V. Someshwar, and G. Warawdekar, "Treatment of acute lower gastrointestinal hemorrhage by superselective transcatheter embolization," Indian Journal of Gastroenterology, vol. 25, no. 6, pp. 290–294, 2006.

[9] G. R. Zuckerman and C. Prakash, "Acute lower intestinal bleeding. Part I: clinical presentation and diagnosis," Gastrointestinal Endoscopy, vol. 48, no. 6, pp. 606–616, 1998.

[10] L. Fisher, M. Lee Krinsky, M. A. Anderson et al., "The role of endoscopy in the management of obscure GI bleeding," Gastrointestinal Endoscopy, vol. 72, no. 3, pp. 471–479, 2010.

[11] T. C. L. Wong, K.-T. Wong, P. W. Y. Chiu et al., "A comparison of angiographic embolization with surgery after failed endoscopic hemostasis to bleeding peptic ulcers," Gastrointestinal Endoscopy, vol. 73, no. 5, pp. 900–908, 2011.

[12] M. Miller Jr. and T. P. Smith, "Angiographic diagnosis and endovascular management of nonvariceal gastrointestinal hemorrhage," Gastroenterology Clinics of North America, vol. 34, no. 4, pp. 735–752, 2005.

[13] M. Nusbaum and S. Baum, "Radiographic demonstration of unknown sites of gastrointestinal bleeding," Surgical forum, vol. 14, pp. 374–375, 1963.

[14] J. Rösch, C. T. Dotter, and M. J. Brown, "Selective arterial embolization. A new method for control of acute gastrointestinal bleeding," Radiology, vol. 102, no. 2, pp. 303–306, 1972.

[15] S. Mirsadraee, P. Tirukonda, A. Nicholson, S. M. Everett, and S. J. McPherson, "Embolization for non-variceal upper gastrointestinal tract haemorrhage: a systematic review," Clinical Radiology, vol. 66, no. 6, pp. 500–509, 2011.

[16] J. F. Angle, N. H. Siddiqi, M. J. Wallace et al., "Quality improvement guidelines for percutaneous transcatheter embolization: society of interventional radiology standards of practice committee," Journal of Vascular and Interventional Radiology, vol. 21, no. 10, pp. 1479–1486, 2010.

[17] R. Kickuth, H. Rattunde, J. Gschossmann, D. Inderbitzin, K. Ludwig, and J. Triller, "Acute lower gastrointestinal hemorrhage: minimally invasive management with microcatheter embolization," Journal of Vascular and Interventional Radiology, vol. 19, no. 9, pp. 1289–1296, 2008.

[18] A. N. Barkun, M. Bardou, E. J. Kuipers et al., "International consensus recommendations on the management of patients with nonvariceal upper gastrointestinal bleeding," Annals of Internal Medicine, vol. 152, no. 2, pp. 101–113, 2010.

[19] R. Loffroy, P. Rao, S. Ota, M. De Lin, B.-K. Kwak, and J.-F. Geschwind, "Embolization of acute nonvariceal upper gastrointestinal hemorrhage resistant to endoscopic treatment: results and predictors of recurrent bleeding," CardioVascular and Interventional Radiology, vol. 33, no. 6, pp. 1088–1100, 2010.

[20] S. F. Kerr and S. Puppala, "Acute gastrointestinal haemorrhage: the role of the radiologist," Postgraduate Medical Journal, vol. 87, no. 1027, pp. 362–368, 2011.

[21] P. Chevallier, S. Novellas, G. Vanbiervliet et al., "Transcatheter embolization for endoscopically unmanageable acute nonvariceal upper gastrointestinal hemorrhage," Journal de Radiologie, vol. 88, no. 2, pp. 251–258, 2007.

[22] L. Defreyne, P. Vanlangenhove, M. De Vos et al., "Embolization as a first approach with endoscopically unmanageable acute nonvariceal gastrointestinal hemorrhage," *Radiology*, vol. 218, no. 3, pp. 739–748, 2001.

[23] G. A. Poultsides, C. J. Kim, R. Orlando III, G. Peros, M. J. Hallisey, and P. V. Vignati, "Angiographic embolization for gastroduodenal hemorrhage: safety, efficacy, and predictors of outcome," *Archives of Surgery*, vol. 143, no. 5, pp. 457–461, 2008.

[24] R. Aina, V. L. Oliva, E. Therasse et al., "Arterial embolotherapy for upper gastrointestinal hemorrhage: outcome assessment," *Journal of Vascular and Interventional Radiology*, vol. 12, no. 2, pp. 195–200, 2001.

6

Congenital Extrahepatic Portosystemic Shunts: Spectrum of Findings on Ultrasound, Computed Tomography, and Magnetic Resonance Imaging

Pankaj Gupta,[1] **Anindita Sinha,**[1] **Kushaljit Singh Sodhi,**[1] **Anupam Lal,**[1] **Uma Debi,**[1]
Babu R. Thapa,[2] **and Niranjan Khandelwal**[1]

[1]*Department of Radiodiagnosis and Imaging, Post Graduate Institute of Medical Education and Research (PGIMER), Chandigarh 160012, India*
[2]*Pediatric Gastroenterology, Post Graduate Institute of Medical Education and Research (PGIMER), Chandigarh 160012, India*

Correspondence should be addressed to Anindita Sinha; dranindita@gmail.com

Academic Editor: Henrique M. Lederman

Congenital extrahepatic portosystemic shunt (CEPS) is a rare disorder characterised by partial or complete diversion of portomesenteric blood into systemic veins via congenital shunts. Type I is characterised by complete lack of intrahepatic portal venous blood flow due to an end to side fistula between main portal vein and the inferior vena cava. Type II on the other hand is characterised by partial preservation of portal blood supply to liver and side to side fistula between main portal vein or its branches and mesenteric, splenic, gastric, and systemic veins. The presentation of these patients is variable. Focal liver lesions, most commonly nodular regenerative hyperplasia, are an important clue to the underlying condition. This pictorial essay covers imaging characteristics in abdominopelvic region.

1. Introduction

Abernethy described the first case of congenital extrahepatic portosystemic shunt on autopsy on a 10-month-old female who died of unknown cause [1]. He demonstrated the absence of portal vein and existence of a mesentericocaval shunt. This is the classic description of congenital extrahepatic portosystemic shunt type I. These cases are characterised by complete absence of intrahepatic portal blood flow [2]. Type II shunts are more varied in their anatomy and are characterised by partial interruption of portal venous flow to the liver caused by portocaval, gastrorenal, mesenterico-renal, splenorenal, or mesenterico-iliac shunts [3]. The embryogenesis of this congenital anomaly is complex. Clinical presentation is variable and complex. Cases of incidental detection during imaging for evaluation of unrelated complaints are described. Adults may be diagnosed on evaluation of hepatic encephalopathy [4]. Imaging plays an important role in establishing diagnosis and detection of associated focal liver lesions and malformations that are commonly encountered in type I

malformation. Biopsy is indicated in cases where findings for type I malformation are equivocal on imaging and when benign nature of the focal liver lesions cannot be established with certainty on imaging [5]. Management is guided by the type of malformation and clinical presentation. Type I malformations are not amenable to surgical or endovascular procedures. Liver transplant is the only potential therapy in patients presenting with medically recalcitrant signs and symptoms [6]. Type II malformations can be corrected by surgical ligation or endovascular occlusion [7].

2. Classification

Classification is based on the presence or the lack of intrahepatic portal venous flow. In type I congenital extrahepatic portosystemic shunt, there is complete shunting of the portal blood via a fistulous communication between main portal vein and inferior vena cava [2]. Intrahepatic portal venous branches are not developed. Two subtypes have been

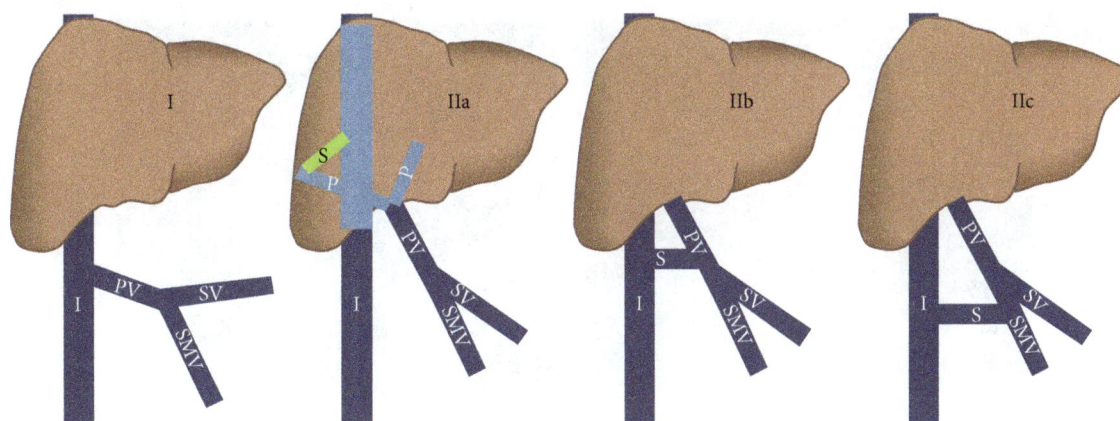

FIGURE 1: Schematic diagram showing various types of CEPS. I: IVC, P: portal vein branches, PV: portal vein, S: shunt, SMV: superior mesenteric vein, and SV: splenic vein.

described: type Ia, where splenic vein and superior mesenteric vein drain separately into the systemic veins, and type Ib, where a splenic vein and SMV form a common channel before draining into the inferior vena cava [2, 8]. Type II congenital extrahepatic portosystemic shunt is characterised by partial diversion of the portal blood flow into the systemic veins [3]. The main portal vein may be attenuated; however, the intrahepatic portal vein branches are present. Based on the level of abnormal communication, three subtypes have been described. Type IIa shunts arise from portal vein branches and include the patent ductus venous in addition to other shunts [9]. In type IIb congenital extrahepatic portosystemic shunt, the shunts arise from the main portal vein, its bifurcation, or portomesenteric confluence. Type IIc shunts are peripheral shunts arising from gastric, mesenteric, or splenic veins. Overall, type I congenital extrahepatic portosystemic shunt is more common than type II [10]. Spontaneous closure has not been described except in patent ductus venosus [11]. Various types of shunts are depicted in Figure 1.

3. Embryogenesis

Congenital extrahepatic portosystemic shunt is highly complex as is the development of the portal venous system and inferior vena cava [12]. Portal vein develops from paired vitelline ducts on the anterior surface of the yolk sac. It joins primitive sinus venosus. Inferior vena cava develops from several venous channels. Hepatic segment of the inferior vena cava develops from the right end of the primitive sinus venosus. Thus, there is an embryological communication between portal vein and inferior vena cava [12].

4. Clinical Presentation

The clinical presentation of congenital extrahepatic portosystemic shunt is highly variable and nonspecific. There is a striking female predilection for type I congenital extrahepatic portosystemic shunt [13]. Presentation can be related to abnormal hepatic development or function: portosystemic shunt or associated congenital anomalies. Diversion of nutrient rich portal venous blood away from liver causes fatty degeneration and liver atrophy. Liver enlargement can however be noted in the presence of focal liver lesions. Most common liver masses in the setting of congenital extrahepatic portosystemic shunt are secondary to nodular regenerative hyperplasia [14]. Less commonly, focal nodular hyperplasia and hepatic adenoma may be present. The differentiation between these lesions is based on the evaluation of serum alpha-fetoprotein level, CT, and MRI. Features favouring nodular regenerative hyperplasia include multifocality, homogeneity, T1-W hyperintensity, and retention of contrast on portal venous and delayed images. Focal nodular hyperplasia and hepatic adenoma, like nodular regenerative hyperplasia, are arterial hyperenhancing lesions; however, the former characteristically shows a central T2-W hyperintense scar and the latter occurs in the setting of hormone stimulation and shows intracellular fat that can be demonstrated with chemical shift imaging. Haemorrhage is also common in hepatic adenoma and is well demonstrated with noncontrast CT and MRI. Malignant transformation in nodular regenerative hyperplasia lesions is extremely rare [15]. The basic pathogenetic mechanism for focal liver lesions is vascular derangement comprising hepatic ischemia and increased hepatic arterial flow.

Toxic metabolites bypass liver and directly enter systemic circulation in the setting of congenital extrahepatic portosystemic shunt. Toxic metabolites can result in hepatic encephalopathy, though it is rare in infants and children as the brain is relatively resistant at this age. Hepatopulmonary syndrome and digital clubbing are other manifestations in type I congenital extrahepatic portosystemic shunt. Rarely, children can present with psychiatric manifestations [8]. Serum levels of ammonia, galactose, and other toxic metabolites are elevated. Elevated galactose levels can be used for screening of neonates for CEPS. On examination, there may be liver atrophy or hepatomegaly secondary to regenerative nodules. Intermittent obstructive jaundice may be observed due to mass effect caused by regenerative nodules. Liver cirrhosis is a rare complication of CEPS type I. Ascites, splenomegaly, and varices are not a feature of CEPS.

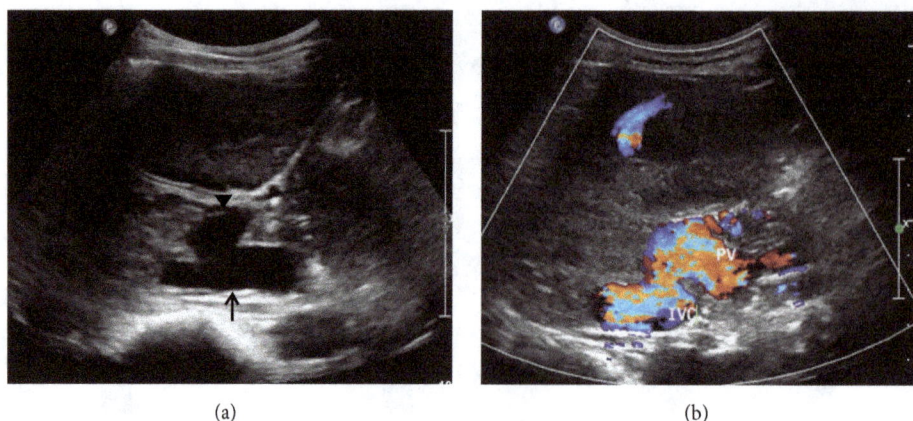

(a)   (b)

FIGURE 2: A 4-year-old boy with vague upper abdominal pain and abdominal distension since he was 2 years old. Gray-scale image (a) shows an abnormal communication between inferior vena cava (arrow) and main portal vein (arrow head). Color Doppler (b) image confirms the abnormal communication by demonstrating flow between inferior vena cava (IVC) and main portal vein (PV).

Peripheral congenital extrahepatic portosystemic shunt can present with bleeding manifestations including vaginal or rectal bleeding [3]. Associated anomalies are consistently detected in type I congenital extrahepatic portosystemic shunt. Most common among these include cardiovascular, gastrointestinal (including polysplenia, annular pancreas, and malrotation), genitourinary, and skeletal malformations [10].

5. Imaging Findings

Imaging plays a crucial role in diagnosis and follow-up of patients with congenital extrahepatic portosystemic shunt.

Ultrasound (US) with color Doppler is the initial imaging modality. It allows the evaluation of the shunt and liver status including liver lesions. In most cases, an absence of portal vein is detected on US in type I congenital extra-hepatic portosystemic shunt. In addition, a direct fistulous communication between main portal vein and IVC may be detected (Figure 2). In type II congenital extrahepatic portosystemic shunt, the main portal vein is hypoplastic owing to the diversion of the portal blood flow. Liver size is variable and may be enlarged or atrophic. Liver echogenicity is also variable. Liver lesions in the setting of congenital extrahepatic portosystemic shunt are typically nodular regen-erative hyperplasia; however, association with focal nodular hyperplasia and hepatocellular carcinoma is also known. The US appearance of these lesions is variable and may appear hyperechoic or hypoechoic (Figure 3). A characteris-tic finding described on gray-scale US in nodular regenerative hyperplasia is a coral atoll-like appearance. This refers to a peripheral hyperechoic rim (Figure 4) surrounding a focal liver lesion [16]. On the contrary, a halo sign, characterised by a hypoechoic rim, has also been reported (Figure 3). The role of contrast enhanced US has not been described in the setting of congenital extrahepatic portosystemic shunt. Contrast enhanced US involves intravenous administration of phospholipid shelled microbubbles (e.g., SonoVue, Bracco, Milan). Microbubbles enhance the signal of both B-mode and

Doppler US. Being a blood pool agent, it does not diffuse into the interstitial spaces, unlike the iodinated contrast agent. A low mechanical index (low US power resulting in symmetrical oscillations) is utilised in general, including imaging of liver lesions. Three-phase approach studying the arterial, portal, and sinusoidal sequence is used. This parallels that employed for dynamic contrast enhanced CT or MRI. Based on the behaviour of the focal liver lesions on three phases, contrast enhanced US has been shown to accurately characterise the lesions [17]. We found contrast enhanced US useful in real-time demonstration of shunt and characterisation of liver lesions (Figures 5(a)–5(c)). In the late phase, the microbubbles are retained in the sinusoidal spaces and hence lesions containing normal hepatocytes (e.g., focal nodular hyperplasia and nodular regenerative hyperplasia) achieve similar echogenicity as the background liver parenchyma and hence disappear. However, contrast enhanced US demands an older child. The role of contrast enhanced US in congenital extrahepatic portosystemic shunt can be a subject of considerable interest for future research.

Diagnosis of congenital extrahepatic portosystemic shunt is confirmed by contrast enhanced MRI or CT. MRI must be preferred over CT as the latter exposes the child to ionising radiations. Besides, MRI is better for characterisation of liver lesions. Both MR angiography and CT angiography allow accurate mapping of the course of the portosystemic shunt (Figures 6 and 7). There may be nonvisualisation of intrahepatic portal vein branches; however, this does not always employ absence. Angiography (as described later) is the modality of choice for confirming the absence of portal vein branches and hence typing the shunt. Besides portosystemic shunt, shunting at other levels including mesenteric vein is also depicted well (Figures 7–9). In type II congenital extrahepatic portosystemic shunt, portal vein is typically hypoplastic (Figure 10). Nodular regenerative hyperplasia lesions have rather characteristic appearance on MRI, allowing a noninvasive diagnosis [5]. The lesions are homogeneous and well defined and are frequently mul-tiple. T1-W images reveal the lesions to be hyperintense

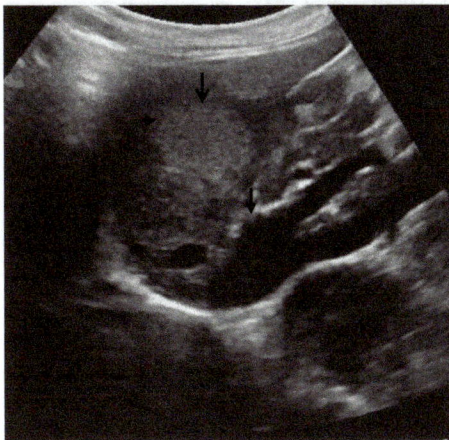

FIGURE 3: A 12-year-old female with complaints of vague upper abdominal discomfort. A well-defined hyperechoic liver lesion (arrow) with peripheral hypoechoic rim (short arrow) is seen. Thick arrow head indicates abnormal communication between main portal vein and inferior vena cava.

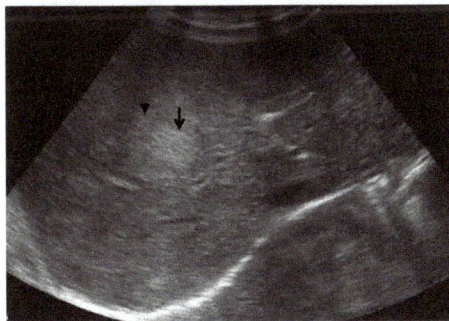

FIGURE 4: A 9-year-old boy with bleeding per rectum since he was 1 year old. A well-defined slightly hyperechoic lesion (arrow) with subtle hyperechoic rim (arrow head) is seen. This refers to carol atoll sign in nodular regenerative hyperplasia.

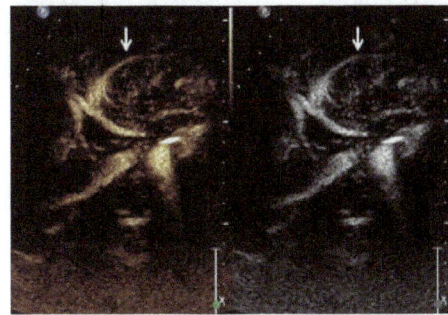

(a)

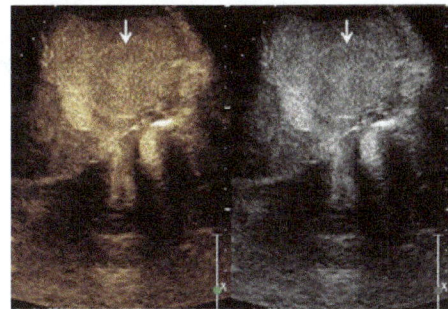

(b)

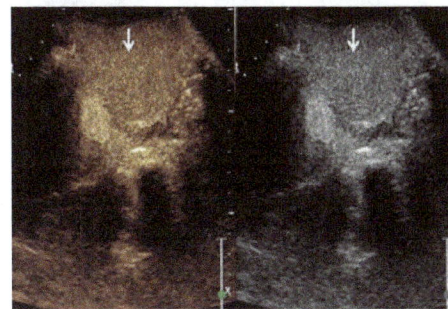

(c)

FIGURE 5: A 4-year-old boy with vague upper abdominal pain and abdominal distension since he was 2 years old. Peripheral enhancement of the lesion (a, arrow) is seen in the arterial phase of contrast enhanced US. The lesion becomes isoechoic to the adjacent liver parenchyma (b, arrow) in the venous phase of contrast enhanced US. The lesion retains contrast (c, arrow) in the delayed phase of contrast enhanced US. Points favouring nodular regenerative hyperplasia include arterial hyperenhancement and retention of contrast in the portal venous and delayed phases.

(Figure 11(a)) while T2-W signal characteristics are more variable (Figure 11(b)). Most lesions are isointense to slightly hyperintense on T2-W images. The lesions show arterial hyperenhancement (Figure 11(c)) and remain isointense to slightly hyperintense on portal venous, equilibrium, and delayed phase images (Figure 11(d)). Contrast enhanced MRI adds to the diagnostic confidence in lesion characterisation and has become standard protocol in evaluation of focal liver lesions. Arterial hyperenhancement reflects the vascular supply of the nodular regenerative hyperplasia lesions from the hepatic artery. Tendency for these lesions to remain hyperintense on portal venous and delayed phases is different from other benign lesions that become isointense in these phases as well as from hepatocellular carcinoma that shows venous phase washout and appears hypointense relative to the liver parenchyma. Liver specific MRI contrast agents including gadobenate dimeglumine (MultiHance, Bracco, Milan) have unique property of hepatocyte uptake and biliary excretion. This adds to the lesion characterisation as lesions containing functioning hepatocytes are expected to retain contrast and appear isointense to the liver parenchyma on the hepatobiliary phase images. This was demonstrated in one of our patients (Figure 11(e)). The more commonly employed extracellular agents, for example, gadopentetate dimeglumine (Magnevist, Bayer, NJ), have no biliary excretion. Disadvantage of using MultiHance is the need for repeat imaging and hence repeat sedation/anaesthesia in a young child. Similar behaviour of the lesions is expected following administration of contrast in CT. Fat, calcification, and haemorrhage are not the imaging features of nodular regenerative hyperplasia.

Transrectal portal scintigraphy (with 123 I-Iodoamphetamine) is a nuclear medicine study that allows calculation of

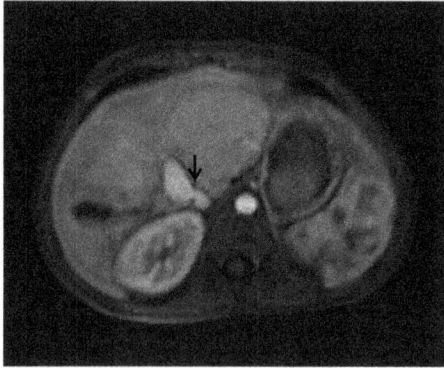

FIGURE 6: A 12-year-old female with complaints of vague upper abdominal discomfort. Axial image of MR angiography reveals an abnormal communication between main portal vein and inferior vena cava (arrow).

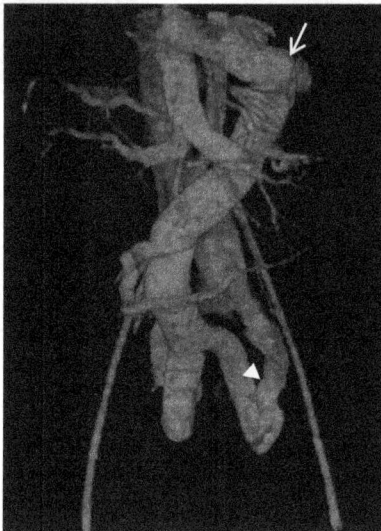

FIGURE 9: A 9-year-old boy with bleeding per rectum since he was 1 year old. Axial MR image of the same patient as above reveals abnormal perirectal vascular channels (arrows).

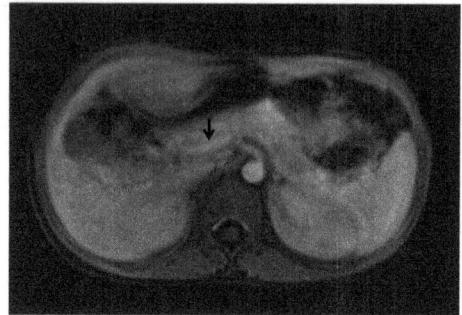

FIGURE 7: A 9-year-old boy with bleeding per rectum since he was 1 year old. Volume rendered CT image reveals dilatation of superior mesenteric vein and inferior mesenteric vein (arrow) with abnormal communication between iliac vein and branches of inferior mesenteric vein (arrow head).

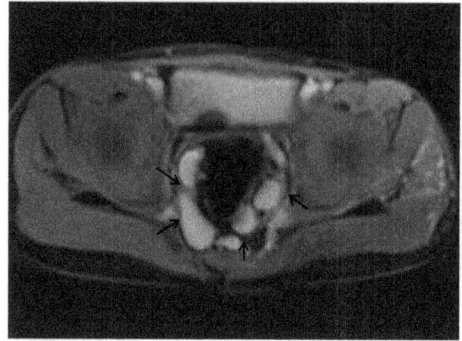

FIGURE 10: A 9-year-old boy with bleeding per rectum since he was 1 year old. Axial contrast enhanced MR image indicates hypoplastic main portal vein (arrow).

the shunt ratio in type II congenital extrahepatic portosystemic shunt [18]. This information is useful in formulating management plan in type II congenital extrahepatic portosystemic shunt.

Accurate typing of the shunt is essential for precise management. In this context, angiography should be regarded as one of the initial investigations in all patients suspected of having CEPS. Besides the transarterial portography, shunt demonstration and typing can also be achieved by direct contrast injection into the shunt with balloon occlusion. Angiography allows the measurement of portal venous pressures required for monitoring following occlusion of shunt [19].

6. Differential Diagnosis

Few important differential diagnoses must be considered. These include acquired portosystemic shunt, portal vein thrombosis, and intrahepatic portosystemic shunt [8]. Absence of ascites, splenomegaly, and specific collateral veins allows confident exclusion of acquired portosystemic shunt. Absence of intraluminal filling defect (in acute thrombosis) and lack of collateral veins, expansion, and wall calcification

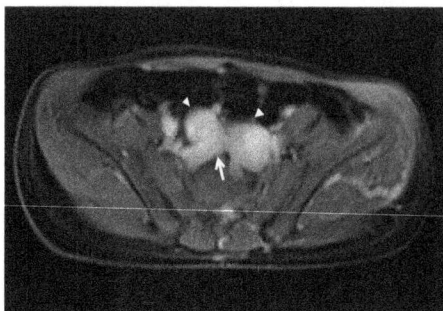

FIGURE 8: A 9-year-old boy with bleeding per rectum since he was 1 year old. Axial MR image reveals abnormal vascular channels in the pelvis suggesting a communication between tributaries of superior mesenteric vein (arrow head) and iliac veins (arrow).

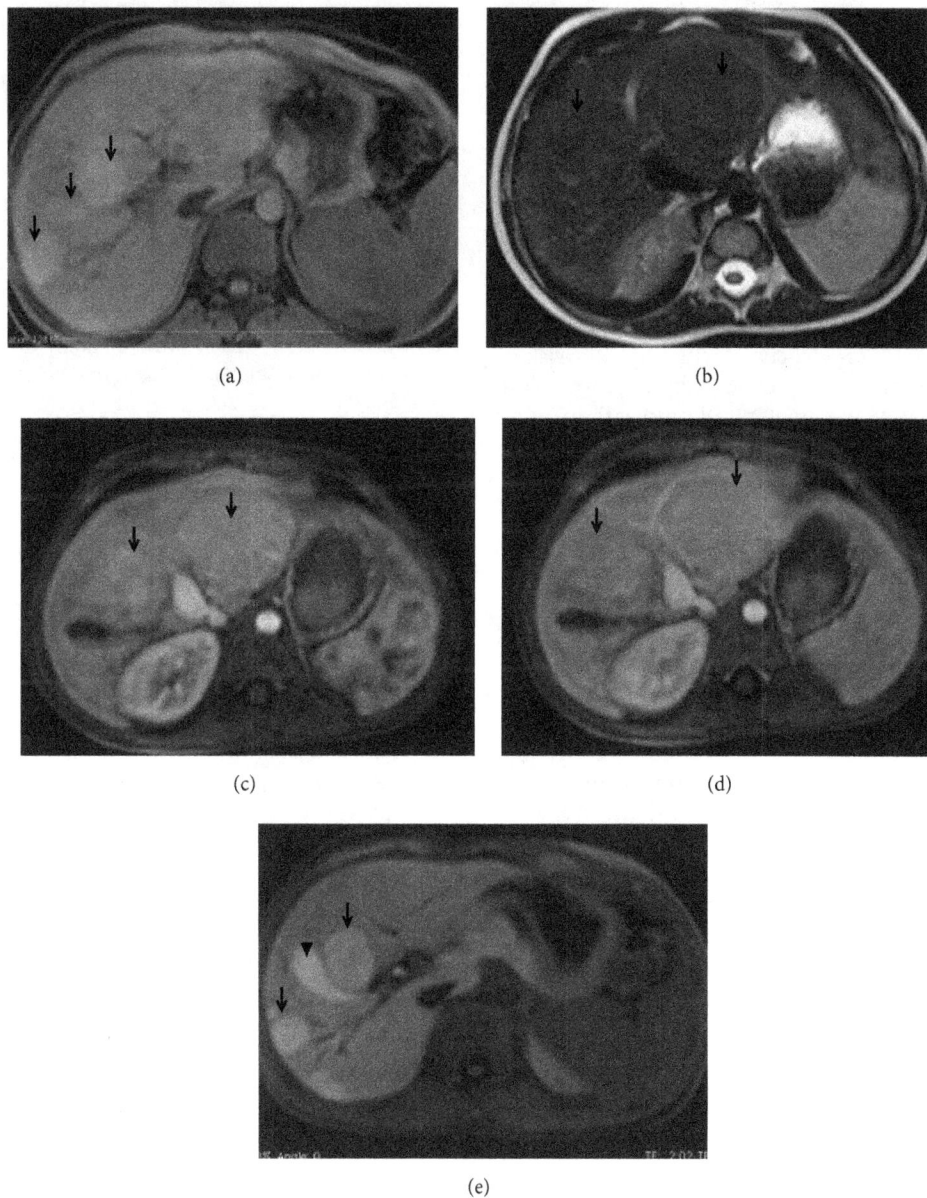

(a)

(b)

(c)

(d)

(e)

FIGURE 11: A 4-year-old boy with vague upper abdominal pain and abdominal distension since he was 2 years old. Axial T1-W image (a) shows multiple well-defined hyperintense lesions (arrows). The lesions are hypointense on T2-W images (b, arrows). Slight arterial hyperenhancement is seen with the lesions (c, arrows). There is retention of contrast in the portal venous phase (d, arrows). Hepatobiliary phase image (e) shows retention of contrast (arrows). Arrow head points to biliary excretion of contrast into gallbladder. Imaging features favouring nodular regenerative hyperplasia include multiple lesions, T1-W hyperintensity, arterial hyperenhancement, and retention of contrast on portal venous and equilibrium phases.

(in chronic thrombosis) rule out the possibility of portal vein thrombosis. The key to differentiation between intrahepatic portosystemic shunts and congenital extrahepatic portosystemic shunt is the location of shunt. While intrahepatic portosystemic shunts are characterised by abnormal connections between branches of the portal vein and the inferior vena cava or hepatic veins, in congenital extrahepatic portosystemic shunt, such shunting involves main portal vein or more peripheral veins.

7. Management

Management depends on the type of congenital extrahepatic portosystemic shunt. No definite curative surgical or endovascular therapy can be employed in type I congenital extrahepatic portosystemic shunt as the shunt is the only route for drainage of the portal blood and hence this shunt cannot be blocked. Only therapeutic option in such cases is liver transplant [6]. This treatment is reserved for patients developing features of hepatic encephalopathy. However, recently a more aggressive approach has been suggested. In a study by Blanc et al., twenty-three patients with congenital portosystemic shunts were evaluated [20]. Two patients had extrahepatic shunt; the rest have intrahepatic shunts classified on the basis of ending of the shunt in the caval system. In both patients with extrahepatic portosystemic shunts, a single stage ligation was performed. On follow-up, both the patients were alive and did not require liver transplantation. Type II shunts are amenable to surgical or endovascular treatment [7]. These therapies are guided by the shunt ratio. A shunt ratio of greater than 60% is associated with a greater risk of development of spontaneous encephalopathy. Asymptomatic patients are typically followed up clinically and with imaging studies.

8. Conclusion

Congenital extrahepatic portosystemic shunt should be considered clinically in children presenting with nonspecific liver dysfunction. On imaging, this vascular anomaly should be suspected when there are multiple liver lesions and lack of imaging signs of portal hypertension. Primary diagnosis can be offered with US and Doppler. MRI and CT allow classification of the shunt and evaluation of the associated congenital anomalies. Definitive management is liver transplant in type I and surgical or endovascular closure of the shunt in type II.

Conflict of Interests

The authors declare that there is no conflict of interests regarding the publication of this paper.

References

[1] A. A. Konstas, S. R. Digumarthy, L. L. Avery et al., "Congenital portosystemic shunts: imaging findings and clinical presentations in 11 patients," *European Journal of Radiology*, vol. 80, no. 2, pp. 175–181, 2011.

[2] G. Morgan and R. Superina, "Congenital absence of the portal vein: two cases and a proposed classification system for portosystemic vascular anomalies," *Journal of Pediatric Surgery*, vol. 29, no. 9, pp. 1239–1241, 1994.

[3] T. B. Lautz, N. Tantemsapya, E. Rowell, and R. A. Superina, "Management and classification of type II congenital portosystemic shunts," *Journal of Pediatric Surgery*, vol. 46, no. 2, pp. 308–314, 2011.

[4] H. Kandpal, R. Sharma, N. K. Arora, and S. D. Gupta, "Congenital extrahepatic portosystemic venous shunt: imaging features," *Singapore Medical Journal*, vol. 48, no. 9, pp. e258–e261, 2007.

[5] C. P. Murray, S.-J. Yoo, and P. S. Babyn, "Congenital extrahepatic portosystemic shunts," *Pediatric Radiology*, vol. 33, no. 9, pp. 614–620, 2003.

[6] E. S. Woodle, J. R. Thistlethwaite, J. C. Emond et al., "Successful hepatic transplantation in congenital absence of recipient portal vein," *Surgery*, vol. 107, no. 4, pp. 475–479, 1990.

[7] G.-H. Hu, L.-G. Shen, J. Yang, J.-H. Mei, and Y.-F. Zhu, "Insight into congenital absence of the portal vein: is it rare?" *World Journal of Gastroenterology*, vol. 14, no. 39, pp. 5969–5979, 2008.

[8] E. Alonso-Gamarra, M. Parrón, A. Pérez, C. Prieto, L. Hierro, and M. López-Santamaría, "Clinical and radiologic manifestations of congenital extrahepatic portosystemic shunts: a comprehensive review," *Radiographics*, vol. 31, no. 3, pp. 707–723, 2011.

[9] W. W. Meyer and J. Lind, "The ductus venosus and the mechanism of its closure," *Archives of Disease in Childhood*, vol. 41, no. 220, pp. 597–605, 1966.

[10] E. R. Howard and M. Davenport, "Congenital extrahepatic portocaval shunts—the Abernethy malformation," *Journal of Pediatric Surgery*, vol. 32, no. 3, pp. 494–497, 1997.

[11] M. D. Stringer, "The clinical anatomy of congenital portosystemic venous shunts," *Clinical Anatomy*, vol. 21, no. 2, pp. 147–157, 2008.

[12] R. S. Loomba, M. Frommelt, D. Moe, and A. J. Shillingford, "Agenesis of the venous duct: two cases of extrahepatic drainage of the umbilical vein and extrahepatic portosystemic shunt with a review of the literature," *Cardiology in the Young*, vol. 25, no. 2, pp. 208–217, 2014.

[13] L. Grazioli, D. Alberti, L. Olivetti et al., "Congenital absence of portal vein with nodular regenerative hyperplasia of the liver," *European Radiology*, vol. 10, no. 5, pp. 820–825, 2000.

[14] E. Arana, L. Martí-Bonmatí, V. Martínez, M. Hoyos, and H. Montes, "Portal vein absence and nodular regenerative hyperplasia of the liver with giant inferior mesenteric vein," *Abdominal Imaging*, vol. 22, no. 5, pp. 506–508, 1997.

[15] S. Kawano, S. Hasegawa, N. Urushihara et al., "Hepatoblastoma with congenital absence of the portal vein—a case report," *European Journal of Pediatric Surgery*, vol. 17, no. 4, pp. 292–294, 2007.

[16] E. Caturelli, G. Ghittoni, T. V. Ranalli, and V. V. Gomes, "Nodular regenerative hyperplasia of the liver: coral atoll-like lesions on ultrasound are characteristic in predisposed patients," *British Journal of Radiology*, vol. 84, no. 1003, pp. e129–e134, 2011.

[17] C. Bartolozzi and R. Lencioni, "Contrast-specific ultrasound imaging of focal liver lesions. Prologue to a promising future," *European Radiology*, vol. 11, supplement 3, pp. E13–E14, 2001.

[18] P. Vajro, L. Celentano, F. Manguso et al., "Per-rectal portal scintigraphy is complementary to ultrasonography and endoscopy in the assessment of portal hypertension in children with chronic cholestasis," *Journal of Nuclear Medicine*, vol. 45, no. 10, pp. 1705–1711, 2004.

[19] O. Bernard, S. Franchi-Abella, S. Branchereau, D. Pariente, F. Gauthier, and E. Jacquemin, "Congenital portosystemic shunts in children: recognition, evaluation, and management," *Seminars in Liver Disease*, vol. 32, no. 4, pp. 273–287, 2012.

[20] T. Blanc, F. Guerin, S. Franchi-Abella et al., "Congenital portosystemic shunts in children: a new anatomical classification correlated with surgical strategy," *Annals of Surgery*, vol. 260, no. 1, pp. 188–198, 2014.

7

Lumbar Facet Joint Arthritis is Associated with More Coronal Orientation of the Facet Joints at the Upper Lumbar Spine

Thorsten Jentzsch,[1] James Geiger,[1] Stefan M. Zimmermann,[1] Ksenija Slankamenac,[1] Thi Dan Linh Nguyen-Kim,[2] and Clément M. L. Werner[1]

[1] *Division of Trauma Surgery, Department of Surgery, University Hospital Zürich, Rämistrasse 100, 8091 Zürich, Switzerland*
[2] *Institute of Diagnostic and Interventional Radiology, University Hospital Zürich, Rämistrasse 100, 8091 Zürich, Switzerland*

Correspondence should be addressed to Thorsten Jentzsch; thorsten.jentzsch@usz.ch

Academic Editor: David Maintz

We retrospectively analyzed CT scans of 620 individuals, who presented to our traumatology department between 2008 and 2010. Facet joint (FJ) arthritis was present in 308 (49.7%) individuals with a mean grade of 1. It was seen in 27% of individuals ≤40 years and in 75% of individuals ≥41 years ($P < 0.0001$) as well as in 52% of females and 49% of males ($P = 0.61$). Mean FJ orientation was 30.4° at L2/3, 38.7° at L3/4, 47° at L4/5, and 47.3° at L5/S1. FJ arthritis was significantly associated with more coronal (increased degree) FJ orientation at L2/3 ($P = 0.03$) with a cutoff point at ≥32°. FJs were more coronally oriented (48.8°) in individuals ≤40 years and more sagittally oriented (45.6°) in individuals ≥41 years at L5/S1 ($P = 0.01$). Mean FJ asymmetry was 4.89° at L2/3, 6.01° at L3/4, 6.67° at L4/5, and 7.27° at L5/S1, without a significant difference for FJ arthritis. FJ arthritis is common, increases with age, and affects both genders equally. More coronally oriented FJs (≥32°) in the upper lumbar spine may be an individual risk factor for development of FJ arthritis.

1. Introduction

A functional spinal unit consists of anteriorly located adjacent vertebrae separated by an intervertebral disc and posteriorly located facet (zygapophyseal) joints (FJ) [1]. FJs are composed of an inferior articular process, facing anteriorly, and a superior articular process, facing posteriorly, of two adjacent vertebrae [2]. Being synovial-lined, diarthrodial, and freely moveable functional units, they transmit shear forces and help the intervertebral discs in carrying about 16% of the vertical load [3, 4]. FJ orientation planes differ at various levels, with a more sagittal and curved orientation for resistance against axial rotation in the upper compared to a more coronal and flat orientation for resistance against flexion and shearing forces in the lower lumbar segments [5, 6]. FJ asymmetry or tropism describes the asymmetry of the left and right FJ angle [7, 8].

Low back pain is one of the most common health problems [9]. It affects up to 85% of people at least once during their lifetime and up to 5% chronically [10]. Even though etiologies of low back pain are multifactorial [11], FJ arthritis is common and affects at least 50% of the population [12]. After Ghormley [13] first described a facet syndrome in 1933, there has been an ongoing debate [14, 15] about the possible association low back pain and FJ pathology [16]. FJs are synovial covered joints with hyaline cartilage [17] and innervated by the medial branches of the dorsal rami from two levels [18, 19]. Recently, it has been shown that inflammatory chemical mediators are increased in degenerated FJs [20]. In order to investigate the association of low back pain and FJ pathology, most studies [21–25] successfully utilized FJ (nerve) blocks and its associated pain relief. Thus, there is convincing evidence that FJ pain plays an important role in low back pain [26, 27] and occurs in up to 45% of individuals [25].

However, controversies still exist in the following issues. In general, study samples have been rather small for FJ arthritis on CT scans, which is especially true for the prevalence of FJ arthritis, particularly in younger individuals [28–36]. Gender predilection has not been reported consistently [12, 15, 29, 37]. It also remains unclear whether FJ arthritis is associated with FJ orientation and/or FJ asymmetry, and if so, at which level [1, 6–8, 32, 38–48]. Previous studies [32, 49] have only reported an increase in FJ arthritis with more sagittally oriented FJs at the lower lumbar spine. Yet, it is unknown if changes in FJ orientation at the upper lumbar spine lead to FJ orientation at the lumbar spine. Therefore, our goal was to clarify these remaining issues by quantifying the degree of radiographically detectable (1) FJ arthritis on CT scans of the lumbar spine from L2-S1 in regards to (2) age, (3) gender, (4) FJ orientation, and (5) FJ asymmetry.

2. Materials and Methods

The study has been approved by the institutional review board (ethical committee no. KEK-ZH-Nr.2011-0507). We retrospectively analyzed CT scans of 620 individuals (2480 functional units), with a mean age of 42.5 (range, 14–94) years, who presented to our traumatology department and underwent a whole body CT scan, including the pelvis and lumbar spine, between 2008 and 2010. A dual-source computed tomography scanner (Somatom Definition, Siemens Healthcare, Forchheim, Germany) was used [50]. Our study utilized CT scans instead of plain radiographs or magnetic resonance imaging, because they are more accurate in displaying FJs on axial planes [51, 52]. FJs of the lumbar spine were evaluated between the second lumbar and the first sacral level [53]. Axial planes with the largest intersecting set of the superior and inferior FJ process were chosen.

(1) Assessment of FJ arthritis was carried out as previously described in similar studies, where a grading scale described by Pathria [29, 54] was used. Grade 0 (normal) indicates a normal facet joint, whereas grades 1–3 display increasing signs of FJ arthritis with each grade including signs of the lower grade. Grade 1 (mild) shows joint space narrowing, grade 2 (moderate) demonstrates sclerosis, and grade 3 (severe) reveals osteophytes [55] (Figure 1). (2) Individuals were grouped into those ≤40 and ≥41 years. (3) Gender was also evaluated. (4) FJ orientation in the axial plane was evaluated by measuring the angle between the midline of the sagittal plane and the midline of the FJ as described by Schuller et al. [56, 57] (Figure 2). FJ orientation (Figure 2) was determined on axial CT planes of the lumbar spine using the AGFA Impax viewer. The midline of the sagittal planes corresponds to a line drawn through the center of the vertebral body and spinous process. Therefore, each FJ was compared against this line. The midline of FJs was evaluated on axial cross-sections where the largest part of the joint, that is, most parts of the superior and inferior articular facets were visible. The overall FJ orientation was calculated by averaging the angles between the right and left side of the FJs. We used absolute angles, indicating that we did not consider rotation in one direction as positive and rotation in the opposite direction as negative. The FJ orientation was labeled as coronal if angles were >45°, sagittal if angles were ≤45°, and anisotropic if one side was over and the other side under 45° [58]. (5) FJ asymmetry was determined as the absolute

difference between the right and left FJ angle and categorized into four groups determined according to their 50th, 75th, and 95th percentile, for example, group one includes 50% of the sample, group two 25%, group three 20%, and group four 5%.

All statistical analyses were performed by the Institute for Social and Preventive Medicine, Division of Biostatistics at the University of Zürich, using the R program [59]. Several different statistical approaches were applied to test the null hypothesis [60]. This study is an observational study, which means that analysis follows a descriptive and exploratory form. Therefore, P values are interpreted as a quantitative measure of the evidence against the null hypothesis. As a rough guideline, we assumed weak evidence against the null hypothesis for P-values ≥0.01 and <0.1, modest evidence against the null hypothesis for P values between ≥0.001 and <0.01, and strong evidence against the null hypothesis for P values <0.001. Therefore, correction for multiple comparisons has been assessed. The G_2 test was used for the following models: FJ arthritis, versus (2) age (categorized), (3) gender and (5) FJ asymmetry. The G_2-test was used to test the association between ordinal outcomes and nominal explanatory variables. Besides the usual properties of a statistical test, the G_2 test also provides a decomposition of the total test value G_2 into the ordinal levels of the outcome variable, and can therefore be used to determine the threshold of the ordinal levels. For example, the decomposition of the G_2-value for the 4 degrees of FJ arthritis, which is an ordinal measure, is as follows: $G_2 = G_20; 1 + G_201; 2 + G_2012; 3$, which means that the total G_2-value can be written as G_2-value of a comparison between FJ arthritis 0 and 1, plus a G_2-value of a comparison between FJ arthritis 0 + 1 and 2, plus a G_2-value of a comparison between FJ arthritis 0 + 1 + 2 and 3. If the equation would be 100 = 10 + 30 + 100 for a certain explanatory variable, the largest difference occurs between 30 and 100. Therefore, patients with a degree of 3 in regard to FJ arthritis show the largest difference with respect to this explanatory variable. A χ^2-test was applied to test the association between a nominal outcome and a nominal explanatory variable. The χ^2-test was used for the following models: (4) FJ orientation (categorized) versus age (categorized) and gender, as well as (5) FJ asymmetry versus age (categorized) and gender. The proportional odds model was used for (1) FJ arthritis versus (4) FJ orientation. We also calculated the cut-off point for FJ arthritis by using the ROC curves analysis. Afterwards we performed a univariate as well as a multivariate logistic regression analysis by grouping the patient population according to the cut-off point. Age and gender were defined as potential confounder for the multivariate regression analysis.

3. Results

(1) Arthritis. Of our 620 individuals, who were evaluated for radiological FJ arthritis on axial planes of CT scans from L2-S1, 308 (49.7%) individuals showed signs of FJ arthritis. The mean grade of FJ arthritis was 1.310 (50.0%); individuals were not affected by FJ arthritis (grade 0), 103 (16.6%) individuals presented with grade 1, 107 (17.3%) individuals with grade 2,

Grade 0   Grade 1

Grade 2   Grade 3

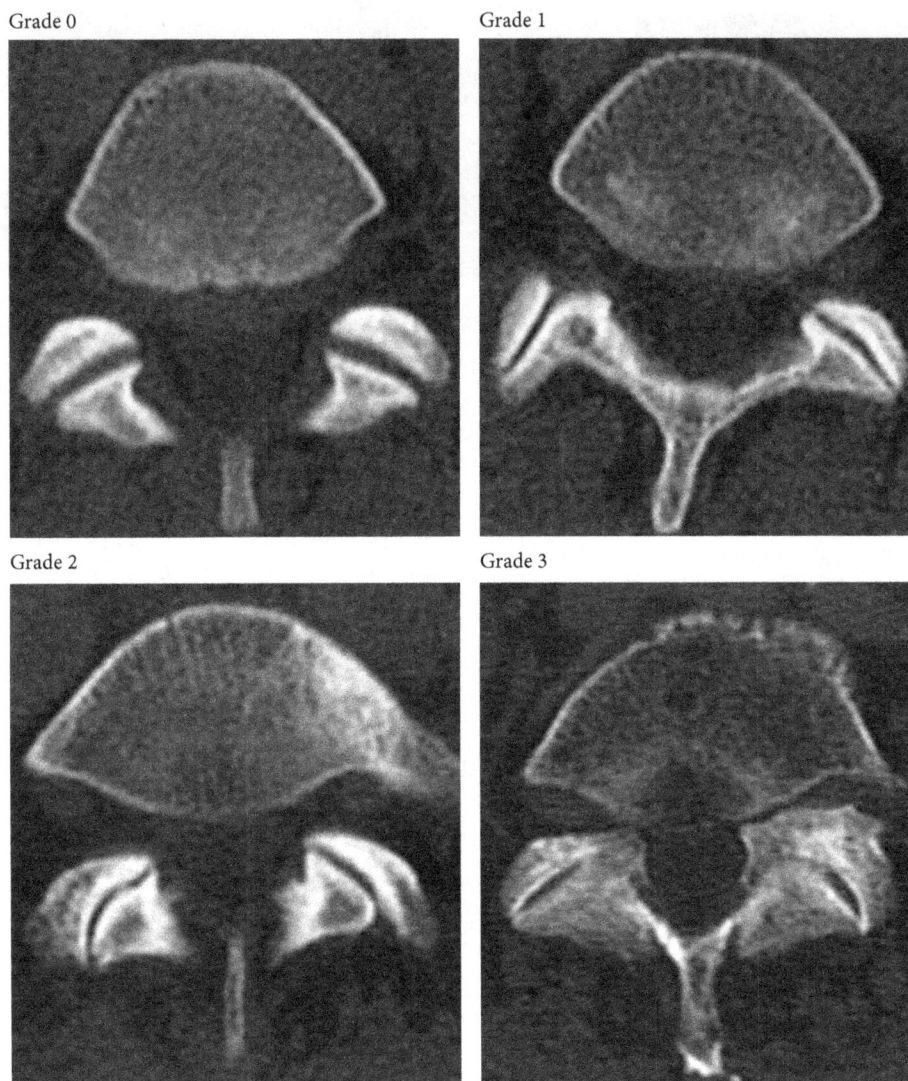

FIGURE 1: Grading scale for FJ arthritis. Grade 0 = normal FJ. Grade 1 (mild) = joint space narrowing, grade 2 (moderate) = sclerosis, and grade 3 (severe) = osteophytes.

and 98 (15.8%) individuals with grade 3 (Table 1). Two (0.3%) individuals could not be evaluated for FJ arthritis because spondylodesis had been performed or appropriate planes had not been reconstructed adequately.

(2) Age. Separated into two age groups, our study included 330 (53.2%) individuals ≤40 years and 290 (46.8%) individuals >40 years. FJ arthritis significantly differed between age groups, with elderly individuals being more commonly affected ($P < 0.0001$) (Figure 3). All 4 degrees of FJ arthritis were found in both age groups (≤40 years, >40 years) but with different proportions. FJ arthritis was present in 27% of individuals in the age group ≤40 years. In contrast, FJ arthritis was found 75% of individuals in the age group >40 years. Furthermore, FJ arthritis manifested in 95% of individuals in the age group ≥65 years, which included 97 individuals. The $G_20,12$; 3-value indicates that comparison of the first 3 groups of FJ arthritis with a degree of 0, 1, and 2 to the most severe

group of FJA with a degree of 3 showed the largest gap in age (207 = 30 + 58 + 119). This suggests that severe FJ arthritis seemed to be more likely in elderly individuals.

(3) Gender. There were 202 females (32.6%) and 418 males (67.4%). FJ arthritis did not show significant gender predilection, even if separated into age groups. 52% of females and 49% of males displayed signs of FJ arthritis ($P = 0.61$). Females presented with a mean FJ arthritis of 1.07, compared to 0.95 in males. Each grade of FJ arthritis included a similar number of females and males. Grade 0 affected 48% of females and 51% of males, grade 1 affected 15% of females and 17% of males, grade 2 affected 19% of females and 17% of males, and grade 3 affected 18% of females and 15% of males.

(4) Orientation. Mean FJ orientation was measured as 30.4° (SD 7.7°, range 7.4–66°) at L2/3, 38.7° (SD 9.6°, range 4.5–73.7°) at L3/4.47° (SD 9.8°, range 16.2–76.4°) at L4/5 and

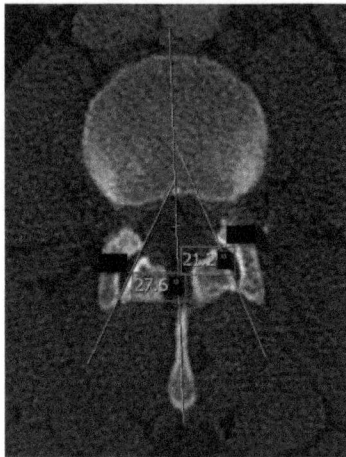

FIGURE 2: Measuring technique for FJ orientation. FJ orientation in the axial plane was evaluated by measuring the angle between the midline of the sagittal plane and the midline of the FJ. Coronal FJ orientation is shown on the left side, whereas sagittal orientation including measurement of FJ orientation is shown on the right side. The red box indicates the value for FJ orientation. The blacked out numbers were disregarded because they were created automatically by our software and contained irrelevant information.

TABLE 1: Prevalence of facet joint (FJ) arthritis.

Grade	Patients (absolute number)	Patients (percentage)
0	310	50
1	103	16.6
2	107	17.3
3	98	15.8

between FJ arthritis and FJ orientation could be established at the other levels. There was a significant difference for FJ orientation in our age groups at L5/S1 ($P = 0.01$), where more coronal FJ orientation (48.8°) manifested in individuals ≤40 years and a more sagittal FJ orientation (45.6°) was present in individuals >40 years. No significant difference was found in FJ orientation and age groups at other levels (30.0° versus 31.00° ($P = 0.61$) for L2/3, 43.6° versus 42.1° ($P = 0.41$) for L3/4 and 48.1° versus 45.9° ($P = 0.13$) for L4/5). There were no significant differences for FJ orientation and gender ($P = 0.13$–0.73).

(5) Asymmetry. The mean values for FJ asymmetry were calculated as 4.89° at L2/3, 6.01° at L3/4, 6.67° at L4/5, and 7.27° at L5/S1. There was no difference between FJ arthritis and FJ asymmetry (P values = 0.11 for L5/S1, 0.26 for L4/5, 0.10 for L3/4 and 0.17 for L2/3). There were no significant differences in age groups for each level ($P = 0.35$ at L2/3, 0.23 at L3/4, 0.27 at L4/5, 0.28 at L5/S1). However, there was modest evidence that FJ asymmetry is more common in females than in males at L5/S1 ($P = 0.01$) but not at the other levels ($P = 0.47$, 0.91 and 0.33 for L2/3, L3/4 and L5/S1). FJ asymmetry also increased in a craniocaudal fashion.

4. Discussion

Our study investigated one of the largest samples of CT scans with regard to FJ arthritis in the literature. As hypothesized we were able to show that (1) radiological appearance of FJ arthritis is a very common entity, affecting nearly half of all individuals, (2) increases with age, (3) does not display gender predilection, (4) was significantly associated with coronal, that is, increased degree of FJ orientation at L2/3, and (5) is not correlated with FJ asymmetry.

Limitations of our study attribute to the fact that all individuals presented to a trauma department. Even though a selection bias may be assumed, we did not include individuals with a fracture of the lumbar spine. We were not able to check for intra- or interrater reliability, but measurements were carried out by two trained specialists in this field. Furthermore, the measuring technique has been described before and did not require validation. We did not pay special attention to degenerative disc disease since this has been investigated in previous studies [7, 34, 49]. Another problem is caused by the parallax effect. It has been advocated [61, 62] that the spinous process may be an unreliable anatomic midline marker because anatomic variations, such as scoliosis, in the relationship between the anterior vertebral body and posterior spinous process may skew the interpreter's view on X-rays. However, this

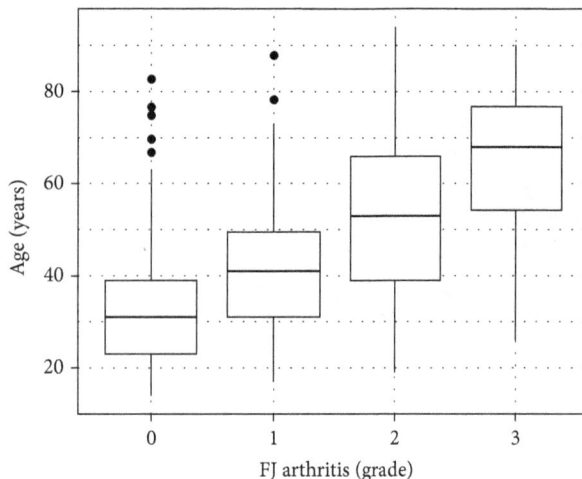

FIGURE 3: Grade of FJ arthritis and age. This figure describes the increasing grade of FJ arthritis with age.

47.3° (SD 9.9°, range 19.6–84.4°) at L5/S1. FJs of the proximal lumbar levels were more sagittally oriented compared to those at distal lumbar levels, which were more coronally oriented (Figures 4 and 5). Thus, there was a cephalocaudal trend of an increasing degree of FJ orientation.

FJ arthritis was significantly associated with more coronal, that is, increased degree of FJ orientation at L2/3 (mean FJ orientation of 30.1° without FJ arthritis (grade 0) versus mean FJ orientation of 32.1° with FJ arthritis (grade 3) ($P = 0.03$, OR 1.021 (95%-CI 1.002–1.014))) (Figure 4). The cutoff point was ≥32°. This means that more coronally oriented FJs, that is, ≥32°, at this level were associated with a higher radiological degree of FJ arthritis. No significant association

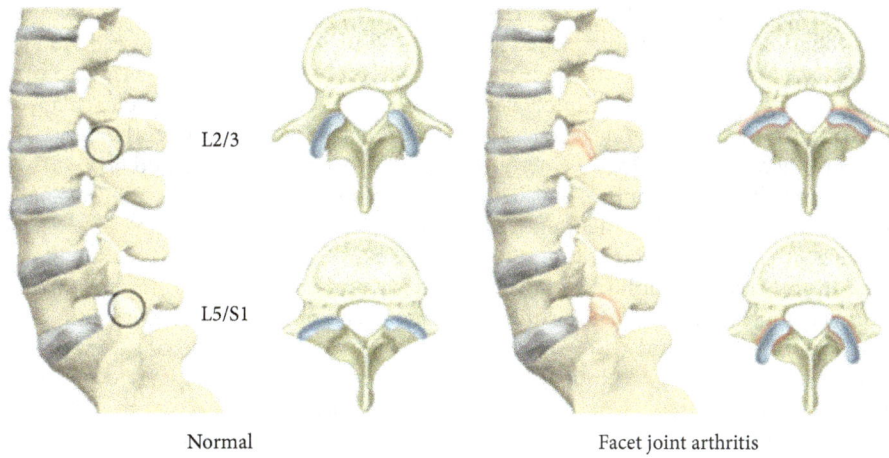

FIGURE 4: FJ arthritis and FJ orientation. On the left side, sagittally oriented FJs at L2/3 and coronally oriented FJ at L5/S1 are associated with normal FJs at the lumbar spine. The right side illustrates inversely oriented FJs with arthritic FJs at the lumbar spine, namely, coronals oriented FJs at L2/3 and sagittally oriented FJs at L5/S1.

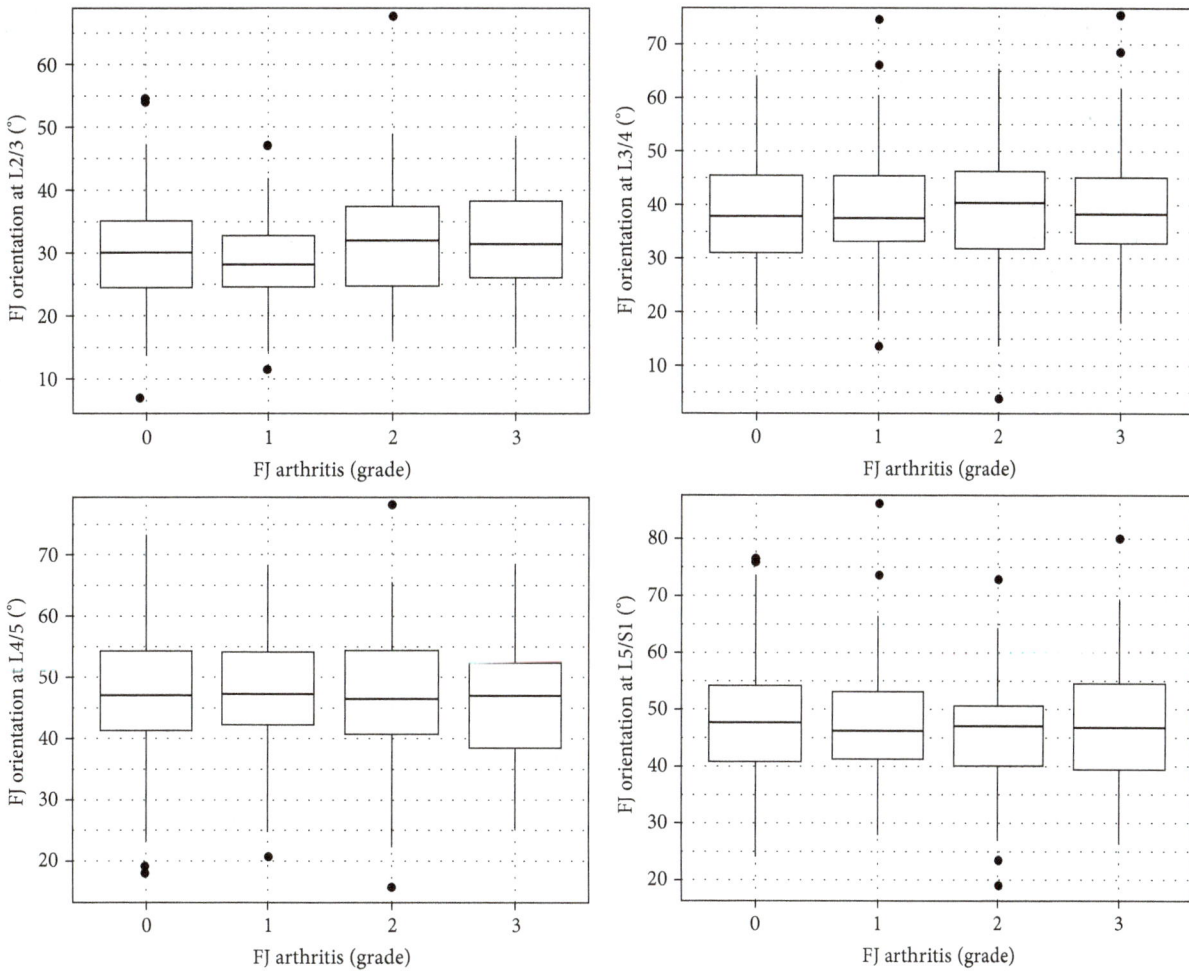

FIGURE 5: Cephalocaudal change in FJ orientation. There was a steady progress from a sagittal toward a more coronal FJ orientation at the lumbar spine in a cephalocaudal fashion, namely, 30° at L2/3 and 47° at L5/S1.

parallax effect is much smaller for more accurate images of CT scans, which we used for our evaluation. The measuring technique used in our study has been well established in previous studies [6, 32, 38, 42]. Anyhow, this issue does not affect our evaluation of FJ orientation because we calculated the mean of both sides and did not interpret each side independently. We do acknowledge that setting of a wrong midline may pose a problem in regard to FJ tropism, but so far no solution to this issue has been presented in the literature. The interesting finding that the interpedicular midpoint is the most accurate guide to the coronal midline by Mistry and Robertson. [62] could be implemented in future studies. Due to the retrospective nature of this study, we were not able to investigate which individuals showed clinical signs of FJ arthritis. Anyway, even though there is an ongoing debate [14–16, 21–25] whether radiologic proof of FJ arthritis is clearly associated with back pain, it was not the purpose of our study. Due to the cross-sectional design, we were unable to determine whether more coronally oriented FJs at L2/3 lead to FJ arthritis or the other way around. However, we believe that these changes in FJ orientation go along with FJ arthritis rather than being a manifestation of aging, because we did not find a significant association between changes in FJ orientation at L2/3, and age, or a combined significant association at the other levels. This interesting topic may be evaluated in future longitudinal studies. We did not specify the exact level or side of FJ arthritis since all levels and sides seemed to be affected in a similar fashion, with lower levels being slightly more frequently affected [12]. Even though our study included a similar number of individuals under and over 40 years, it comprised nearly twice as many males, which may be attributed to the fact that males are injured more often and are overrepresented in a trauma population [60].

(1) Arthritis. FJ arthritis was found in almost 50% of individuals in our study. This is similar to previous studies. Eubanks et al. [12] studied 647 cadavers and reported the following prevalence of FJ arthritis: 53% at L1/2, 66% at L2/3, 72% at L3/4, 79% at L4/5, and 59% at L5/S1. Kalichman et al. [28] also reported a high prevalence of FJ arthritis, namely, 64.5%, in a study 187 individuals from the 3,529 participants enrolled in the Framingham Heart Study who were assessed for aortic calcification with CT scans. Looking at 361 patients, Suri et al. [29], found an even higher prevalence of FJ arthritis, where 22% presented with isolated posterior (FJ) arthritis and 57% showed signs of posterior and anterior arthritis. Our results support the fact that FJ arthritis is a common pathology of the spine. The individuals in our study displayed a lower mean age of 42.5 years compared to the mean age of 52.6 years and 58.0 years in previously mentioned studies by Kalichman et al. [28] and Suri et al. [29] respectively, whereby Eubanks et al. [12] did not report a mean age. This explains why our results for FJ arthritis affect a smaller number of individuals.

(2) Age. We showed that FJ arthritis was present in 27% of individuals ≤40 years. Our results also illustrated a significant association of FJ arthritis and increasing age (Figure 3). 75% of our individuals ≥41 years and 95% ≥65 years presented with FJ arthritis. Likewise, previous studies [30, 31, 33, 35, 36] have revealed that FJ arthritis arises at a young age and is found in more than 50% of individuals over 40 years. In a study by Swanepoel et al. [34], who investigated individuals under 30 years, macroscopic cartilage fibrillation was more pronounced in FJs than in other joints, such as hip, knee, and ankle. In Eubanks' et al. study [12], FJ arthritis was present in 57% of individuals between 20–29 years, 82% between 30–39 years, 93% between 40–49 years, 97% between 50–59 years, and 100% over 60 years. In an ancillary to the Framingham study, Suri et al. [29] investigated 361 individuals and reported a correlation of FJ arthritis with age (OR 1.09). 89% of individuals over 65 years suffered from FJ arthritis. In a different study of 57 cadaveric specimens of spinal-disease-free organ donors, Li et al. [33] stated that FJ arthritis increased with age and no spine was completely spared by FJ arthritis over the age 42 years. These results all report the same fact and are not surprising since FJs transmit shear forces, carry about 16% of the vertical load, and tend to be subject to wear and tear [3, 4].

(3) Gender. Our study did not find a significant association of FJ arthritis and gender, even though females were slightly more commonly affected (52%) than males (49%). Similarly, in a study by Abbas et al. [37], FJ arthritis did not show gender predilection in 215 individuals, which was investigated from L3-S1 on CT scans. In a study of 188 individuals by Kalichman et al. [15], females were slightly more commonly affected by FJ arthritis than men, namely, 67% versus 60%. However, this difference was not significant. According to Suri et al. [29] females (OR 1.86) were more commonly affected, too. On the other hand, men had a higher prevalence of FJ arthritis in a cadaveric study of 645 spines ($P < 0.001$) by Eubanks et al. [12], but unfortunately, no percentages were stated. Overall, there is more evidence that gender cannot be counted on as a risk factor for FJ arthritis. This is surprising, because most of the males, especially those presenting to our traumatology department, are working in hard labor jobs. Being synovial-lined, diarthrodial, and freely moveable functional units, they transmit shear forces and help the intervertebral discs in carrying about 16% of the vertical load. Therefore, most of the weight is carried by the intervertebral disc. Even though hard labor may mainly affect arthritis of the intervertebral disc, a recent study has shown that estrogen also leads to arthritis of the intervertebral disc [63]. In conclusion, these two factors may balance each other out. Other potential factors that cause increased shear forces in women may play a role as well, such as scoliosis, weaker musculature, and carrying heavier weights in relation to their muscle strength, including pregnancy and carrying shopping bags [64].

(4) Orientation. Our results point out that increased FJ arthritis was significantly associated with a higher degree of FJ orientation, indicating a more coronal FJ orientation, at the upper lumbar spine, namely, L2/3 ($P = 0.03$). Interestingly, the cut-off point was ≥32°, indicating that more coronally oriented FJs, that is, ≥32° were associated with a higher radiological degree of FJ arthritis at this level. Even though

not significant, the same trend was observed for L3/4 (OR 1.009), while our results were equivocal for the lower lumbar spine. Therefore, coronally oriented FJs at L2/3 may present a surrogate for FJ arthritis later on in life.

The correlation of FJ arthritis and FJ orientation has only been reported for the lower part of the lumbar spine. A significant association between FJ arthritis and sagittal FJ orientation of the lower lumbar spine was found in a study of CT scans with 188 individuals by Kalichman et al. [6] and a MRI study if 111 individuals by Fujiwara et al. [38]. Likewise, a recent CT study of 123 individuals by Liu et al. [32] linked FJ arthritis to more sagittally oriented FJs at L4/5 and L5/S1. Our novel finding of increased FJ arthritis with more coronally oriented FJs at the upper lumbar spine might be attributed to the specific function of FJs at different lumbar levels. Normal FJ orientation planes differ at various levels, with a more sagittal and curved orientation for resistance against axial rotation in the upper compared to a more coronal and flat orientation for resistance against flexion and shearing forces in the lower lumbar segments [5, 6]. If the upper lumbar segments display more coronally oriented FJs, they are more prone to FJ arthritis because they are not designed to withstand repeating axial rotation. Another theory by Dunlop et al. [65] hypothesizes that aging leads to increased stress in the anteromedial part of the FJ due to repetitive abrasion during flexion and rotation and therefore changes the morphology of FJs, resulting in increased sagittal orientation [42]. Importantly, inverse orientation of the normal state, namely, coronally oriented FJs at the upper and sagittaly oriented FJs at the lower lumbar spine may be independent risk factors for FJ arthritis (Figure 4).

In our study, more coronal FJ orientation was present in individuals ≤40 years, and a more sagittal FJ orientation manifested in individuals ≥41 years at L5/S1. This is in line to previous study by Wang and Yang [42], who noted that degenerative spondylolisthesis, which has been associated with sagittal FJ orientation in several reports [6, 40, 41], was accompanied by a negative correlation of age and coronally oriented FJs ($r = -0.4555$) through investigation of the orientation of FJs at L4/5 in 300 individuals at different age groups. Masharawi et al. [43] did not find an association between FJ orientation and age studying 240 human vertebral columns. These FJ changes may be attributed to degenerative wear and tear, either at the FJs or at the intervertebral disc, and resulting traumatic change FJ orientation into a more sagittal alignment [38]. Like previous studies by Wang and Yang [42] and Masharawi et al. [43], we also did not find an association between gender and FJ orientation. Besides, we were able to show a significant steady progress from a sagittal toward a more coronal FJ orientation in a cephalocaudal fashion, namely, 30° at L2/3 and 47° at L5/S1 (Figures 4 and 5). This is in line with an ancillary CT study of the Framingham Heart Study with 3529 individuals by Kalichman et al. [6], who also showed an increasing FJO from L3-S1.

(5) Asymmetry. Our values for FJ asymmetry are in line with previous studies [40], where FJ asymmetry was commonly under 7°. We were not able to show a correlation between FJ arthritis and FJ asymmetry. This is in line with most previous studies [6, 7, 40], such as by Boden et al. [7], who studied 140 individuals with CT scans. Likewise, Grogan et al. [40] studied 21 cadavers and a total of 104 FJs with CT scans and did not find an association between FJ arthritis and FJ asymmetry. On the other hand, a single paper by Kong et al. [46] stated that FJ arthritis was associated with FJ asymmetry at L4/5 but not at L3/4, and L5/S1 in an MRI study of 300 individuals. Moreover, there was no association of FJ asymmetry and age in our study. Previous studies [6, 46, 47] have yielded the same results. Overall, we could not find evidence for previous hypotheses, which attributed FJ asymmetry to asymmetric mechanical stress or inborn deformities. Our findings are supported by a study of dried vertebrae of 240 humans by Masharawi et al. [48], where FJ asymmetry was considered a normal characteristic of the thoracolumbar spine.

However, in our study, FJ asymmetry was significantly more common in females than in males at L5/S1, which is in contrast to the study by Kong et al. [46], who did not find a meaningful relationship. Interestingly, there was evidence that FJ asymmetry increases cephalocaudally, with a mean of 4.89° at L2/3 and 7.27° at L5/S1. This indicates that FJ asymmetry is less common in sagittally oriented and more common in coronally oriented FJs, namely, the lower lumbar levels. Accordingly, Cassidy et al. [8] and Masharawi et al. [44] stated that FJ asymmetry is more commonly found in coronally oriented FJs. This may be explained by the increased load and degenerative changes at the lower lumbar spine [66], which may lead to uncontrolled changes of the FJs. This may affect women more commonly due to changes in estrogen or other unknown factors [63].

5. Conclusion

In conclusion, FJ arthritis is common affecting about half of individuals, increases with age, and affects both genders equally. Coronally oriented FJs (≥32°) in the upper lumbar spine, namely, at L2/3 may be an individual risk factor and surrogate for development of FJ arthritis in the entire lumbar spine, which is worth further investigations. Besides, coronal FJ orientation increases craniocaudally, while sagittal orientation at the lower lumbar spine increases with age. FJ asymmetry is not associated with FJ arthritis, is more common in females at the lower lumbar spine, and also increases in a craniocaudal fashion.

6. Disclosure

Each author certifies that he or a member of his or her immediate family has no funding or commercial associations that might pose a conflict of interest in connection with the submitted paper. Each author certifies that his institution approved the human protocol for this investigation and that all investigations were conducted in conformity with ethical principles of research.

Acknowledgments

The authors would like to thank Ms. Carol De-Simio-Hilton for her help with the preparation of the figures and Ms. Sina

Rüeger, MSc, from the Institute for Social and Preventive Medicine, Division of Biostatistics at the University of Zurich and for her help with statistical analysis.

References

[1] M. Benoist, "Natural history of the aging spine," *European Spine Journal*, vol. 12, supplement 2, pp. S86–S89, 2003.

[2] B. L. Laplante and M. J. DePalma, "Spine osteoarthritis," *PM&R*, vol. 4, supplement 5, pp. S28–S36, 2012.

[3] M. A. Adams and W. C. Hutton, "The effect of posture on the role of the apophysial joints in resisting intervertebral compressive forces," *Journal of Bone and Joint Surgery. British*, vol. 62, no. 3, pp. 358–362, 1980.

[4] L. Kalichman and D. J. Hunter, "Lumbar facet joint osteoarthritis: a review," *Seminars in Arthritis and Rheumatism*, vol. 37, no. 2, pp. 69–80, 2007.

[5] S. P. Cohen and S. N. Raja, "Pathogenesis, diagnosis, and treatment of lumbar zygapophysial (facet) joint pain," *Anesthesiology*, vol. 106, no. 3, pp. 591–614, 2007.

[6] L. Kalichman, P. Suri, A. Guermazi, L. Li, and D. J. Hunter, "Facet orientation and tropism: associations with facet joint osteoarthritis and degeneratives," *Spine*, vol. 34, no. 16, pp. E579–E585, 2009.

[7] S. D. Boden, K. D. Riew, K. Yamaguchi, T. P. Branch, D. Schellinger, and S. W. Wiesel, "Orientation of the lumbar facet joints: association with degenerative disc disease," *Journal of Bone and Joint Surgery. American*, vol. 78, no. 3, pp. 403–411, 1996.

[8] J. D. Cassidy, D. Loback, K. Yong-Hing, and S. Tchang, "Lumbar facet joint asymmetry: intervertebral disc herniation," *Spine*, vol. 17, no. 5, pp. 570–574, 1992.

[9] D. Hoy, C. Bain, G. Williams et al., "A systematic review of the global prevalence of low back pain," *Arthritis & Rheumatism*, vol. 64, no. 6, pp. 2028–2037, 2012.

[10] D. Hoy, P. Brooks, F. Blyth, and R. Buchbinder, "The epidemiology of low back pain," *Best Practice & Research Clinical Rheumatology*, vol. 24, no. 6, pp. 769–781, 2010.

[11] D. S. Binder and D. E. Nampiaparampil, "The provocative lumbar facet joint," *Current Reviews in Musculoskeletal Medicine*, vol. 2, no. 1, pp. 15–24, 2009.

[12] J. D. Eubanks, M. J. Lee, E. Cassinelli, and N. U. Ahn, "Prevalence of lumbar facet arthrosis and its relationship to age, sex, and race: an anatomic study of cadaveric specimens," *Spine*, vol. 32, no. 19, pp. 2058–2062, 2007.

[13] R. Ghormley, "Low back pain with special reference to the articular facets, with presentation of an operative procedure," *JAMA*, vol. 101, no. 23, pp. 1773–1777, 1933.

[14] A. C. Schwarzer, C. N. April, R. Derby, J. Fortin, G. Kine, and N. Bogduk, "Clinical features of patients with pain stemming from the lumbar zygapophysial joints: is the lumbar facet syndrome a clinical entity?" *Spine*, vol. 19, no. 10, pp. 1132–1137, 1994.

[15] L. Kalichman, L. Li, D. H. Kim et al., "Facet joint osteoarthritis and low back pain in the community-based population," *Spine*, vol. 33, no. 23, pp. 2560–2565, 2008.

[16] S. M. Eisenstein and C. R. Parry, "The lumbar facet arthrosis syndrome. Clinical presentation and articular surface changes," *Journal of Bone and Joint Surgery. British*, vol. 69, no. 1, pp. 3–7, 1987.

[17] N. Bogduk and R. Engel, "The menisci of the lumbar zygapophyseal joints. A review of their anatomy and clinical significance," *Spine*, vol. 9, no. 5, pp. 454–460, 1984.

[18] N. Bogduk, A. S. Wilson, and W. Tynan, "The human lumbar dorsal rami," *Journal of Anatomy*, vol. 134, part 2, pp. 383–397, 1982.

[19] N. Bogduk, "The innervation of the lumbar spine," *Spine*, vol. 8, no. 3, pp. 286–293, 1983.

[20] A. Igarashi, S. Kikuchi, S. Konno, and K. Olmarker, "Inflammatory cytokines released from the facet joint tissue in degenerative lumbar spinal disorders," *Spine*, vol. 29, no. 19, pp. 2091–2095, 2004.

[21] M. V. Boswell, J. D. Colson, N. Sehgal, E. E. Dunbar, and R. Epter, "A systematic review of therapeutic facet joint interventions in chronic spinal pain," *Pain Physician*, vol. 10, no. 1, pp. 229–253, 2007.

[22] M. V. Boswell, V. Singh, P. S. Staats, and J. A. Hirsch, "Accuracy of precision diagnostic blocks in the diagnosis of chronic spinal pain of facet or zygapophysial joint origin: a systematic review," *Pain Physician*, vol. 6, no. 4, pp. 449–456, 2003.

[23] J. van Zundert, N. Mekhail, P. Vanelderen, and M. van Kleef, "Diagnostic medial branch blocks before lumbar radiofrequency zygapophysial (Facet) joint denervation: benefit or burden?" *Anesthesiology*, vol. 113, no. 2, pp. 276–278, 2010.

[24] S. P. Cohen, K. A. Williams, C. Kurihara et al., "Multicenter, randomized, comparative cost-effectiveness study comparing 0, 1, and 2 diagnostic medial branch (facet joint nerve) block treatment paradigms before lumbar facet radiofrequency denervation," *Anesthesiology*, vol. 113, no. 2, pp. 395–405, 2010.

[25] L. Manchikanti, V. Singh, V. Pampati et al., "Evaluation of the relative contributions of various structures in chronic low back pain," *Pain Physician*, vol. 4, no. 4, pp. 308–316, 2001.

[26] P. Suri, D. J. Hunter, J. Rainville, A. Guermazi, and J. N. Katz, "Presence and extent of severe facet joint osteoarthritis are associated with back pain in older adults," *Osteoarthritis Cartilage*, vol. 21, no. 9, pp. 1199–1206, 2013.

[27] L. F. Czervionke and D. S. Fenton, "Fat-saturated MR imaging in the detection of inflammatory facet arthropathy (facet synovitis) in the lumbar spine," *Pain Medicine*, vol. 9, no. 4, pp. 400–406, 2008.

[28] L. Kalichman, D. H. Kim, L. Li, A. Guermazi, and D. J. Hunter, "Computed tomography-evaluated features of spinal degeneration: prevalence, intercorrelation, and association with self-reported low back pain," *Spine Journal*, vol. 10, no. 3, pp. 200–208, 2010.

[29] P. Suri, A. Miyakoshi, D. J. Hunter et al., "Does lumbar spinal degeneration begin with the anterior structures? A study of the observed epidemiology in a community-based population," *BMC Musculoskeletal Disorders*, vol. 12, article 202, 2011.

[30] T. Tischer, T. Aktas, S. Milz, and R. V. Putz, "Detailed pathological changes of human lumbar facet joints L1-L5 in elderly individuals," *European Spine Journal*, vol. 15, no. 3, pp. 308–315, 2006.

[31] N. C. Gries, U. Berlemann, R. J. Moore, and B. Vernon-Roberts, "Early histologic changes in lower lumbar discs and facet joints and their correlation," *European Spine Journal*, vol. 9, no. 1, pp. 23–29, 2000.

[32] H. X. Liu, Y. Shen, P. Shang, Y. X. Ma, X. J. Cheng, and H. Z. Xu, "Asymmetric facet joint osteoarthritis and its relationships to facet orientation, facet tropism and ligamentum flavum thickening," *Journal of Spinal Disorders & Techniques*, 2012.

[33] J. Li, C. Muehleman, Y. Abe, and K. Masuda, "Prevalence of facet joint degeneration in association with intervertebral joint degeneration in a sample of organ donors," *Journal of Orthopaedic Research*, vol. 29, no. 8, pp. 1267–1274, 2011.

[34] M. W. Swanepoel, L. M. Adams, and J. E. Smeathers, "Human lumbar apophyseal joint damage and intervertebral disc degeneration," *Annals of the Rheumatic Diseases*, vol. 54, no. 3, pp. 182–188, 1995.

[35] D. Weishaupt, M. Zanetti, J. Hodler, and N. Boos, "MR imaging of the lumbar spine: prevalence of intervertebral disk extrusion and sequestration, nerve root compression, end plate abnormalities, and osteoarthritis of the facet joints in asymptomatic volunteers," *Radiology*, vol. 209, no. 3, pp. 661–666, 1998.

[36] S. W. Wiesel, N. Tsourmas, H. L. Feffer, C. M. Citrin, and N. Patronas, "A study of computer-assisted tomography. I. The incidence of positive CAT scans in an asymptomatic group of patients," *Spine*, vol. 9, no. 6, pp. 549–551, 1984.

[37] J. Abbas, K. Hamoud, S. Peleg et al., "Facet joints arthrosis in normal and stenotic lumbar spines," *Spine*, vol. 36, no. 24, pp. E1541–E1546, 2011.

[38] A. Fujiwara, K. Tamai, H. S. An et al., "Orientation and osteoarthritis of the lumbar facet joint," *Clinical Orthopaedics and Related Research*, no. 385, pp. 88–94, 2001.

[39] W. Tassanawipas, P. Chansriwong, and S. Mokkhavesa, "The orientation of facet joints and transverse articular dimension in degenerative spondylolisthesis," *Journal of the Medical Association of Thailand*, vol. 88, supplement 3, pp. S31–S34, 2005.

[40] J. Grogan, B. H. Nowicki, T. A. Schmidt, and V. M. Haughton, "Lumbar facet joint tropism does not accelerate degeneration of the facet joints," *American Journal of Neuroradiology*, vol. 18, no. 7, pp. 1325–1329, 1997.

[41] L. Y. Dai, "Orientation and tropism of lumbar facet joints in degenerative spondylolisthesis," *International Orthopaedics*, vol. 25, no. 1, pp. 40–42, 2001.

[42] J. Wang and X. Yang, "Age-related changes in the orientation of lumbar facet joints," *Spine*, vol. 34, no. 17, pp. E596–E598, 2009.

[43] Y. Masharawi, B. Rothschild, G. Dar et al., "Facet orientation in the thoracolumbar spine: three-dimensional anatomic and biomechanical analysis," *Spine*, vol. 29, no. 16, pp. 1755–1763, 2004.

[44] Y. M. Masharawi, D. Alperovitch-Najenson, N. Steinberg et al., "Lumbar facet orientation in spondylolysis: a skeletal study," *Spine*, vol. 32, no. 6, pp. E176–E180, 2007.

[45] A. S. Don and P. A. Robertson, "Facet joint orientation in spondylolysis and isthmic spondylolisthesis," *Journal of Spinal Disorders and Techniques*, vol. 21, no. 2, pp. 112–115, 2008.

[46] M. H. Kong, W. He, Y.-D. Tsai et al., "Relationship of facet tropism with degeneration and stability of functional spinal unit," *Yonsei Medical Journal*, vol. 50, no. 5, pp. 624–629, 2009.

[47] L. Kalichman, A. Guermazi, L. Li, and D. J. Hunter, "Association between age, sex, BMI and CT-evaluated spinal degeneration features," *Journal of Back and Musculoskeletal Rehabilitation*, vol. 22, no. 4, pp. 189–195, 2009.

[48] Y. Masharawi, B. Rothschild, K. Salame, G. Dar, S. Peleg, and I. Hershkovitz, "Facet tropism and interfacet shape in the thoracolumbar vertebrae: characterization and biomechanical interpretation," *Spine*, vol. 30, no. 11, pp. E281–E292, 2005.

[49] A. Fujiwara, K. Tamai, M. Yamato et al., "The relationship between facet joint osteoarthritis and disc degeneration of the lumbar spine: an MRI study," *European Spine Journal*, vol. 8, no. 5, pp. 396–401, 1999.

[50] C. Karlo, R. Gnannt, T. Frauenfelder et al., "Whole-body CT in polytrauma patients: effect of arm positioning on thoracic and abdominal image quality," *Emergency Radiology*, vol. 18, no. 4, pp. 285–293, 2011.

[51] G. F. Carrera, V. M. Haughton, A. Syvertsen, and A. L. Williams, "Computed tomography of the lumbar facet joints," *Radiology*, vol. 134, no. 1, pp. 145–148, 1980.

[52] M. T. Modic, W. Pavlicek, M. A. Weinstein et al., "Magnetic resonance imaging of intervertebral disk disease. Clinical and pulse sequence considerations," *Radiology*, vol. 152, no. 1, pp. 103–111, 1984.

[53] F. Holdsworth, "Fractures, dislocations, and fracture-dislocations of the spine," *Journal of Bone and Joint Surgery. American*, vol. 52, no. 8, pp. 1534–1551, 1970.

[54] M. Pathria, D. J. Sartoris, and D. Resnick, "Osteoarthritis of the facet joints: accuracy of oblique radiographic assessment," *Radiology*, vol. 164, no. 1, pp. 227–230, 1987.

[55] A. Kettler and H.-J. Wilke, "Review of existing grading systems for cervical or lumbar disc and facet joint degeneration," *European Spine Journal*, vol. 15, no. 6, pp. 705–718, 2006.

[56] S. Schuller, Y. P. Charles, and J.-P. Steib, "Sagittal spinopelvic alignment and body mass index in patients with degenerative spondylolisthesis," *European Spine Journal*, vol. 20, no. 5, pp. 713–719, 2011.

[57] N. K. Mahato, "Facet dimensions, orientation, and symmetry at L5-S1 junction in lumbosacral transitional states," *Spine*, vol. 36, no. 9, pp. E569–E573, 2011.

[58] K. Hasegawa, H. Shimoda, K. Kitahara, K. Sasaki, and T. Homma, "What are the reliable radiological indicators of lumbar segmental instability?" *Journal of Bone and Joint Surgery. British*, vol. 93, no. 5, pp. 650–657, 2011.

[59] R Development Core Team, *R: A Language and Environment for Statistical Computing*, The R Foundation for Statistical Computing, Vienna, Austria, 2009.

[60] American College of Surgeons Committee on Trauma, *National Trauma Data Bank Annual Report*, 2010.

[61] J. Petilon, M. Hardenbrook, and W. Sukovich, "The effect of parallax on intraoperative positioning of the Charité artificial disc," *Journal of Spinal Disorders and Techniques*, vol. 21, no. 6, pp. 422–429, 2008.

[62] D. N. Mistry and P. A. Robertson, "Radiologic landmark accuracy for optimum coronal placement of total disc arthroplasty in the lumbar spine," *Journal of Spinal Disorders and Techniques*, vol. 19, no. 4, pp. 231–236, 2006.

[63] Y.-X. J. Wang and J. F. Griffith, "Effect of menopause on lumbar disk degeneration: potential etiology," *Radiology*, vol. 257, no. 2, pp. 318–320, 2010.

[64] Y. X. Wang, J. F. Griffith, X. J. Zeng et al., "Prevalence and sex difference of lumbar disc space narrowing in elderly chinese men and women: osteoporotic fractures in men (Hong Kong) and osteoporotic fractures in women (Hong Kong) studies," *Arthritis & Rheumatism*, vol. 65, no. 4, pp. 1004–1010, 2013.

[65] R. B. Dunlop, M. A. Adams, and W. C. Hutton, "Disc space narrowing and the lumbar facet joints," *Journal of Bone and Joint Surgery. British*, vol. 66, no. 5, pp. 706–710, 1984.

[66] Y. Otsuka, H. S. An, R. S. Ochia, G. B. J. Andersson, A. A. Espinoza Orías, and N. Inoue, "In vivo measurement of lumbar facet joint area in asymptomatic and chronic low back pain subjects," *Spine*, vol. 35, no. 8, pp. 924–928, 2010.

8

Geriatric Chest Imaging: When and How to Image the Elderly Lung, Age-Related Changes, and Common Pathologies

J. Gossner[1] and R. Nau[2]

[1] *Department of Clinical Radiology, Göttingen-Weende Hospital, An der Lutter 24, 37074 Göttingen, Germany*
[2] *Department of Geriatric Medicine, Göttingen-Weende Hospital, An der Lutter 24, 37074 Göttingen, Germany*

Correspondence should be addressed to J. Gossner; johannesgossner@gmx.de

Academic Editor: Paul Sijens

Even in a global perspective, societies are getting older. We think that diagnostic lung imaging of older patients requires special knowledge. Imaging strategies have to be adjusted to the needs of frail patients, for example, immobility, impossibility for long breath holds, renal insufficiency, or poor peripheral venous access. Beside conventional radiography, modern multislice computed tomography is the method of choice in lung imaging. It is especially important to separate the process of ageing from the disease itself. Pathologies with a special relevance for the elderly patient are discussed in detail: pneumonia, aspiration pneumonia, congestive heart failure, chronic obstructive pulmonary disease, the problem of overlapping heart failure and chronic obstructive pulmonary disease, pulmonary drug toxicity, incidental pulmonary embolism pulmonary nodules, and thoracic trauma.

1. Introduction

The population in many societies is getting older. The United Nations estimate that the number of people older than 65 years will increase from 743 million in 2009 to 2 billions in 2050. At this time, there will be more people older than 65 years than children younger than 15 years [1]. In fact, around 15% of patients treated in German hospitals are already older than 80 years [2]. With age, the frequency of multimorbidity increases. Geriatric medicine uses the term frailty to describe the process of progredient loss of mental and physical performance making the patients more vulnerable to further disease [3]. Sometimes it is difficult to separate the process of ageing from disease itself. Therefore, diagnostic imaging of older patients requires special knowledge. In this review, after a short description of imaging strategies, ethical considerations, and the normal ageing processes of the lung, distinct pathologies with a special relevance for the elderly patient are discussed.

2. Imaging Strategies

In contrast to younger people, handling of elderly patients is different and usually takes more time. In most cases, elderly patients have to be transferred to the radiology department and may need supervision while waiting. Positioning requires more time, and often patients need assistance. With bedridden patients, more than one person is needed for proper positioning. This need for more time and staff has to be kept in mind but is in most cases not reimbursed [4]. The ideal imaging test for elderly patient is fast and needs few changes in positioning.

2.1. Chest Radiography. The standard examination in imaging of the lung is chest radiography with a posterior-anterior and a lateral projection. Chest radiography is easy to perform, cheap, and, according to the ACR Appropriateness Criteria, in most scenarios the initial test when lung disease is suspected [5]. In frail patients, standard projections of the chest often cannot be obtained, and a chest radiograph in supine position has to be taken with well-known limitations.

2.2. Computed Tomography. In addition to conventional X-ray, the ideal test in more complex cases is computed tomography (CT). With modern multislice CT scanners, the lung can be examined in a few seconds. But even with modern CT scanners, motion artifacts due to breathing may be a problem in the elderly. Strategies to reduce these motion artifacts include the caudal start of the scan, where motion artifacts due to breathing are pronounced, and the use of a higher pitch. If there are still marked motion artifacts causing problems with image interpretation, we are adding several axial slices in classical high resolution CT technique (Figure 1).

Imaging of the lung parenchyma is possible without contrast media, but for imaging of lung vessels with computed tomographic pulmonary angiography (CTPA) or tumor staging, contrast media are mandatory. Elderly patients are at higher risk for contrast medium-induced nephropathy (CIN). In some cases, renal function is already impaired and there are other risk factors like diabetes, high blood pressure, heart insufficiency, hypovolemia, and atherosclerosis. Age > 75 years is also an independent risk factor for CIN [6]. It has to be considered, however, that only a very small part of patients with CIN require hemodialysis [6]. The most important prophylaxis is adequate hydration, which is especially important in elderly patients who often drink too little. The incidence of CIN is also related to the amount of used contrast media [7]. Interestingly, it has been reported that even thoracic CT scans with 15 mL iodinated contrast media showed satisfactory diagnostic quality for routine chest scans, for example, in the staging of mediastinal lymph nodes [8]. CTPA requires optimal opacification of the lung vessels, and therefore a minimum of 60 mL contrast media should be used. A high flow rate is usually recommended to obtain a good vascular enhancement. Unfortunately, poor peripheral venous access is common in the elderly and sometimes only small bore cannulas can be placed. We have shown that even with low flow rates (2.0 or 2.5 mL/s) and 60 mL of contrast media, sufficient vascular enhancement can be obtained [9]. Another strategy to minimize the dose of contrast media is the use of low kV settings [10].

2.3. Transthoracic Ultrasound. Transthoracic ultrasound may offer additional information to conventional chest radiography [11]. In the frail patient, it is easy to use bedside test. In the case of pleural effusion, it is more sensitive than radiography (especially compared to supine radiographs) and adds further information about the composition of the pleural fluid [11]. For example, it may show septations, a major cause for insufficient drainage after pleural tube placement. With transthoracic ultrasound, further information about congestive heart failure, pneumothorax, or pleura-based consolidations can be obtained [11].

2.4. Nuclear Medicine. Ventilation-perfusion scintigraphy has been replaced in the imaging of acute pulmonary embolism (PE) by CTPA in most departments. In elderly patients, prevalence of existing lung disease and therefore abnormal chest X-ray is relatively high, and therefore in this patient group, the sensitivity for scintigraphy in diagnosing PE is impaired [12]. In the elderly patient, CT scanning should be the preferred test, especially as in a substantial number of patients, diagnosis other than PE can be found (pneumonia, congestive heart failure). In patients with known allergy to iodinated contrast media, nephropathy or manifest hyperthyroidism scintigraphy is a good alternative.

2.5. Magnet Resonance Imaging (MRI). Although recent advances with lung MRI are not used in everyday imaging of the lung, an exception is the detailed imaging in Pancoast tumors. If lung imaging with MRI is performed in the elderly, a comprehensive examination to avoid excessive examination times should be used, for example, a combination of fast spin echo T2-weighted coronal images and diffusion weighted images [13]. With poor renal function, the use of contrast media is also of concern because of possible nephrogenic systemic fibrosis. A lot of older patients have contraindications for MRI like cardiac pace makers or older ferromagnetic surgical material.

2.6. A Practical Approach of Lung Imaging in the Elderly. The basic examination is chest radiography. If further workup is needed (suspected pulmonary embolism, immunocompromised patient, consolidation without clinical or laboratory signs of inflammation, and mass or complex effusion), a chest CT should be performed. A thin collimated scan (1 mm slice thickness) in caudocranial direction is recommended. Contrast media should be administered only if necessary. In the followup, the modality should be chosen conidering the underlying disease. A possible imaging algorhithm is provided in Scheme 1.

3. Ethical Considerations

Ethical considerations are important in the care of the elderly. Treating physicians always need to consider if a potential diagnosis obtained by imaging may alter treatment. Otherwise, the test should not be done. Even in cases where an exact diagnosis, for example, staging in a malignant disease, may help to plan further optimal treatment, it has to be accepted that patients may refuse imaging and insist on palliation only towards the end of their life. In particular, elderly patients should not feel to be obliged to agree with further diagnostics [14].

4. Changes of the Lungs with Ageing

With ageing, an enlargement of the distal airspaces due to the loss of supporting tissue can be found, a condition for which the terms "senile lung," "senile hyperinflation," or "senile emphysema" have been proposed [15, 16] (Figure 2).

Histologically, a homogeneous dilatation of the airspaces without signs of inflammation, fibrosis, or other architectural distortions can be seen [15]. As a result, signs of hyperinflation can be seen on conventional chest radiography [17]. In a recent study, there were more elderly asymptomatic adults (age > 75 years) with centrilobular emphysematous changes in CT imaging compared to a younger control group (age < 55 years) [18]. In the same study, interstitial changes of the lung with a subpleural reticular pattern could be found in 60% of the elderly patients. Bronchial wall thickening was shown in 50%. In another study, 25% of the elderly asymptomatic

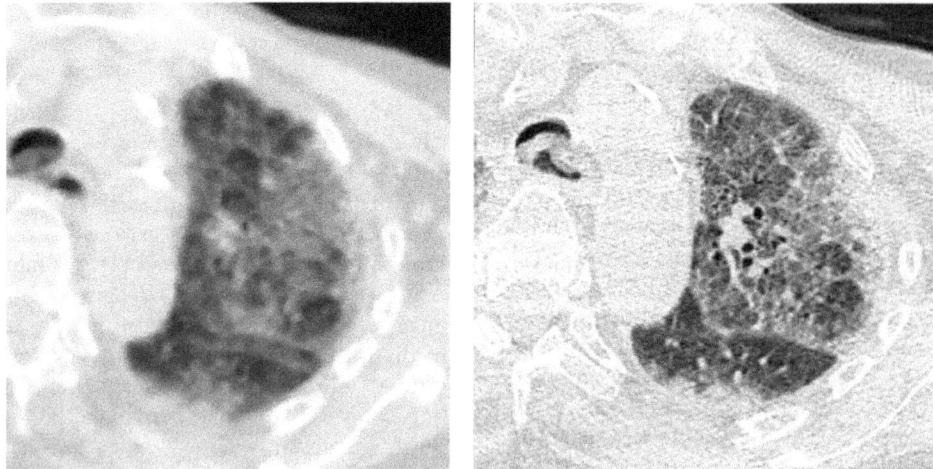

FIGURE 1: Motion artifacts due to breathing in an elderly patient impairing interpretation of the interstitial changes. An additional scan with the use of a standard high resolution technique is substantially improving diagnostic performance.

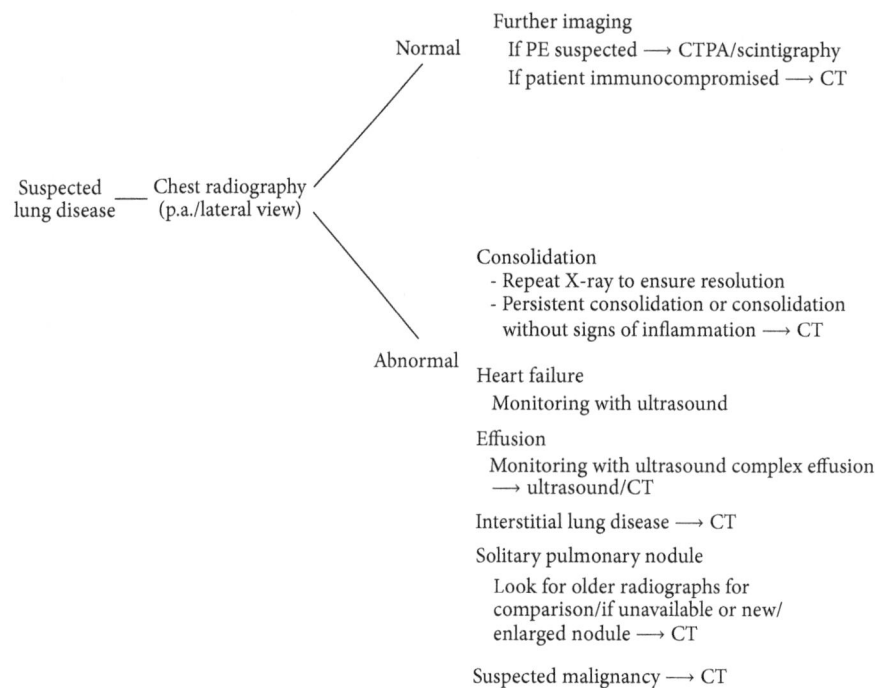

SCHEME 1

patients showed small cysts [17]. Lee et al. showed an increased air trapping with age [19]. The frequent finding of small basal atelectasis in asymptomatic elderly patients has been reported [20]. Further morphological changes with ageing are progressive calcifications of the airways and the rib cage [15, 16, 20] (Figure 3).

Like other muscles, there is a loss of diaphragmatic muscle mass [16], but in an older CT study, no measurable decrease in muscle thickness of the diaphragm could be found [21]. The reduced mass of other thoracic muscles has been described but has not been studied in detail [20].

5. Borderlands of the Normal: Possible Problems in Differentiation between Age-Related Changes and Pathology

As described previously, it has been shown that emphysematous changes and basal fibrotic changes are a common finding in elderly patients, especially on CT. There are no normative values described in the literature, but age-related changes are usually described to be moderate. So, it is obvious that differentiation may be difficult to early changes in chronic obstructive lung disease or interstitial lung disease.

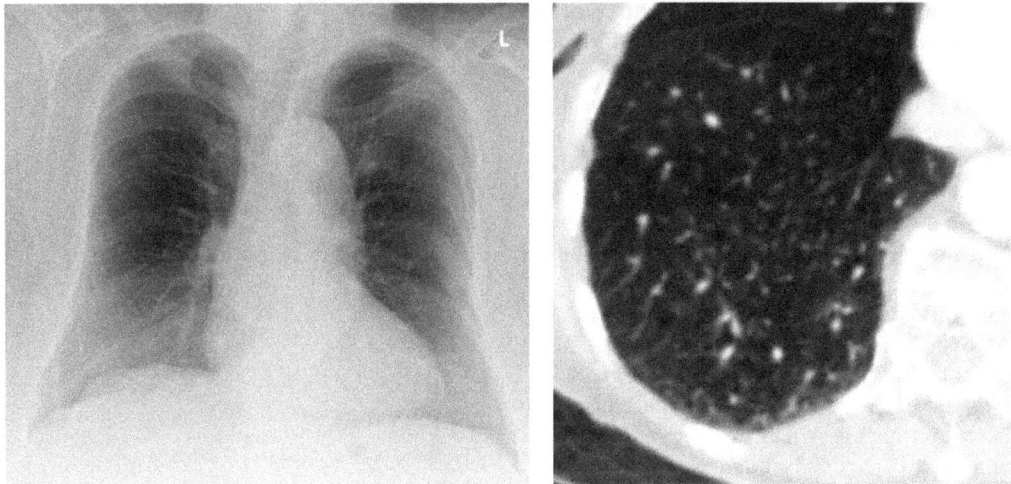

FIGURE 2: Senile emphysema in an 88-year-old patient. Chest X-ray (on the left) and centrilobular emphysematous changes on computed tomography (on the right). Imaging was ordered because of suspected mesenterial ischemia.

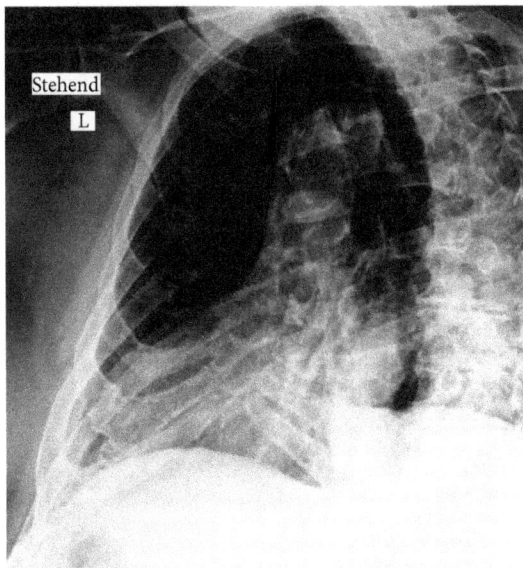

FIGURE 3: Extensive calcifications of the cartilaginous parts of the rib cage in an 85-year-old patient (suspected fracture).

For example, the finding of a moderate basal lung fibrosis may be due to age-related changes or findings of interstitial lung disease (usual interstitial pneumonia (UIP) or non-specific interstitial pneumonia (NSIP)), which can be found along with autoimmune disease or idiopathic interstitial lung disease. A differentiation is important as the latter two need specific treatment in opposition to age-related changes. Therefore, close correlation between the morphological extent of the fibrotic changes, clinical history (i.e., known autoimmune disease), and observation of associated changes is crucial. Extensive changes as well as marked honeycombing or traction bronchiectasis are unlikely to be only age-related associated signs like ground glass opacities which have not been reported with age-related changes

but may be due to congestive heart failure or infection. Correlation with preexisting imaging should be performed to assess disease progression.

The finding of senile emphysema is usually not accompanied by the clinical findings of chronic obstructive pulmonary disease like cough and sputum production.

In some cases, differentiation may be not possible and follow-up imaging is needed.

6. Pathologies with a Special Relevance in the Geriatric Population

6.1. Pneumonia. Pneumonia still is one of the leading causes of death from infection and is most commonly at the extreme of ages, that is, in the very young and in the elderly population [22]. In elderly patients, the immune system is often compromised. Beside an age-related decrease in immune activity, there are medications altering immune function. For example, long-term use of systemic corticosteroids in rheumatic disease significantly increases the risk of severe pneumonias with need for hospitalization [23]. Clinically, pneumonia can be divided into typical or atypical presentation, and in accordance to history in community acquired, nosocomial or infections in the immunocompromised. The most important imaging tool is conventional chest radiography. The role of radiography is to detect or rule out infiltrates, to show the extent of disease and possible complications, and to show response to treatment [24]. If pneumonia is suspected in an immunocompromised patient, a negative X-ray is not adequate to rule out infection and a CT should be advocated. Complications like empyema or abscesses are shown superiorly by CT [24]. There is a considerable overlap in the radiological morphology due to different pathogenic agents, so the morphological type of pneumonia is only a weak indicator of certain pathogens [25]. But in synopsis with clinical history and findings, chest X-ray will restrict the spectrum of possible pathogens and guide the calculated use of antibiotics. It has to be stressed that without clinical information, the differentiation between infectious infiltrates and other consolidating lung processes like cryptogenic organizing pneumonia is not possible [24]. If there are persistent infiltrations, bronchioalveolar carcinoma, now known as lepidic type of adenocarcinoma, should be included in the differential diagnosis. Clearance of pneumonic infiltration in the elderly takes usually more time. It has been shown that 15% of elderly patients still showed radiographic abnormalities beyond 3 months. Delayed clearance could be correlated to existing comorbidity [26]. We recommend a minimum interval of 3 months for the follow-up X-ray to to rule out preceeding malignant changes. Attention should be paid to the reactivation of tuberculosis. Many elderly patients are showing posttuberculotic changes on imaging. In reactivated pulmonary tuberculosis, patchy consolidations in the upper lobes or the superior segments of the lower lobes are the most common finding. Cavitations with a predilection in the upper lung zones can be found in up to 45% of patients [27].

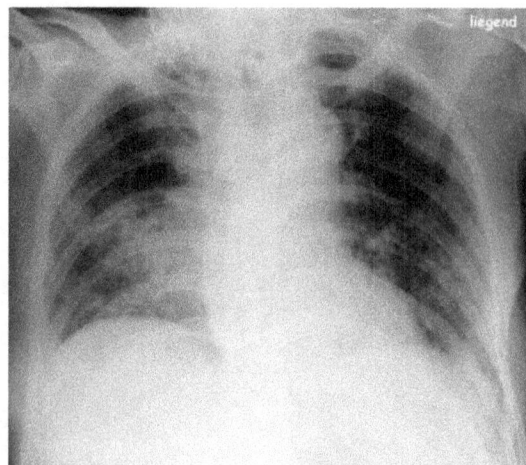

FIGURE 4: Consolidation in the right lower lobe due to aspiration in an 85-year-old patient (aspiration was confirmed using fluoroscopy).

6.2. Aspiration Pneumonia. Oropharyngeal contents or gastric acid which is misdirected to the lower airways can cause severe inflammation. In addition to the chemical pneumonitis pathogens from the oral flora, reaching the lower respiratory tract may cause difficult-to-treat bacterial pneumonia [28]. It has been shown that even healthy elderly people are swallowing more slowly than younger persons and the cough reflex is impaired. This may lead to pharyngeal colonisation with pathogenic bacteria [29, 30]. Aspiration of small amounts is common during sleep even in healthy young adults [31]. In conclusion to this, it seems that the amount of aspiration and/or colonization of the pharynx or gastric content by bacteria is important. It should be kept in mind that proton pump inhibitors and H_2 antagonists cause an increase in gastric pH which supports bacterial colonisation of the stomach. In everyday practice, the major cause of dysphagia is stroke and Parkinson's syndrome [28]. In a study by Nakagawa et al. [32], in the followup after stroke, 24% of patients with dysphagia developed pneumonia within one year. In contrast, none of the stroke patients without dysphagia developed pneumonia. Radiologically, recurrently found infiltrates involving the right lower lobe or the upper lobes in elderly patients should raise the suspicion of aspiration pneumonia (Figure 4).

If aspiration is suspected, we perform a fluoroscopic swallowing study with the use of barium in different formed boluses (thick liquids, semithick liquids, semisolid food, or solid food). This may guide dietary modifications, which are the most common management approach [28]. A commonly found phenomenon in elderly patients is laryngeal penetration, which means that small amounts of contrast media are entering the larynx. Only if the barium passes, the glottis aspiration can be diagnosed (Figure 5).

Another problem to be kept in mind is reflux in patients with percutaneous gastroenterostomy feeding tubes. In these patients, reflux may ultimately lead to aspiration. The diagnostic approach of choice is also fluoroscopy. The change to a jejunal position of the tip of the feeding tube can solve

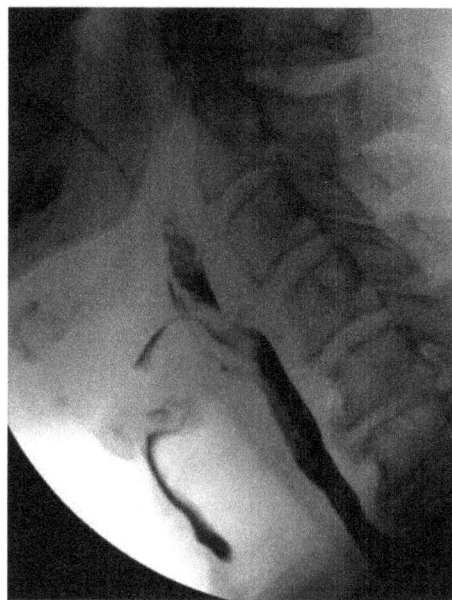

FIGURE 5: Spot view from a fluoroscopic examination in a 76-year-old patient after stroke showing aspiration.

this problem, but it has to be kept in mind that jejunal tubes are easily congested making the clinical handling of these patients problematic. At last, the side effects of medications should be remembered. Neuroleptics may cause dyskinesia of the muscles needed for swallowing with consecutive aspiration. In one study, the use of neuroleptic medication was associated with a higher risk of aspiration pneumonia [33].

6.3. Lung Changes with Congestive Heart Failure. Cardiac disease, especially left heart failure, is a major differential diagnosis for dyspnea in the elderly. With pulmonary venous, hypertension hydrostatic edema of the lungs occurs with a well-known appearance on conventional chest X-ray: cranialization of the pulmonary blood flow, increased vascular and interstitial markings with Kerley B lines, peribronchial cuffing, heart enlargement, and pleural effusions. With progression, alveolar edema occurs which in most cases can be differentiated from edema of noncardiogenic causes, like renal edema or capillary permeability edema (e.g., ARDS) [34]. From our experience, the diagnosis of early stages of congestive heart failure may be complicated by concomitant fibrotic changes. Correlation with already existing images or serial imaging will help to solve this problem. In patients with emphysema due to chronic obstructive pulmonary disease (COPD) the distribution relies on the remaining intact parenchyma, so atypical findings are common. Pulmonary edema in the right upper lobe can occur in patients with severe mitral regurgitation. Pulmonary venous hypertension has typical features on CT imaging (enlargement of the upper lobe pulmonary vessels, thickening of the bronchial walls, diffuse smooth thickening of the interlobular septae, and ground glass opacities accompanied by effusions and heart enlargement, Figure 6) [35].

In particular, in elderly patients with dyspnea undergoing CTPA for pulmonary embolism, we often find signs of congestive heart failure

6.4. The Problem of Overlapping Pathology in COPD/Congestive Heart Failure.

Beside the difficulty in discriminating age-related changes from pathology, there is the problem of clinical overlapping pathology with multimorbidity. With respect to imaging of the lung, the distinction between heart failure and COPD is a major concern. Up to 50% of patients with heart failure have concomitant COPD, and in most studies the prevalence was around 20%. On the other hand, about 20% of patients with COPD also have signs of left heart failure [36]. Heart failure mimics any clinical sign of COPD and vice versa, like cough, breathlessness, and exercise fatigue. Lung function tests may be misleading, and there is no established laboratory marker for differentiation between these two diseases. Therefore, in the case of acute dyspnea, it is a clinical routine to order a chest X-ray for further differential diagnosis. The major problem is that signs of heart failure may be atypical and asymmetric according to the areas with preserved normal pulmonary structure in patients with emphysematous lung changes in consequence to COPD. This may easily be confounded with peribronchial infiltrations, which are common during exacerbations of COPD. For a systematic differentiation, it is important to look for signs of COPD first. Theoretically, two extreme forms of COPD may be constructed: "pure" chronic bronchitis and "pure" emphysema. In clinical practice, as can be seen on CT, a mixture of these components is found in almost all patients with COPD. The pure forms are showing distinct changes in imaging. With "pure chronic bronchitis," there is the finding of a "dirty chest" with increased interstitial lung markings and bronchial wall thickening. With further disease, progression signs of right heart enlargement and pulmonary arterial hypertension can be found. The value of chest radiography in chronic bronchitis has undergone

considerable debate, but most authors state that the findings of a "dirty chest" are insensitive and have the problem of low reproducibility and interobserver variability [37]. The imaging of emphysema with chest radiography has undergone less debate, because the signs of hyperinflation of the lungs are obvious and objective measurements can be made [37]. The lateral view is of special importance, and it shows widening of the retrosternal space (>2.5 cm) and the flattening of the diaphragm (the angle between the chest wall and diaphragm is becoming larger than 90 degrees). If hyperinflation is found, atypical forms of pulmonary edema should be expected and kept in mind. Patients with initial emphysematous changes or senile emphysematous changes are normally not showing signs of significant hyperinflation on conventional X-ray. Our observations suggest that the destruction of normal pulmonary vascularity in these early stages is not marked enough to show noticeable asymmetric edematous changes with congestive heart failure. Because of the flattened costophrenic angles and scarring changes, ultrasound is often needed to make the diagnosis of small pleural effusion in patients with emphysema.

6.5. Pulmonary Drug Toxicity.

Pulmonary drug toxicity has recently received increased attention. Once believed to occur only with a few drugs, the list of causative agents is steadily growing. In a 2001 review, already about 150 causative drugs were mentioned and even more can be found in an internet database (PneumoTox) [38, 39]. The incidence is unclear, because systematic studies are lacking [40]. Age is not a risk factor per se, but as an effect of their multimorbidity, elderly people often take a variety of drugs. So, they are exposed to a wider range of possible causative agents and drug interactions (e.g., degradation via similar enzymatic mechanisms) which may cause an enhanced pulmonary toxicity [40]. If pulmonary drug toxicity is suggested or is a potential differential diagnosis, imaging with high resolution chest CT should be performed because of its superior sensitivity over plain radiography [41]. On imaging, common forms of toxic changes are fibrosing alveolitis (with a pattern often resembling findings in nonspecific interstitial pneumonia), predominantly subpleural consolidations (resembling cryptogenic organizing pneumonia or eosinophilic pneumonia), and in the more acute setting hypersensitivity reactions with imaging findings ranging from ground glass opacities and alveolar consolidations to severe diffuse alveolar damage indistinguishable from ARDS [38, 40] (Figure 7).

Different clusters of drugs according to the radiological presentation have been proposed [39], but in general, the most important point is to consider the possibility of drug-induced lung disease in the elderly.

6.6. Incidental Pulmonary Embolism.

With the evolution of multislice CT, incidental PE has been shown to be an incidental finding in up to 6% of inpatients undergoing imaging of the chest with CT [42]. Incidental PE is more common in patients with known malignancy. Interestingly, in a study by Ritchie et al. [42], an increased prevalence with age was found. It is known that elderly people have a

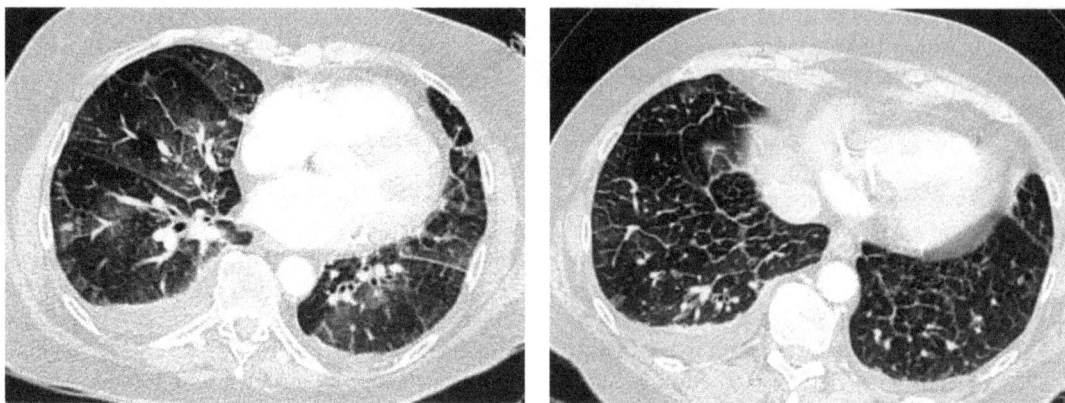

FIGURE 6: Computed tomography in 77-year-old patients showing signs of congestive heart failure with ground glass opacities, smooth thickening of interlobular septae, and bilateral effusions.

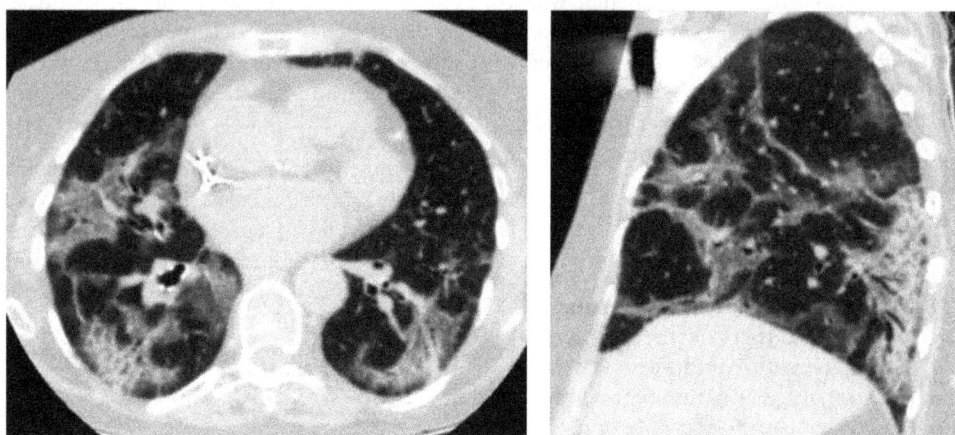

FIGURE 7: Drug induces lung changes with the use of amiodarone in an 81-year-old patient. Computed tomography shows the pattern of cryptogenic organizing pneumonia.

higher incidence of thromboembolic disease (symptomatic as well as asymptomatic). This may be explained by an elevated incidence of risk factors such as malignancy or immobility. In most cases, these incidental PEs are found on the subsegmental level. The clinical significance of incidental PE is unclear. As reviewed by Desai, currently available data suggests that even without treatment, mortality is not elevated [43]. Some authors argue that the lung acts as a filter, and the clearance of small emboli is a physiological process [44].

6.7. *The Problem of Pulmonary Nodules.* With the development of thin-section helical CT, the detection of small nodules, especially when using maximum intensity projections, has become routine. On chest X-ray, pulmonary nodules could be found in about 0.2% of patients [45]. In contrast, with multislice CT especially in lung cancer screening studies, the majority of patients showed pulmonary nodules [45]. There is a wide differential diagnosis, and the vast majority (over 80%) are granulomas or intrapulmonary lymph nodes with another 10% being hamartomas [46]. Morphologically,

only benign forms of calcifications are a clear sign of nonmalignant nodules, these include complete, central, or popcorn-like calcifications. As the chance of malignancy increases with size, this is the major criterium for the need of further assessment and is central part of current guidelines [47]. Recently, special attention has been paid to the subset of subsolid nodules, because of the close correlation to the spectrum of adenocarcinoma dedicated guidelines by the Fleischner Society have been proposed. If possible, the comparison with older X-ray images is recommended as a large portion of nodules can be detected retrospectively, and a constant size over 2 years indicates benignancy [46]. In daily practice, small solid nodules are found in the majority of elderly patients. In our department, the following strategy is used in these cases: first we are looking for morphological signs of benignancy: benign forms of calcifications, the presence of fat, the configuration of typical intrapulmonary lymph nodes, and cluster-like appearance in bronchiolitis with the typical "tree-in-bud" pattern. If none of these previously mentioned applies to the nodules, we are using adjusted guidelines of the Fleischner Society; that is, prolonged follow-up intervals (minimum 6 months) are recommended in close correlation with the clinical state of the patient [47]. It is important to remember that even in patients with known malignancy only a small portion of nodules smaller than 10 mm are in fact metastasis [48]. Therefore, follow-up imaging is also the method of choice in oncologic elderly patients with small pulmonary nodules.

6.8. Trauma. The increasing risk of falls with ageing is an everyday topic in geriatric medicine. Ojo et al. studied the type of injuries with falls in elderly people and found chest injuries in 6.9% of patients [49]. In this group, the vast majority suffered from rib fractures (86%). The primary imaging test in suspected rib fracture is radiography, but even with dedicated oblique views, it has been reported that up to 50% of fractures are missed. In our department, with minor blunt trauma, we are performing a single oblique view of the affected side of the chest together with a standard radiography of the lung (single view, p.a.) to search for complications of the trauma (effusion, lung contusion, and pneumothorax) [50]. If there are uncertainties or there is major trauma, CT is the imaging of choice. Ultrasound has shown a high sensitivity for diagnosing rib fractures, but its use is time consuming and operator dependent. It may be reserved for selected cases, for example, further workup of suspected rib fracture in minor chest trauma despite negative radiographs [50].

7. Teaching Points/Conclusion

(i) The basic examination of the lung is chest radiography. If further workup is needed, chest CT should be performed. To minimize motion artifacts due to breathing, a caudocranial scan direction is recommended. If there are still motion artifacts hindering interpretation add some classical HR-CT scans.

(ii) Common age-related changes include basal fibrotic changes, senile emphysema, and progressive calcification of the airways and rib cage.

(iii) In particular, age-related fibrotic changes may be difficult to differentiate from early fibrotic changes with UIP/NSIP. Extensive changes as well as marked honeycombing, traction bronchiectasis, and ground glass opacities are unlikely in "pure" age-related changes.

(iv) Resolution of pneumonic infiltrations is slower in the elderly, therefore recommend follow-up imaging after 3 months.

(v) If aspiration is suspected, fluoroscopic examinations may establish diagnosis.

(vi) Congestive heart failure may show an atypical or asymmetric pattern in patients with preexisting lung disease which always includes heart failure in the differential diagnosis of dyspnea.

(vii) Think of pulmonary drug toxicity.

(viii) Follow-up imaging is usually the appropriate management strategy with pulmonary nodules.

(ix) If in doubt, look out for existing radiographs for comparison.

Conflict of Interests

The authors have no conflict of interests to declare.

References

[1] United Nations, "Commission on Population and Development. 42nd Session: programme implementation and future work of the secretariat in the field of demographic trends," Geneva, Switzerland, 2009.

[2] Statistisches Bundesamt, *Diagnosedaten der Patienten und Patientinnen in Krankenhäusern*, Statistisches Bundesamt, Wiesbaden, Germany, 2011.

[3] J. E. Morley, H. M. Perry III, and D. K. Miller, "Something about frailty," *Journals of Gerontology. Series A*, vol. 57, no. 11, pp. M698–M704, 2002.

[4] S. L. Torres, A. G. Dutton, and T. A. Linn-Watson, *Patient Care in Imaging Technology*, Lippincott Williams & Wilkins, Philadelphia, Pa, USA, 2010.

[5] ACR Appropiateness criteria, http://www.acr.org/Quality-Safety/Appropriateness-Criteria/.

[6] O. Toprak and M. Cirit, "Risk factors for contrast-induced nephropathy," *Kidney and Blood Pressure Research*, vol. 29, no. 2, pp. 84–93, 2006.

[7] R. G. Cigarroa, R. A. Lange, R. H. Williams, and L. D. Hillis, "Dosing of contrast material to prevent contrast nephropathy in patients with renal disease," *American Journal of Medicine*, vol. 86, no. 6, pp. 649–652, 1989.

[8] D. R. Engelkemier, A. Tadros, and A. Karimi, "Lower iodine load in routine contrast-enhanced CT: an alternative imaging strategy," *Journal of Computer Assisted Tomography*, vol. 36, no. 2, pp. 191–195, 2012.

[9] J. Gossner, "Feasibility of computed tomography pulmoary angiography with low flow rates," *Journal of Clinical Imaging Science*, vol. 2, p. 57, 2012.

[10] Z. Szucs-Farkas, F. Schibler, J. Cullmann et al., "Diagnostic accuracy of pulmonary CT angiography at low tube voltage: intraindividual comparison of a normal-dose protocol at 120 kVp and a low-dose protocol at 80 kVp using reduced amount of contrast medium in a simulation study," *American Journal of Roentgenology*, vol. 197, no. 5, pp. W852–W859, 2011.

[11] S. Sartori and P. Tombesi, "Emerging roles for transthoracic ultrasonography in pleuropulmonary pathology," *World Journal of Radiology*, vol. 2, pp. 83–90, 2010.

[12] L. M. Freeman, E. G. Stein, S. Sprayregen, M. Chamarthy, and L. B. Haramati, "The current and continuing important role of ventilation-perfusion scintigraphy in evaluating patients with suspected pulmonary embolism," *Seminars in Nuclear Medicine*, vol. 38, no. 6, pp. 432–440, 2008.

[13] M. Wielpütz and H. U. Kauczor, "MRI of the lung: state of the art," *Diagnostic and Interventional Radiology*, vol. 18, pp. 344–355, 2012.

[14] P. S. Mueller, C. C. Hook, and K. C. Fleming, "Ethical issues in geriatrics: a guide for clinicians," *Mayo Clinic Proceedings*, vol. 79, no. 4, pp. 554–562, 2004.

[15] E. K. Verbeken, M. Cauberghs, I. Mertens, J. Clement, J. M. Lauweryns, and K. P. van de Woestijne, "The senile lung; Comparison with normal and emphysematous lungs. 1. Structural aspects," *Chest*, vol. 101, no. 3, pp. 793–799, 1992.

[16] G. Sharma and J. Goodwin, "Effect of aging on respiratory system physiology and immunology," *Clinical Interventions in Aging*, vol. 1, no. 3, pp. 253–260, 2006.

[17] A. Heinrich, *Alternsvorgänge im Röntgenbild*, Leipzig, 1941.

[18] S. J. Copley, A. U. Wells, K. E. Hawtin et al., "Lung morphology in the elderly: comparative CT study of subjects over 75 years old versus those under 55 years old," *Radiology*, vol. 251, no. 2, pp. 566–573, 2009.

[19] K. W. Lee, S. Y. Chung, I. Yang, Y. Lee, E. Y. Ko, and M. J. Park, "Correlation of aging and smoking with air trapping at thin-section CT of the lung in asymptomatic subjects," *Radiology*, vol. 214, no. 3, pp. 831–836, 2000.

[20] B. Hochhegger, G. Pontes de Mereiles, K. Irion et al., "The chest and ageing: radiological findings," *Jornal Brasileiro de Pneumologia*, vol. 38, no. 5, pp. 656–665, 2012.

[21] C. I. Caskey, E. A. Zerhouni, E. K. Fishman, and A. D. Rahmouni, "Aging of the diaphragm: a CT study," *Radiology*, vol. 171, no. 2, pp. 385–389, 1989.

[22] J. H. Reynolds, G. McDonald, H. Alton, and S. B. Gordon, "Pneumonia in the immunocompetent patient," *British Journal of Radiology*, vol. 83, no. 996, pp. 998–1009, 2010.

[23] S. Bernatsky, M. Hudson, and S. Suissa, "Anti-rheumatic drug use and risk of serious infections in rheumatoid arthritis," *Rheumatology*, vol. 46, no. 7, pp. 1157–1160, 2007.

[24] T. Franquet, "Imaging of pneumonia: trends and algorithms," *European Respiratory Journal*, vol. 18, no. 1, pp. 196–208, 2001.

[25] R. D. Tarver, S. D. Teague, D. E. Heitkamp, and D. J. Conces Jr., "Radiology of community-acquired pneumonia," *Radiologic Clinics of North America*, vol. 43, no. 3, pp. 497–512, 2005.

[26] A. A. El Solh, A. T. Aquilina, H. Gunen, and F. Ramadan, "Radiographic resolution of community-acquired bacterial pneumonia in the elderly," *Journal of the American Geriatrics Society*, vol. 52, no. 2, pp. 224–229, 2004.

[27] Y. J. Jeong and K. S. Lee, "Pulmonary tuberculosis: up-to-date imaging and management," *American Journal of Roentgenology*, vol. 191, no. 3, pp. 834–844, 2008.

[28] P. E. Marik and D. Kaplan, "Aspiration pneumonia and dysphagia in the elderly," *Chest*, vol. 124, no. 1, pp. 328–336, 2003.

[29] T. Nagatake, "Aspiration and aspiration pneumonia," *The Japan Medical Association Journal*, vol. 46, pp. 12–18, 2003.

[30] J. Robbins, J. W. Hamilton, G. L. Lof, and G. B. Kempster, "Oropharyngeal swallowing in normal adults of different ages," *Gastroenterology*, vol. 103, no. 3, pp. 823–829, 1992.

[31] K. Gleeson, D. F. Eggli, and S. L. Maxwell, "Quantitative aspiration during sleep in normal subjects," *Chest*, vol. 111, no. 5, pp. 1266–1272, 1997.

[32] T. Nakagawa, K. Sekizawa, K. Nakajoh, H. Tanji, H. Arai, and H. Sasaki, "Silent cerebral infarction: a potential risk for pneumonia in the elderly," *Journal of Internal Medicine*, vol. 247, no. 2, pp. 255–259, 2000.

[33] H. Wada, K. Nakajoh, T. Satoh-Nakagawa et al., "Risk factors of aspiration pneumonia in Alzheimer's disease patients," *Gerontology*, vol. 47, no. 5, pp. 271–276, 2001.

[34] E. N. C. Milne, M. Pistolesi, M. Miniati, and C. Giuntini, "The radiologic distinction of cardiogenic and noncardiogenic edema," *American Journal of Roentgenology*, vol. 144, no. 5, pp. 879–894, 1985.

[35] M. L. Storto, S. T. Kee, J. A. Golden, and W. R. Webb, "Hydrostatic pulmonary edema: high-resolution CT findings," *American Journal of Roentgenology*, vol. 165, no. 4, pp. 817–820, 1995.

[36] N. M. Hawkins, M. C. Petrie, P. S. Jhund, G. W. Chalmers, F. G. Dunn, and J. J. V. McMurray, "Heart failure and chronic obstructive pulmonary disease: diagnostic pitfalls and epidemiology," *European Journal of Heart Failure*, vol. 11, no. 2, pp. 130–139, 2009.

[37] N. L. Müller and H. Coxson, "Chronic obstructive pulmonary disease • 4: imaging the lungs in patients with chronic obstructive pulmonary disease," *Thorax*, vol. 57, no. 11, pp. 982–985, 2002.

[38] M. Özkan, R. A. Dweik, and M. Ahmad, "Drug- induced lung disease," *Cleveland Clinic Journal of Medicine*, vol. 68, pp. 782–795, 2001.

[39] Pneumotox online, http://www.pneumotox.com/.

[40] P. Camus, P. Foucher, P. Bonniaud, and K. Ask, "Drug-induced infiltrative lung disease," *European Respiratory Journal*, vol. 18, supplement 32, pp. 93S–100S, 2001.

[41] J. E. Ellis, J. R. Cleverly, and N. L. Müller, "Drug- induced lung disease: high resolution CT findings," *American Journal of Roentgenology*, vol. 175, no. 4, pp. 1019–1024, 2000.

[42] G. Ritchie, S. McGurk, C. McCreath, C. Graham, and J. T. Murchison, "Prospective evaluation of unsuspected pulmonary embolism on contrast enhanced multidetector CT (MDCT) scanning," *Thorax*, vol. 62, no. 6, pp. 536–540, 2007.

[43] S. R. Desai, "Unsuspected pulmonary embolism on CT scanning: yet another headache for clinicians?" *Thorax*, vol. 62, no. 6, pp. 470–472, 2007.

[44] J. W. Gurney, "No fooling around: direct visualization of pulmonary embolism," *Radiology*, vol. 188, no. 3, pp. 618–619, 1993.

[45] S. M. Holin, R. E. Dwork, S. Glaser, A. E. Rikli, and J. B. Stocklen, "Solitary pulmonary nodules found in a community-wide chest roentgenographic survey; a five-year follow-up study," *American Review of Tuberculosis*, vol. 79, no. 4, pp. 427–439, 1959.

[46] C. Beigelman-Aubry, C. Hill, and P. A. Grenier, "Management of an incidentally found pulmonary nodule," *European Radiology*, vol. 17, no. 2, pp. 449–466, 2007.

[47] H. MacMahon, J. H. M. Austin, G. Gamsu et al., "Guidelines for management of small pulmonary nodules detected on CT scans: a statement from the Fleischner Society," *Radiology*, vol. 237, no. 2, pp. 395–400, 2005.

[48] M. Hanamiya, T. Aoki, Y. Yamashita, S. Kawanami, and Y. Korogi, "Frequency and significance of pulmonary nodules on thin-section CT in patients with extrapulmonary malignant neoplasms," *European Journal of Radiology*, vol. 81, no. 1, pp. 152–157, 2012.

[49] P. Ojo, J. O'Connor, D. Kim, K. Ciardiello, and J. Bonadies, "Patterns of injury in geriatric falls," *Connecticut Medicine*, vol. 73, no. 3, pp. 139–145, 2009.

[50] S. J. Bhavnagri and T.-L. H. Mohammed, "When and how to image a suspected broken rib," *Cleveland Clinic Journal of Medicine*, vol. 76, no. 5, pp. 309–314, 2009.

9

Gestational Trophoblastic Disease: A Multimodality Imaging Approach with Impact on Diagnosis and Management

Sunita Dhanda,[1,2] Subhash Ramani,[2] and Meenkashi Thakur[2]

[1] Department of Diagnostic Imaging, National University Hospital, Level 2, Main Building, 5 Lower Kent Ridge Road, Singapore 119074
[2] Tata Memorial Hospital, Dr. E. Borges Marg, Parel, Mumbai, Maharashtra 400012, India

Correspondence should be addressed to Sunita Dhanda; sunitadhanda63@gmail.com

Academic Editor: Andreas H. Mahnken

Gestational trophoblastic disease is a condition of uncertain etiology, comprised of hydatiform mole (complete and partial), invasive mole, choriocarcinoma, and placental site trophoblastic tumor. It arises from abnormal proliferation of trophoblastic tissue. Early diagnosis of gestational trophoblastic disease and its potential complications is important for timely and successful management of the condition with preservation of fertility. Initial diagnosis is based on a multimodality approach: encompassing clinical features, serial quantitative β-hCG titers, and pelvic ultrasonography. Pelvic magnetic resonance imaging (MRI) is sometimes used as a problem-solving tool to assess the depth of myometrial invasion and extrauterine disease spread in equivocal and complicated cases. Chest radiography, body computed tomography (CT), and brain MRI have been recommended as investigative tools for overall disease staging. Angiography has a role in management of disease complications and metastases. Efficacy of PET (positron emission tomography) and PET/CT in the evaluation of recurrent or metastatic disease has not been adequately investigated yet. This paper discusses the imaging features of gestational trophoblastic disease on various imaging modalities and the role of different imaging techniques in the diagnosis and management of this entity.

1. Introduction

Gestational trophoblastic disease (GTD) refers to an abnormal trophoblastic proliferation composed of a broad spectrum of lesions ranging from benign, albeit premalignant hydatiform mole (complete and partial), through to the aggressive invasive mole, choriocarcinoma, and placental site trophoblastic tumor (PSTT). Gestational trophoblastic neoplasia (GTN) refers to the aggressive subset that has a capability for independent growth and metastases and requires chemotherapy. It includes invasive mole, choriocarcinoma, and PSTT. GTN may arise following evacuation of a molar pregnancy as well as after a normal term or preterm pregnancy, abortion, or ectopic pregnancy. Hence, it is also referred to as persistent trophoblastic neoplasia (PTN). These lesions vary considerably in clinicopathologic behavior and propensity for local invasion and metastases. Although GTD may occur as a pregnancy complication in women of any age, it is more common at teenage or advanced maternal age (40–50 years) [1, 2]. Early detection of GTN is important as it has

an excellent prognosis following treatment due to exquisite chemosensitivity of most of these lesions [1, 2]. In this paper, we describe the role of various imaging techniques in the diagnosis and management of GTD. A brief overview of the underlying pathophysiology, clinical features, classification, and posttreatment surveillance of the disease is also provided.

2. Pathophysiology

Trophoblast is a gestational tissue which covers the blastocyst and provides route for nourishment between the maternal endometrium and the developing embryo in early pregnancy. Ultimately, it covers the surface of chorionic villi and forms the fetal portion of the placenta. Trophoblast is comprised of cytotrophoblast, syncytiotrophoblast, and intermediate trophoblast. Cytotrophoblast shows high mitotic activity; however, it lacks hormone synthesis. Syncytiotrophoblast forms the chorionic villi, has low mitotic activity, and synthesizes beta-human chorionic gonadotrophin (β-hCG), which is used as a tumor marker. Intermediate trophoblast has features of the other two components and is responsible for endometrial invasion and implantation. In the various forms of GTD, different components of trophoblast show abnormal proliferation to a variable extent [1]. Although most GTNs secrete β-hCG hormone with abnormal elevation of β-hCG titers being one of their diagnostic features of GTD, the titers vary in different tumor types. Some choriocarcinomas and bimorphic tumor types secrete only low levels of β-hCG [3]. PSTT represents a neoplastic proliferation of intermediate trophoblasts [2]. Unlike other forms of GTD, it is characterized by low β-hCG levels due to lack of syncytiotrophoblastic proliferation [2–4]. However, it shows increased expression of tissue as well as serum human placental lactogen (hPL) [4].

Hydatiform mole results from an aberrant fertilization process. It includes complete and partial mole, the former being more common. Complete hydatiform mole arises when a single haploid sperm (23X) fertilizes a chromosomally empty ovum followed by chromosomal duplication and formation of a zygote with no maternal contribution. This leads to a genetically diploid pattern (more commonly 46XX) in a complete mole. Similar fertilization and duplication with a 23Y sperm do not produce a viable (46YY) zygote. Rarely, 46XY pattern may result due to fertilization of a chromosomally empty ovum by two different sperms. In contrast, partial hydatiform mole usually has a triploid chromosomal pattern (46XXX, 46XXY, and 46XYY), resulting from fertilization of a normal egg by two sperms [1, 2, 5, 6].

Pathologically, hydatiform mole is composed of abnormally proliferating syncytiotrophoblastic and cytotrophoblastic cells resulting in generalized swelling of chorionic villi. Complete mole shows severe villous swelling, resembling a bunch of grapes and usually an absence of embryo. Villous swelling is less intense in a partial mole and an embryo is usually present. The embryo may survive up to early second trimester [1, 2]. Complete or partial hydatiform mole invading the myometrium is called invasive mole. Hydatiform mole is a premalignant condition with 16% of complete and 0.5% partial moles undergoing transformation into malignant forms (invasive mole, choriocarcinoma, or PSTT) [1, 2]. Choriocarcinoma consists of malignant proliferation of cytotrophoblast and syncytiotrophoblast in various proportions; however, it is histopathologically distinct from invasive mole in that it lacks chorionic villous formations. It may arise following hydatiform mole, term pregnancy, miscarriage, or ectopic pregnancy. Choriocarcinoma is a highly malignant, necrotic, hemorrhagic, and locally invasive form of GTN. Early and extensive vascular invasion results in metastases even when the primary tumor is quite small [1, 2]. Choriocarcinoma arising after miscarriage or term pregnancy may present after several years, directly as metastases, elevated β-hCG levels, and normal pelvic sonography findings [2, 6]. PSTT is the rarest form of GTN with uncertain biological behavior [2, 4, 7]. It arises from the placental implantation site following a normal pregnancy, abortion, or hydatiform mole, most commonly from an antecedent normal pregnancy. It is generally a slow growing tumor with a tendency for local and lymph nodal metastases before distant metastases (a very rare feature in choriocarcinoma) [2].

3. Clinical and Laboratory Features

Initial diagnosis of GTD is based on a combination of history, examination, quantitative β-hCG titers, and pelvic sonography. Diagnosis of hydatiform mole based on clinical features may be difficult due to nonspecificity of signs and symptoms. Patients present with irregular vaginal bleeding, excessive vomiting, transvaginal expulsion of grape-like vesicles, abnormally enlarged uterus, and features of preeclampsia, anemia, or hyperthyroidism [1, 5, 8]. β-hCG levels show large variation in normal, multiple, and abnormal gestations and when considered in isolation may be misleading for diagnosis of hydatiform mole. Hence, early first trimester sonography remains the investigation of choice for initial diagnosis of hydatiform mole [1, 8].

The standard treatment for hydatiform form is suction evacuation, resulting in approximately 84% cure rate for complete moles and 99.5% for partial moles [1, 2]. It is difficult to predict patient outcome at the time of initial diagnosis. Hence, all patients are followed up with serial quantitative serum β-hCG measurements following suction evacuation, to allow early diagnosis of persistent trophoblastic neoplasia [1, 5, 9]. β-hCG levels should decline following suction evacuation. As per the latest FIGO guidelines [10], posthydatiform mole GTN may be diagnosed based on any of the following criteria:

(1) β-hCG level plateau for 4 measurements over a period of 3 weeks or longer, that is, for days 1, 7, 14, and 21;

(2) a rise in β-hCG levels for 3 consecutive measurements or longer over a period of at least 2 weeks or more, that is, on days 1, 7, and 14;

(3) histological diagnosis of choriocarcinoma;

(4) elevated β-hCG levels for 6 months or more after evacuation.

Although β-hCG is useful for diagnosis of PTN, imaging studies may play a confirmatory role in early disease or patients with confusing clinical picture. The most important role of ultrasound in patients with suspected PTN is to exclude a normal gestation as a cause of elevated β-hCG level [1].

Nonmetastatic GTN presents as a localized uterine tumor with abnormal vaginal bleeding. Uterine perforation may result in intraperitoneal bleed, presenting as an acute abdomen. Metastases have been reported in 19% of cases, most commonly from choriocarcinoma [2]. Hematogenous dissemination is the principal route of spread, most commonly to lung (80%) followed by vagina (30%), brain (10%), and liver (10%). It may also metastasize to kidney, gastrointestinal tract, skin, or fetus (from choriocarcinoma). Isolated metastasis to other sites is rare in the absence of lung and vaginal metastases [2, 6, 9]. Hypervascular metastases may present with features of hemorrhage. Lung metastases may be asymptomatic or present with hemoptysis, dyspnea, chest pain, or pulmonary artery hypertension. Vaginal metastases may result in torrential vaginal bleeding. Hence, a biopsy should be avoided. Brain metastases may present with headache, seizures, motor, or sensory deficit. Liver metastases are usually asymptomatic [2, 9].

4. Imaging Features of the Uterine Disease

4.1. Ultrasound. Grey-scale ultrasound with color and spectral Doppler imaging is a very useful tool for diagnosing GTD, determining presence of invasive disease, predicting response to chemotherapy, postchemotherapy follow-up, and detection of recurrence [2, 6].

4.1.1. Ultrasonographic Features of Hydatiform Mole. Ultrasound is the first line imaging investigation for diagnosis of a clinically suspected hydatiform mole since a single abnormally elevated serum β-hCG level measured at the time of patient presentation is not diagnostic and may be seen in a multiple gestation as well [2, 6, 8, 11, 12]. Pelvic sonography is performed as a routine investigation during early pregnancy to accurately date the gestation and determine any abnormalities [6, 11]. Ultrasound can be done by transabdominal or transvaginal approach. Transvaginal sonography provides better details of the lesion due to its superior spatial resolution and proximity to the anatomy of interest. On the contrary, transabdominal approach needs the patient to hold urine resulting in patient discomfort and provides fewer details. On first trimester transabdominal ultrasound, hydatiform mole which constitutes 80% cases of GTD will be seen most frequently as an enlarged uterus with a heterogeneous endometrial mass of variable echogenicity (predominantly echogenic) [1, 2, 6, 12]. Ultrasound appearance of the lesion has been classically described earlier as "snowstorm" or "granular" due to multiple echogenic foci [1]. Transvaginal sonography (TVS) can better demonstrate the lesion morphology and any myometrial invasion. Fluid-filled molar vesicles, representing hydropic, and swollen villi are typically seen as multiple small anechoic spaces varying in size from 1–30 mm throughout the lesion on first trimester transvaginal sonography (Figure 1). With increasing gestational age, the anechoic spaces become larger and more numerous due to presence of prominent villi, making sonographic diagnosis of hydatiform mole easier in second trimester than in the first trimester even by transabdominal approach [2, 6]. Uterine volume should also be accurately estimated on ultrasound as it correlates with the tumor burden and hence determines risk stratification [2].

A fetus or fetal parts are not seen in a complete hydatiform mole except in 1-2% of cases with coexistent dizygotic diploid twin pregnancy [1]. In contrast, partial mole is usually associated with a fetus which is growth retarded or anomalous and an enlarged, thickened placenta with numerous anechoic cystic lesions. A dizygotic diploid twin pregnancy coexistent with a complete mole can be differentiated from a triploid partial mole on ultrasound by identifying a separate normal placenta in the former [1, 2, 6]. Placental appearance similar to partial mole may result from hydropic placental degeneration associated with first trimester embryonic demise of any cause [2, 6].

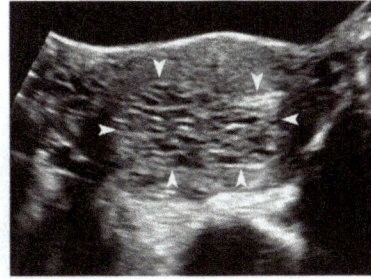

FIGURE 1: Complete hydatiform mole. Transverse transabdominal sonography (TAS) image of the uterus shows distension of the uterine cavity by echogenic material with numerous small, irregular cystic spaces within (arrowheads). The normal hypoechoic myometrium can be seen stretched at the periphery. There is no identifiable fetal tissue.

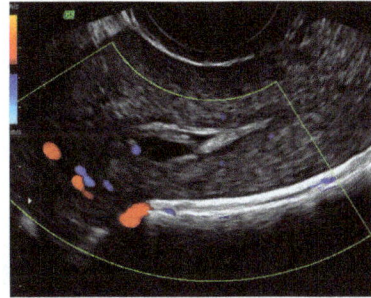

FIGURE 2: Complete mole in a patient with 8-week amenorrhoea resembling a blighted ovum. Sagittal transvaginal sonography (TVS) shows an anechoic empty gestational sac-like structure with thin echogenic lining and a size smaller than expected for the gestational age.

Differentiation of the complete and partial moles can be difficult but is of limited clinical significance, as the management is similar [6].

Although ultrasound is very useful for suggesting a molar pregnancy, final diagnosis still rests with the pathology [2]. Ultrasound finding of a heterogeneous endometrial mass is nonspecific and may also be seen in retained products of conception [2, 8]. Sometimes, it may appear as a large, central fluid collection, mimicking an anembryonic gestation or miscarriage (Figure 2) [1]. However, correlation with clinical features and β-hCG will be useful in making the distinction.

Ovaries may show theca lutein cysts due to hyperstimulation by high circulating gonadotropin levels in up to 40% of cases. The cysts are multilocular and usually bilateral. Rarely, these may hemorrhage or rupture leading to an acute abdomen. They usually resolve within a few months after treatment of the intrauterine process [1].

4.1.2. Ultrasonographic Features of Invasive Disease (GTN). Myometrial invasion is best appreciated on TVS due to superior demonstration of the interface between trophoblastic tissue and myometrium [2]. Invasive mole, choriocarcinoma, and PSTT are seen on grey-scale ultrasound as nonspecific focal masses (Figures 3(a)–3(f)) with myometrial epicenter

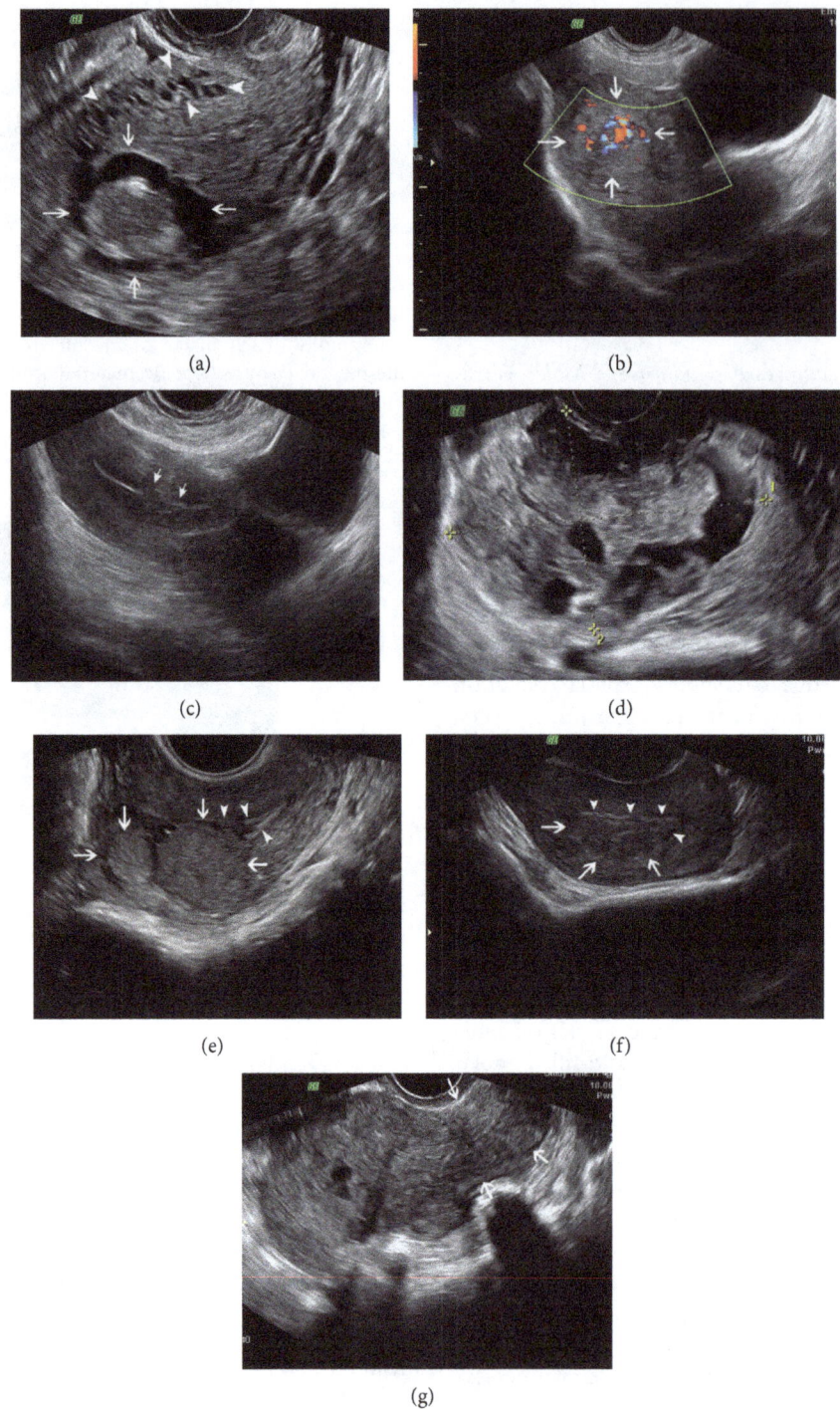

(a)

(b)

(c)

(d)

(e)

(f)

(g)

FIGURE 3: Sonographic spectrum of GTN. (a) Complex solid-cystic mass in the uterine fundus with myometrial epicenter (arrows) on sagittal TVS. Anechoic serpiginous structures in the adjoining myometrium represent increased vascularity (arrowheads). (b) Predominantly echogenic myometrial mass (arrows) effacing the zonal anatomy of uterus on Sagittal TAS. Color flow Doppler ultrasound reveals prominent vascularity in the lesion. (c) Small hypoechoic lesion (arrows) with irregular margins in the lower uterine body, disrupting the endometrial stripe and invading the adjoining myometrium on Sagittal TAS. (d) Ill-defined multicystic myometrial mass (between cursors) on transverse TVS. (e) Two round well-defined submucosal myometrial GTN lesions (arrows) with homogeneous isoechoic to hyperechoic echotexture, indenting the endometrial stripe (arrowheads) and partially effacing it on sagittal TVS, resembling submucosal fibroids. (f) An ovoid isoechoic mass with irregular margins (arrows) at endomyometrial interface on sagittal TVS simulating an adenomyoma or a submucosal fibroid. Arrowheads = endometrium (g) Enlarged uterus with a lobulated contour and heterogeneous echotexture on sagittal TVS. Arrows = cervix.

and are sonographically indistinguishable from one another. The mass may be echogenic, hypoechoic, complex, or multicystic. It may show anechoic spaces which represent hemorrhage, necrosis, cysts, or vascular spaces. More extensive disease may appear as a heterogeneously enlarged uterus with lobulated contour or large pelvic mass which may extend to involve other pelvic organs (Figure 3(g)) [12]. These masses may be potentially confused with fibroids or adenomyosis. Adenomyosis typically appears as a diffuse disease process causing enlarged uterus with a diffuse heterogeneous echo texture. It can also manifest as asymmetrical myometrial thickening, myometrial cysts, indistinct endometrial-myometrial junction, polyploid lesion, or focal mass within the myometrium with poorly defined margins that blend with the surrounding myometrium. Typical fibroid usually presents as a well-circumscribed hypoechoic myometrial lesion, although echogenicity may vary. The various ultrasound presentations of gestational trophoblastic neoplasia may overlap with these imaging findings of fibroids and adenomyosis. However, correlation with serum β-hCG levels, clinical history, and lack of extreme vascularity on Doppler sonography aid in their differentiation [12, 13].

Persistent trophoblastic neoplasia is presumed to be invasive mole unless there is presence of metastases to suggest choriocarcinoma. Since both invasive mole and choriocarcinoma are usually treated with chemotherapy, histological differentiation of the two types is not needed routinely [1]. With effective chemotherapy, the lesions usually become progressively smaller and hypoechoic on ultrasound [12]. However, differentiation of PSTT from invasive mole or choriocarcinoma is important because it is relatively chemoresistant and often requires hysterectomy for treatment [2, 6]. Although invasive mole, choriocarcinoma and PSTT are indistinguishable sonographically, the diagnosis of PSTT is strongly suggested when there are sonographic features of GTN with very low levels of β-hCG [6].

4.1.3. Role of Doppler Imaging. Color flow and spectral Doppler are routinely performed in addition to grey-scale ultrasound for diagnosis of the primary or recurrent GTD and posttreatment follow-up. In a normal pregnancy, first trimester Doppler study of the intrauterine arteries shows high resistance flow with low diastolic velocities except at the implantation site [2, 6]. The flow resistance reduces in the second and third trimesters with increasing physiological arterial invasion by trophoblastic tissue. In contrast, molar pregnancy shows high velocity, low impedance waveforms in the first and early second trimesters themselves due to high degree of arterial invasion by abnormally proliferating trophoblast. Arterio-venous shunts associated with neovascularization within the invasive myometrial mass result in an appearance of chaotic vasculature with color aliasing and loss of vascular discreteness on Color Doppler imaging (Figure 4). This extreme vascularity appears as high velocity and low impedance flow [2, 6, 12]. Vascular impedance can be quantified using indices derived from the uterine artery waveform known as pulsatility index (PI) and resistive index (RI). High resistance flow produces high PI and RI, and

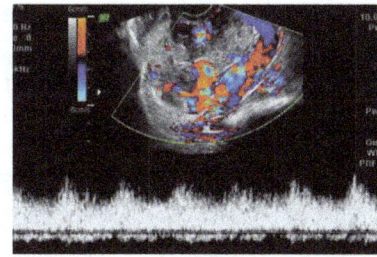

FIGURE 4: Color flow Doppler of the same patient as in Figure 3(d) reveals a mosaic pattern of color signal within the cystic spaces representing turbulent flow. Spectral analysis of the abnormal vasculature reveals high velocity low impedance pulsatile flow.

vice versa. Although there are no unanimously agreed cut-off values for these indices, an RI of less than 0.4 and a PI of less than 1.5 indicative of low uterine artery resistance have been observed in gestational trophoblastic neoplasia [2, 14, 15]. Doppler ultrasound can help determine presence of invasive disease by demonstrating extension of this abnormal vascularity into the myometrium [6].

These Doppler ultrasound features may also be seen due to any cause of increased pelvic blood flow such as retained products of conception, ectopic pregnancy, pelvic inflammation, nontrophoblastic pelvic malignancy, or uterine arterio-venous malformation [12]. Zhou et al. [14] observed lower resistive indices (RI) in invasive mole and choriocarcinoma than complete or partial hydatiform mole indicative of greater degree of vascular invasion in the first two.

PSTT may be hypovascular or hypervascular, with the former form being not associated with prominent vascularity on Doppler ultrasound [2, 12].

Studies by Long et al. [16] and Agarwal et al. [15] have suggested PI to be a potential surrogate marker to predict response of GTN to chemotherapy. Patients with low pulsatility index (PI) have been shown to be more likely to become chemoresistant to single drug therapy with methotrexate.

Recently published studies by Agarwal et al. [17] and Sita-Lumsden [18] have revalidated the usefulness of uterine artery PI (UAPI) as a predictor of methotrexate resistance (MTX-R) independent of Charing Cross Hospital and FIGO scores. The risk of MTX-R in patients with a FIGO score of 6 and UAPI was shown to be 100% versus 20% in patients with PI > 1 (χ^2 P < 0.0001) by Agarwal et al. Sita-Lumsden et al. showed that UAPI $\leq$ 1 predicted MTX-R independent of the FIGO score (hazard ratio 2.9, P = 0.04), with an absolute risk of MTX-R in women with a UAPI $\leq$ 1 of 67% (95% CI 53–79%) compared with 42% (95% CI 24–61%) with a UAPI > 1 (P = 0.036).

Doppler ultrasound also has a potential for following disease response to chemotherapy. Cystic vascular spaces in the myometrial mass of invasive disease show regression during successful chemotherapy. These changes follow decline in serum β-hCG levels [2, 6].

GTN is the commonest cause of uterine vascular malformations (arterio-venous shunts and pseudoaneurysms) and Doppler ultrasound can be a useful tool for demonstrating them (Figures 5 and 6) [2, 6, 19]. These vascular abnormalities

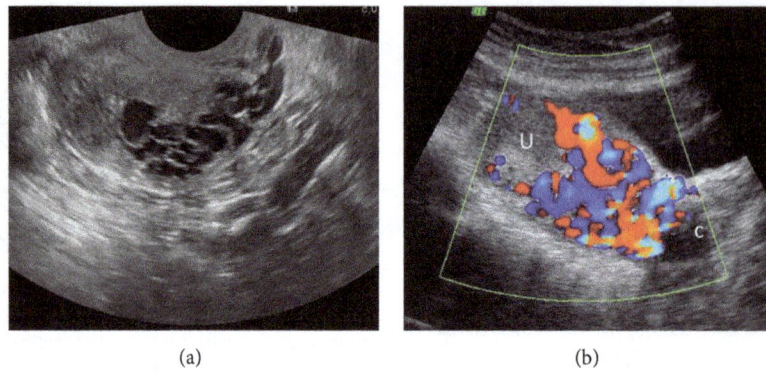

(a)   (b)

FIGURE 5: Uterine vascular malformation presenting with recurrent vaginal bleeding following successful treatment of invasive mole. Sagittal TVS image (a) of the uterus reveals multiple tortuous, serpiginous anechoic spaces in the myometrium. Color Doppler TAS (b) reveals a mosaic pattern of color signal within the spaces. U = uterus; C = cervix. No evidence of any myometrial mass is seen to suggest a residual GTN.

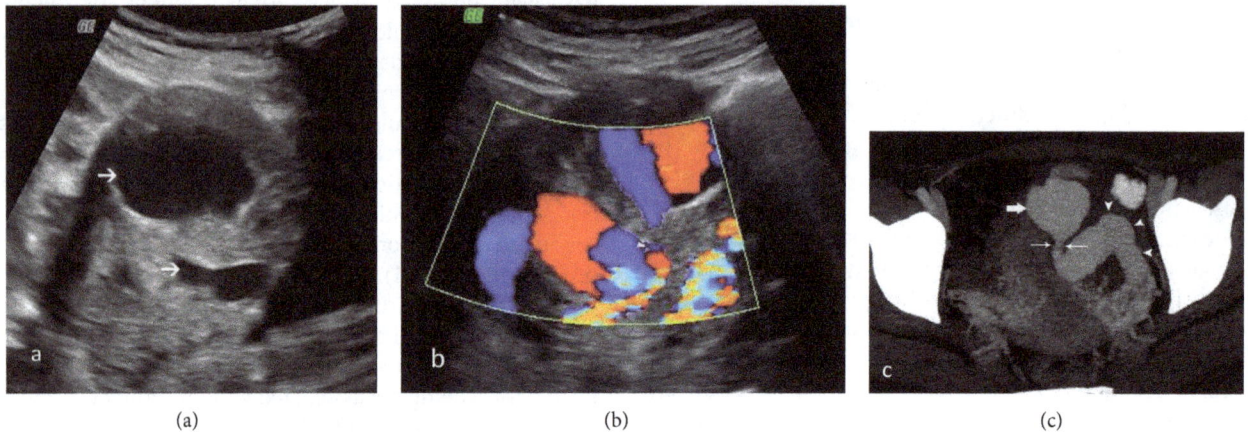

(a)   (b)   (c)

FIGURE 6: A 25-year-old patient presenting with episodic torrential vaginal bleeding, 3 months after completion of chemotherapy for choriocarcinoma. β-hCG levels were not raised. Grey-scale TAS (a) shows two large anechoic lesions in the myometrium (arrows). Color Doppler (b) demonstrates a whirled to-and-fro color flow in these cystic spaces. CT angiogram image (c) reveals a grossly dilated left uterine artery (arrowheads) with a saccular pseudoaneurysm (thick arrow) showing a narrow neck (thin arrows) arising from it and protruding into the adjoining myometrium.

may persist in up to 15% of cases following complete response to chemotherapy as a result of residual scarring. These are not considered to be significant if asymptomatic and associated with normal serum and urinary β-hCG levels. The abnormalities may regress spontaneously on follow-up imaging. However, rising β-hCG levels should prompt search for a recurrent GTN with whole-body imaging [2].

4.2. Computed Tomography (CT). CT is principally used for detection of metastatic disease (discussed in a later section). Uterine disease is seen as an enlarged uterus with focal irregular low attenuation lesions (Figure 7) on CT pelvis, which may also demonstrate bilateral ovarian enlargement with multiple theca lutein cysts. Parametrial disease spread is seen as enhancing tissue in this region (Figure 8) [2]. CT can also identify vascular malformations resulting from GTN (Figure 6(c)) [20].

4.3. Magnetic Resonance Imaging (MRI). MRI does not have a role in routine assessment of pelvic disease. It is sometimes used as a problem-solving tool to assess the depth of myometrial invasion and extrauterine disease spread in equivocal and complicated cases, suspected PSTT, and recurrent GTN [1, 2]. MRI appearance of molar pregnancy can be relatively nonspecific and difficult to distinguish from retained products of conception or ectopic pregnancy [21, 22]. First trimester MRI may reveal little or no abnormality. In the second trimester, hydatiform mole is visualized as a heterogeneously hyperintense tumor distorting the normal zonal architecture on T2-weighted images which may show numerous characteristic cystic spaces. It causes uterine enlargement and distension of the endometrial cavity with indistinct boundary between the endometrium and myometrium. On T1-weighted images, it is isointense or mildly hyperintense to the myometrium with areas of hemorrhage, seen as focal signal hyperintensity [23, 24].

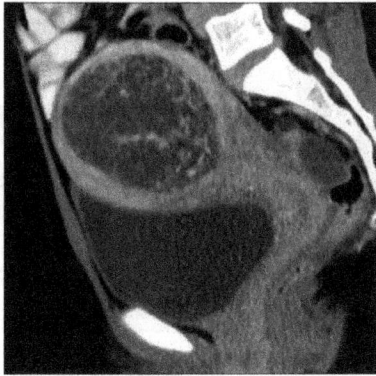

FIGURE 7: Sagittal reformation of contrast enhanced CT in a patient with complete hydatiform mole shows a large low attenuation, central uterine mass with intact surrounding myometrium.

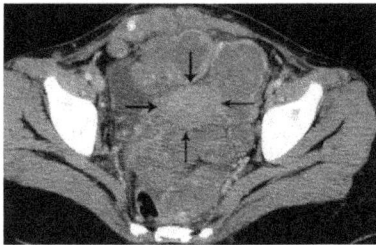

FIGURE 8: Choriocarcinoma in a 23-year-old patient who presented 2 years after a normal pregnancy with abdominal distension and markedly raised β-hCG levels. Axial contrast enhanced CT image of the pelvis reveals extensive, heterogeneously enhancing extrauterine tumor deposits in the pelvis involving pouch of Douglas, left parametrium, anterior peritoneum, and both recti (asterisk). Uterus is marked with black arrows.

Diffuse myometrial involvement by the tumor is seen as diffuse myometrial signal hyperintensity with obliteration of the normal zonal anatomy. Invasive GTN has similar signal characteristics however with a myometrial epicenter (Figure 9), invasion into parametrium (Figure 10), and more frequent hemorrhage and necrosis [23]. MRI is superior to ultrasound for identification of parametrial invasion, which is seen as heterogeneous T2 hyperintense masses beyond the confines of the uterus (Figure 10) [2, 25].

On contrast enhanced dynamic MRI, viable trophoblastic tissue with surrounding inflammatory response is seen as marked enhancement on early arterial phase [26]. Tumor hypervascularity is also seen as prominent tortuous flow voids in the tumor and adjoining myometrium, parametrium, and adnexae on both T1 and T2-weighted images with engorgement of internal iliac and arcuate vessels with respect to the external iliac artery (Figure 9) [24]. However, the hypovascular form of PSTT has been demonstrated to be hyperintense to myometrium on both T1- and T2-weighted images with absence of prominent vascularity or flow voids and poor enhancement on postcontrast images [2].

With successful treatment, uterine volume and tumor hypervascularity decrease with restoration of normal zonal

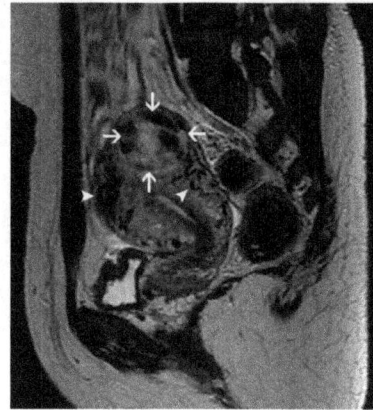

FIGURE 9: Sagittal T2-weighted MR image in a patient with invasive mole demonstrates a heterogeneous, hyperintense uterine mass in the fundus with a myometrial epicenter (arrows). Tortuous flow voids (arrowheads) consistent with vessels are seen in the adjoining myometrium, indicative of tumor hypervascularity.

anatomy on T2-weighted images and reduction of heterogeneous appearance (Figure 10). Intralesional hemorrhage may occur (Figure 10(c)). MRI findings usually normalize at 6–9 months following effective chemotherapy. Persistent uterine vascular malformations are seen as residual tortuous and coiled vessels within a thickened myometrium [2, 20, 24].

Bulky necrotic trophoblastic tissue in the uterine wall may serve as a nidus for infection and cause severe uterine sepsis. If untreated, GTN may penetrate into myometrium with resultant uterine perforation and serious intraperitoneal hemorrhage (Figure 11) [6].

4.4. Conventional Angiography. Although color Doppler ultrasound is the modality of choice for diagnosing uterine vascular malformations, angiography is the preferred method in patients who may potentially undergo embolization for management of the vascular malformations persisting despite complete response to chemotherapy and complicated by refractory, life threatening vaginal, or intraperitoneal hemorrhage (seen in only 2% of cases) [19, 27]. Traditionally, these cases have been managed surgically with uterine artery ligation or hysterectomy. However, selective uterine artery catheterization and embolization are a safe and effective alternative treatment with preservation of fertility in these patients of reproductive age group (Figure 12) [2, 6, 19, 27]. Therapeutic target is 80% or more reduction in the size of the malformation [27]. Repeated embolotherapy may be required for recurrent bleeding [6]. Chances of uterine infarction are low due to extensive pelvic collateralization [2]. Pain requiring opiate analgesia is a frequent complication of treatment [27].

Other indications for conventional angiography in GTN include selective embolization of isolated vaginal metastases and chemoembolization of hepatic metastases. Angiography characteristically demonstrates the hepatic metastasis as a hypervascular mass with aneurysmal dilatation of peripheral ends of hepatic arteries in the arterial phase and persistent vascular lakes in the venous phase [2].

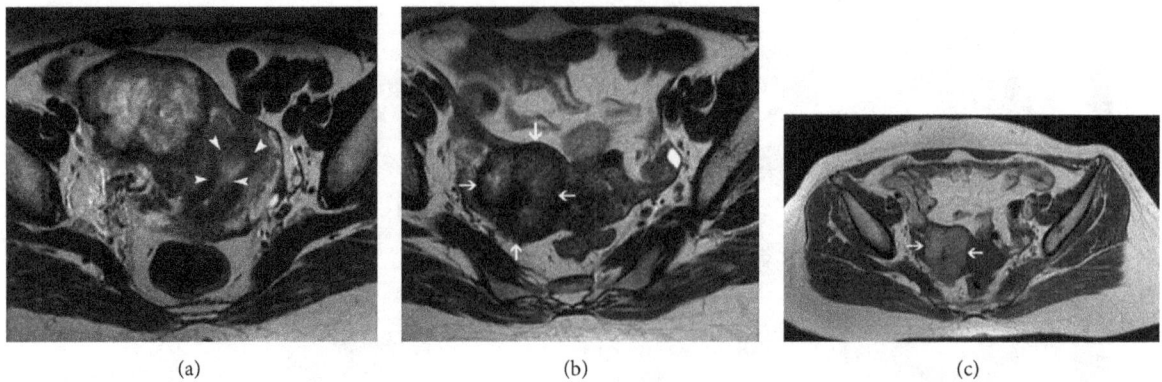

FIGURE 10: Choriocarcinoma in a 22-year-old patient with extremely raised β-hCG levels, 3 months after an abortion. Axial T2-weighted MR image (a) reveals a heterogeneous, hyperintense mass in the right lateral myometrium with parametrial extension. Note is made of a relatively preserved endometrial cavity (arrowheads). Postchemotherapy follow-up MRI ((b), (c)) demonstrates interval regression of the trophoblastic tumor (arrows) with reduction in its size, heterogeneity, and signal hyperintensity on T2-weighted image (b). Hyperintense signal of the lesion (arrows) on T1-weighted image (c) indicates intralesional hemorrhage, a known occurrence following chemotherapy.

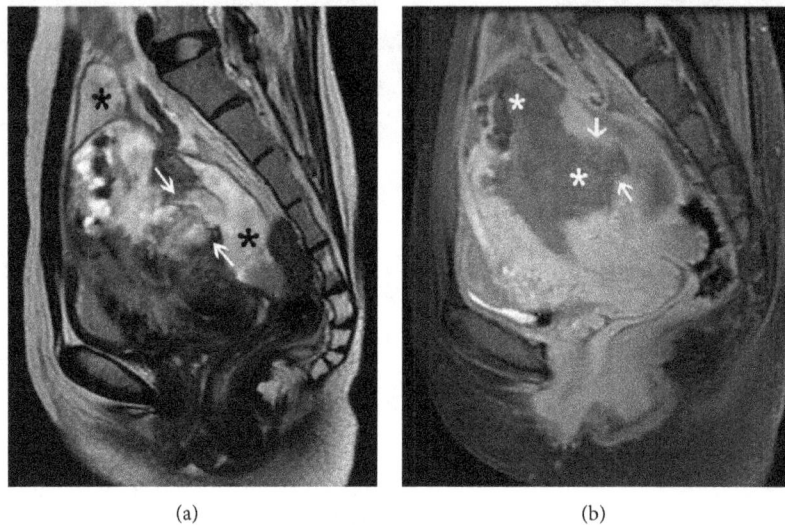

FIGURE 11: Bulky choriocarcinoma with myometrial rupture. Sagittal T2-weighted image (a) shows an ill-defined heterogeneous mass in the uterine fundus and posterior corpus with full thickness myometrial penetration (arrows) and associated fluid collection (black asterisk) around the uterus. Sagittal contrast-enhanced fat-suppressed T1-weighted MR image (b) demonstrates the mass to be completely necrotic with a large myometrial perforation showing focal continuity (arrows) with the collection in the pouch of Douglas.

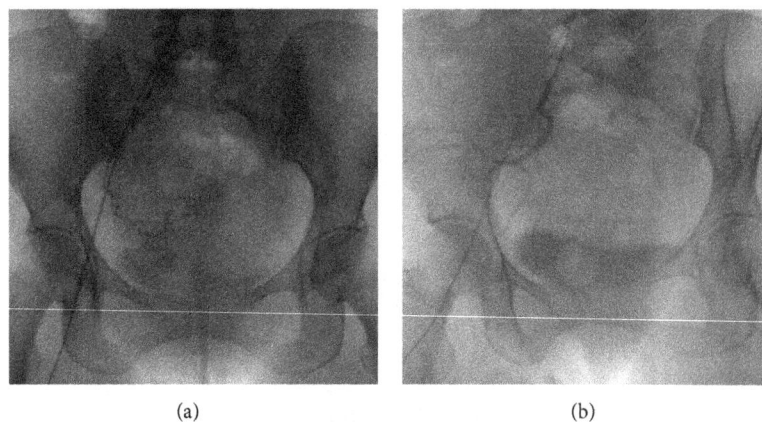

FIGURE 12: Conventional angiogram (a) in a 23-year-old nulliparous woman with GTN and recurrent massive intraperitoneal bleed showing a uterine vascular malformation on the right side. Selective right uterine artery catheterization was performed via right common iliac artery approach followed by embolization with polyvinyl alcohol gel foam. Postembolization angiogram (b) demonstrates complete obliteration of the vascular malformation.

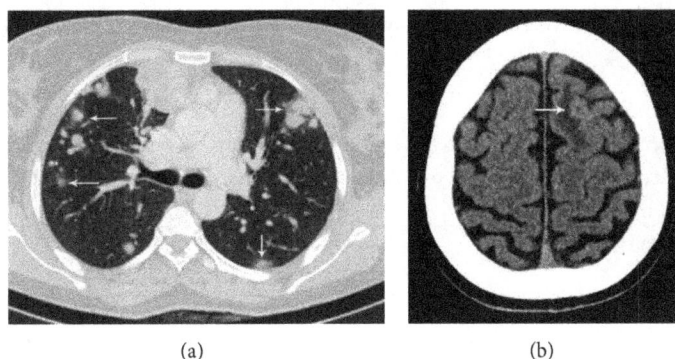

(a)   (b)

FIGURE 13: Choriocarcinoma with widespread metastases, presenting with seizures. CT chest (a) shows multiple metastatic lung nodules. Ground glass halo (arrows) around many of these nodules represents hemorrhage. Noncontrast CT brain (b) demonstrates a round, mildly hyperdense lesion (arrow) at gray-white matter junction in the left frontal lobe with surrounding vasogenic edema suggestive of hemorrhagic brain metastasis.

4.5. Metastatic Work-Up. CT scan is more sensitive than chest radiograph for diagnosing lung metastases. Parenchymal lung metastases are seen as multiple, rounded, soft tissue density lesions, usually up to 3 cm in size. The lesions may be solitary, miliary and may rarely show cavitation. A large amount of trophoblastic tissue embolized into the pulmonary vasculature may result in features of acute pulmonary artery hypertension. CT may demonstrate large intravascular tumor thrombus and resultant lung infarct. Both parenchymal and intravascular metastases may show hemorrhage due to their hypervascular nature, resulting in air space shadowing or ground glass opacity (Figure 13(a)). Less common endobronchial tumors may present with endobronchial obstruction. Pleural effusion may result from bleeding of lung nodules into pleural space [2].

Asymptomatic patients without lung metastases are unlikely to have brain metastases and do not require brain MRI or CT. However, patients with known lung or vaginal metastases are at significant risk of central nervous system involvement and should be screened with MRI or CT to exclude brain metastases [2, 9]. Brain metastases are usually multiple, located at grey-white matter junction, and associated with hemorrhage and surrounding edema. Due to hemorrhage, the lesions appear hyperdense on unenhanced CT (Figure 13(b)) and show variable signal intensity on MRI depending on the age of the intralesional hemorrhage. Owing to their hypervascular nature, the lesions usually enhance well [1, 2, 12].

Vaginal disease usually results from contiguous spread from the uterine lesion. Vaginal metastases are usually evaluated with MRI which demonstrates T2 hyperintense vaginal wall lesion with indistinct margins (Figure 14) [2, 24]. Isolated vaginal metastases may be effectively managed with selective embolization [2].

Liver metastases mark poor prognosis and occur later in the course of disease. Ultrasound screening of the liver may be carried out at the time of pelvic assessment. However, patients with known lung or vaginal metastases or high risk factors should be staged with CT abdomen. Liver metastases

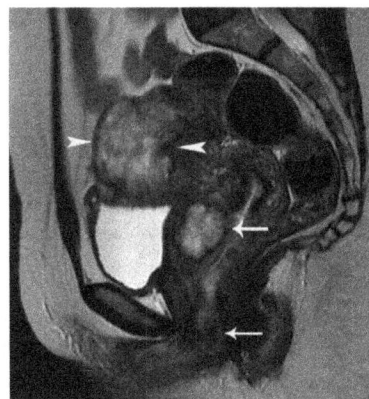

FIGURE 14: GTN with vaginal metastases. Sagittal T2-weighted MR image shows a lobulated heterogeneously hyperintense myometrial mass with ill-defined margins (arrowheads) and effacement of normal zonal anatomy of uterus. Two morphologically similar lesions (arrows) are seen in the vaginal wall consistent with metastases, which were missed on initial ultrasound.

are typically seen as multiple hypervascular lesions on both CT and MRI, showing avid contrast enhancement in the arterial phase and sometimes hemorrhagic transformation. These are indistinguishable from other hypervascular hepatic tumors on CT and should never be biopsied due to a risk of fatal hemorrhage [2].

Potential role of FDG PET (18-fluoro-deoxy-glucose positron emission tomography) and PET/CT in the evaluation of recurrent or metastatic disease is a topic of active interest. Preliminary studies suggest that FDG PET is potentially useful in providing precise mapping of metastases and tumour extent, monitoring treatment response, and detecting recurrent or residual disease after chemotherapy. It may be used as problem-solving tool in cases with diagnostic ambiguity on conventional imaging techniques and laboratory tests. However, careful evaluation in combination with other imaging modalities needs to be done to reduce the risk of false positive and negative results [28–33].

TABLE 1: (a) FIGO 2000 classification for GTN-staging system. (b) FIGO 2000 classification for GTN-risk scoring system.

(a)

Stage I	Disease confined to the uterus.
Stage II	GTN extends outside the uterus but is limited to the genital structures (adnexa, vagina, and broad ligament).
Stage III	GTN extends to the lungs, with or without known genital tract involvement.
Stage IV	All other metastatic sites.

Source: FIGO Oncology Committee (2003) [10].

(b)

Score	0	1	2	4
Age (years)	<40	≥40	—	—
Antecedent pregnancy	Mole	Abortion	Term	—
Interval months from index pregnancy	<4	4–<7	7–<13	≥13
Pretreatment serum β-hCG (iu/mL)	$<10^3$	$10^3 - <10^4$	$10^4 - <10^5$	$\geq 10^5$
Largest tumor size (cm) (including uterus)	<3	3–<5	≥5	—
Site of metastases	Lung	Spleen, kidney	Gastrointestinal	Liver, brain
Number of metastases	—	1–4	5–8	>8
Previous failed chemotherapy	—	—	Single drug	Two or more drugs

Source: FIGO Oncology Committee (2003) [10].

4.6. Staging and Classification of GTN with Impact on Management. Various staging systems and classifications based on morphology, anatomy, and clinical prognostic scoring of GTN are followed across the world. No single system has gained a universal acceptance. Treatment selection criteria are not uniform everywhere [34–45]. In order to address these issues, the International Society for the Study of Trophoblastic diseases, the International Gynecologic Cancer Society, and International Federation of Gynecology and Obstetrics (FIGO) recommended a new FIGO staging (Table 1(a)) and risk scoring system (Table 1(b)) for GTN after much deliberation and discussions. This is comprised of a combination of basic FIGO stages and simplified WHO scoring system which was adopted in 2000 [3, 9].

Chemotherapy is the mainstay of the management of invasive mole and choriocarcinoma due to exquisite chemosensitivity of most of these lesions, especially if detected early and classified correctly [1–3, 6]. It has been suggested that low risk groups (WHO score ≤ 6) should be managed with a single agent chemotherapy (methotrexate or actinomycin-D) to maximize the cure rates while minimizing toxicity [3, 9, 46–48]. The treatment of choice for high-risk group is combination chemotherapy. Currently, the most widely used combination is EMA-CO (etoposide, methotrexate, actinomycin-D, cyclophosphamide, and vincristine) [3, 9, 49, 50]. Appropriate management results in overall high cure rates (100% for low risk and 80–90% for high-risk group) [2, 9].

4.7. Posttreatment Follow-Up. After completion of chemotherapy and normalization of β-hCG levels, patients are followed up with serial β-hCG levels for one year, although follow-up protocols vary at different institutes [2, 9]. Contraception should be maintained during this period to optimize the chance of detecting a relapse, thus allowing prompt treatment, and to allow DNA repair or apoptosis of the developing ova, potentially damaged by the teratogenic effect of chemotherapy [2, 9]. Follow-up imaging after chemotherapy is performed in case of a rise in β-hCG levels to differentiate a normal gestation from disease relapse and to diagnose any complications. Vast majority of patients of GTN treated with chemotherapy can anticipate normal reproductive function [2, 9, 51–53]. Subsequent pregnancy should be evaluated with early ultrasound to confirm normality. β-hCG levels should be obtained at 6 and 12 weeks after the subsequent pregnancy [2, 9, 52] to exclude occult trophoblastic disease. Also, patients should be warned against possibility of an early menopause and risk of developing second tumors, such as acute myeloid leukemia (reported with etoposide) as an adverse effect of chemotherapy [9].

5. Conclusion

Radiologist plays a key role in the initial diagnosis of GTD and guiding disease management and early detection of its complications. Although serum β-hCG is a useful biochemical marker for GTD, it is not diagnostic when considered in isolation. Ultrasound is the first line radiological investigation in confirming the diagnosis of GTD in a case suspected on the basis of clinical findings and β-hCG levels. Ultrasound in combination with Doppler is also a useful tool for diagnosing invasive disease, assessing treatment response, and detecting local recurrence. MRI is invaluable to assess extrauterine disease spread and complications. Chest radiograph, brain MRI, and body CT are primarily used to rule out metastatic disease. Conventional angiography can be used to manage patients with heavy bleeding or for chemoembolization of hepatic metastases. PET/CT is fast emerging as a promising tool for disease mapping, monitoring treatment response, and identifying recurrent or residual disease after chemotherapy. Prudent use of these imaging techniques permits early diagnosis and appropriate management, contributing to excellent cure rates of the disease.

Conflict of Interests

The authors declared no conflict of interests.

References

[1] B. J. Wagner, P. J. Woodward, and G. E. Dickey, "From the archives of the AFIP. Gestational trophoblastic disease: radiologic-pathologic correlation," *Radiographics*, vol. 16, no. 1, pp. 131–148, 1996.

[2] S. D. Allen, A. K. Lim, M. J. Seckl, D. M. Blunt, and A. W. Mitchell, "Radiology of gestational trophoblastic neoplasia," *Clinical Radiology*, vol. 61, no. 4, pp. 301–313, 2006.

[3] B. W. Hancock, "Staging and classification of gestational trophoblastic disease," *Bailliere's Best Practice and Research in Clinical Obstetrics and Gynaecology*, vol. 17, no. 6, pp. 869–883, 2003.

[4] S. J. Kim, "Placental site trophoblastic tumour," *Bailliere's Best Practice and Research in Clinical Obstetrics and Gynaecology*, vol. 17, no. 6, pp. 969–984, 2003.

[5] K. M. Elsayes, A. T. Trout, A. M. Friedkin et al., "Imaging of the placenta: a multimodality pictorial review," *Radiographics*, vol. 29, no. 5, pp. 1371–1391, 2009.

[6] K. A. Jain, "Gestational trophoblastic disease: pictorial review," *Ultrasound Quarterly*, vol. 21, no. 4, pp. 245–253, 2005.

[7] C. M. Feltmate, D. R. Genest, L. Wise, M. R. Bernstein, D. P. Goldstein, and R. S. Berkowitz, "Placental site trophoblastic tumor: a 17-year experience at the New England Trophoblastic Disease Center," *Gynecologic Oncology*, vol. 82, no. 3, pp. 415–419, 2001.

[8] C. Betel, M. Atri, A. Arenson, M. Khalifa, R. Osborne, and G. Tomlinson, "Sonographic diagnosis of gestational trophoblastic disease and comparison with retained products of conception," *Journal of Ultrasound in Medicine*, vol. 25, no. 8, pp. 985–993, 2006.

[9] T. Y. Ng and L. C. Wong, "Diagnosis and management of gestational trophoblastic neoplasia," *Bailliere's Best Practice and Research in Clinical Obstetrics and Gynaecology*, vol. 17, no. 6, pp. 893–903, 2003.

[10] H. Ngan, H. Bender, J. L. Benedet et al., "Gestational trophoblastic neoplasia, FIGO 2000 staging and classification," *International Journal of Gynecology and Obstetrics*, vol. 83, supplement 1, pp. 175–177, 2003.

[11] A. K. P. Shanbhogue, N. Lalwani, and C. O. Menias, "Gestational trophoblastic disease," *Radiologic Clinics of North America*, vol. 51, no. 6, pp. 1023–1034, 2013.

[12] K. K. Kani, J. H. Lee, M. Dighe, M. Moshiri, O. Kolokythas, and T. Dubinsky, "Gestatational trophoblastic disease: multimodality imaging assessment with special emphasis on spectrum of abnormalities and value of imaging in staging and management of disease," *Current Problems in Diagnostic Radiology*, vol. 41, no. 1, pp. 1–10, 2012.

[13] S. Chopra, A. S. Lev-Toaff, F. Ors, and D. Bergin, "Adenomyosis: common and uncommon manifestations on sonography and magnetic resonance imaging," *Journal of Ultrasound in Medicine*, vol. 25, no. 5, pp. 617–627, 2006.

[14] Q. Zhou, X. Y. Lei, Q. Xie, and J. D. Cardoza, "Sonographic and Doppler imaging in the diagnosis and treatment of gestational trophoblastic disease: a 12-year experience," *Journal of Ultrasound in Medicine*, vol. 24, no. 1, pp. 15–24, 2005.

[15] R. Agarwal, S. Strickland, I. A. McNeish et al., "Doppler ultrasonography of the uterine artery and the response to chemotherapy in patients with gestational trophoblastic tumors," *Clinical Cancer Research*, vol. 8, no. 5, pp. 1142–1147, 2002.

[16] M. G. Long, J. E. Boultbee, R. Langley, E. S. Newlands, R. H. J. Begent, and K. D. Bagshawe, "Doppler assessment of the uterine circulation and the clinical behaviour of gestational trophoblastic tumours requiring chemotherapy," *British Journal of Cancer*, vol. 66, no. 5, pp. 883–887, 1992.

[17] R. Agarwal, V. Harding, D. Short et al., "Uterine artery pulsatility index: a predictor of methotrexate resistance in gestational trophoblastic neoplasia," *British Journal of Cancer*, vol. 106, no. 6, pp. 1089–1094, 2012.

[18] A. Sita-Lumsden, H. Medani, R. Fisher et al., "Uterine artery pulsatility index improves prediction of methotrexate resistance in women with gestational trophoblastic neoplasia with FIGO score 5-6," *BJOG*, vol. 120, no. 8, pp. 1012–1015, 2013.

[19] P. Polat, S. Suma, M. Kantarcý, F. Alper, and A. Levent, "Color Doppler US in the evaluation of uterine vascular abnormalities," *Radiographics*, vol. 22, no. 1, pp. 47–53, 2002.

[20] S. Umeoka, T. Koyama, K. Togashi, H. Kobayashi, and K. Akuta, "Vascular dilatation in the pelvis: Identification with CT and MR imaging," *Radiographics*, vol. 24, no. 1, pp. 193–208, 2004.

[21] J. W. Barton, S. M. McCarthy, E. I. Kohorn, L. M. Scoutt, and R. C. Lange, "Pelvic MR imaging findings in gestational trophoblastic disease, incomplete abortion, and ectopic pregnancy: are they specific?" *Radiology*, vol. 186, no. 1, pp. 163–168, 1993.

[22] E. I. Kohorn, S. M. McCarthy, and J. W. Barton, "Is magnetic resonance imaging a useful aid in confirming the diagnosis of nonmetastatic gestational trophoblastic neoplasia?" *International Journal of Gynecological Cancer*, vol. 6, no. 2, pp. 128–134, 1996.

[23] M. Nagayama, Y. Watanabe, A. Okumura, Y. Amoh, S. Nakashita, and Y. Dodo, "Fast MR imaging in obstetrics," *Radiographics*, vol. 22, no. 3, pp. 563–580, 2002.

[24] H. Hricak, B. E. Demas, C. A. Braga, M. R. Fisher, and M. L. Winkler, "Gestational trophoblastic neoplasm of the uterus: MR assessment," *Radiology*, vol. 161, no. 1, pp. 11–16, 1986.

[25] A. K. P. Lim, D. Patel, N. Patel et al., "Pelvic imaging in gestational trophoblastic neoplasia," *Journal of Reproductive Medicine for the Obstetrician and Gynecologist*, vol. 53, no. 8, pp. 575–578, 2008.

[26] Y. Yamashita, M. Torashima, M. Takahashi et al., "Contrast-enhanced dynamic MR imaging of postmolar gestational trophoblastic disease," *Acta Radiologica*, vol. 36, no. 2, pp. 188–192, 1995.

[27] A. K. P. Lim, R. Agarwal, M. J. Seckl, E. S. Newlands, N. K. Barrett, and A. W. M. Mitchell, "Embolization of bleeding residual uterine vascular malformations in patients with treated gestational trophoblastic tumors," *Radiology*, vol. 222, no. 3, pp. 640–644, 2002.

[28] P. Mapelli, G. Mangili, M. Picchio et al., "Role of 18F-FDG PET in the management of gestational trophoblastic neoplasia," *European Journal of Nuclear Medicine and Molecular Imaging*, vol. 40, no. 4, pp. 505–513, 2013.

[29] R. Cortés-Charry, L. M. Figueira, L. Nieves, and L. Colmenter, "Metastasis detection with 18 FDG-positron emission tomography/computed tomography in gestational trophoblastic neoplasia: a report of 2 cases," *Journal of Reproductive Medicine*, vol. 51, no. 11, pp. 897–901, 2006.

[30] T. C. Chang, T. C. Yen, Y. T. Li et al., "The role of ^{18}F-fluoro-deoxyglucose positron emission tomography in gestational trophoblastic tumours: a pilot study," *European Journal of Nuclear Medicine and Molecular Imaging*, vol. 33, no. 2, pp. 156–163, 2006.

[31] T. Dhillon, C. Palmieri, and N. J. Sebire, "Value of whole body 18FDG-PET to identify the active site of gestational trophoblastic neoplasia," *Journal of Reproductive Medicine*, vol. 51, no. 11, pp. 879–887, Nov 2006.

[32] I. Ak and S. Özalp, "Prognostic relevance of F-18 fluorodeoxyglucose positron emission tomography and computed tomography in molar pregnancy before evacuation," *Journal of Reproductive Medicine for the Obstetrician and Gynecologist*, vol. 54, no. 7, pp. 441–446, 2009.

[33] H. Zhuang, A. J. Yamamoto, N. Ghesani, and A. Alavi, "Detection of choriocarcinoma in the lung by FDG positron emission tomography," *Clinical Nuclear Medicine*, vol. 26, no. 8, article 723, 2001.

[34] N. Ishizuka, J. W. Brewer, M. M. Hreshchyshyn et al., "Choriocarcinoma," in *Transactions of a Conference of the International Union against Cancer*, J. F. Holland and M. M. Hreshchyshyn, Eds., vol. 3 of *UICC Monograph Series*, Appendix 1, Springer, Berlin, Germany, 1967.

[35] Registration Committee for Trophoblastic Disease of the Japan Society of Obstetrics and Gynaecology, "Report of the registration committee for trophoblastic disease," *Acta Obstetricia et Gynaecologica Japonica*, vol. 34, pp. 1805–1812, 1982.

[36] H. C. Song, P. C. Wu, M. Y. Tong, and Y. O. Wang, "Clinical staging," in *Trophoblastic Tumours Diagnosis and Treatment People's Health*, pp. 128–129, 1981.

[37] D. B. Smith, L. Holden, E. S. Newlands, and K. D. Bagshawe, "Correlation between clinical staging (FIGO) and prognostic groups with gestational trophoblastic disease," *British Journal of Obstetrics and Gynaecology*, vol. 100, no. 2, pp. 157–160, 1993.

[38] G. T. Ross, D. P. Goldstein, R. Hertz, M. B. Lipsett, and W. D. Odell, "Sequential use of methotrexate and actinomycin D in the treatment of metastatic choriocarcinoma and related trophoblastic diseases in women," *The American Journal of Obstetrics and Gynecology*, vol. 93, no. 2, pp. 223–229, 1965.

[39] C. B. Hammond, L. G. Borchert, L. Tyrey, W. T. Creasman, and R. T. Parker, "Treatment of metastatic trophoblastic disease: good and poor prognosis," *American Journal of Obstetrics & Gynecology*, vol. 115, no. 4, pp. 451–457, 1973.

[40] H. E. Dijkema, J. G. Aalders, H. W. A. de Bruijn, R. N. Laurini, and P. H. B. Willemse, "Risk factors in gestational trophoblastic disease, and consequences for primary treatment," *European Journal of Obstetrics and Gynecology and Reproductive Biology*, vol. 22, no. 3, pp. 145–152, 1986.

[41] K. D. Bagshawe, "Risk and prognostic factors in trophoblastic neoplasia," *Cancer*, vol. 38, no. 3, pp. 1373–1385, 1976.

[42] World Health Organization, "Gestational trophoblastic disease," WHO Technical Report Senes 692, WHO, Geneva, Switzerland, 1983.

[43] E. S. Newlands, "Investigation and treatment of persistent trophoblastic disease and gestational trophoblastic tumours in the UK," in *Gestational Trophoblastic Disease*, B. W. Hancock, E. S. Newlands, and R. S. Berkowitz, Eds., pp. 173–190, Chapman & Hall, London, UK, 1997.

[44] FIGO Oncology Committee Report, "FIGO news," *International Journal of Gynecology & Obstetrics*, vol. 39, no. 2, pp. 149–150, 1992.

[45] L. H. Sobin and C. Wittekind, *TNM Classification of Malignant Tumours*, Wiley-Liss, New York, NY, USA, 1997.

[46] J. R. Lurain and E. P. Elfstrand, "Single-agent methotrexate chemotherapy for the treatment of nonmetastatic gestational trophoblastic tumors," *The American Journal of Obstetrics and Gynecology*, vol. 172, no. 2, pp. 574–579, 1995.

[47] J. P. Roberts and J. R. Lurain, "Treatment of low-risk metastatic gestational trophoblastic tumors with single-agent chemotherapy," *American Journal of Obstetrics and Gynecology*, vol. 174, no. 6, pp. 1917–1924, 1996.

[48] J. T. Soper, D. L. Clarke-Pearson, A. Berchuck, G. Rodriguez, and C. B. Hammond, "5-Day methotrexate for women with metastatic gestational trophoblastic disease," *Gynecologic Oncology*, vol. 54, no. 1, pp. 76–79, 1994.

[49] M. Bower, E. S. Newlands, L. Holden et al., "EMA/CO for high-risk gestational trophoblastic tumors: results from a cohort of 272 patients," *Journal of Clinical Oncology*, vol. 15, no. 7, pp. 2636–2643, 1997.

[50] S. J. Kim, S. N. Bae, J. H. Kim et al., "Effects of multiagent chemotherapy and independent risk factors in the treatment of high-risk GTT—25 years experiences of KRI-TRD," *International Journal of Gynecology and Obstetrics*, vol. 60, no. 1, pp. S85–S96, 1998.

[51] R. P. Woolas, M. Bower, E. S. Newlands, M. Seckl, D. Short, and L. Holden, "Influence of chemotherapy for gestational trophoblastic disease on subsequent pregnancy outcome," *British Journal of Obstetrics and Gynaecology*, vol. 105, no. 9, pp. 1032–1035, 1998.

[52] R. S. Berkowitz, D. P. Goldstein, M. R. Bernstein, and B. Sablinska, "Subsequent pregnancy outcome in patients with molar pregnancy and gestational trophoblastic tumors," *Journal of Reproductive Medicine for the Obstetrician and Gynecologist*, vol. 32, no. 9, pp. 680–684, 1987.

[53] J. T. Soper, "Gestational trophoblastic disease," *Obstetrics & Gynecology*, vol. 108, no. 1, pp. 176–187, 2006.

10

Evaluation of Contrast Extravasation as a Diagnostic Criterion in the Evaluation of Arthroscopically Proven HAGL/pHAGL Lesions

Catherine Maldjian,[1] Vineet Khanna,[1] James Bradley,[2] and Richard Adam[1]

[1] *Department of Radiology, University of Pittsburgh, Pittsburgh, PA 15213-2582, USA*
[2] *Department of Orthopedic Surgery, UPMC, Pittsburgh, PA 15213-2582, USA*

Correspondence should be addressed to Catherine Maldjian; cmaldjian@gmail.com

Academic Editor: Ali Guermazi

Purpose. The validity of preoperative MRI in diagnosing HAGL lesions is debated. Various investigations have produced mixed results with regard to the utility of MRI. The purpose of this investigation is to apply a novel method of diagnosing HAGL/pHAGL lesions by looking at contrast extravasation and to evaluate the reliability of such extravasation of contrast into an extra-articular space as a sign of HAGL/pHAGL lesion. *Methods.* We utilized specific criteria to define contrast extravasation. We evaluated these criteria in 12 patients with arthroscopically proven HAGL/pHAGL lesion. We also evaluated these criteria in a control group. *Results.* Contrast extravasation occurred in over 83% of arthroscopically positive cases. Contrast extravasation as a diagnostic criterion in the evaluation of HAGL/pHAGL lesions demonstrated a high interobserver degree of agreement. *Conclusions.* In conclusion, extra-articular contrast extravasation may serve as a valid and reliable sign of HAGL and pHAGL lesions, provided stringent criteria are maintained to assure that the contrast lies in an extra-articular location. In cases where extravasation is not present, the "J" sign, though nonspecific, may be the only evidence of subtle HAGL and pHAGL lesions. *Level of Evidence.* Level IV, Retrospective Case-Control series.

1. Introduction

Current knowledge is mixed with regard to the reliability of MRI for diagnosing HAGL/pHAGL lesions. Specific findings on MRI that have been discussed previously include direct identification of the disrupted ligament, contrast extravasation medial to the humerus, and the "J" sign. This investigation looks at areas of contrast extravasation into anatomical spaces not previously studied, such as the quadrilateral space and intra/paramuscular spaces. This greatly enhanced the diagnostic capability of MRI. While contrast extravasation medial to the humerus has previously been elucidated, this is the first study to prescribe rigorous MRI criteria in order to differentiate true extravasation of contrast from a low-lying axillary pouch or "J" sign. While the "J" sign is not specific for HAGL/pHAGL, it was the only finding in 2 patients in our HAGL/pHAGL cohort, and it may be the only finding in subtle cases. This constitutes the largest series of arthroscopically proven HAGL lesions reported thus far. This is also the only series that evaluates interobserver variability for diagnosing HAGL/pHAGL by MRI criteria and the only study that evaluates a cohort of control patients for comparison to validate the use of an MRI sign of HAGL/pHAGL lesion. Our hypothesis is that extra-articular contrast extravasation will serve as a reliable diagnostic marker in the detection of HAGL/pHAGL lesions.

2. Methods

This study was performed retrospectively with internal institutional review board approval. Informed consent by the IRB was waived since this was a retrospective study. A list of exams performed during a seven-year period was extracted from the institutional database conforming to the following criteria: arthroscopically proven HAGL lesion with preoperative MRI.

12 cases were retrieved that satisfied these criteria. 11 of these studies were performed as MR arthrograms. One was performed as a nonarthrographic, conventional MRI. A control cohort of 23 patients was retrieved from the institutional database over a one-year period that had MR arthrogram and in addition had available arthroscopic data confirming that there was no evidence of HAGL or pHAGL. Arthrographic technique was performed with an anterior approach, instilling 12 mL of highly diluted gadolinium based contrast (0.1 mL/20 mL or 5 parts per 10,000). The mixture contained 10 mL of saline, 5 cc of iodinated contrast (Isovue 300, (iopamidol)), 5 cc of 1% lidocaine, and 0.1 mL of gadobenate dimeglumine (Multihance, Bracco Diagnostics, Princeton, NJ). MRI exams were all performed on 1.5 Tesla units. Examinations were performed supine using a dedicated shoulder coil. Standard oblique sagittal T1 and fat saturated axial and oblique coronal T1 weighted pulse sequences were obtained. Fat suppressed T2 weighted acquisitions in all 3 imaging planes were also obtained in all arthrographic cases. In the one nonarthrographic case, axial PD, oblique coronal PD and fat suppressed T2, and oblique sagittal T1 and fat suppressed T2 imaging was performed. The images were evaluated retrospectively, independently by 2 fellowship trained musculoskeletal radiologists, each with over 10 years of experience, for extravasation of contrast into an extra-articular space. Criteria for extravasation would normally include any space that does not communicate with the joint; however, we excluded bursal spaces in our analysis, such as the subdeltoid/subacromial bursa and subcoracoid bursa, which would have other clinical ramifications, and we ensured that none of the cases demonstrated overdistension of the joint where anterior leakage could obfuscate the diagnosis of true pathological extravasation. Criteria for extravasation included visualization of contrast in intramuscular spaces, inter/paramuscular spaces, the quadrilateral space, and the juxta-diaphyseal region along the humeral shaft. Extravasation into the latter space was defined more rigorously than on prior studies and consisted of contrast extending along the medial humeral shaft beyond the field of view, such that no pouch like structure maintaining the contrast was present in the field of view. This was done intentionally in order to explicitly differentiate such extravasation from the "J" sign as well as from possible overdistension, both of which preserve an axillary pouch structure. In the one patient with a nonarthrographic exam, joint fluid extending off the field of view constituted criteria for juxtahumeral leakage. Fluid in the quadrilateral space was designated as positive criteria for "extravasation," since this is not normally seen after trauma. Intramuscular or paramuscular edema, on the other hand, can be seen after trauma; therefore "extravasation" for this parameter in the nonarthrographic case was defined as intra- or paramuscular fluid confluent with and communicating with joint fluid. The presence or absence of extravasation was recorded for each reader and compared for agreement. The location of extravasation(s) was also specified independently by each reader.

After independent analysis of all 12 cases by 2 fellowship trained musculoskeletal radiologists, any disagreement between the 2 readers was resolved by consensus between both readers as a final analysis. We also evaluated for the presence of a "J" sign, which we defined as a low-lying axillary pouch. Since there is no method to quantify this in the current literature, we adhered to a qualitative analysis. Devising a method to quantify a low-lying axillary pouch with which we define the "J" sign would be beyond the scope of this paper, which seeks to address the usefulness of contrast extravasation for diagnosing IGL ruptures. Furthermore, this sign is very nonspecific as there are several etiologies for ligamentous laxity and stretching other than IGL tear, including injury without frank tear, and theoretically connective tissue disorders such as Marfan syndrome and Ehlers-Danlos syndrome, and idiopathic or genetic hypermobility. No correlative gold standard on arthroscopy exists with which we gauge the accuracy of a hypothetical quantitative measurement made on MRI to differentiate between these possibilities.

3. Results

The age range for the patient population with HAGL/pHAGL injuries was 15–44. The mean age was 21.5. There were 6 males and 6 females. 8 of the lesions were right-sided and 4 were left-sided. At arthroscopy 7 HAGL lesions and 4 pHAGL were identified and one patient's shoulder exhibited both HAGL and pHAGL. 10 patients demonstrated extra-articular extravasation in at least one space according to both readers and 2 patients did not, with 100% agreement between both readers as to general extravasation in at least one space (Tables 1 and 2). Therefore the diagnosis of ligament rupture based on extravasation was achieved with excellent interobserver reliability with Kappa = 1. Further analysis of the discrete locations of extravasation demonstrated complete agreement for all except for one instance of quadrilateral space extravasation, with interobserver reliability by kappa statistics of 1 for juxtahumeral extravasation, kappa statistic of 1 for intramuscular extravasation, kappa statistic of 1 for paramuscular extravasation, and kappa statistic of 0.883 for the quadrilateral space. The one case of discordant readings involved extravasation into the quadrilateral space in the one nonarthrographic case (Table 2). The correct diagnosis of ligament rupture was achieved by both readers in this case due to the concomitant presence of juxta-diaphyseal leakage. Reanalysis of this case by consensus resulted in a final agreement of extravasation of fluid into the QL space. Juxta-diaphyseal contrast was seen in 2 cases and juxta-diaphyseal fluid communicating with the joint was seen in the one nonarthrographic case where it was deemed the equivalent of extravasation, yielding a total of 3 cases of juxta-diaphyseal leakage (Figure 1).

Paramuscular/intramuscular extravasation was seen in 3 patients (Figure 2). All three patients had pHAGL. 2 demonstrated teres minor muscle extravasation, one with and one without intermuscular involvement between the teres minor and infraspinatus. The 3rd patient demonstrated leakage anterior to the subscapularis, remote from the typical location of extravasation through the anterior capsule from overdistension of the joint. Quadrilateral space extravasation was identified in 7 instances with one of these being the nonarthrographic study where the presence of fluid in the quadrilateral space was deemed the equivalent of contrast by one

TABLE 1: Cohort group (all patients arthroscopically proven HAGL tears).

Age	Gender	Laterality of IGL	Anterior or posterior HAGL	Extravasation to any site		Juxtahumeral space		Quadrilateral space		Paramuscular space		Intramuscular space	
				Reader 1	Reader 2	Reader 1	Reader 2	Reader 1	Reader 2	Reader 1	Reader 2	Reader 1	Reader 2
44	Female	Right	Anterior	Yes	Yes	No	No	Yes	Yes	No	No	No	No
16	Female	Left	Anterior	No	No	No	No	No	No	No	No	No	No
32	Female	Right	Anterior and Posterior	Yes	Yes	No	No	Yes	Yes	No	No	No	No
21	Male	Left	Anterior	Yes	Yes	No	No	Yes	Yes	No	No	No	No
15	Female	Right	Anterior	Yes	Yes	Yes	Yes	Yes	Yes	No	No	No	No
19	Male	Left	Posterior*	Yes	Yes	No	No	No	No	Yes (IS-TM)	Yes (IS-TM)	Yes (TM)	Yes (TM)
21	Male	Left	Posterior*	Yes	Yes	Yes	Yes	No	No	No	No	Yes (TM)	Yes (TM)
21	Male	Right	Anterior*	Yes	Yes	No	No	No	No	No	No	No	No
16	Female	Right	Anterior*	Yes	Yes	No	No	Yes	Yes	No	No	No	No
18	Male	Right	Posterior	Yes	Yes	Yes	Yes	Yes	Yes	Yes (Ant SS)	Yes (Ant SS)	No	No
21	Male	Right	Anterior*	Yes	Yes	No	No	No	Yes	No	No	No	No
15	Female	Right	Posterior	No	No	No	No	No	No	No	No	No	No

TM = Teres minor.
IS-TM = Paramuscular space between infraspinatus and teres minor.
Ant SS = Paramuscular space anterior to subscapularis.
* = Torn ligament was directly visualized on MR arthrogram also.
Sensitivity of extravasation to any site in detecting HAGL lesions: 83%.

TABLE 2: To measure the agreement between reader 1 and reader 2 in interpreting extravasation to any site, and to a particular site, kappa statistic was used, with excellent agreement between readers amongst all sites of extravasation. Excellent agreement was defined as Kappa > 0.81 [1].

	Extravasation to any site	Juxtahumeral space	Quadrilateral space	Paramuscular space	Intramuscular space
Kappa (reader 1, reader 2)	1	1	0.833	1	1

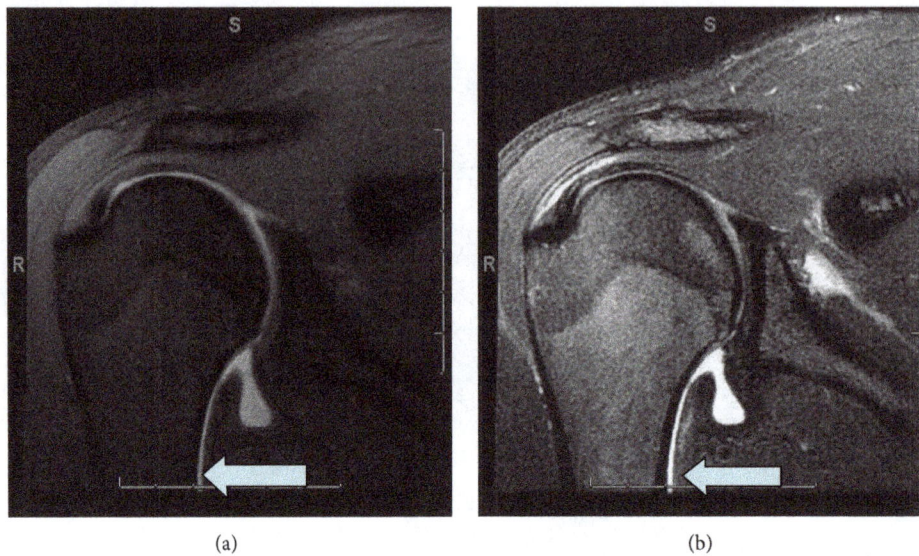

(a)   (b)

FIGURE 1: Case 8. Oblique coronal T1 and T2 demonstrating contrast/fluid extending along the medial humerus and off the field of view (arrow), consistent with extra-articular extravasation.

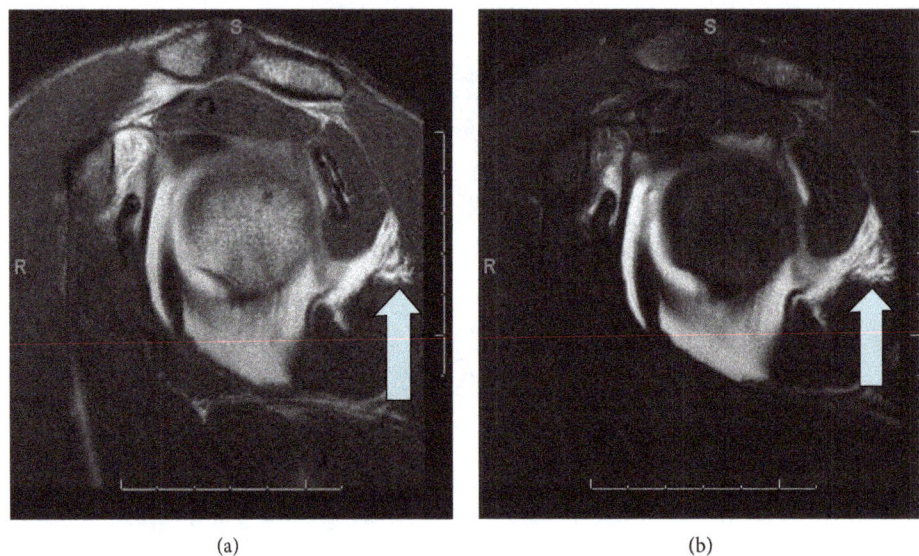

(a)   (b)

FIGURE 2: Case 6. Oblique sagittal T1 and T2 demonstrate contrast/fluid extravasating between muscle fibers of teres minor (arrow).

reader and subsequently by consensus by both readers (Figure 3). One of the 4 patients with pHAGL exhibited this finding. 5 of the 7 patients with HAGL exhibited this finding. The sole patient with both pHAGL and HAGL also exhibited this finding. Of the three locations (juxta-diaphyseal, para/intermuscular, and quadrilateral space) there was more

than one location involved in any given patient in 3 patients of the 10 that showed extravasation, or 30%, and in 3 of the total patients with HAGL/pHAGL or 25%. If the spaces are further subdivided into juxta-diaphyseal, paramuscular, intermuscular, and quadrilateral space, more than one location of extravasation were seen in 4 of 10 patients with

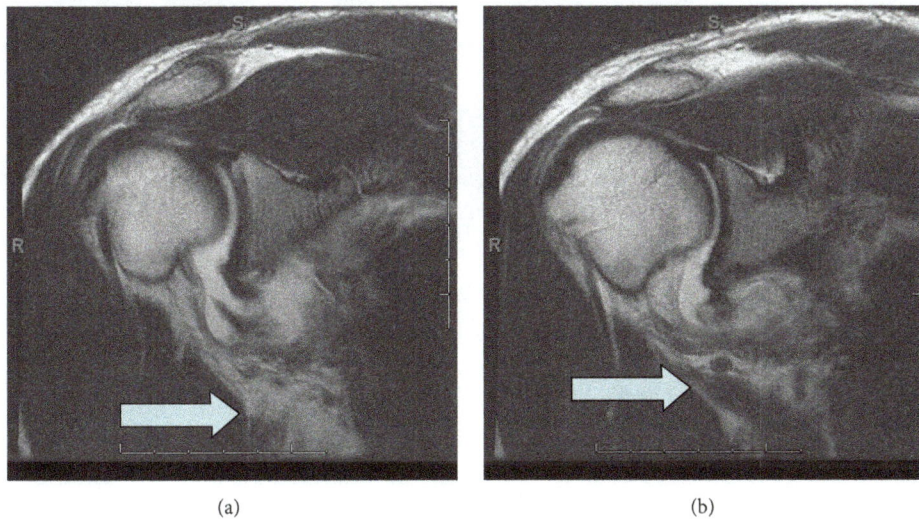

FIGURE 3: Case 11. Oblique coronal T2 demonstrates joint fluid extending into quadrilateral space (arrow).

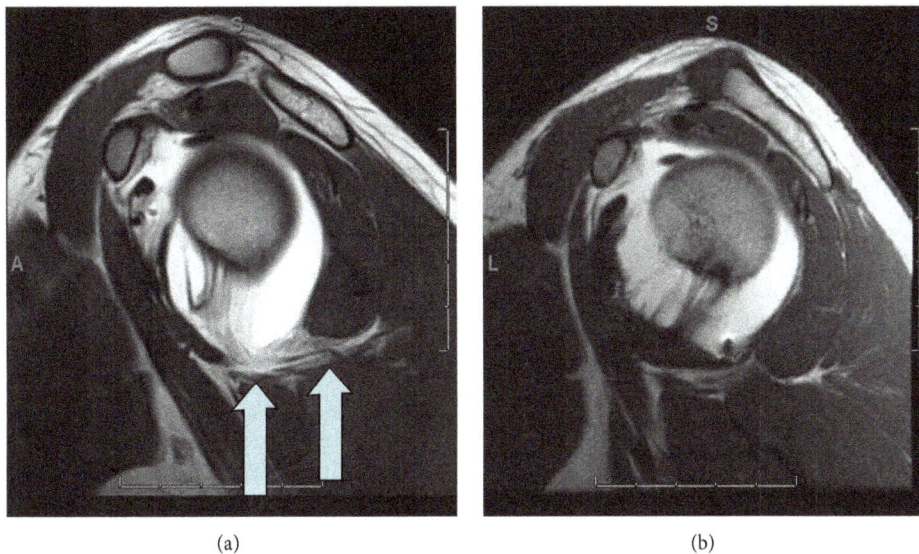

FIGURE 4: Case 9. Oblique sagittal T1 before and after HAGL repair: (a) prerepair shows contrast/fluid in quadrilateral space. (b) shows no extra-articular extravasation 2 years after repair. The intermuscular distance between the teres major and teres minor is increased on (a) (arrows) with an apparent gap at the axillary pouch in this area, which is no longer seen after repair.

extravasation (40%) and in 4 of the total cohort of patients with HAGL/pHAGL or 33%. The most common site of extravasation overall was in the quadrilateral space, where it occurred in 7 of 10 patients who demonstrated extravasation or 70% and in 7 of the 12 patients with HAGL and/or pHAGL lesions or 58% (Figure 4). 3 of these also showed additional site of leakage, one in an inter/paramuscular space (anterior to the subscapularis) (Figure 5) and two in a juxta-diaphyseal location. Juxta-diaphyseal leakage occurred in 3 patients, two being in conjunction with quadrilateral space involvement and one occurring as an isolated finding. In all three patients, arthroscopy identified HAGL lesions. None of the patients with pHAGL exhibited this finding. There were 3 cases of

para- or intramuscular involvement. As stated above, one of these 3 cases occurred in conjunction with quadrilateral space leakage. The other 2 cases were isolated findings, both demonstrating teres minor muscle infiltration.

Correlation with the initial MRI reports at the time of the exams revealed that the diagnosis of HAGL/pHAGL was originally missed in 4 of the 12 cases. On retrospective review all 4 cases demonstrated extravasation and/or "J" sign. 2 of these had isolated "J" sign (Figure 6). 2 of these had a "J" sign in conjunction with quadrilateral space involvement.

Overall detection based on leakage of contrast/fluid was 10 out of the 12 patients or 83%. Direct visualization of a ruptured ligament was seen in 5 of the 12 patients with HAGL or

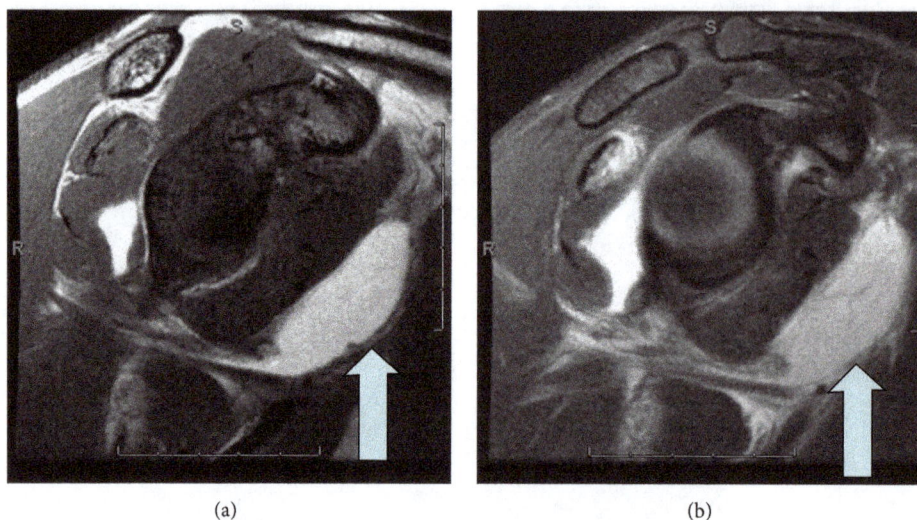

(a)

(b)

FIGURE 5: Case 10. Oblique sagittal T1 and T2 demonstrate contrast/fluid in the quadrilateral space and extending anterior to the subscapularis muscle (arrow).

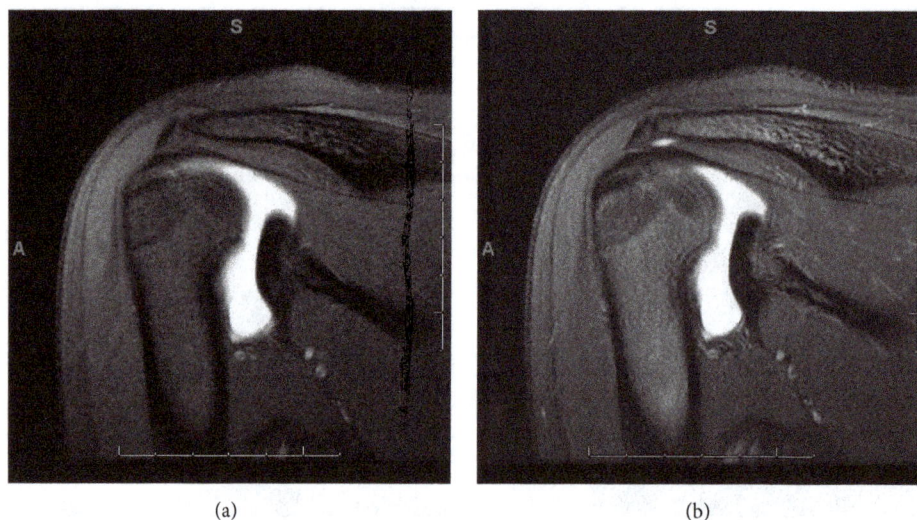

(a)

(b)

FIGURE 6: Case 12. HAGL not identified on initial report. Oblique coronal T1 fat saturated and oblique coronal T2 fat saturated images demonstrate J sign of MR arthrogram. No other findings were seen.

pHAGL or 42% (Figure 7) and all of these cases demonstrated some form of extra-articular contrast extravasation. Therefore detection based on extra-articular contrast extravasation proved to be a superior method in comparison to the direct sign of ligament tear.

4. Control Cohort

The age range of the control population was 17 to 79. The mean age of the control population was 37.5. There were 10 females and 13 males. There were 12 right and 11 left shoulders evaluated. Results of MR arthrography analysis for both readers demonstrated no extravasation into the spaces designated for this study in the control population patients. There was 100% agreement between readers (Table 3).

5. Discussion

The IGL is the main anterior stabilizer of the shoulder at 90 degrees of abduction and external rotation and has an important role for glenohumeral joint stability [2]. Humeral avulsion of the inferior glenohumeral ligament was originally described by Nicola in 1942 [3]. HAGL contribute to anterior instability in less than 10% of cases [4, 5]. Nonetheless, they are important to recognize as they are accompanied by additional arthroscopic abnormalities in most cases [6]. Knowledge of a potential HAGL lesion prior to arthroscopy may be useful for preoperative planning and treatment [6]. If these lesions are not recognized and addressed when coexisting with other causes of instability, treatment of the other causes alone may result in unremitting instability [6]. Several

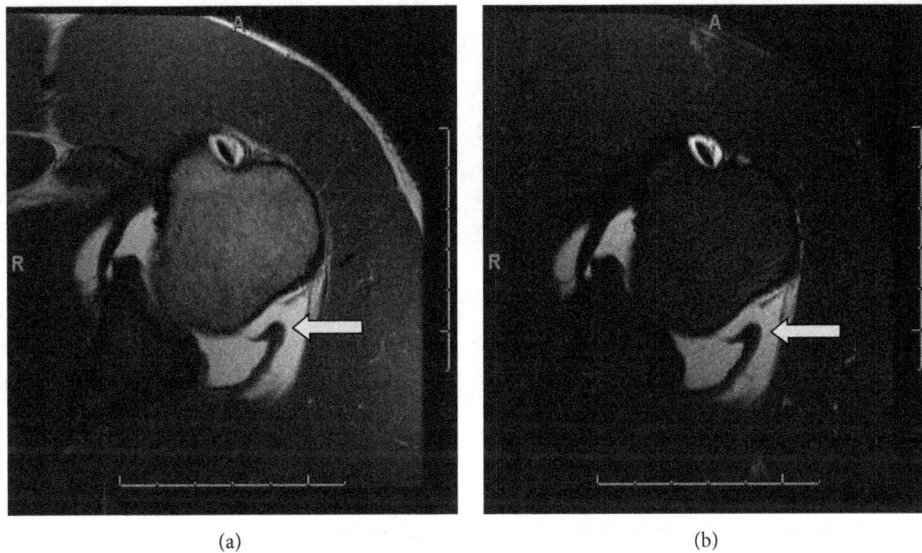

(a)   (b)

FIGURE 7: Case 7. Axial T1 and fat saturated T2 images demonstrate posterior band of IGL with thickening and retraction of ligament (arrow) and contrast on both intra- and extra-articular sides of the ligament.

TABLE 3: Control group (all patients arthroscopically negative for HAGL tear).

Age	Gender	Laterality of IGL tear	Extravasation to any site	
			Reader 1	Reader 2
20	Female	Right	No	No
35	Female	Right	No	No
20	Female	Right	No	No
39	Male	Right	No	No
41	Male	Right	No	No
57	Female	Right	No	No
63	Female	Right	No	No
79	Female	Left	No	No
46	Male	Left	No	No
42	Male	Left	No	No
55	Female	Left	No	No
44	Male	Left	No	No
18	Male	Left	No	No
47	Female	Left	No	No
19	Female	Right	No	No
41	Male	Right	No	No
18	Male	Left	No	No
17	Male	Left	No	No
46	Female	Left	No	No
20	Male	Right	No	No
36	Male	Right	No	No
42	Male	Right	No	No
18	Male	Right	No	No

investigators have expounded on imaging findings of HAGL lesions. Bone avulsion from the medial aspect of the humeral neck has been described as a radiographic finding [7]. This is reported to occur in 20% of cases [8]. Therefore, radiography is not sufficiently sensitive for diagnosing these lesions. Findings on MRI include extravasation of contrast through the defect, extravasation along the medial humeral shaft, [8, 9] and the J sign. The "J" sign refers to the appearance of the axillary pouch. When avulsion occurs in HAGL/pHAGL the detached end of the IGL falls inferiorly and converts the axillary pouch from its usual "U" shape to a "J" shaped morphology [8, 9].

The reliability of MRI to establish the diagnosis of HAGL varies widely from study to study. This apparent wide divergence in the reported reliability of MRI for diagnosing HAGL lesions was the impetus for our study.

The largest MRI study to date describes posterior HAGL lesions in 17 pts, 8 of which had arthroscopic confirmation [10]. Criteria for positive cases on MRI were detachment of the ligament with or without abnormal distribution of contrast along the humeral shaft based on coronal and sagittal images. All 8 lesions that had arthroscopy were confirmed [10]. Their study did not evaluate patterns of contrast extravasation in the 8 arthroscopically proven cases. In addition, the MR images were read by 2 radiologists in consensus, so that interobserver reliability is not established. No control cohort was utilized in their study to test for validity. Bui-Mansfield et al. reported on 4 patients with arthroscopy and MRI data, with 2 of the 4 positive cases being missed on MRI [8]. In addition, false positive MRIs were reported by these investigators. The MRI exams were not reported as MR arthrograms; therefore it is assumed that they were performed without intra-articular contrast. Castagna et al. reported on 9 de novo arthroscopically proven posterior HAGL lesions, with inclusion criteria consisting of no history of prior shoulder surgery [11]. Despite 77% of their patients undergoing MRI (7/9), pHAGL lesion was not detected on any of the preoperative MRI exams. All 7 of these MRIs were performed as MR arthrograms. None of the MRIs were diagnosed as pHAGL preoperatively. Interestingly, the authors reported that on retrospective review 6 of the 7 MRIs demonstrated findings consistent with pHAGL. No MRI criteria were stated for establishing the diagnosis of pHAGL lesions for the initial interpretation or for the retrospective review, but once the diagnosis was known arthroscopically, the findings became apparent in retrospective review. Therefore, it would seem that the diagnosis is attainable; however the criteria for achieving the proper diagnosis need to be better elucidated.

Melvin et al. reported on 4 cases which were deemed HAGL lesions on MRI but arthroscopically did not have HAGL [12]. 3 of the 4 MRI were performed as MR arthrograms and these 3 had capsular rents on arthroscopy. These authors state that the diagnosis of HAGL lesions should be reserved for arthroscopy. While certain familiar MRI criteria were utilized in that study, the application of these criteria was somewhat lax. In one illustration the authors use contrast alongside the medial humeral neck as a false positive diagnosis for HAGL. In that case the contrast appears to be suspended by an irregular pouch and is not free flowing down the humeral diaphysis and off the field of view. The investigators found a hole in the IGL on arthroscopy but no HAGL lesion with those imaging findings. We applied more stringent criteria for our definition of extra-articular extravasation of contrast along the humeral shaft in which we required the contrast to be free flowing off the field of view with no discernible pouch like structure maintaining the contrast, thereby assuring that the ligament was torn. In 2 additional cases those investigators state that the MRI demonstrates a tear of the IGL where both these images demonstrate low signal strands of tissue in the axillary pouch. One of these 2 cases had a posterior capsular rent without a HAGL lesion. One of the cases depicted what appeared to be a J sign. The finding of "disruption" of the ligament was unreliable in that study for diagnosing HAGL. Part of the problem is that the criteria for ligamentous disruption are not clearly defined and can be subjective. Relying solely on the appearance of what one believes is the ligament is problematic because non-HAGL capsular injuries may be difficult to differentiate from ligamentous tears on MRI.

In our study, we amassed arthroscopically proven cases of HAGL lesions, the largest such series to date. We applied specific criteria to these cases, placing our emphasis on extravasation of contrast into extra-articular spaces as a novel method to ensure that the ligament is truly disrupted. This is the first study to test interobserver reliability of an MR sign of HAGL/pHAGL injury.

When we embarked upon this study, we sought signs that would be more straightforward than the current methods for diagnosing IGL injuries. Contrast extravasation would be one such clearly definable, easily discernible, objective, and reproducible method of doing so. It is therefore not surprising that our study showed excellent interobserver variability, establishing this as a reliable method. The fact that no extravasation was seen in any of the control patients establishes validity of using contrast extravasation as a sign of HAGL or pHAGL injury and justifies this novel approach. No prior investigation has tested the reliability or validity of any

MRI sign of HAGL/pHAGL lesions. Extravasation of contrast into anatomical spaces such as the quadrilateral and intra/paramuscular spaces has not been previously investigated for HAGL/pHAGL lesions. Furthermore, classical findings in anatomical spaces that have been previously described were classified more rigorously than on prior studies. Extension along the humeral diaphysis was deemed extra-articular extravasation only if it extended inferiorly beyond the field of view such that no pouch like structure could be seen restricting the free flow of contrast. Persistence of a low-lying pouch like structure was designated as a "J" sign and was classified as a separate and distinct finding from extravasation.

On the original MRI reports, 8 of the 12 cases were correctly diagnosed. Using our criteria for extravasation into an extra-articular anatomical space, 10 of the 12 cases could be diagnosed correctly. Extravasation of contrast into the QL space enabled us to detect 2 cases retrospectively that were missed on the original readings. These 2 cases also demonstrated a "J" sign. In the one case where contrast was not injected, both readers arrived at the correct diagnosis of HAGL lesion due to contrast extravasation along the humeral shaft; however there was initial discordance as to whether contrast extended into the quadrilateral space which was resolved on reanalysis. We hypothesize that had this been performed as an MR arthrogram, the presence of contrast would have been readily discerned and the initial discrepancy would have been avoided. Because there was fluid along the humeral shaft and extending off the field of view, the case was correctly diagnosed as HAGL, demonstrating the diagnostic utility of extravasation, which exploits the multiplicity of spaces through which fluid/contrast can escape the joint. In 2 cases, no extra-articular contrast was discerned in our study. Both of these cases showed the "J" sign. While the "J" sign is not diagnostic, it may be the only manifestation of such injuries and therefore should not be dismissed, particularly in the proper clinical setting.

Juxta-diaphyseal extravasation was seen only in patients with HAGL, intramuscular or paramuscular extravasation occurred only in patients with pHAGL, and QL space leakage could be seen in patients with HAGL or pHAGL lesions. While this data might suggest a propensity for leakage in certain sites for specific types of IGL injuries, we advise caution against drawing such conclusions based on this small cohort of 12 patients.

Only 5 of our 12 cases, or 42%, clearly depicted a disrupted ligament. Ideally one might expect disruption of the humeral attachment of the IGL to be diagnostic for HAGL/pHAGL on MRI; yet studies have given rise to mixed data with regard to the reliability of this finding in and of itself. This may be because investigators are using different diagnostic criteria for disruption of the ligament or because differentiation of the ligament from a portion of the capsule can be problematic. In the most recent MRI study of HAGL lesions this finding came under attack as it gave rise to false positives in both cases where it was invoked [12]. We propose a method for diagnosing HAGL lesions based on extra-articular dissemination of contrast. This analysis may be more straightforward and reproducible than attempting to differentiate a capsular rent from ligament avulsion. We further subdivided these extra-articular spaces into para/intramuscular spaces, the quadrilateral space, or the juxta-diaphyseal space with extension beyond the field of view. We excluded spaces such as the subdeltoid/subacromial bursa and subcoracoid bursa, which would have other clinical ramifications. These criteria for contrast extravasation proved to be sensitive for HAGL and one or more were observed in 83% (10 of 12) of cases.

6. Limitations

Limitations to this study include a relatively small cohort group of 12 patients, limiting the statistical power of our conclusions. While interobserver interpretation was studied between two musculoskeletal radiologists, a larger study could include a greater number of musculoskeletal radiologists and measure interobserver variability amongst this larger group. Other proposed ideas in a larger study could also include both musculoskeletal and nonmusculoskeletal radiologists to assess differences in interobserver variability between these two groups.

7. Conclusion

In conclusion, our study examined extra-articular extravasation as a method for diagnosing HAGL/pHAGL lesions. Using this analysis the positive detection rate in a cohort of arthroscopically proven HAGL/pHAGL was 83% (10 of 12). Interobserver reliability was excellent. In cases where extravasation is not present, the "J" sign, though nonspecific, may be the only evidence of subtle HAGL and pHAGL lesions.

Conflict of Interests

The authors declare that there is no conflict of interests regarding the publication of this paper.

References

[1] J. R. Landis and G. G. Koch, "The measurement of observer agreement for categorical data," *Biometrics*, vol. 33, no. 1, pp. 159–174, 1977.

[2] L. D. Field, D. J. Bokor, and F. H. Savoie III, "Humeral and glenoid detachment of the anterior inferior glenohumeral ligament: a cause of anterior shoulder instability," *Journal of Shoulder and Elbow Surgery*, vol. 6, no. 1, pp. 6–10, 1997.

[3] T. Nicola, "Anterior dislocation of the shoulder: the role of the articular capsule," *Journal of Bone & Joint Surgery*, vol. 25, pp. 614–616, 1942.

[4] D. J. Bokor, V. B. Conboy, and C. Olson, "Anterior instability of the glenohumeral joint with humeral avulsion of the glenohumeral ligament," *The Journal of Bone and Joint Surgery, British*, vol. 81, no. 1, pp. 93–96, 1999.

[5] E. M. Wolf, J. C. Cheng, and K. Dickson, "Humeral avulsion of glenohumeral ligaments as a cause of anterior shoulder instability," *Arthroscopy*, vol. 11, no. 5, pp. 600–607, 1995.

[6] L. T. Bui-Mansfield, K. P. Banks, and D. C. Taylor, "Humeral avulsion of the glenohumeral ligaments: the HAGL lesion," *The American Journal of Sports Medicine*, vol. 35, no. 11, pp. 1960–1966, 2007.

[7] B. R. Bach, R. F. Warren, and J. Fronek, "Disruption of the lateral capsule of the shoulder. A cause of recurrent dislocation," *Journal of Bone and Joint Surgery, British*, vol. 70, no. 2, pp. 274–276, 1988.

[8] L. T. Bui-Mansfield, D. C. Taylor, J. M. Uhorchak, and J. J. Tenuta, "Humeral avulsions of the glenohumeral ligament: imaging features and a review of the literature," *American Journal of Roentgenology*, vol. 179, no. 3, pp. 649–655, 2002.

[9] D. W. Stoller, "MR arthrography of the glenohumeral joint," *Radiologic Clinics of North America*, vol. 35, no. 1, pp. 97–116, 1997.

[10] C. B. Chung, S. Sorenson, J. R. Dwek, and D. Resnick, "Humeral avulsion of the posterior band of the inferior glenohumeral ligament: MR arthrography and clinical correlation in 17 patients," *American Journal of Roentgenology*, vol. 183, no. 2, pp. 355–359, 2004.

[11] A. Castagna, S. J. Snyder, M. Conti, M. Borroni, G. Massazza, and R. Garofalo, "Posterior humeral avulsion of the glenohumeral ligament: a clinical review of 9 cases," *Arthroscopy*, vol. 23, no. 8, pp. 809–815, 2007.

[12] J. S. Melvin, J. D. MacKenzie, E. Nacke, B. J. Sennett, and L. Wells, "MRI of HAGL lesions: four arthroscopically confirmed cases of false-positive diagnosis," *The American Journal of Roentgenology*, vol. 191, no. 3, pp. 730–734, 2008.

11

^{18}F-Fluorodeoxyglucose Positron Emission Tomography/Computed Tomography Accuracy in the Staging of Non-Small Cell Lung Cancer

Nieves Gómez León,[1] **Sofía Escalona,**[2] **Beatriz Bandrés,**[1] **Cristobal Belda,**[3] **Daniel Callejo,**[2] **and Juan Antonio Blasco**[2,4]

[1] Department of Radiology, Research Institute La Princesa, La Princesa University Hospital, C/Diego de León 62, 28006 Madrid, Spain
[2] Health Technology Assessment Unit, Lain Entralgo Agency, C/Gran Vía 27, 28013 Madrid, Spain
[3] National School of Health, Sinesio Delgado 4, 28029 Madrid, Spain
[4] Institute for Health and Consumer Protection, Joint Research Centre, European Commission, Via E. Fermi 2749, 21027 Ispra, Italy

Correspondence should be addressed to Nieves Gómez León; ngomezl@salud.madrid.org

Academic Editor: Paul Sijens

Aim of the performed clinical study was to compare the accuracy and cost-effectiveness of PET/CT in the staging of non-small cell lung cancer (NSCLC). *Material and Methods.* Cross-sectional and prospective study including 103 patients with histologically confirmed NSCLC. All patients were examined using PET/CT with intravenous contrast medium. Those with disease stage ≤IIB underwent surgery (n = 40). Disease stage was confirmed based on histology results, which were compared with those of PET/CT and positron emission tomography (PET) and computed tomography (CT) separately. 63 patients classified with ≥IIIA disease stage by PET/CT did not undergo surgery. The cost-effectiveness of PET/CT for disease classification was examined using a decision tree analysis. *Results.* Compared with histology, the accuracy of PET/CT for disease staging has a positive predictive value of 80%, a negative predictive value of 95%, a sensitivity of 94%, and a specificity of 82%. For PET alone, these values are 53%, 66%, 60%, and 50%, whereas for CT alone they are 68%, 86%, 76%, and 72%, respectively. Incremental cost-effectiveness of PET/CT over CT alone was €17,412 quality-adjusted life-year (QALY). *Conclusion.* In our clinical study, PET/CT using intravenous contrast medium was an accurate and cost-effective method for staging of patients with NSCLC.

1. Introduction

Lung cancer is the most common fatal neoplasm in developed countries. Non-small cell lung cancer (NSCLC) is responsible for 80% of all deaths from this neoplasm [1]. Despite all efforts to improve early diagnosis, survival rates remain very low (about 18% at 5 years) [2]. The stage at which NSCLC is detected is the most important of all prognostic factors and the only one that determined treatment options in our study before targeted therapy was administered. The TNM classification of malignant tumors [3] for staging NSCLC is internationally accepted and validated.

CT is currently the most commonly used technique in tumor staging. However, results, which are based on normal lymph node size, have limited value. In contrast, PET provides valuable functional information because it can detect metabolically active tumor cells.

Over the last 10 years, PET has become an important tool for staging lung cancer, given its high sensitivity in the detection of lymph node involvement and distant metastasis [4] and its current use in presurgical stratification of NSCLC [5]. The combination of CT and PET makes it possible to visualize anatomical and metabolic images together, thus minimising the limitations and maximising the benefits of each technique individually.

The aims of the present study were as follows: (1) to compare the accuracy of PET/CT and of PET and CT alone for staging NSCLC, with histological examination as the gold standard; and (2) to determine the cost-effectiveness of PET/CT in staging of NSCLC.

2. Material and Methods

2.1. Patient Sample. This prospective study involved 103 patients with a clinical and histological diagnosis of NSCLC (confirmed by fine-needle aspiration and biopsy of the tumor) whose disease stage was not known and who had not yet received treatment.

All patients gave their written informed consent to participate in the study in accordance with the regulations of the institutional review board.

The patients' medical histories were examined before decisions on treatment were taken. Demographic data, histological diagnosis, and clinical status were recorded, and all patients underwent PET/CT.

2.2. PET/CT Protocol. All images were acquired with a combined in-line PET/CT system (Discovery LS; GE Healthcare, Milwaukee, Wisconsin, USA) that integrates a 4-detector row spiral CT (LightSpeed Plus; GE Healthcare) with a PET scanner (Advance NXi; GE Healthcare).

A standard dose of 370 MBq of ^{18}F-FDG was intravenously injected 45–60 minutes before imaging. Scanning was performed from the base of the skull to the midthigh while patients were in the supine position. To obtain a precise anatomic correlation between PET and CT images, whole-body scanning was performed with the arms in the upright position for both PET and CT.

Diagnostic contrast-enhanced CT was initially performed at 140 KV and with automatic current adjustment (maximum, 300 mA) according to the patient's weight.

A volume of 140 mL of iodinated contrast agent (iobitridol[Xenetix 300], 300 mg of iodine per milliliter; Guerbet) was first administered intravenously at 3 mL/s using an automated injector (model XD 5500; Ulrich Medical Systems). PET emission scanning was performed immediately after CT, with an identical transverse field of view and in the caudocranial direction.

Coregistered scans were displayed using Entegra or Xeleris software (GE Healthcare).

2.3. Interpretation of Isolated PET Images. A specialist in nuclear medicine interpreted PET images. Abnormal ^{18}F-FDG uptake was defined as accumulation outside the normal anatomic structures and of greater intensity than background activity inside the normal structures. Any visual focus of ^{18}F-FDG uptake over that of the background was deemed to represent tumor tissue.

The uptake of the radiotracer was also assessed semiquantitatively using the standardized uptake value (SUV) method.

However, the SUV is also limited in that it is affected by many factors, including blood sugar level, body weight, time elapsed since administration of the radiotracer, and the size and heterogeneity of the area of interest. Most authors, therefore, agree with visual interpretation of the results,

although an SUV higher than 2.5/3 is considered pathological [14]. Currently, we apply the recommendations described by the Dutch F18-FDG-PET standard (NEDPAS). A conclusion was recorded for each patient in agreement with the TNM classification system.

2.4. Interpretation of Isolated CT Images. CT images were interpreted by a radiologist. Lymph nodes with a shorter axis >10 mm were deemed positive. Chest lymph nodes were located according to the criteria of the American Thoracic Society [15].

2.5. Interpretation of Combined PET and CT Images. PET/CT images were assessed by the nuclear medicine specialist and radiologist working as a team. Lymph nodes were considered diseased when they showed pathological ^{18}F-FDG activity, irrespective of their size. Those showing no such activity were considered disease-free. The patient was considered to have extranodal disease when ^{18}F-FDG activity in the tumor was greater than that of the background organ and the SUV was higher than 2.5/3.

2.6. Classification of Disease by PET/CT, CT, and PET. Disease stage was assigned according to the PET/CT results and to the PET and CT results taken separately following the criteria of the 7th edition of the TNM system [3].

Patients were then classified as candidates for surgery (stage ≤IIB) or for other treatments (≥IIIA).

2.7. Classification of Disease by Histological Examination. All primary lung tumors of the 103 patients were studied histologically, either by bronchoscopy or CT-guided fine needle aspiration.

A histological evaluation was performed for the tumor samples of all 103 patients (43 patients with adenocarcinoma, 29 with large-cell carcinoma, and 31 with epidermoid carcinoma). Of these patients, only 40 were candidates for surgery.

2.8. Gold Standard Reference. Mediastinoscopy was carried out during surgery, and each node or lesion was histologically confirmed. If the stage was IIIB and/or IV, the gold standard was also the histological confirmation in samples taken using biopsy, CT-guided PAAF, and/or fibrobronchoscopy, as in the case of surgical patients. Mediastinal nodes were not studied when the result had no impact on treatment decisions. Endoscopic ultrasound (EUS) and endobronchial ultrasound (EBUS) are used to reach mediastinal nodes. EUS involves upper gastrointestinal endoscopy and enables visualization and sampling of the posterior mediastinal nodes. A similar ultrasound system is used in bronchoscopy, with which most of the mediastinal nodes are accessible. However, at the time our patients were recruited these techniques were not available at our hospital. A 5-year clinical follow-up revealed that no stage IIIB and IV patients survived.

In cases with suspicion of adrenal metastasis, other tests (e.g., magnetic resonance imaging) were performed and biopsy specimens were taken. All suspicious lesions in

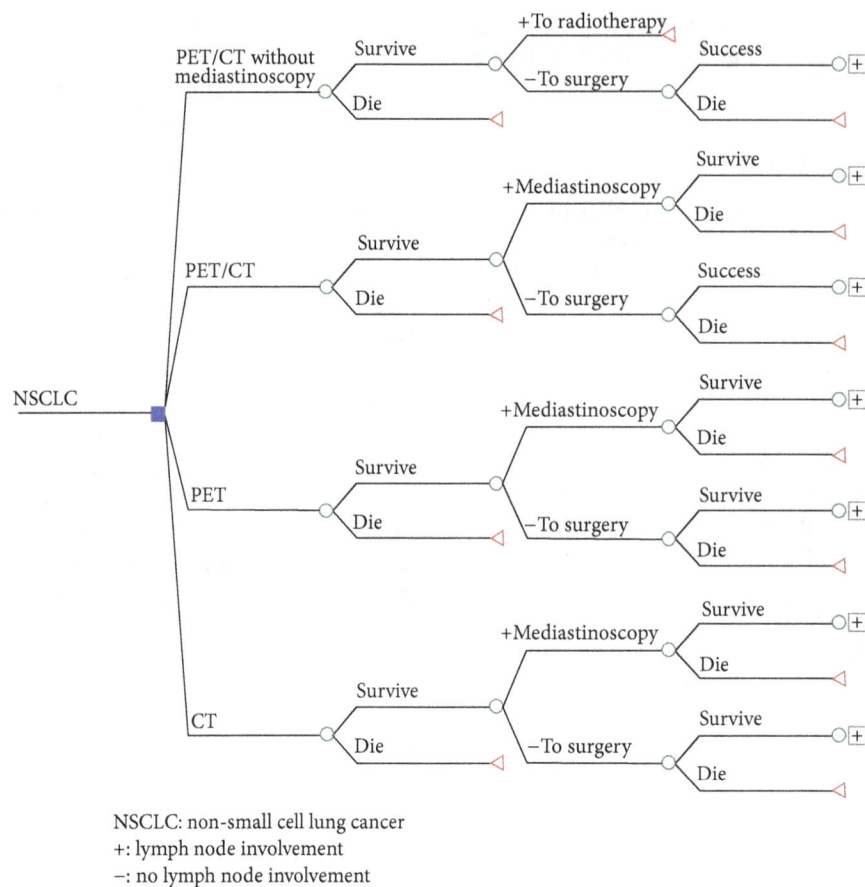

NSCLC: non-small cell lung cancer
+: lymph node involvement
−: no lymph node involvement

FIGURE 1: Structure of the decision tree for assessing the cost-effectiveness of the different staging alternatives examined.

the liver or bone were biopsied. Patients were treated with chemotherapy and/or radiotherapy.

2.9. Interpretation of Results: Statistical Analysis. All calculations were performed using IBM SPSS v.19.0 software. Significance was set at $P < 0.05$.

Kappa indices were determined to estimate the degree of agreement between the staging results of the histological examination and those of PET/CT, CT alone, and PET alone for the different subgroups of patients and tumors.

2.10. Cost-Effectiveness. A cost-effectiveness analysis was performed to determine which method (PET/CT, PET, or CT) should be the approach of choice [16] for staging of NSCLC and to select the treatment strategy [17].

A decision tree model (Figure 1) was constructed for determination of disease stage in patients with NSCLC using each of the three techniques [18].

Health benefits for patients were summarized as quality-adjusted life-years (QALYs). Patient survival was predicted according to disease stage and treatment provided based on the criteria of the SEER Cancer Statistics Review [10].

The DEALE model [19] was used to calculate life expectancy from the 5-year survival value. Utilities used to estimate QALYs were retrieved from the literature [6]. The unit costs included in the model were taken from the official

Spanish National Health System data for 2010 [8, 9] and are expressed in euros.

The variables used in the model are summarized in Table 1 [6–13].

2.11. Economic Sensitivity Analysis. The sensitivity analysis also included a branch in the decision tree that considered those treatment decisions based exclusively on PET/CT data (i.e., without histological confirmation).

Once the value for the base case (QALYs) was calculated, univariate sensitivity analysis was performed [20] to identify the effect of uncertainty on the values of the different variables in the decision tree. The upper and lower limits of the 95% confidence intervals for these values were calculated. Costs were included at ±20% of their value (Table 1).

A probabilistic sensitivity analysis based on 10,000 Monte Carlo simulations was performed to analyze the joint effect of uncertainty on the values of the variables included in the decision tree. The most commonly reported distributions of the values were used in all calculations [21].

3. Results

The study included 103 patients (90 men [87.4%] and 13 women [12.6%]) with a mean age of 68 years (SD 10, range 46 to 83). The initial histological analysis revealed that

TABLE 1: Variables used in the cost-effectiveness analysis.

Variable	Value	Lower limit	Upper limit	Source
Sensitivity of mediastinoscopy	0.72	0.63	0.81	[6, 7]
Specificity of PET	0.50	0.40	0.60	Present study
Specificity of CT	0.72	0.63	0.81	Present study
Specificity of PET/CT	0.82	0.75	0.89	Present study
Sensitivity of PET/CT	0.94	0.89	0.99	Present study
Sensitivity of PET	0.60	0.51	0.69	Present study
Sensitivity of CT	0.72	0.63	0.81	Present study
Prevalence	0.61	0.52	0.71	Present study
Costs				
Surgery cost	9917.83	7934.26	11901.37	DRG SNS [8]
PET cost	1091	872.8	1309.2	DRG CM [9]
PET/CT cost	1290	400	1500	DRG CM [9]
Radio + chemo cost	12807.33	10245.86	15368.80	DRG SNS [8]
CT cost	199	159.2	238.8	DRG CM [9]
Mediastinoscopy cost	4043.06	3234.44	4851.67	DRG SNS [8]
Outcomes				
Life expectancy after surgery	7.85	4.5	11.20	[10]
Life expectancy after radiotherapy	3.50	1.80	5.20	[10]
U after curative surgery	0.88	0.82	0.94	[6, 11]
U during surgery recovery period	−0.15	−0.30	0	[6, 11]
U with progressive disease	0.473	0.273	0.673	[12, 13]
U after palliative radiotherapy	0.673	0.65	0.70	[12, 13]

PET = positron emission tomography; CT = computed tomography; DRG = disease-related group; SNS = Spanish National Health system; CM = "Comunidad de Madrid" (Autonomous Region of Madrid); U = patient-valued utility with respect to disease stage.

41 patients had adenocarcinoma, two had bronchoalveolar carcinoma, 31 had epidermoid carcinoma, and 29 had large-cell carcinoma.

Forty of the 103 patients (38.8%, 36 men and four women) were classified by PET/CT and histology as candidates for surgery; nine of these patients had stage IA disease, 11 had stage IB disease, six had stage IIB disease,12 had stage IIIA disease, and two had stage IIIB disease (Figure 2).

Twenty-three nonsurgical patients had stage IV (metastatic) disease (10 with adrenal gland involvement, one with trapezius muscle involvement (Figure 3), one with bone involvement, and 11 with multiple metastases, including liver involvement). An additional two suspicious bone biopsies revealed false-positive results; one was a posttraumatic injury, and the other was compatible with fibrous dysplasia.

3.1. TNM Staging Performance. The concordance of each diagnostic technique (CT, PET, and PET/CT) in the TNM staging of patients with a histologically proven stage is shown in Table 2. The concordance of each diagnostic technique with the final histology results for tumor size, nodes, and metastasis is shown in Table 3.

Compared to the histology results, PET/CT more accurately staged disease in all 103 patients (kappa = 0.83) than CT (kappa = 0.694) and PET (kappa = 0.614).

TABLE 2: Concordance between the three diagnostic techniques and TNM staging ($n = 63$; 40 surgical patients and 23 with metastases).

	CT	PET	PET/CT	HP* gold standard
IA	9	5	8	9
IB	17	11	8	11
IIA	0	2	1	0
IIB	7	3	8	6
IIIA	7	16	13	12
IIIB	2	5	2	2
IV	21	21	23	23
Kappa	0.694	0.614	0.836	
Stratified kappa	0.065	0.069	0.053	

HP: histopathology.

3.2. T Staging. Primary tumor (T) staging based on PET/CT data sets was more accurate than staging based on individual CT or PET (Table 4).

3.3. N Staging. Concordance for staging the lymph node involvement (N) between PET/CT and histological examination was good (kappa = 0.75, $P < 0.001$). Five patients were incorrectly classified (false positives) by PET/CT as having

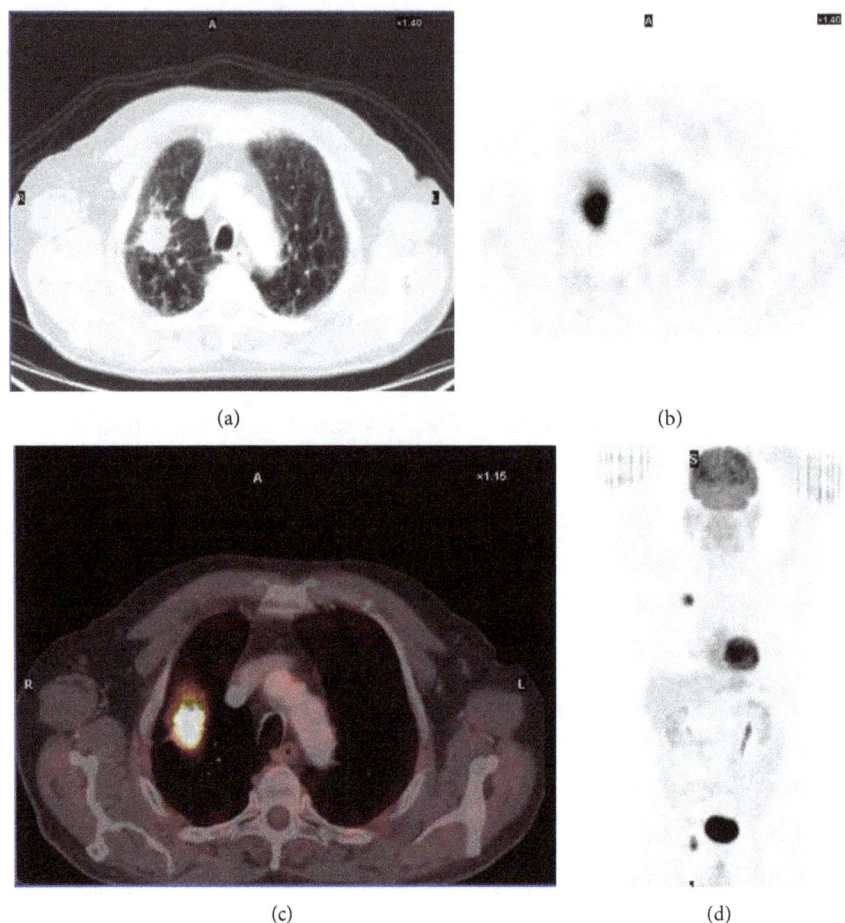

FIGURE 2: Images for a 60-year-old man. (a) CT image of an NSCLC primary tumor (epidermoid carcinoma) in the right upper lobe. (b) PET image showing intense ^{18}F-FDG uptake. (c) PET/CT image showing tumor localisation and radiotracer uptake. (d) Coronal whole-body PET image.

grade N1 ($n = 4$) or N2 ($n = 1$) lymph node involvement; histological examination yielded a classification of grade N0 involvement (these lymph nodes only showed anthracosis and/or lymphoid hyperplasia). Agreement between PET and histological examination was moderate (kappa = 0.57, $P <$ 0.001). CT alone classified 18 patients incorrectly, thus showing very poor agreement with the histological classification.

Good concordance was observed between PET/CT and the final node assessment (kappa = 0.75, $P < 0.001$), thus indicating that PET/CT is the best of the three diagnostic techniques.

3.4. M Staging. Concordance for metastatic disease (M) classification observed between PET/CT and histological examination was good (kappa = 0.90, $P < 0.001$) when the latter was deemed medically necessary. Agreement between PET and histological examination was also good (kappa = 0.78, $P < 0.001$), as it was for CT alone (kappa = 0.81, $P < 0.001$). Compared with histological examination, PET/CT accurately staged disease in the 103 patients (kappa = 0.83); compared with CT (kappa = 0.694) and PET (kappa = 0.614). The two false-positive results recorded in two patients with

bone involvement (see above) due to traumatic injury and fibrous dysplasia.

3.5. Overall Disease Staging Accuracy. Staging accuracy was calculated for the three approaches. PET/CT showed a sensitivity of 94% (95% CI, 86.1–98.3), specificity of 82% (95% CI, 72.2–93.3), positive predictive value (PPV) of 80%, and negative predictive value (NPV) of 95%. CT alone showed a sensitivity of 76% (95% CI, 63.0–81.0), specificity of 72% (95% CI, 63.0–81.0), PPV of 68%, and NPV of 86%. PET alone showed a sensitivity of 60% (95% CI, 51.0–69.0), specificity of 50% (95% CI, 40.0–60.0), PPV of 53%, and NPV of 66% (Table 5).

3.6. Cost-Effectiveness Analysis. Disease staging using CT alone correctly classified 73% of the study patients. The associated mortality associated with a lack of accuracy in disease staging was 2.7%. For PET alone these values were 57.7% and 2.8%, respectively. With PET/CT, disease was classified correctly in 89.8% of cases, and associated mortality fell to 1.4%. Thus, PET/CT shows greater disease staging accuracy and leads to reduced mortality. Medium-term survival was similar for all three alternatives.

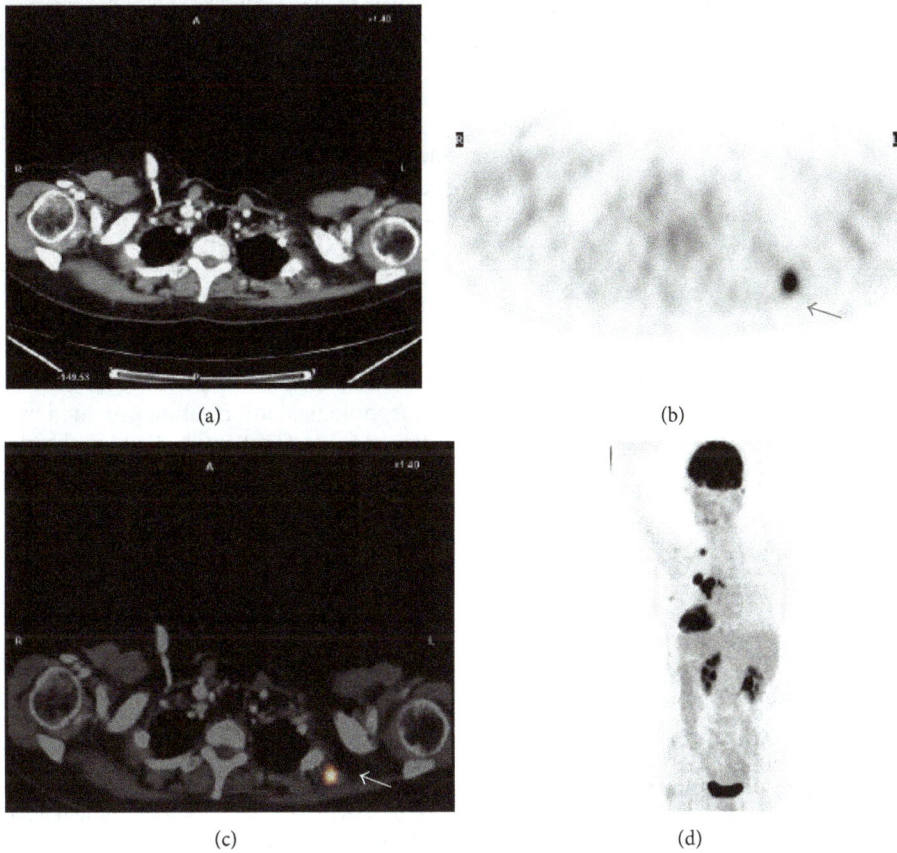

FIGURE 3: Images for a 55-year-old woman with stage IIIB NSCLC (adenocarcinoma). (a) CT imaging failed to detect any metastatic tumor. (b) PET image showing intense, nonlocalised uptake of ^{18}F-FDG. (c) PET/CT image showing ^{18}F-FDG uptake in a metastatic tumor in the trapezius muscle. Histological confirmation of the metastatic nature of the lesion. (d) Coronal whole-body PET image showing primary and metastatic lesions (arrowheads). PET = positron emission tomography; CT = computed tomography.

TABLE 3: Concordance between the three diagnostic techniques and histology.

		CT	PET	PET/CT	HP *gold standard*	Total biopsies
Size	T0	1	5	6	12	
	T1	21	15	16	12	
	T2	39	37	41	39	103
	T3	29	32	26	26	
	T4	13	14	14	14	
Kappa		0.726	0.596	0.882		
Stratified kappa		0.051	0.061	0.037		
Nodes	N0	59	39	43	24	
	N1	8	19	16	4	
	N2	23	28	24	10	40
	N3	13	17	20	2	
	Nx				63	
Kappa ($n = 40$)		0.332	0.566	0.756		40
Stratified kappa		0.121	0.105	0.092		
Metastases	M0	81	78	78	80	25
	M1	22	25	25	23	
Kappa		0.8915	0.783	0.910		
Stratified kappa		0.048	0073	0.053		

HP: histopathology.

TABLE 4: Concordance of each diagnostic technique with the "T" of the surgical patients.

Site	CT	PET	PET/CT	HP *gold standard*
Left upper lobe	$k = 0.90^*$	$k = 0.70^*$	$k = 1^*$	17
Right upper lobe	$k = 0.64^*$	$k = 0.56^*$	$k = 0.73^*$	11
Middle lobe	$k = 0.65^*$	No agreement	$k = 1^*$	1
Lingula	$k = 0.6^*$	No agreement	$k = 1^*$	1
Left lower lobe	$k = 0.95^*$	No agreement	$k = 0.96^*$	5
Right lower lobe	$k = 0.95^*$	No agreement	$k = 0.96^*$	5

$^*P < 0.001$.

TABLE 5: Patient-based analysis of diagnostic accuracy of PET/CT, CT, and PET ($n = 103$).

	Sensitivity	Specificity	PPV	NPV
PET/CT	94 (86.1–98.3)	82 (72.2–93.3)	80 (ND)	95 (ND)
CT	76 (63.0–81.0)	72 (63.0–81.0)	68 (ND)	86 (ND)
PET	60 (51.0–69.0)	50 (40.0–60.0)	53 (ND)	66 (ND)

PPV: positive predictive value and NPV: negative predictive value. ND: no data.

CT, PET, and PET/CT achieved 3.739, 3.710, and 3.771 QALYs with a total cost of €16,877, €17,425, and €17,438, respectively. PET/CT led to savings by reducing the number of mediastinoscopies required to determine whether surgery was indicated, thus reducing the number of unnecessary procedures.

Disease staging by CT alone is superior to that of PET alone, which is associated with greater use of resources from the healthcare system and leads to more unnecessary procedures and fewer QALYs. With PET/CT, each year of life gained with respect to the use of CT alone would cost €45,374, and each QALY would cost €17,412.

The tornado chart (Figure 4) shows the variation in cost-effectiveness of PET/TC and CT depending on the variables included in the decision tree.

The variable that showed the greatest influence in the incremental cost-effectiveness ratio was the low disease staging sensitivity of CT alone. This was associated with an incremental cost ratio ranging from €9,500 to €32,500 per QALY. The cost of PET/CT also had considerable influence; at a cost of €400, PET/CT would be superior to CT.

The results of the cost-effectiveness acceptability curve can be seen in Figure 5.

4. Discussion

The results of the present prospective study are consistent with those reported elsewhere [22–25]. PET/CT showed the highest sensitivity and specificity (94% and 82%, resp.) of the techniques assessed.

The PPV of PET/CT was 80% and the NPV was 95%. PET alone was the least accurate technique, owing to its poor anatomical resolution. All these studies reported significant differences between PET/CT and PET alone [22]. CT was more accurate in patients who underwent surgery in the present study than in the studies cited above.

The benefits of PET/CT over PET alone stem from the morphological information provided by CT, which improves detection of focal infiltration of the thoracic wall and the invasion of the mediastinum or vasculature. This information is not available with PET alone [22, 26]. CT performed using iodine contrast medium is, therefore, an important partner in this combined technique, enabling better characterization of the primary tumor and understanding of its relationship with the adjacent anatomical structures.

PET/CT enabled better differentiation between hypermetabolic tumors and atelectatic lung parenchyma or areas of adjacent pneumonitis, as previously reported [27] (Figures 6(a) and 6(b)).

In lymph node disease staging, PET/CT provides good results with respect to histological examination (kappa = 0.756, $P < 0.001$). PET alone shows only moderate agreement (kappa = 0.566, $P < 0.001$), although detection of disease is less dependent on tumor size than CT alone, as reported by other authors [23, 24].

The overall sensitivity of PET has been reported to be 79–85% with a specificity of 89–92%. The values were significantly greater than those reported for CT alone (57–61% and 77–82% resp.) [28, 29]. However, both the sensitivity and specificity of PET and PET/CT vary with lymph node size; namely, they are very sensitive (100%) but less specific (78%) with large lymph nodes and fairly sensitive (82%) and specific (93%) with nodes of normal size [30].

The NPV of 90% reported for PET/CT in the literature [31] is a key finding. In contrast, PPV is much lower (70%), owing to false positives caused by inflammation. In our study, five false positives were recorded with PET/CT; four classifications of N1 and one of N2 were scored as N0 in the histology examination. These corresponded to nodes affected by anthracosis and/or lymphoid hyperplasia [30, 32]. False positives have been associated with a background of inflammatory disorders, such as tuberculosis, silicosis, and interstitial pneumonitis [32].

PET/CT results should be interpreted with caution [33]. The ACCP [34] recommends confirmation by histopathology in patients without distant metastases but with well defined, enlarged mediastinal nodes and in patients with normal-sized mediastinal lymph nodes and a central tumor. It is also recommended in patients with primary tumors in stage I but whose mediastinal lymph nodes show uptake in PET tests.

Yang et al. [32] showed that PET/CT correctly classified 81% of false negatives by CT (radiotracer uptake was detected

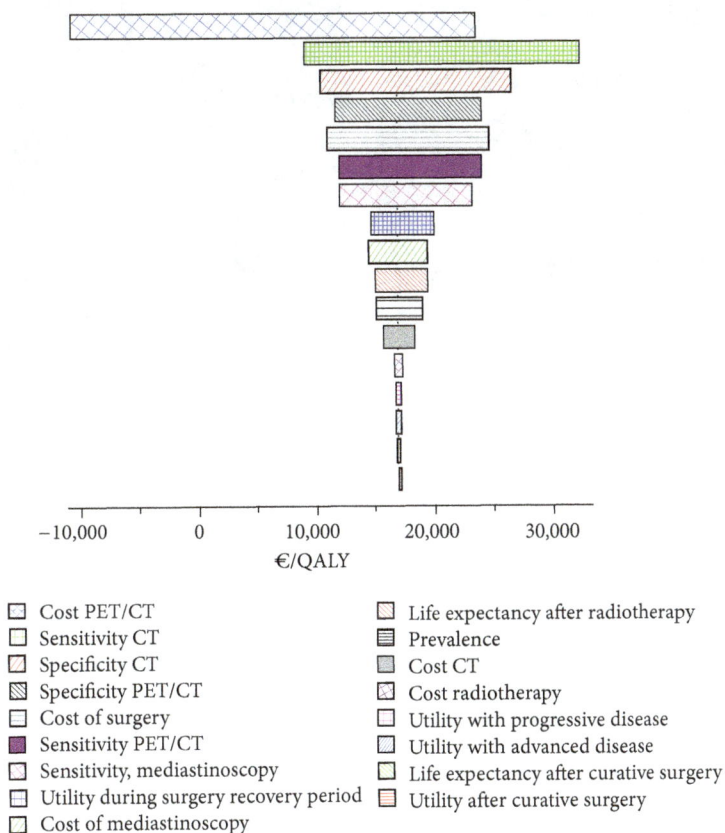

Cost PET/CT
Sensitivity CT
Specificity CT
Specificity PET/CT
Cost of surgery
Sensitivity PET/CT
Sensitivity, mediastinoscopy
Utility during surgery recovery period
Cost of mediastinoscopy

Life expectancy after radiotherapy
Prevalence
Cost CT
Cost radiotherapy
Utility with progressive disease
Utility with advanced disease
Life expectancy after curative surgery
Utility after curative surgery

FIGURE 4: Tornado chart showing the variation in cost-effectiveness of PET/TC and CT depending on the variables included in the decision tree.

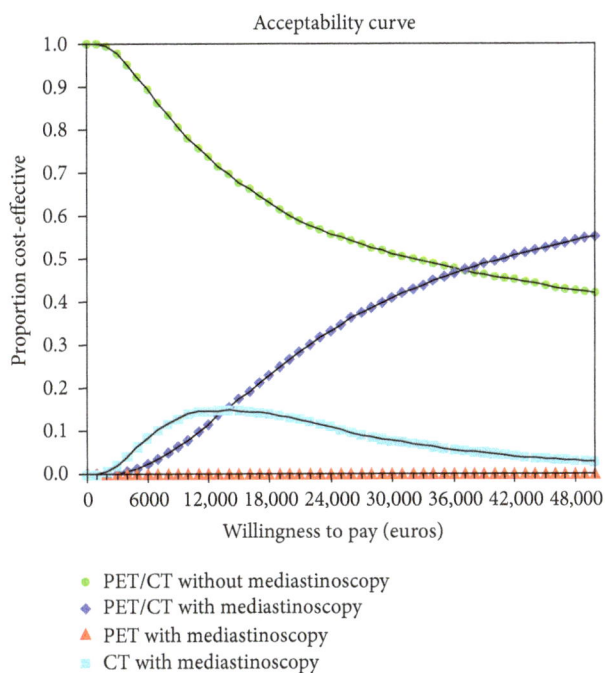

- PET/CT without mediastinoscopy
- PET/CT with mediastinoscopy
- PET with mediastinoscopy
- CT with mediastinoscopy

FIGURE 5: Cost-effectiveness acceptability curve.

(a)

(b)

(c)

(d)

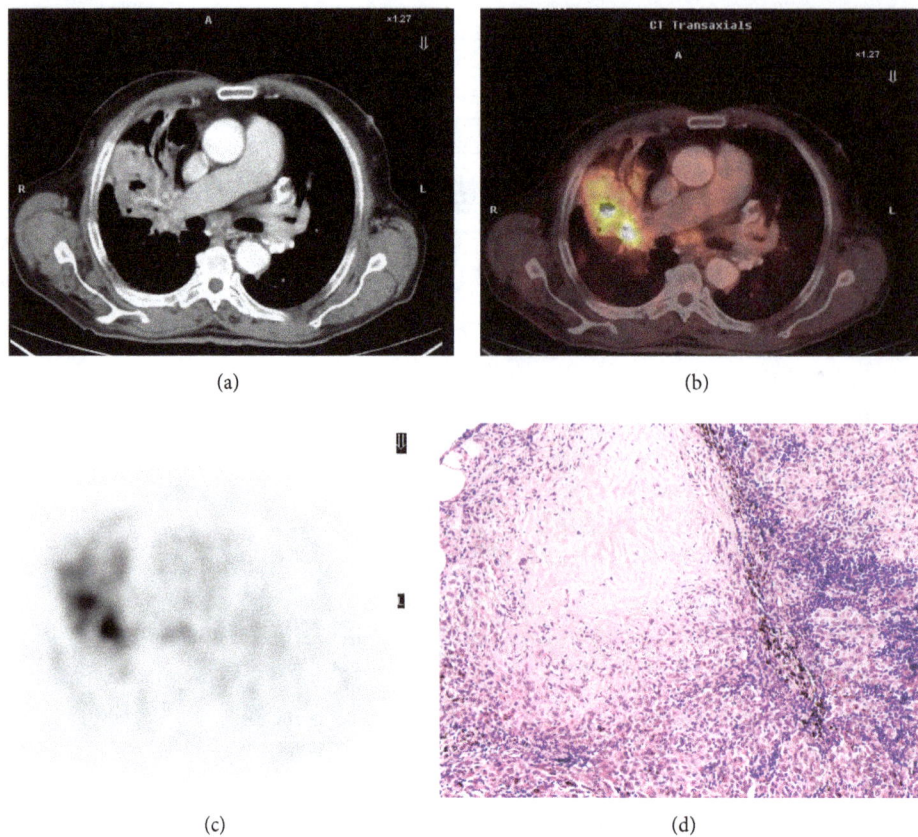

FIGURE 6: Images for a 62-year-old man with stage T2b and N1 NSCLC (epidermoid) in the right upper lobe. (a) CT image showing a lesion in the right upper lobe with adenopathy in space 7. (b) PET image showing ^{18}F-FDG uptake (maximum SUV 9). (c) PET/CT image showing ^{18}F-FDG uptake in the primary lesion and affected lymph node. (d) Histological analysis revealed the lymph node lesion not to be a tumor but rather hyperplastic anthracoid inflammation. Thus PET/CT provided a false-positive result.

in normal-sized lymph nodes) and 72% of false positives (lymph nodes of pathological size with no uptake). Twenty-seven of the patients included had metastatic disease: ten adrenal metastases, 15 generalised metastases (including liver and brain), and two bone metastases. Up to 40% of patients with NSCLC have metastases at diagnosis [35], mainly at the above-mentioned sites. Detection of these metastases is crucial when selecting treatment, since their presence rules out any curative intent.

PET/CT enables more precise localization and better characterization of tumors scored as uncertain by CT alone [22, 23] and is useful in the assessment of adrenal nodules in patients with NSCLC, showing greater accuracy in the detection of metastases (84–92%) than PET, as well as greater specificity. The sensitivity of PET is close to 100% when the adrenal uptake of ^{18}F-FDG is greater than that of the liver [35] (Figure 7).

The better disease staging achieved with PET/CT has been associated with changes in treatment in 9–15% of patients [23] in terms of curative intent, treatment type (chemotherapy, radiotherapy, or surgery), and planning of radiotherapy. In one randomized study [36], the inclusion of PET in the examination of patients with NSCLC led

to a significant reduction in the number of unnecessary thoracotomies (from 41% to 21%).

The lack of a reference standard for PET/CT with respect to node involvement in nonsurgical patients is a limitation of this study. Histological examination of the anomalies detected by imaging methods in patients who are not candidates for surgery are currently performed using EUS and EBUS, which are included in the guidelines for staging lung cancer, mainly N2. As with the remaining techniques; they also generate false-positive results in lymph node stations that require mediastinoscopy [37]. A five-year follow-up revealed that none of the patients in stages IIIB and IV survived. The maximum survival was three years (one stage IIIB patient). However, the results obtained indicate that PET/CT should be the method of choice when staging disease in patients with NSCLC, given that complementary tests cannot provide more information.

The incremental cost-effectiveness of PET/CT was around €17,500 per QALY compared to CT alone. This figure is higher than that estimated by other healthcare systems [6–9], which considered PET and CT separately before analyzing their combined costs.

(a)

(b)

(c)

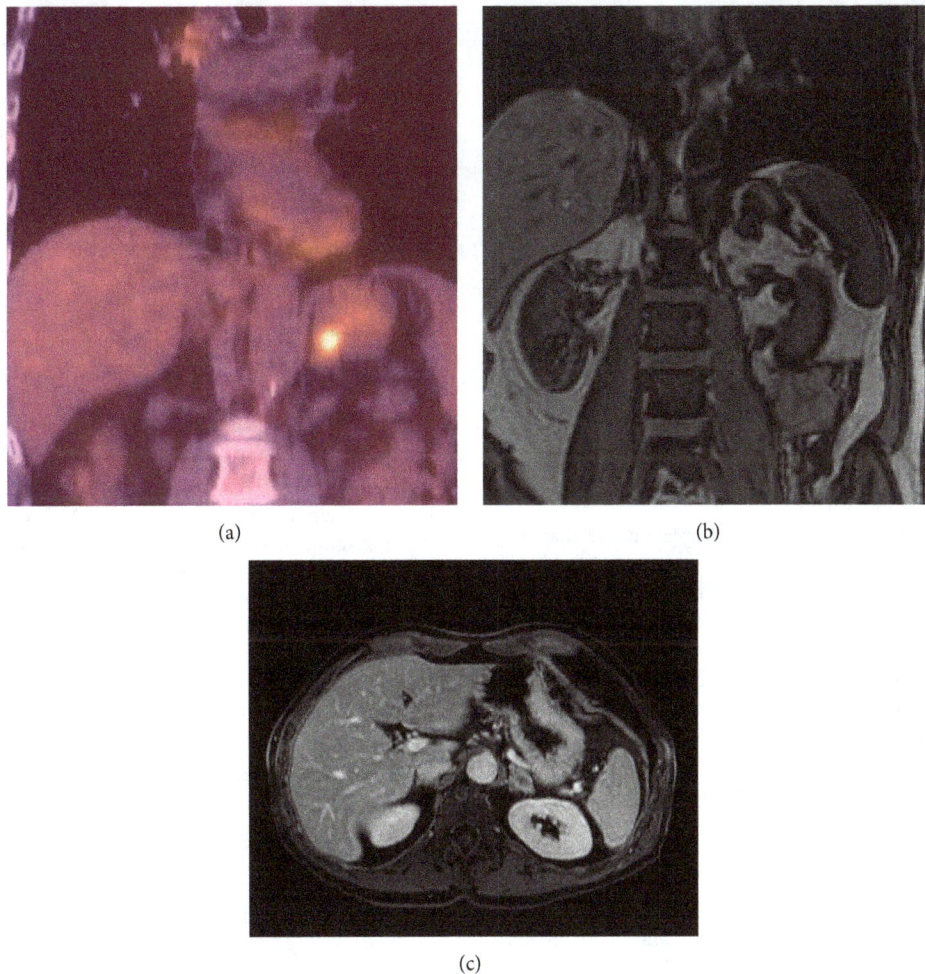

FIGURE 7: Images for a 70-year-old man with NSCLC (adenocarcinoma). (a) PET/CT showed intense ^{18}F-FDG uptake by an adrenal metastasis. (b) Coronal out-of-phase image and (c) axial MR image with contrast medium confirming adrenal metastasis.

The present results showed that staging NSCLC by PET alone provided no benefit over staging by CT alone and required more resources. Our findings indicate that PET/CT is the most accurate strategy for disease staging. When willingness to pay is low (under €30,000 per QALY) [38], PET/CT is probably a more efficient strategy without mediastinoscopy, and treatment decisions can be adopted in accordance with the result. However, when willingness to pay is high (>€40,000 per QALY), PET/CT plus confirmatory mediastinoscopy is the most efficient strategy.

The strengths of the present study include its prospective design and the analysis of key variables (per life years gained and QALYs). This is the first cost-effectiveness analysis of these three techniques in Spain.

The cost-effectiveness analysis is limited in that it was based on costs obtained from the literature, which may not accurately reflect the costs associated with the Spanish Health System; unfortunately, local cost figures were not available.

In conclusion, PET/CT with intravenous contrast medium was found to be an accurate and cost-effective method for staging patients with NSCLC. Therefore, it should be the method of choice for staging in patients with this disease.

Conflict of Interests

The authors declare that there is no conflict of interests regarding the publication of this paper.

References

[1] A. Jemal, R. Siegel, E. Ward et al., "Cancer statistics, 2008," CA Cancer Journal for Clinicians, vol. 58, no. 2, pp. 71–96, 2008.

[2] P. Yang, M. S. Allen, M. C. Aubry et al., "Clinical features of 5,628 primary lung cancer patients: experience at Mayo Clinic from 1997 to 2003," Chest, vol. 128, no. 1, pp. 452–462, 2005.

[3] L. H. Sobin, M. K. Gospodarowicz, and C. Wittekind, "Lung (ICD-O C34)," in TNM Classification of Mali gnant Tumors, L. H. Sobin, M. K. Gospodarowicz, and C. Wittekind, Eds., pp. 138–146, Blackwell Publishing, Chichester, UK, 7th edition, 2010.

[4] B. A. Dwamena, S. S. Sonnad, J. O. Angobaldo, and R. L. Wahl, "Metastases from non-small cell lung cancer: mediastinal staging in the 1990s—Meta-analytic comparison of PET and CT," *Radiology*, vol. 213, no. 2, pp. 530–536, 1999.

[5] J. W. Fletcher, B. Djulbegovic, H. P. Soares et al., "Recommendations on the use of ^{18}F-FDG PET in oncology," *Journal of Nuclear Medicine*, vol. 49, no. 3, pp. 480–508, 2008.

[6] I. Bradbury, E. Bonell, J. Boynton et al., "Positron emission tomography (PET) imaging in cancer management," Health Technology Assessment Report 2, Health Technology Board for Scotland, Glasgow, Scotland, 2002.

[7] NICE and National Collaborating Centre for Acute Care, *Diagnosis and Treatment of Lung Cancer*, National Collaborating Centre for Acute Care, London, UK, 2005, http://www.rcseng.ac.uk/.

[8] Ministerio de Sanidad, Política Social e Igualdad. Pesos y costes de los GRDs del Sistema Nacional de Salud, http://www.msssi.gob.es/estadEstudios/estadisticas/.

[9] "ORDEN 629/2009, de 31 de agosto, por la que se fijan los precios públicos por la prestación de los servicios y actividades de naturaleza sanitaria de la red de centros de la Comunidad de Madrid," *Boletín Oficial de la Comunidad de Madrid*, no. 215, 2009.

[10] S. F. Altekruse, C. L. Kosary, M. Krapcho et al., *SEER Cancer Statistics Review, 1975–2007*, National Cancer Institute, Bethesda, Md, USA, 2010, http://seer.cancer.gov/csr/1975_2007.

[11] S. S. Gambhir, C. K. Hoh, M. E. Phelps, I. Madar, and J. Maddahi, "Decision tree sensitivity analysis for cost-effectiveness of FDG-PET in the staging and management of non-small-cell lung carcinoma," *Journal of Nuclear Medicine*, vol. 37, no. 9, pp. 1428–1436, 1996.

[12] B. Nafees, M. Stafford, S. Gavriel, S. Bhalla, and J. Watkins, "Health state utilities for non small cell lung cancer," *Health and Quality of Life Outcomes*, vol. 6, article 84, 2008.

[13] Y. Asukai, A. Valladares, C. Camps et al., "Cost-effectiveness analysis of pemetrexed versus docetaxel in the second-line treatment of non-small cell lung cancer in Spain: Results for the non-squamous histology population," *BMC Cancer*, vol. 10, article 26, 2010.

[14] W. A. Weber, "Use of PET for monitoring cancer therapy and for predicting outcome," *Journal of Nuclear Medicine*, vol. 46, no. 6, pp. 983–995, 2005.

[15] S. J. Uybico, C. C. Wu, R. D. Suh, N. H. Le, K. Brown, and M. S. Krishnam, "Lung cancer staging essentials: the new TNM staging system and potential imaging pitfalls," *Radiographics*, vol. 30, no. 5, pp. 1163–1181, 2010.

[16] P. J. Neumann, C.-H. Fang, and J. T. Cohen, "30 years of pharmaceutical cost-utility analyses: growth, diversity and methodological improvement," *PharmacoEconomics*, vol. 27, no. 10, pp. 861–872, 2009.

[17] M. F. Drummond and T. O. Jefferson, "Guidelines for authors and peer reviewers of economic submissions to the BMJ. The BMJ Economic Evaluation Working Party," *The British Medical Journal*, vol. 313, pp. 275–283, 1996.

[18] R. Goeree, B. J. O'Brien, and G. Blackhouse, "Principles of good modeling practice in healthcare cost-effectiveness studies," *Expert Review of Pharmacoeconomics and Outcomes Research*, vol. 4, no. 2, pp. 189–198, 2004.

[19] J. R. Beck, S. G. Pauker, J. E. Gottlieb, K. Klein, and J. P. Kassirer, "A convenient approximation of life expectancy (The "DEALE"). II. Use in medical decision-making," *The American Journal of Medicine*, vol. 73, no. 6, pp. 889–897, 1982.

[20] B. J. O'Brien and A. H. Briggs, "Analysis of uncertainty in health care cost-effectiveness studies: an introduction to statistical issues and methods," *Statistical Methods in Medical Research*, vol. 11, no. 6, pp. 455–468, 2002.

[21] K. Claxton, M. Sculpher, C. McCabe et al., "Probabilistic sensitivity analysis for NICE technology assessment: not an optional extra," *Health Economics*, vol. 14, no. 4, pp. 339–347, 2005.

[22] D. Lardinois, W. Weder, T. F. Hany et al., "Staging of non-small-cell lung cancer with integrated positron-emission tomography and computed tomography," *The New England Journal of Medicine*, vol. 348, no. 25, pp. 2500–2507, 2003.

[23] R. J. Cerfolio, B. Ojha, A. S. Bryant, V. Raghuveer, J. M. Mountz, and A. A. Bartolucci, "The accuracy of integrated PET-CT compared with dedicated PET alone for the staging of patients with nonsmall cell lung cancer," *Annals of Thoracic Surgery*, vol. 78, no. 3, pp. 1017–1023, 2004.

[24] B. S. Halpern, C. Schiepers, W. A. Weber et al., "Presurgical staging of non-small cell lung cancer: positron emission tomography, integrated positron emission tomography/CT, and software image fusion," *Chest*, vol. 128, no. 4, pp. 2289–2297, 2005.

[25] S. L. Aquino, J. C. Asmuth, N. M. Alpert, E. F. Halpern, and A. J. Fischman, "Improved radiologic staging of lung cancer with 2-[18F]-fluoro-2-deoxy-D-glucose-positron emission tomography and computed tomography registration," *Journal of Computer Assisted Tomography*, vol. 27, no. 4, pp. 479–484, 2003.

[26] A. C. Pfannenberg, P. Aschoff, K. Brechtel et al., "Low dose non-enhanced CT versus standard dose contrast-enhanced CT in combined PET/CT protocols for staging and therapy planning in non-small cell lung cancer," *European Journal of Nuclear Medicine and Molecular Imaging*, vol. 34, no. 1, pp. 36–44, 2007.

[27] V. H. Gerbaudo and B. Julius, "Anatomo-metabolic characteristics of atelectasis in F-18 FDG-PET/CT imaging," *European Journal of Radiology*, vol. 64, no. 3, pp. 401–405, 2007.

[28] B. A. Dwamena, S. S. Sonnad, J. O. Angobaldo, and R. L. Wahl, "Metastases from non-small cell lung cancer: mediastinal staging in the 1990s—meta-analytic comparison of PET and CT," *Radiology*, vol. 213, no. 2, pp. 530–536, 1999.

[29] O. Birim, A. P. Kappetein, T. Stijnen, and A. J. Bogers, "Meta-analysis of positron emission tomographic and computed tomographic imaging in detecting mediastinal lymph node metastases in nonsmall cell lung cancer," *Annals of Thoracic Surgery*, vol. 79, no. 1, pp. 375–382, 2005.

[30] N. Al-Sarraf, K. Gately, J. Lucey, L. Wilson, E. McGovern, and V. Young, "Lymph node staging by means of positron emission tomography is less accurate in non-small cell lung cancer patients with enlarged lymph nodes: analysis of 1145 lymph nodes," *Lung Cancer*, vol. 60, no. 1, pp. 62–68, 2008.

[31] R. M. Pieterman, J. W. G. van Putten, J. J. Meuzelaar et al., "Preoperative staging of non-small-cell lung cancer with positron-emission tomography," *The New England Journal of Medicine*, vol. 343, no. 4, pp. 254–261, 2000.

[32] W. Yang, Z. Fu, J. Yu et al., "Value of PET/CT versus enhanced CT for locoregional lymph nodes in non-small cell lung cancer," *Lung Cancer*, vol. 61, no. 1, pp. 35–43, 2008.

[33] Y. K. Kim, K. S. Lee, B. T. Kim et al., "Mediastinal nodal staging of nonsmall cell lung cancer using integrated ^{18}F-FDG PET/CT in a tuberculosis-endemic country: diagnostic efficacy in 674 patients," *Cancer*, vol. 109, no. 6, pp. 1068–1077, 2007.

[34] F. C. Detterbeck, M. A. Jantz, M. Wallace, J. Vansteenkiste, and G. A. Silvestri, "Invasive mediastinal staging of lung cancer: ACCP evidence-based clinical practice guidelines (2nd edition)," *Chest*, vol. 132, supplement 3, pp. 202S–220S, 2007.

[35] L. E. Quint, S. Tummala, L. J. Brisson et al., "Distribution of distant metastases from newly diagnosed non-small cell lung cancer," *The Annals of Thoracic Surgery*, vol. 62, no. 1, pp. 246–250, 1996.

[36] H. van Tinteren, O. S. Hoekstra, E. F. Smit et al., "Effectiveness of positron emission tomography in the preoperative assessment of patients with suspected non-small-cell lung cancer: the PLUS multicentre randomised trial," *The Lancet*, vol. 359, no. 9315, pp. 1388–1392, 2002.

[37] R. J. Cerfolio, A. S. Bryant, M. A. Eloubeidi et al., "The true false negative rates of esophageal and endobronchial ultrasound in the staging of mediastinal lymph nodes in patients with non-small cell lung cancer," *Annals of Thoracic Surgery*, vol. 90, no. 2, pp. 427–434, 2010.

[38] V. Ortún, "30.000 euros por AVAC," *Economía y Salud*, vol. 49, pp. 1–2, 2004.

12

Multisite Kinetic Modeling of ^{13}C Metabolic MR Using [1-^{13}C]Pyruvate

Pedro A. Gómez Damián,[1,2,3] **Jonathan I. Sperl,**[1] **Martin A. Janich,**[1,4,5] **Oleksandr Khegai,**[1,5] **Florian Wiesinger,**[1] **Steffen J. Glaser,**[5] **Axel Haase,**[3] **Markus Schwaiger,**[4] **Rolf F. Schulte,**[1] **and Marion I. Menzel**[1]

[1]*GE Global Research, 85748 Garching bei München, Germany*
[2]*Medical Engineering, Tecnológico de Monterrey, 64849 Monterrey, NL, Mexico*
[3]*Medical Engineering, Technische Universität München, 85748 Garching bei München, Germany*
[4]*Nuclear Medicine, Technische Universität München, 81675 Munich, Germany*
[5]*Chemistry, Technische Universität München, 85748 Garching bei München, Germany*

Correspondence should be addressed to Marion I. Menzel; menzel@ge.com

Academic Editor: David Maintz

Hyperpolarized ^{13}C imaging allows real-time *in vivo* measurements of metabolite levels. Quantification of metabolite conversion between [1-^{13}C]pyruvate and downstream metabolites [1-^{13}C]alanine, [1-^{13}C]lactate, and [^{13}C]bicarbonate can be achieved through kinetic modeling. Since pyruvate interacts dynamically and simultaneously with its downstream metabolites, the purpose of this work is the determination of parameter values through a multisite, dynamic model involving possible biochemical pathways present in MR spectroscopy. Kinetic modeling parameters were determined by fitting the multisite model to time-domain dynamic metabolite data. The results for different pyruvate doses were compared with those of different two-site models to evaluate the hypothesis that for identical data the uncertainty of a model and the signal-to-noise ratio determine the sensitivity in detecting small physiological differences in the target metabolism. In comparison to the two-site exchange models, the multisite model yielded metabolic conversion rates with smaller bias and smaller standard deviation, as demonstrated in simulations with different signal-to-noise ratio. Pyruvate dose effects observed previously were confirmed and quantified through metabolic conversion rate values. Parameter interdependency allowed an accurate quantification and can therefore be useful for monitoring metabolic activity in different tissues.

1. Introduction

While ^{13}C magnetic resonance spectroscopy (MRS) has been utilized for *in vivo* imaging and spectroscopy of metabolism [1] for a long time, only the development of dynamic nuclear polarization (DNP) helped to overcome the inherent sensitivity limit; as through hyperpolarization using DNP followed by rapid dissolution, the ^{13}C MR signal can be amplified by more than 10,000-fold [2].

One of the most common and viable agents for *in vivo* use is [1-^{13}C]pyruvate (PYR) [3]. After intravenous injection, it is transported to the observed tissue or organ under observation, where it is enzymatically metabolized to its downstream metabolites [1-^{13}C]alanine (ALA) by alanine transaminase (ALT), [1-^{13}C]lactate (LAC) by lactate dehydrogenase (LDH), and [^{13}C]bicarbonate (BC) by pyruvate dehydrogenase (PDH) to varying extent, depending on tissue type and predominant metabolic activity. At the same time PYR is in chemical exchange with [1-^{13}C]pyruvate-hydrate (PYRH). As part of gluconeogenesis, PYR may also be carboxylated to oxaloacetate [4].

In order to quantify the metabolic exchange between PYR and its downstream metabolites, MRS data acquired over a certain time period after injection first require assignment of spectral peaks [5] in the spectral domain and second require quantification of these peaks over time. Several different methods have been used for this time-domain analysis, and among these the most simple and robust method is the determination of metabolite signal ratios. These ratios are usually obtained from the peak metabolite signals [6] or through integrating over time [5]. The latter approach has been employed in our previous study, conducted by Janich et al. [5], where hyperpolarized PYR spectra were quantified for different PYR doses and subsequently used to determine the dose effects on Wistar rats based on time integrated metabolite signal ratios.

Although the approach of obtaining relative metabolite signal ratios, LAC to PYR or ALA to PYR, is straightforward and robust, independently if obtained from peak signal or time integrals, the results suffer from an increasingly strong T_1 weighting of the integral, which skews the resulting ratios. Furthermore, although time-domain visualization and signal ratio determination is an effective tool for assessing the effect of different PYR doses, it provides no quantitative kinetic data of metabolic exchange.

In order to achieve this quantification, different methods for kinetic modeling of hyperpolarized ^{13}C MR data have been reported. Most approaches, derived from the modified Bloch equations, represent a two-site interaction between PYR and one specific downstream metabolite, for example, either LAC or ALA [7–14]. Modeling can be extended to include more sites (intra- and extracellular) or more metabolites [9, 12] (for a comprehensive comparison, see [15]). Even so, presumably for robustness, previous work focuses primarily on fitting data with just one downstream metabolite, keeping most parameters fixed, or even model free, based on signal ratios [5, 16, 17]. When PYR is injected and the corresponding metabolic reactions begin to take place, PYR is not metabolized exclusively into ALA (or LAC), but it changes dynamically into all of the aforementioned downstream metabolites [18]. There is furthermore some skepticism, if the implicit assumption of rate constant stability holds in all applications [17] and there are few analyses on model parameter dependence on SNR [19]. In particular, metabolic conversion in the heart predominantly follows the PDH path producing BC [6, 20]. We therefore hypothesize that the simultaneous consideration of various metabolic pathways is necessary to obtain an accurate evaluation of *in vivo* metabolic conversion rates. On this basis, we propose using a mathematical framework for multisite modeling (similar to [8, 21, 22]) by simultaneously fitting different possible ^{13}C metabolic pathways for PYR, which can typically be observed after injection of pyruvate labeled in the [1-^{13}C] position.

Additionally, although our prior work [5] evaluates quantification of spectra and employed a semiquantitative method to investigate metabolic conversion under different PYR doses (based on metabolite to PYR ratios), it does not provide fully quantitative kinetic data. Therefore, in this subsequent work we employ the experimental data obtained in [5] and implement the proposed multisite, dynamic model to determine metabolic conversion and signal decay rates for full quantification of the kinetics of metabolic conversion. Furthermore, the proposed model gives access to effective longitudinal relaxation times ($T_{1\mathrm{eff}}$), both for PYR and for the downstream metabolites.

Using the identical biological data, the kinetic parameters estimated by the multisite model are then compared to the parameters obtained using the two-site models proposed both in [8] and in [23]. The estimated parameters of all models are also compared between the three different doses utilized in [5], that is, 20, 40, and 80 mM (corresponding to 0.1, 0.2, and 0.4 mmol/kg bodyweight) of PYR, in order to evaluate the capability of the model for the assessment of dose response. As identical data is used, the evaluation allows for direct assessment of kinetic model stability and quality. Ideally, a successful kinetic model would allow the reduction of data variability due to modeling to a minimum, allowing the visualization of biological variability (i.e., as a response to dose treatment, etc.). In addition, using simulated metabolic data based on exemplary conversion rates, we assessed the variability and stability of the kinetic models under the influence of noise. Here, the expectation towards a model is that both systematic bias and standard deviation of the resulting metabolic conversion rates should be as low as possible over a large range of signal-to-noise ratio (SNR).

2. Theory

In our previous study [5], MRS spectral data after injection of pyruvate was acquired and analyzed utilizing time-domain fitting with AMARES [24], resulting in a time course of metabolite levels. To quantify the metabolic conversion, this previous study employed integrated metabolite signal ratios. In the following paragraphs, we will compare this simple integrative approach to kinetic modeling using three different approaches, which are two-site exchange differential model, two-site exchange integral model, and multisite exchange integral model.

2.1. Two-Site Exchange Differential Model. Using a two-site exchange differential model (2SDM) allows computing metabolic exchange rates $k_{\mathrm{pyr} \to x}$ and the respective metabolite's effective signal decay rates r_x by solving a system of linear equations given in differential form

$$\frac{dM_x(t)}{dt} = -r_x M_x(t) + k_{\mathrm{pyr} \to x} M_{\mathrm{pyr}}(t). \tag{1}$$

The effective metabolite signal decay rate r_x is dominated by T_1 relaxation, the respective backward metabolic exchange rate $k_{x \to \mathrm{pyr}}$, and a flip angle (FA) term, which also depends on the repetition time (TR), accounting for the irreversible consumption of signal after successive excitations:

$$r_x = \frac{1}{T_x} + k_{x \to \mathrm{pyr}} + f(\mathrm{FA}) \tag{2}$$

with

$$f(\mathrm{FA}) = \frac{1 - \cos(\mathrm{FA})}{\mathrm{TR}}. \tag{3}$$

Hence, r_x results in a single, inseparable term of signal decay. However, FA and TR are known from experimentation and can be corrected for. In case the backward exchange rate $k_{x \to \text{pyr}}$ is assumed to be negligible, true T_1 relaxation times can be quantified; however, it remains unclear whether this assumption holds true in all physiological states of the animal.

2SDM does not assume a PYR input function and for that reason the first order differential equation (1) can be solved as a linear system. This approach is independent of the time course of PYR administration and is therefore straightforward to apply.

2.2. Two-Site Exchange Integral Model. Another approach in kinetic modeling, the two-site exchange integral model (2SIM), assumes a PYR input function that represents the PYR signal in time ($M_{\text{pyr}}(t)$). In Zierhut et al. [8] a series of piecewise defined exponential equations were presented:

$$M_{\text{pyr}}(t) = \begin{cases} \dfrac{I_{\text{pyr}}}{r_{\text{pyr}}}\left[1 - e^{-r_{\text{pyr}}(t - t_{\text{arrival}})}\right], & t_{\text{arrival}} \leq t < t_{\text{end}}, \\ M_{\text{pyr}}(t_{\text{end}})\, e^{-r_{\text{pyr}}(t - t_{\text{end}})}, & t \geq t_{\text{end}}. \end{cases} \tag{4}$$

The first part of the equation takes into account PYR signal loss due to r_{pyr} and the injection of PYR with a constant rate I_{pyr} from the arrival time t_{arrival} until t_{end}. It nevertheless assumes that no conversion of PYR takes place during injection. The second part, for all time measurements later than t_{end}, is characterized only by the PYR signal loss. In a similar manner, an assumption on the initial PYR concentration can be made instead of an assumption on the input function, leading to the modeling of only the exponential decay, as shown in [25]. Explicit modeling of M_{pyr} allows for (1) to be solved yielding metabolite signals in time [8]:

$$M_x(t)$$

$$= \begin{cases} \dfrac{k_{\text{pyr} \to x} I_{\text{pyr}}}{r_{\text{pyr}} - r_x}\left[\dfrac{1 - e^{-r_x(t - t_{\text{arrival}})}}{r_x} - \dfrac{1 - e^{-r_{\text{pyr}}(t - t_{\text{arrival}})}}{r_{\text{pyr}}}\right], \\ \qquad\qquad\qquad\qquad\qquad t_{\text{arrival}} \leq t < t_{\text{end}}, \\ \dfrac{M_{\text{pyr}}(t_{\text{end}}) * k_{\text{pyr} \to x}}{r_{\text{pyr}} - r_x}\left[e^{-r_x(t - t_{\text{end}})} - e^{-r_{\text{pyr}}(t - t_{\text{end}})}\right] \\ \quad + M_x(t_{\text{end}})\, e^{-r_x(t - t_{\text{end}})}, \\ \qquad\qquad\qquad\qquad\qquad t \geq t_{\text{end}}. \end{cases} \tag{5}$$

Alongside the parameters characterizing the PYR input function, these equations contain the same parameters ($k_{\text{pyr} \to x}$ and r_x) that were solved for using 2SDM.

2SIM can be considered as a two-step approach. First, t_{arrival}, r_{pyr}, and I_{pyr} are determined by fitting (4) to the measured PYR signal. t_{end} is simply calculated by summing t_{arrival} and the known injection duration. These parameters are then utilized to fit (5) to the LAC and ALA signals. In [6], this model is also utilized to fit the BC signal. Finally the computed metabolic exchange rates $k_{\text{pyr} \to x}$, the decay rate r_{pyr}, and the flip angle correction (3) can be used to estimate apparent T_1 relaxation of PYR.

2.3. Multisite Exchange Integral Model. As described above, the metabolite signal decay rate r_x depends on T_1 relaxation, backward metabolic exchange rates $k_{x \to \text{pyr}}$, and signal loss from flip angle variations. On the other hand, the PYR signal decay r_{pyr} does not depend on backward metabolic exchange, but on forward metabolic exchange rates $k_{\text{pyr} \to x}$. This signifies that the rate of PYR decay is also proportional to the rate of PYR downstream conversion.

Hence, when passing from 2SIM to a multisite exchange integral model (MSIM), the PYR input function (4)—represented in its differential form—needs to include all of the metabolic exchange rates:

$$\dfrac{dM_{\text{pyr}}(t)}{dt} = \begin{cases} -r_{\text{pyr}} M_{\text{pyr}}(t) - \sum\limits_x k_{\text{pyr} \to x} M_{\text{pyr}}(t) + I_{\text{pyr}}, \\ \qquad t_{\text{arrival}} \leq t < t_{\text{end}}, \\ -r_{\text{pyr}} M_{\text{pyr}}(t) - \sum\limits_x k_{\text{pyr} \to x} M_{\text{pyr}}(t), \\ \qquad t \geq t_{\text{end}}. \end{cases} \tag{6}$$

Note that both the PYR signal decay rate r_{pyr} and the sum of all of the metabolic exchange rates $\sum_x k_{\text{pyr} \to x}$ are multiplied by the same term $M_{\text{pyr}}(t)$ and can therefore be grouped into a total PYR signal decay rate:

$$R_{\text{pyr}} = r_{\text{pyr}} + \sum_x k_{\text{pyr} \to x}. \tag{7}$$

By replacing (7) in (6), the integral form of the new PYR input function reads

$$M_{\text{pyr}}(t) = \begin{cases} \dfrac{I_{\text{pyr}}}{R_{\text{pyr}}}\left[1 - e^{-R_{\text{pyr}}(t - t_{\text{arrival}})}\right], & t_{\text{arrival}} \leq t < t_{\text{end}}, \\ M_{\text{pyr}}(t_{\text{end}})\, e^{-R_{\text{pyr}}(t - t_{\text{end}})}, & t \geq t_{\text{end}}. \end{cases} \tag{8}$$

The representation of the total PYR relaxation rate R_{pyr} as the sum of the PYR relaxation rate and the metabolic conversion rates allows for a simultaneous fitting process, where the conversion rates are taken into account also in the PYR input function, creating dependent curves and a parameter interdependency. In addition, the estimation of T_1 values for PYR can be achieved directly using

$$\dfrac{1}{T_{1\text{pyr}}} = r_{\text{pyr}} - f(\text{FA}). \tag{9}$$

Utilizing the same R_{pyr} term for the metabolite signals, (5) becomes

$$M_x(t)$$

$$= \begin{cases} \dfrac{k_{\text{pyr} \to x} I_{\text{pyr}}}{R_{\text{pyr}} - r_x}\left[\dfrac{1 - e^{-r_x(t - t_{\text{arrival}})}}{r_x} - \dfrac{1 - e^{-R_{\text{pyr}}(t - t_{\text{arrival}})}}{R_{\text{pyr}}}\right], \\ \qquad\qquad\qquad\qquad\qquad t_{\text{arrival}} \leq t < t_{\text{end}}, \\ \dfrac{M_{\text{pyr}}(t_{\text{end}}) * k_{\text{pyr} \to x}}{R_{\text{pyr}} - r_x}\left[e^{-r_x(t - t_{\text{end}})} - e^{-R_{\text{pyr}}(t - t_{\text{end}})}\right] \\ \quad + M_x(t_{\text{end}})\, e^{-r_x(t - t_{\text{end}})}, \\ \qquad\qquad\qquad\qquad\qquad t \geq t_{\text{end}}. \end{cases} \tag{10}$$

As seen in (2), the backward exchange rates are inseparably confounded with T_1 in the respective signal decay rate r_x of each metabolite. A nonnegligible backward reaction thus leads to an overestimation of the true T_1 values for all of the downstream metabolites. For LAC, the overestimation might be considered negligible since the backward reaction was reported to have only a very small effect on kinetics [26], although earlier work indicates upregulated gluconeogenesis in liver-metabolism of tumor-bearing rats [27]. The assumption of negligible backward reactions might also not hold for ALA. There is no need to apply a backward exchange to BC; however, depending on pH, it is breathed out as $^{13}CO_2$ and this could lead to an apparent shortening in T_1. This signifies that the T_1 values for ALA and BC obtained utilizing this model can only be considered bounds for the true value.

3. Methods

3.1. Experimental Data. The experimental data was obtained from healthy male Wistar rats through the acquisition of slice-selective FID signals in heart, liver, and kidney tissue. Three different hyperpolarized PYR concentrations (20, 40, and 80 mM, which correspond to an injected dose of 0.1, 0.2, and 0.4 mmol/kg bodyweight) were utilized to measure a total of 15 animals. Each dose was injected into five different animals twice, resulting in a total of 10 measurements for each dose. A flip angle of 5° was utilized and TR was triggered to animal breathing yielding an average value of ~1 s. SNR was calculated by dividing the maximum PYR signal by the average noise for all time steps. More experimental details can be directly found in [5].

Further exemplary data to evaluate modeling performance at presence of pathology were obtained from adult female Fischer 344 rats (Charles River, Sulzfeld, Germany) beating subcutaneous mammary adenocarcinomas. The animals' anesthesia was maintained with 1–3% isoflurane in oxygen starting about 1 h before the first injection. During the experiment, the heart rate, temperature, and breathing signal were monitored using an animal monitoring system (SA Instruments, Stony Brook, NY, USA). All ^{13}C animal experiments were approved by the regional governmental commission for animal protection (Regierung von Oberbayern, Munich, Germany). Two injections were performed using an 80 mM concentration, allowing for direct comparison. For this set of experiments, a flip angle of 10° was utilized and TR was fixed to 1 s.

3.2. Data Processing. The experimental data $y_{m,i}$ with $m \in \{lac, ala, pyr, bc\}$ acquired at time steps t_i was fitted to MSIM in a constrained least-squares sense; that is,

$$\min_\beta f(\beta) \quad \text{s.t. } lb \le \beta \le ub, \quad (11)$$

with cost function

$$f(\beta) = \sum_m \sum_i \left(y_{m,i} - M_m(t_i, \beta) \right)^2, \quad (12)$$

parameters $\beta = [r_{lac}, \dots, r_{bc}, k_{pyr \to lac}, \dots, k_{pyr \to bc}, I_{pyr}, t_{end}]$, and lower and upper bounds lb and ub, respectively. While

$t_{arrival}$ was fixed to the time when the PYR signal reached 10% of its maximum peak value, t_{end} was set as a fitting parameter accounting for various injection times. On the contrary, the implementation in [8] kept t_{end} fixed while fitting for $t_{arrival}$. Even though the duration of the injection was known, fixing $t_{arrival}$ in function of its peak value and calculating t_{end} as a parameter allowed for different delivery and perfusion times. Delivery, perfusion, and export are however not implicitly included in the model. To improve the convergence properties of the optimization, the gradient of the cost function was calculated analytically. The optimization was carried out using the MATLAB function *fmincon* (MathWorks, Natick, MA, USA) employing the *Trust Region Reflective Algorithm* and a function tolerance of $1E - 10$. The utilized bound constraints were set to physically relevant limits: upper bounds of $0.1\,s^{-1}$ for metabolic conversion rates $k_{pyr \to x}$, since they have been reported to be of a smaller order [8, 23], and of $0.005\,s^{-1}$ for the decay rates r_x (equivalent to a 200 s inverse effective signal decay rate) and lower bounds establishing the positivity of all parameters. Note that the optimization always converged far away from the bounds and they were only implemented for numerical improvement. After optimization, T_1 values were estimated for all metabolites from the effective signal decay rate (see (2) and (9)). Initial conditions were fixed to expected normal parameters; however, randomizing the starting guess in between bounds and performing various iterations yielded comparable results.

Pyruvate-hydrate (PYRH), which is also present in spectroscopy, was not included in the minimization process. The reason for this is that conversion between PYR and PYRH is not enzymatic and we are interested in quantifying metabolic rates that lead to a better understanding of enzymatic activity. Additionally, since chemical exchange with PYRH is instantaneous and almost in equilibrium, including PYR would require adding three extra parameters to the minimization without providing additional information regarding metabolic activity. In fact, if PYRH were to be included, the immediate conversion of PYR to PYRH would lead to an overestimation of the apparent metabolic rate, which in turn would decrease all other parameters intrinsic in R_{pyr} leading to an overestimation of T_1 values for PYR.

The same reasoning holds for the exclusion of additional pools. Although the MSIM model can be further extended to include multiple pools [15, 22], including them only adds variables to the minimization with no direct benefit to the determination of enzymatic conversion rates.

4. Results

4.1. Convergence and Quality of Fit. Parameter fitting with MSIM was shown to converge to an optimal point for every set of experimental data. Figures 1(a)–1(c) show the fitted curves of all metabolites for all models. The residuals for every metabolite and every measurement in the time domain were analyzed (Figures 1(d)–1(f)), and the error of the fitted curves and computed parameters was determined based on the parameter covariance matrix [28]. This error was utilized to determine 95% confidence intervals on the fitted data (see Figures 1(a)–1(c)).

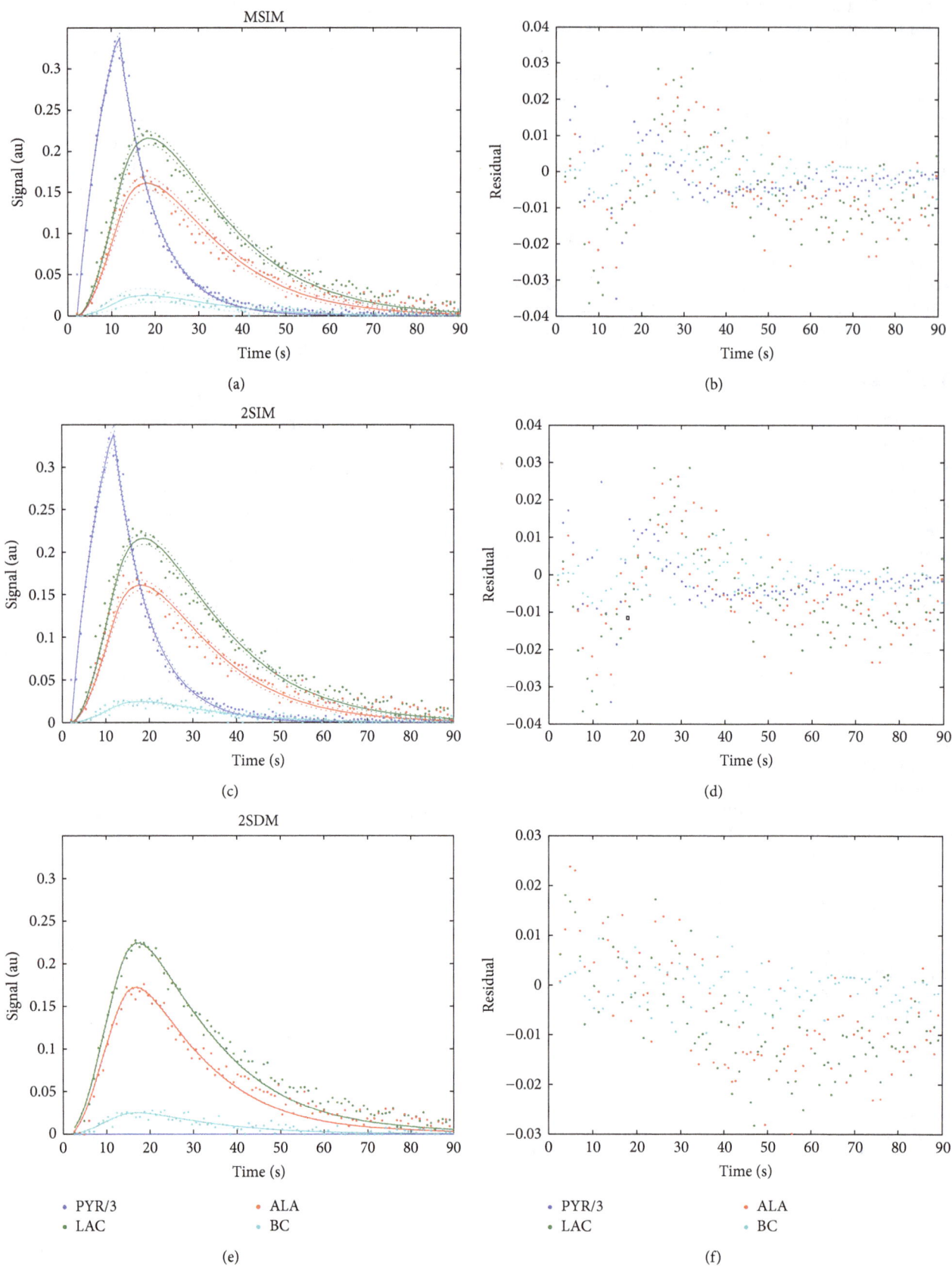

FIGURE 1: Example of metabolic data acquired for a 40 mM (0.2 mmol/kg) dose in kidney predominant tissue, fitted curves (solid lines) using (a) MSIM, (b) 2SIM, and (c) 2SDM and 95% confidence intervals (dotted lines). (d–f) Residuals of fit.

Table 1: Exemplary parameter estimates ($\pm$ standard error) obtained from three different kinetic modeling methods for a $40\,\text{mM}$ ($0.2\,\text{mmol/kg}$) dose of kidney predominant tissue.

Model	MSIM	2SIM	2SDM
$k_{\text{pyr}\rightarrow\text{lac}}$ [s^{-1}]	$0.03194 \pm 9.71E-04$	$0.03202 \pm 7.75E-04$	$0.03448 \pm 1.15E-03$
$k_{\text{pyr}\rightarrow\text{ala}}$ [s^{-1}]	$0.02507 \pm 1.07E-03$	$0.02518 \pm 4.97E-04$	$0.02832 \pm 1.02E-04$
$k_{\text{pyr}\rightarrow\text{bc}}$ [s^{-1}]	$0.00379 \pm 1.51E-03$	$0.00381 \pm 2.67E-04$	$0.00392 \pm 4.48E-04$
$T_{1\text{lac}}$ [s]	16.36 ± 0.620	16.28 ± 0.488	14.13 ± 0.629
$T_{1\text{ala}}$ [s]	14.48 ± 0.752	14.38 ± 0.552	12.18 ± 0.578
$T_{1\text{bc}}$ [s]	14.11 ± 4.78	14.11 ± 1.19	13.46 ± 2.051
$T_{1\text{pyr}}$ [s]	16.67 ± 0.676	16.82 ± 0.845	N/A*

*According to (1), 2SDM only fits for $k_{\text{pyr}\rightarrow x}$ exchange rates and the corresponding T_1 values.

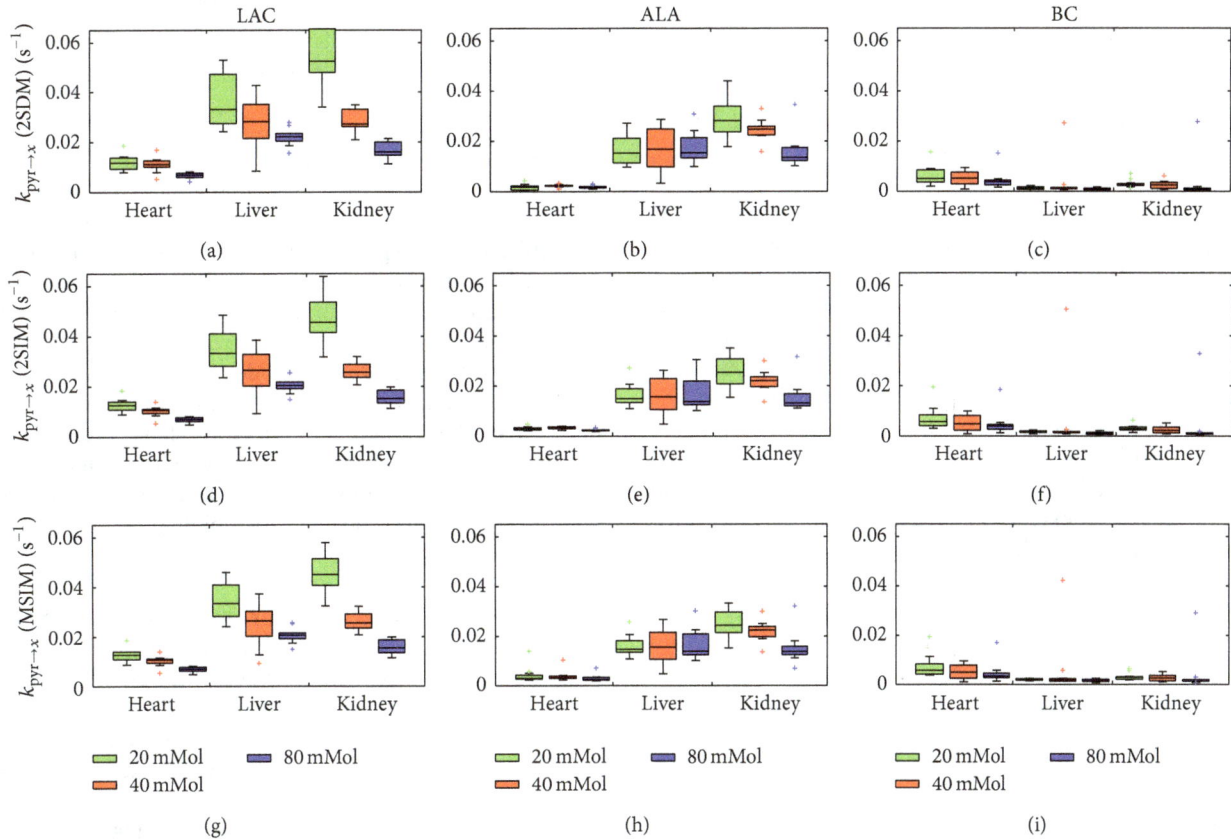

Figure 2: Metabolic conversion rates of LAC (left), ALA (center), and BC (right) obtained for heart, kidney, and liver predominant slices at 20, 40, and 80 mM concentrations (0.1, 0.2, and 0.4 mmol/kg doses) for 2SDM (top), 2SIM (center), and MSIM (bottom). Every box plot displays minima, 25th percentiles, medians, 75th percentiles, maxima, and outliers.

Note that for both MSIM and 2SIM the residuals have a distinct pattern. The pattern indicates that a linear injection rate does not fully model biological activity. In [9], the input function is modeled as a trapezoidal instead of a linear input, but the authors provide no residual analysis. On the other hand, assuming no input function by establishing a fixed initial PYR concentration [25] or solving the differential linear system may not fully account for the entire kinetic time course of the measured signals. In any case, this should be considered as a limitation for both models.

4.2. Model Comparison. For all of the experimental data, parameters were obtained utilizing the 2SDM, the 2SIM, and the MSIM. While a single implementation of MSIM brought

forth parameter values for all downstream metabolites, an independent implementation for LAC, ALA, and BC was necessary in the two-site models. Since all three models were applied on exactly the same experimental data, the comparison between them and to the results obtained for the integrated metabolite signal ratios obtained from Janich et al. [5] directly allows assessing model accuracy separated from biological variability and experiment related inaccuracies like low SNR levels. Results from one exemplary minimization are shown in Table 1; Table 2 displays mean estimated $T_{1\text{pyr}}$ values for all experiments and their respective SNR levels; and Figure 2 details the obtained metabolic conversion rates for all three models.

TABLE 2: T_{1pyr} calculated for MSIM and 2SIM and corresponding SNR levels for all concentrations and slices (mean ± standard deviation).

	T_{1PYR} (MSIM)	T_{1PYR} (2SIM)	SNR
20 mMol			
Heart	8.93 ± 2.68	9.04 ± 2.82	15.52 ± 3.87
Liver	22.14 ± 12.26	24.25 ± 14.28	8.62 ± 2.03
Kidney	27.63 ± 12.11	61.61 ± 91.27	11.63 ± 1.87
40 mMol			
Heart	10.02 ± 2.81	10.17 ± 2.88	44.57 ± 15.56
Liver	20.70 ± 3.72	22.83 ± 8.44	20.14 ± 6.36
Kidney	21.11 ± 7.04	21.73 ± 9.20	27.58 ± 5.38
80 mMol			
Heart	10.85 ± 5.98	10.94 ± 6.11	84.65 ± 32.32
Liver	25.75 ± 7.90	25.88 ± 7.89	23.06 ± 14.60
Kidney	20.69 ± 10.38	20.00 ± 10.33	29.61 ± 12.95

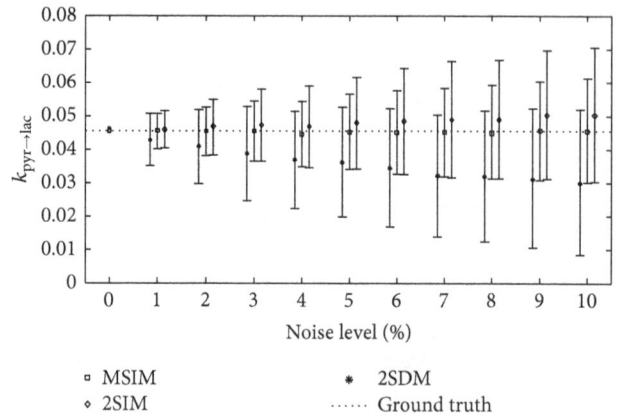

FIGURE 3: Noise level analysis for exemplary simulated data. Error bars show mean ± standard deviation.

Conversion rates and T_{1PYR} values calculated with MSIM tended to be lower than those of 2SIM and these in turn are lower than 2SDM (see Tables 1 and 2). Although performance is very similar for all models, reduced data spread can be observed in PYR to LAC conversion in kidney predominant tissue (Figure 2). Since MSIM fits up to nine parameters simultaneously, estimated error from the parameter covariance matrix was usually higher for MSIM.

Additionally, for an exemplary dataset, a noise analysis of all three models was implemented by adding Gaussian noise to different extent. Parameters were first obtained from an exemplary minimization with MSIM and were then subsequently used for time curve simulation. Every model was then fit 1,000 times with different initial parameters to this simulated time curve to create a model specific ground truth. Finally, based once again on 1,000 iterations, the simulated dataset was corrupted with random Gaussian noise and minimized with each model. Figure 3 displays mean and standard deviation of $k_{pyr \rightarrow lac}$ values up to a 10% noise level.

Figure 3 illustrates that although all models yield the same results in noise-free data, with increasing noise both bias and standard deviation of the two-site models 2SIM and 2SDM increase. As a consequence, the resulting metabolic conversion rates obtained from these two-site models increasingly suffer from systematic under- or overestimation. In contrast, the simulation demonstrates that the MSIM model remains bias-free, even with increased noise level, while exhibiting the smallest standard deviation compared to the two-site models.

From experimental results, it is clear that SNR increases with higher concentrations of injected PYR and that 20 mMol injections in liver and kidney predominant tissue had the lowest SNR (with corresponding noise levels of nearly 10%), whereas SNR in heart was generally higher but had a larger standard deviation (Table 2). According to noise simulations, it is precisely in low SNR regions that MSIM is expected to perform with lower deviations. Standard deviations for T_{1pyr} values and reduced data spread in 20 mMol k_{pyr} quantification, especially in kidney predominant tissue, are indications that this holds.

4.3. Pyruvate Dose Assessment. The effects of PYR dose on Wistar rats were examined through the injection of solutions with concentrations of 20, 40, and 80 mM (doses of 0.1, 0.2, and 0.4 mmol/kg) hyperpolarized PYR. Kinetic data was obtained for all downstream metabolites and visualized with the same box plots used in [5]. With this approach, a direct comparison between the results previously obtained and the results obtained with kinetic modeling could be made, using median values as a distance dimension between the results obtained by the different models, rather than as confirmatory values (see Figure 2). As in [5], all median values suggest saturation effects. A more detailed assessment of the PYR dose effects on metabolism and its biological interpretation can be found in [5].

4.4. Tumor Evaluation. In tumor cells, it is well known that conversion from PYR to LAC is elevated even in the presence of oxygen [29, 30]. Additionally, some tumors show changes in alanine transaminase activity, leading to suppression of conversion of PYR to ALA [31–34]. Both effects were quantified by comparing experimental data obtained from a healthy rat and a rat with mammary carcinoma and using MSIM to obtain conversion rate parameters (see Figure 4). It can be seen that, for the same dose, the $k_{pyr \rightarrow lac}$ conversion rate was more than four times larger in tumor cells than healthy cells and the $k_{pyr \rightarrow ala}$ rate was more than 18 times larger in healthy cells than tumor cells. Therefore, obtained conversion rates provide a quantitative metric of metabolic differences between healthy and tumor cells.

5. Discussion and Conclusion

Three different kinetic modeling methods were implemented and investigated for the quantification of time-dependent metabolite levels. The two-site exchange differential model (2SDM) and two-site exchange integral model (2SIM) assume a two-site interaction between pyruvate (PYR) and one specific metabolite. The proposed multisite exchange integral model (MSIM) takes into account various downstream metabolites in one system and allows fitting in a one-step process. That is, all of the parameters are generated in a single

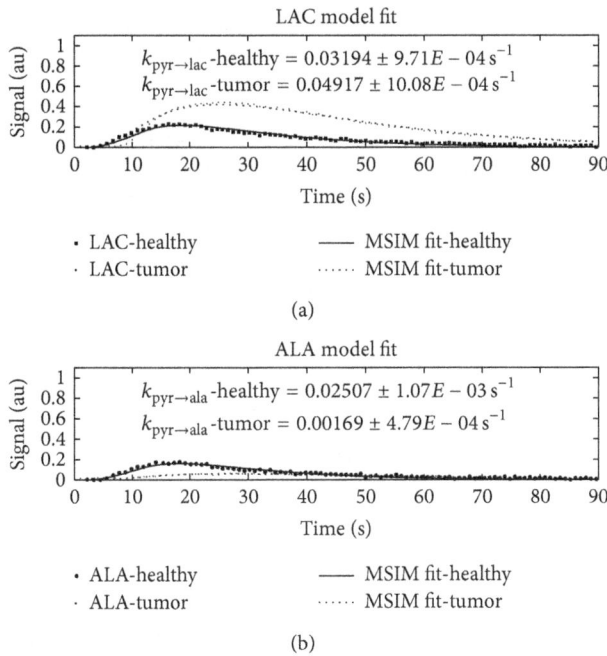

FIGURE 4: Comparison of $k_{\mathrm{pyr}\to\mathrm{lac}}$ and $k_{\mathrm{pyr}\to\mathrm{ala}}$ conversion rates between a healthy rat (from an 80 mM dose in kidney predominant tissue) and a rat with mammary carcinoma.

minimization, avoiding the need for separate implementations for every specific metabolite and resulting in a robust, optimal convergence far from the imposed constraints.

The three models were compared by taking median values as a distance dimension and, using exemplary simulated data, performing a noise analysis. In this analysis, metabolic exchange rate values obtained with 2SDM and 2SIM showed a bias with increasing noise levels. On the other hand, MSIM showed almost no bias, maintaining the average computed value close to the ground truth even at high noise levels, with smaller standard deviations than 2SDM and 2SIM.

Using the experimental data of [5], all kinetic models were compared between different PYR concentrations to assess the effect of increased PYR doses on *in vivo* metabolism. Results obtained from all three kinetic models were very similar; however, MSIM yielded smaller data spread for metabolic conversion in low SNR experiments and more accurate effective T_1 values for PYR as downstream metabolite rates are taken into account during the optimization, while effective T_1-estimation in 2SIM requires postprocessing corrections.

MSIM was then further utilized to evaluate model performance in disease. Obtained conversion rates from MSIM showed significant differences in healthy cells in comparison to tumor cells, where LAC conversion was elevated and ALA conversion, on the other hand, was suppressed.

Extending two-site models into a multisite model yields both biological and numerical insight. Biologically, it has been shown that calculated rates give proof of the saturation effects studied in [5] and can be used to quantify metabolic differences between normal and tumor cells. Numerically, a one-step fitting process with parameter interdependency

performs marginally better than other fitting methods, particularly in regions with low SNR. Further work with the MSIM model will focus on pixelwise metabolic mapping of cellular activity and its application to different metabolic systems.

Abbreviations

x:	Index of downstream metabolites: lactate, alanine, bicarbonate, and pyruvate-hydrate
$k_{\mathrm{pyr}\to x}$:	Metabolic conversion rate from pyruvate to x
LDH:	Lactate dehydrogenase
ALT:	Alanine transaminase
PDH:	Pyruvate dehydrogenase
CA:	Carbonic anhydrase
2SDM:	Two-site differential model
2SIM:	Two-site integral model
MSIM:	Multisite integral model
$M_x(t)$:	Time dependent signal for metabolite x
$M_{\mathrm{pyr}}(t)$:	Time dependent pyruvate signal
$f(\mathrm{FA})$:	Flip angle function
t_{arrival}:	Time of pyruvate arrival
t_{end}:	Time at which pyruvate is no longer injected
I_{pyr}:	Pyruvate injection rate
r_x:	Metabolite signal decay
r_{pyr}:	Pyruvate signal decay rate without metabolic conversion rates
R_{pyr}:	Pyruvate signal decay rate including metabolic conversion rates
lb:	Vector of lower bounds
ub:	Vector of upper bounds
m:	Index of all metabolites (lactate, alanine, pyruvate, and bicarbonate)
t_i:	Sampling times
β:	Vector of optimization parameters
$y_{m,i}$:	Measured data point for metabolite m and time step t_i
$M_m(t,\beta)$:	Time dependent signal of metabolite m as a function of parameters β.

Conflict of Interests

Marion I. Menzel, Jonathan I. Sperl, Martin A. Janich, Florian Wiesinger, and Rolf F. Schulte are employed by GE Global Research. All other authors declare that there is no conflict of interests regarding the publication of this paper.

Acknowledgments

This work was funded by BMBF MOBITUM Grant no. 01EZ0826/7 and BMBF Grant no. 13EZ1114. The authors take responsibility for the content of the paper. Pedro A. Gómez Damián acknowledges the support from the German Academic Exchange Service (DAAD) and the Modality of Professional Experience (MEP) from the Tecnológico de Monterrey.

References

[1] K. M. Brindle, "NMR methods for measuring enzyme kinetics *in vivo*," *Progress in Nuclear Magnetic Resonance Spectroscopy*, vol. 20, no. 3, pp. 257–293, 1988.

[2] J. H. Ardenkjær-Larsen, B. Fridlund, A. Gram et al., "Increase in signal-to-noise ratio of >10,000 times in liquid-state NMR," *Proceedings of the National Academy of Sciences of the United States of America*, vol. 100, no. 18, pp. 10158–10163, 2003.

[3] K. Golman, R. In 't Zandt, and M. Thaning, "Real-time metabolic imaging," *Proceedings of the National Academy of Sciences of the United States of America*, vol. 103, no. 30, pp. 11270–11275, 2006.

[4] M. E. Bizeau, C. Short, J. S. Thresher, S. R. Commerford, W. T. Willis, and M. J. Pagliassotti, "Increased pyruvate flux capacities account for diet-induced increases in gluconeogenesis in vitro," *American Journal of Physiology*, vol. 281, no. 2, pp. R427–R433, 2001.

[5] M. A. Janich, M. I. Menzel, F. Wiesinger et al., "Effects of pyruvate dose on *in vivo* metabolism and quantification of hyperpolarized ^{13}C spectra," *NMR in Biomedicine*, vol. 25, no. 1, pp. 142–151, 2012.

[6] H. J. Atherton, M. A. Schroeder, M. S. Dodd et al., "Validation of the *in vivo* assessment of pyruvate dehydrogenase activity using hyperpolarised ^{13}C MRS," *NMR in Biomedicine*, vol. 24, no. 2, pp. 201–208, 2011.

[7] S. E. Day, M. I. Kettunen, F. A. Gallagher et al., "Detecting tumor response to treatment using hyperpolarized 13C magnetic resonance imaging and spectroscopy," *Nature Medicine*, vol. 13, no. 11, pp. 1382–1387, 2007.

[8] M. L. Zierhut, Y.-F. Yen, A. P. Chen et al., "Kinetic modeling of hyperpolarized ^{13}C$_1$-pyruvate metabolism in normal rats and TRAMP mice," *Journal of Magnetic Resonance*, vol. 202, no. 1, pp. 85–92, 2010.

[9] D. M. Spielman, D. Mayer, Y.-F. Yen, J. Tropp, R. E. Hurd, and A. Pfefferbaum, "In vivo measurement of ethanol metabolism in the rat liver using magnetic resonance spectroscopy of hyperpolarized [1-^{13}C]pyruvate," *Magnetic Resonance in Medicine*, vol. 62, no. 2, pp. 307–313, 2009.

[10] O. Khegai, R. F. Schulte, M. A. Janich et al., "Apparent rate constant mapping using hyperpolarized [1-^{13}C]pyruvate," *NMR in Biomedicine*, vol. 27, no. 10, pp. 1256–1265, 2014.

[11] J. M. Park, S. Josan, T. Jang et al., "Metabolite kinetics in C6 rat glioma model using magnetic resonance spectroscopic imaging of hyperpolarized [1-^{13}C]pyruvate," *Magnetic Resonance in Medicine*, vol. 68, no. 6, pp. 1886–1893, 2012.

[12] S. Josan, D. Spielman, Y.-F. Yen, R. Hurd, A. Pfefferbaum, and D. Mayer, "Fast volumetric imaging of ethanol metabolism in rat liver with hyperpolarized [1-^{13}C]pyruvate," *NMR in Biomedicine*, vol. 25, no. 8, pp. 993–999, 2012.

[13] M. I. Kettunen, D.-E. Hu, T. H. Witney et al., "Magnetization transfer Measurements of exchange between hyperpolarized [1-^{13}C]pyruvate and [1-^{13}C]lactate in a murine lymphoma," *Magnetic Resonance in Medicine*, vol. 63, no. 4, pp. 872–880, 2010.

[14] P. E. Z. Larson, A. B. Kerr, C. Leon Swisher, J. M. Pauly, and D. B. Vigneron, "A rapid method for direct detection of metabolic conversion and magnetization exchange with application to hyperpolarized substrates," *Journal of Magnetic Resonance*, vol. 225, pp. 71–80, 2012.

[15] C. Harrison, C. Yang, A. Jindal et al., "Comparison of kinetic models for analysis of pyruvate-to-lactate exchange by hyperpolarized ^{13}C NMR," *NMR in Biomedicine*, vol. 25, no. 11, pp. 1286–1294, 2012.

[16] D. K. Hill, M. R. Orton, E. Mariotti et al., "Model free approach to kinetic analysis of real-time hyperpolarized ^{13}C magnetic resonance spectroscopy data," *PLoS ONE*, vol. 8, no. 9, Article ID e71996, 2013.

[17] L. Z. Li, S. Kadlececk, H. N. Xu et al., "Ratiometric analysis in hyperpolarized NMR (I): test of the two-site exchange model and the quantification of reaction rate constants," *NMR in Biomedicine*, vol. 26, no. 10, pp. 1308–1320, 2013.

[18] F. A. Gallagher, M. I. Kettunen, and K. M. Brindle, "Biomedical applications of hyperpolarized ^{13}C magnetic resonance imaging," *Progress in Nuclear Magnetic Resonance Spectroscopy*, vol. 55, no. 4, pp. 285–295, 2009.

[19] M. F. Santarelli, V. Positano, G. Giovannetti et al., "How the signal-to-noise ratio influences hyperpolarized ^{13}C dynamic MRS data fitting and parameter estimation," *NMR in Biomedicine*, vol. 25, no. 7, pp. 925–934, 2012.

[20] M. E. Merritt, C. Harrison, C. Storey, F. M. Jeffrey, A. D. Sherry, and C. R. Malloy, "Hyperpolarized ^{13}C allows a direct measure of flux through a single enzyme-catalyzed step by NMR," *Proceedings of the National Academy of Sciences of the United States of America*, vol. 104, no. 50, pp. 19772–19777, 2007.

[21] S. M. Kazan, S. Reynolds, A. Kennerley et al., "Kinetic modeling of hyperpolarized 13C pyruvate metabolism in tumors using a measured arterial input function," *Magnetic Resonance in Medicine*, vol. 70, no. 4, pp. 943–953, 2013.

[22] C. Yang, C. Harrison, E. S. Jin et al., "Simultaneous steady-state and dynamic ^{13}C NMR can differentiate alternative routes of pyruvate metabolism in living cancer cells," *The Journal of Biological Chemistry*, vol. 289, no. 9, pp. 6212–6224, 2014.

[23] F. Wiesinger, I. Miederer, M. I. Menzel et al., "Metabolic rate constant mapping of hyperpolarized 13C pyruvate," ISMRM 3282, 2010.

[24] L. Vanhamme, A. van den Boogaart, and S. van Huffel, "Improved method for accurate and efficient quantification of mrs data with use of prior knowledge," *Journal of Magnetic Resonance*, vol. 129, no. 1, pp. 35–43, 1997.

[25] T. Harris, G. Eliyahu, L. Frydman, and H. Degani, "Kinetics of hyperpolarized ^{13}C$_1$-pyruvate transport and metabolism in living human breast cancer cells," *Proceedings of the National Academy of Sciences of the United States of America*, vol. 106, no. 43, pp. 18131–18136, 2009.

[26] T. Xu, D. Mayer, M. Gu et al., "Quantification of in vivo metabolic kinetics of hyperpolarized pyruvate in rat kidneys using dynamic ^{13}C MRSI," *NMR in Biomedicine*, vol. 24, no. 8, pp. 997–1005, 2011.

[27] J. D. Shearer, G. P. Buzby, J. L. Mullen, E. Miller, and M. D. Caldwell, "Alteration in pyruvate metabolism in the liver of tumor-bearing rats," *Cancer Research*, vol. 44, no. 10, pp. 4443–4446, 1984.

[28] D. M. Bates and D. G. Watts, *Nonlinear Regression Analysis and Its Applications*, John Wiley & Sons, New York, NY, USA, 2008.

[29] O. Warburg, "On the origin of cancer cells," *Science*, vol. 123, no. 3191, pp. 309–314, 1956.

[30] H. Lu, R. A. Forbes, and A. Verma, "Hypoxia-inducible factor 1 activation by aerobic glycolysis implicates the Warburg effect in carcinogenesis," *The Journal of Biological Chemistry*, vol. 277, no. 26, pp. 23111–23115, 2002.

[31] W. Droge, H.-P. Eck, H. Kriegbaum, and S. Mihm, "Release of L-alanine by tumor cells," *The Journal of Immunology*, vol. 137, no. 4, pp. 1383–1386, 1986.

[32] L. Brennan, C. Hewage, J. P. G. Malthouse, and G. J. McBean, "Gliotoxins disrupt alanine metabolism and glutathione production in C6 glioma cells: a ^{13}C NMR spectroscopic study," *Neurochemistry International*, vol. 45, no. 8, pp. 1155–1165, 2004.

[33] H. R. Harding, F. Rosen, and C. A. Nichol, "Depression of Alanine Transaminase Activity in the Liver of Rats Bearing Walker Carcinoma 256," *Cancer Research*, vol. 24, pp. 1318–1323, 1964.

[34] S. M. Ronen, A. Volk, and J. Mispelter, "Comparative NMR study of a differentiated rat hepatoma and its dedifferentiated subclone cultured as spheroids and as implanted tumors," *NMR in Biomedicine*, vol. 7, no. 6, pp. 278–286, 1994.

13

Technical Considerations of Phosphorous-32 Bremsstrahlung SPECT Imaging after Radioembolization of Hepatic Tumors

Elahe Pirayesh,[1] Mahasti Amoui,[1] Shahram Akhlaghpoor,[2] Shahnaz Tolooee,[3] Maryam Khorrami,[1] Hossain PoorBeigi,[3] Shahab Sheibani,[3] and Majid Assadi[4]

[1] Department of Nuclear Medicine, Shohada-e-Tajrish Medical Center, Shahid Beheshti University of Medical Sciences, Tehran, Iran
[2] Department of Interventional Radiology, Noor Medical Imaging Center, Tehran, Iran
[3] Department of Nuclear Sciences, Iranian Atomic Energy Organization, Tehran, Iran
[4] The Persian Gulf Nuclear Medicine Research Center, Bushehr University of Medical Sciences, Bushehr, Iran

Correspondence should be addressed to Majid Assadi; assadipoya@yahoo.com

Academic Editor: David Maintz

Background. Bremsstrahlung (BS) imaging during radioembolization (RE) confirms the deposition of radiotracer in hepatic/extrahepatic tumors. The aim of this study is to demonstrate ^{32}P images and to optimize the imaging parameters. *Materials and Methods.* Thirty-nine patients with variable types of hepatic tumors, treated with the intra-arterial injection of ^{32}P, were included. All patients underwent BS SPECT imaging 24–72 h after tracer administration, using low energy high resolution (LEHR) (18 patients) or medium energy general purpose (MEGP) (21 patients) collimators. A grading scale from 1 to 4 was used to express the compatibility of the ^{32}P images with those obtained from CT/MRI. *Results.* Although the image quality obtained with the MEGP collimator was visually and quantitatively better than with the LEHR (76% concordance score versus 71%, resp.), there was no statistically significant difference between them. *Conclusion.* The MEGP collimator is the first choice for BS SPECT imaging. However, if the collimator change is time consuming (as in a busy center) or an MEGP collimator is not available, the LEHR collimator could be practical with acceptable images, especially in a SPECT study. In addition, BS imaging is a useful method to confirm the proper distribution of radiotherapeutic agents and has good correlation with anatomical findings.

1. Introduction

Radioembolization (RE) is a promising therapeutic modality for patients with unresectable hepatic tumors. In this procedure, radioisotopes preferentially localize in the peritumoral and intratumoral arterial vasculature, while exposure to the normal hepatic parenchyma remains within tolerable limits. RE is based on the predominant arterial blood supply of hepatic tumoral lesions by the hepatic artery, in contrast to normal liver parenchyma, which is mainly supplied by the portal vein [1, 2]. Therapeutic agents are properly sized pharmaceuticals which incorporate the β radiating isotopes, such as ^{90}Y, ^{188}Re, and ^{166}Ho [3–5]. The clinical applications of these β+ emitters for the treatment of different kinds

of malignant and nonmalignant diseases are increasing [6]. Posttreatment imaging confirms the distribution of radiotracers within the target organ, or an additional unexpected deposition [7]. These data help the physician to predict the patient's response to RE therapy or the probable side effects [7].

In this study, phosphorus-32 (^{32}P) particles were used for the RE of hepatic tumors. Phospherous-32, a pure β+ emitter available as a therapeutic radiopharmaceutical since the 1960s, has many suitable features for radioembolization therapy, such as a long half-life (14.3 days) and a maximum energy of 1.7 MeV. However, secondary photon emissions, called Bremsstrahlung (BS), produce a broad spectrum of limited energies and, therefore, compromise the selection of energy windows and collimation, as well as the reconstruction of the SPECT images [8, 9].

Most studies which assess the parameters for the BS imaging of pure β emitters (e.g., ^{32}P or ^{90}Y) have used phantoms [9–16], and there is a gap in the comprehensive research to evaluate these factors in clinical practice. This study was designed to optimize the imaging parameters, including the energy window and collimator type for BS imaging. In addition, we evaluated the correlation of this technique with the anatomical findings in patients with hepatic tumors being treated with RE.

2. Materials and Methods

A total of 39 patients with unresectable hepatic or metastatic tumors of any origin, which were candidates for RE [17] with ^{32}P particles, were included in this study. The chromic phosphate ^{32}P radiopharmaceutical, with a mean size of 50–150 μm and a mean injected activity of 260 MBq (75–450 MBq), was produced locally at the research reactor (IAEO, Iran). Calculations of the appropriate radiation dose were undertaken according to the following formula: dose (Gy) = 7.3 × activity (mCi)/hepatic mass (kg) [18].

This study complies with the declaration of Helsinki and was approved by the institutional ethics committee of the Shahid Beheshti University of Medical Sciences, and all patients provided written informed consent.

2.1. Anatomical Imaging. Cross-sectional imaging with a CT or MRI was accomplished for all patients in order to determine the size and location of the lesions as numerical segments consistent with the physiological division of Couinaud [19]. The findings were reported by a radiologist, and the liver volume was calculated.

2.2. Radioembolization Procedure. The standard angiographic method for the assessment of the femoral artery was used [20]. The celiac and superior mesenteric arteries were catheterized using a Cordis Simon I catheter, and DSA angiography was prepared using a Siemens' C-Arm Angiography Unit. Superselective catheterization was done using Cook's 3F microcatheter and ^{32}P particles were injected into the artery. Afterwards, a postembolization angiogram was obtained [21].

2.3. Bremsstrahlung Imaging. Imaging was conducted 24–72 hours after the RE of the hepatic tumors. The imaging system consisted of a Siemens single head e.cam gamma camera equipped with a low energy high resolution (LEHR) or a medium energy general purpose (MEGP) collimator. In order to select the window setting, the BS energy spectra with the LEHR and MEGP collimators were obtained using a 37 MBq ^{32}P point source, in a glass vial placed at a distance of 10 cm from the collimator in the center of the field of view (FOV). An energy window setting of 100 keV ± 25% was chosen.

All patients were randomly divided into two groups, A and B. In group A, planar and SPECT imaging were done with the LEHR collimator, whereas an MEGP collimator was used in group B. Planar imaging was performed in the anterior and posterior projections of the upper abdomen for 10 minutes, using a 64 × 64 matrix. In the SPECT study, the data were acquired in a 64 × 64 matrix for 64 projections over 360°, for a period of 30 seconds per projection. Raw data were reconstructed from either filtered-back projections or iterative (ordered subsets expectation maximization (OSEM)) methods [22]. The OSEM method with four iterations and two subsets was selected as the method of choice for the reconstruction due to fewer image distortions. The images were reconstructed in transaxial, sagittal, and coronal slices.

2.4. Image Interpretation. The images obtained from the SPECT and CT/MRI were evaluated visually by two nuclear medicine specialists and one radiologist in a blinded and independent fashion. A linear black and white scale with a lower and upper threshold of 0% and 100%, respectively, was used for all planar and SPECT images. The distribution of ^{32}P in the liver was assessed and reported as focal or multifocal lesions in the involved segments. Based on the compatibility of the ^{32}P images with anatomical findings (CT/MRI), a grading system proposed by Boan et al. [23] was applied per patient as grade 4 for poor correlation, grade 3 for intermediate correlation, grade 2 for good correlation, and grade 1 for a perfect match. In cases of disagreement between the physicians, a consensus was reached. The extrahepatic activity was also reported.

2.5. Statistical Analysis. Continuous variables were expressed as the mean ± SD, and categorical variables were expressed as absolute values and percentages. A 2-tailed t-test was used to compare the mean values between the groups. The Mann-Whitney U test was used to compare the statistical differences between the LEHR and the MEGP collimators as a grading system. A P value of less than 0.05 was considered statistically significant. All statistical analyses were performed using an IBM computer and the SPSS Inc. PASW software, version 18.0.

3. Results

Thirty-nine patients with a variety of hepatic tumoral lesions were treated with RE and evaluated (Table 1). The choice of energy window shows the ^{32}P BS energy spectra taken with a gamma camera equipped with the LEHR and MEGP collimators (Figure 1). In contrast to the standard gamma emitters, the energy spectrum of the BS is very complex, with no pronounced photopeak. The lowest detectable energy in the spectra is about 25 keV, with a peak of around 75 and 150 keV. Considering these spectra, the energy window was set at 100 keV ± 25% for all measurements. The number of measured photons was significantly reduced with the MEGP resulting in a reduced sensitivity.

Regarding the effect of the collimator type, 18 patients in group A were imaged with the LEHR collimator and 21 patients in group B, with the MEGP collimator. In addition, the planar and SPECT images from the LEHR and MEGP collimators were obtained (Figure 2). A comparison of the

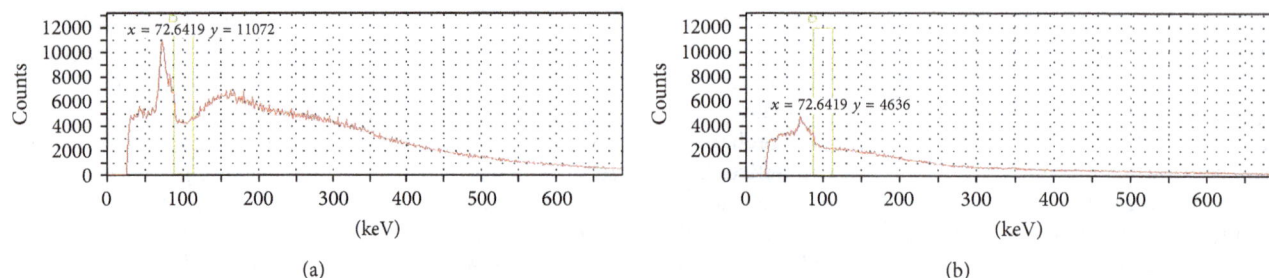

FIGURE 1: P-32 Bremsstrahlung energy spectra with (a) LEHR collimator and (b) MEGP collimator, obtained using a 37 MBq ^{32}P point source, in a glass vial, at a distance of 10 cm from the collimator.

TABLE 1: Characteristics of patients treated with RE.

Age	54 yr. (27–78)
Sex	$n = 39$
Male	20
Female	19
Primary cancer	
Colon	25
Breast	5
HCC	3
Carcinoid	3
Pancreas	1
Lung	2

TABLE 2: Correlation grading for compatibility of ^{32}P images obtained by the LEHR collimator and the MEGP collimator, with anatomical findings.

	LEAP	MEGP	Total
Score 1	1	2	3
Score 2	4	3	7
Score 3	6	8	14
Score 4	7	8	15
Total	18	21	39

CT/MRI and BS SPECT images as the correlative grading score between the MEGP and LEAP collimators is summarized in Table 2. There is a good or perfect correlation with the anatomical findings (scores 1 and 2) in 13 (71%) BS images from group A (LEHR collimator), and in 16 (76%) from group B (MEGP collimator). However, this difference is not statistically significant (P value = 0.9). Taken as a whole, in 29 patients (74%) the BS images have a satisfactory concordance (Figure 3). A perfect concordance of the SPECT and CT images of a necrotic tumor is demonstrated in Figure 4.

Some unusual findings were also recorded. The extrahepatic accumulation of the radiotracer was observed in the spleen of two patients, duodenum of one patient, and the pancreas of one patient (see Figure 5).

4. Discussion

The application of the β+ emitting radionuclides for the treatment of malignant and nonmalignant conditions is increasing [6]. In these cases, imaging can be performed by measuring the BS photons emitted from the β particles as they lose their energy in the body [24]. BS radiation is not ideal for diagnostic purposes, because of the continuous energy range, interseptal penetration of high energy photons, and the creation of photons far from the radiation emission site [9, 10]. Despite these problems, BS imaging is important in confirming the satisfactory delivery, pharmacokinetics, and potential abnormal deposition of the radiotracer [16, 25–29]. Furthermore, it has been demonstrated that BS imaging

is useful for the direct quantification and dosimetry of β-emitter isotopes in clinical practice [4, 30–32]. We evaluated optimized parameters for ^{32}P BS imaging after the RE of the hepatic tumors, and to our knowledge, this is the first clinical study to assess these factors to improve image quality.

As a result of the complexity of the spectrum and the absence of a pronounced photopeak, the task of selecting a suitable energy window was particularly difficult. Furthermore, the optimal energy window for a particular beta emitter is still a matter of debate within the research community [24]. Considering the ^{32}P BS spectrum (Figure 1) and the results of other studies [26, 30, 33, 34], the energy window of 100 keV + 25% was selected. As shown in Figure 1, the lower energy (about 75 keV) of the ^{32}P BS energy spectra is compatible with the X-ray characteristics due to the interaction of the high energy BS photons which lead the septa of the collimator. The rise in the spectrum of about 150 keV reflects the penetration of the septa of the collimators by higher energy. The same phenomenon has been previously reported in ^{32}P, ^{90}Y, and ^{89}Sr BS measurements with a gamma camera [9–11, 13, 15, 27]. Although the maximum energies of ^{32}P and ^{90}Y are different (1.7 MeV vs. 2.27 MeV), their BS spectra appear to be similar. Ito et al. [11] compared different energy windows for BS ^{90}Y imaging and concluded that images obtained with an energy window of 120 keV + 15% provided the highest resolution and lowest uncertainty. Shen et al. [9] showed that the best and most practical selection is an energy window of 55–285 keV. Therefore, the selection of the energy window varies with each study. Some researchers select narrow energy windows [16, 26, 34, 35], while others prefer wider ranges [7, 10, 29] depending on the purpose of the imaging; if the goal is

Anterior 205 K duration: 600 s 64 × 64   Anterior 72 K duration: 600 s 64 × 64

(a)

(b)

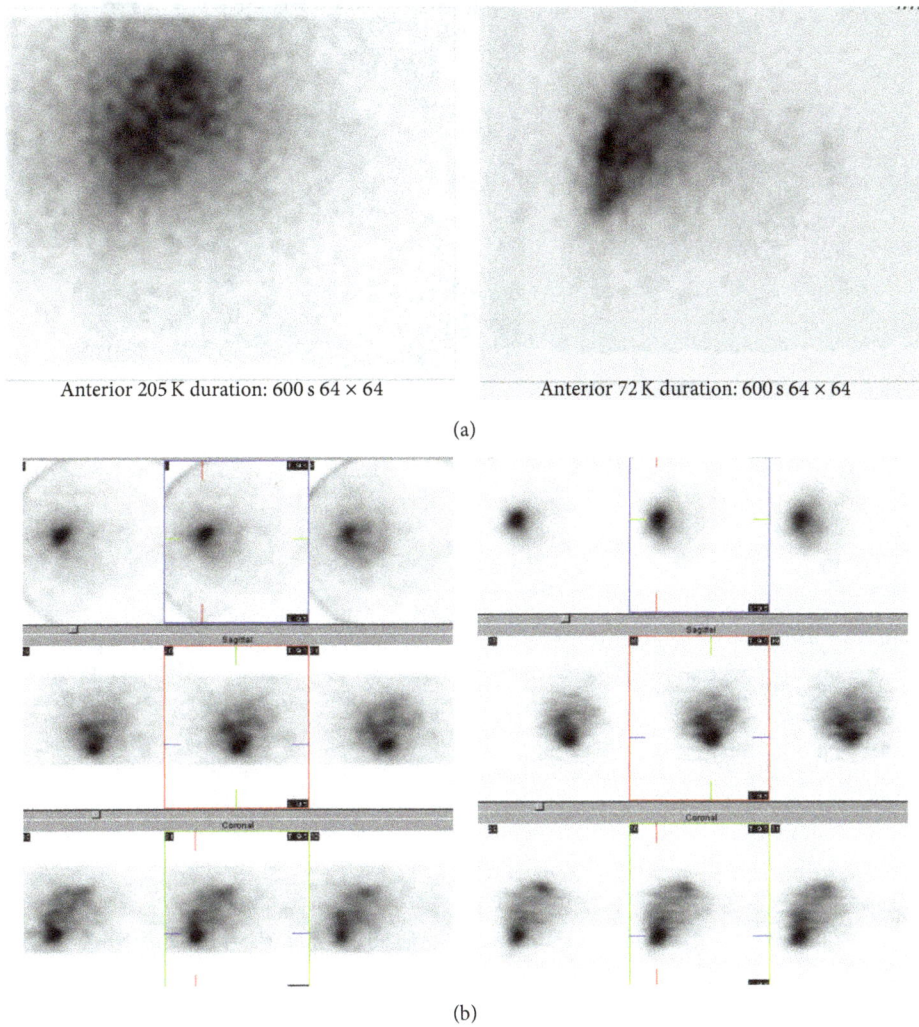

FIGURE 2: A patient with metastatic colon cancer treated with 333 MBq ^{32}P particles. (a) Bremsstrahlung ^{32}P images in planar study with LEHR and MEGP collimators. (b) Bremsstrahlung ^{32}P images in SPECT study with LEHR and MEGP collimators.

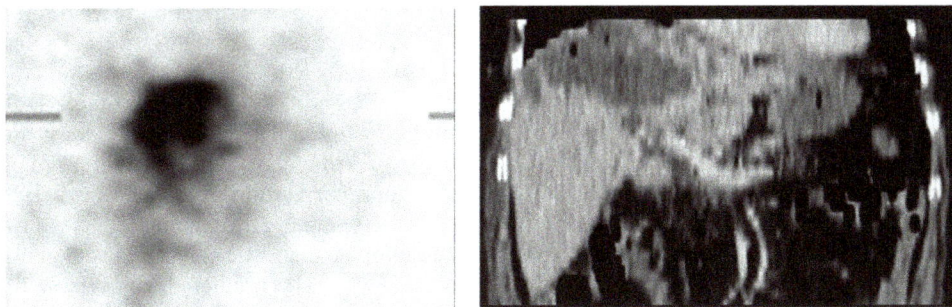

FIGURE 3: A patient with metastatic colon cancer treated with 296 MBq ^{32}P particles. It shows a perfect concordance of Bremsstrahlung and CT images (grade 1).

accurate localization of distributed activity, a narrower range is ideal.

In this study, we examined the collimator type for ^{32}P BS imaging. Thirty-nine patients were divided into two groups, with an LEHR collimator in group A and an MEGP collimator in group B. The other imaging parameters were similar in both groups. In comparison to the anatomical images, the concordance scores of the SPECT images in groups A and B were statistically insignificant. The MEGP collimator created higher quality images because of lower septal penetration background activity, compared to the LEHR. Meanwhile, the LEHR collimator did create acceptable images, particularly

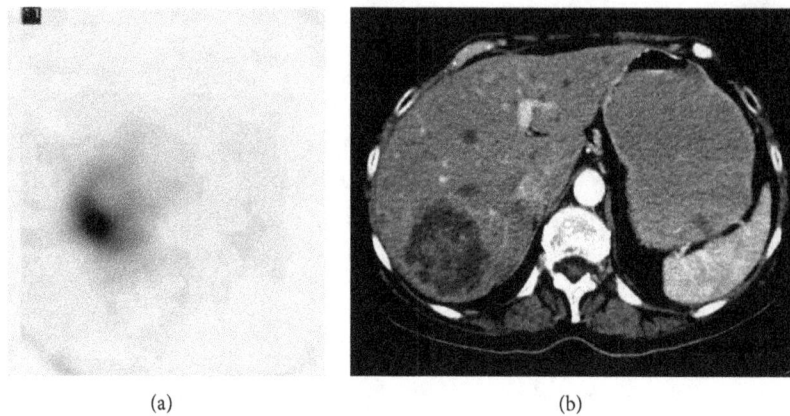

(a)   (b)

FIGURE 4: (a) Enlarged necrotic tissue secondary to previous chemoembolization (nonradioactive lipiodol) and (b) correlated CT slice.

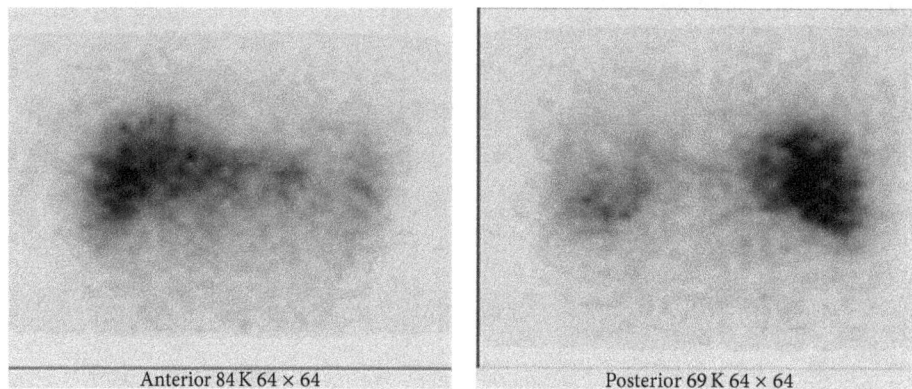

Anterior 84 K 64 × 64   Posterior 69 K 64 × 64

FIGURE 5: Unusual findings of splenic activity visualized after RE with ^{32}P particles.

in the SPECT study (Figures 2 and 3). In a quantitative study on the planar images using the phantom, Shen et al. [9] showed that the sensitivity of the LEAP collimator was three times better than that of the MEGP collimator, whereas the system resolution of the MEGP collimator was three times better than that of the LEAP collimator. Similar results were obtained by Cipriani et al. [15] and Shukla et al. [13]. Therefore, most researchers working on BS imaging have used ME [7, 10, 11, 15, 25–30, 33–37] or HE collimators [16, 32].

In this study, we selected the narrow energy window and used the LEHR collimator (instead of the LEAP), which relatively improved the system resolution. In addition, compared to planar images, the SPECT method improves lesion contrast and anatomical clarity by the removal of superimposed radioactivity [38]. These factors influenced lesion detectability; thus, it could be concluded that the MEGP collimator is the best choice for BS SPECT imaging. However, if the collimator change is time-consuming (as in a busy center) or the MEGP collimator is not available, the LEHR collimator could be practical as it creates acceptable images, especially in SPECT studies.

Despite the inherently poor resolution of BS imaging, as our previous study showed, there is a relatively good correlation between BS imaging and the CT/MRI or other nuclear medicine studies [39]. Mansberg et al. [28] showed that BS

images have anatomical correlations with sites containing maximum tumor density. Similarly, Tehranipour et al. [37] described concordant findings from the ^{18}F-FDG PET and ^{90}Y-Bremsstrahlung scans after the RE of a hepatic tumor in one case report. The correspondence of the ^{99}mTc-MDP and ^{89}Sr BS images was also reported [15, 35, 40].

Our study showed a relatively good correlation between the SPECT and CT/MRI images (Table 2). The results of this study reveal that BS SPECT images have adequate resolution for posttreatment evaluations, and that 74 percent of patients have good correlation or a perfect match with the CT/MRI images, confirming the technically appropriate localization of the radiopharmaceuticals. As such, a potential good response to therapy can be predicted. Conversely, a poor correlation could be due to small metastatic lesions undetectable in BS images because of an inherently low spatial resolution. Furthermore, the distribution of particles could be affected during intra-arterial injections by vessel selection, the flow in a selected vessel, or the size and amount of the injected particles. Discordant findings can also be related to technical errors (such as a superselective intra-arterial injection) during the RE, or poor vascularized hepatic tumors, thereby leading to the accumulation of radiotracers in normal tissues [26, 33, 41]. In contrast to concordance cases, the therapeutic response will not be ideal in discordant cases because of inadequate radiation to the target [26]. We will, however, evaluate the clinical applications of the anticipated grading system in an ongoing study.

The potential advantage of ^{32}P scintigraphy is its ability to depict the vascularity of viable tumor cells rather than the necrotic tissue of a tumor mass (Figure 5). Therefore, BS imaging of P-32 after the RE of the hepatic tumors can be reflective of vascularized and viable tumoral tissues [33].

The extrahepatic deposition of radiotracers is an important finding, which can assist physicians in subsequent treatment planning. The extrahepatic activity in the spleen (Figure 4), lung, and GI tract can have probable unwanted complications. In addition, because of the lower delivered radiation dose to the target, failure in the treatment can be predicted. Ahmadzadehfar et al. demonstrated the importance of BS imaging to predict RE-induced extrahepatic side effects [29]. Sebastian et al. [26] have also reported gastric ulcerations as a result of microspheres entering into an aberrant gastric artery.

It should be mentioned that the current study had some limitations. One of the most important drawbacks is its small sample size. Another limitation is that we did not perform an angiogram with Tc-MAA to rule out a possible high lung shunt; however, further evidence needs to be acquired.

5. Conclusion

Despite the shortcomings of BS imaging, good quality images can be obtained by the optimization of the energy window and collimator type. BS imaging of ^{32}P, after the RE of hepatic tumors, can confirm the hepatic and extrahepatic distribution of radiotracers to predict the patient's response to RE therapy. This study shows that an LEHR collimator may produce acceptable images, especially for the SPECT.

Conflict of Interests

The authors declare that there is no conflict of interests regarding the publication of this paper.

References

[1] C. van de Wiele, L. Defreyne, M. Peeters, and B. Lambert, "Yttrium-90 labelled resin microspheres for treatment of primary and secondary malignant liver tumors," *Quarterly Journal of Nuclear Medicine and Molecular Imaging*, vol. 53, no. 3, pp. 317–324, 2009.

[2] R. J. Lewandowski, J.-F. Geschwind, E. Liapi, and R. Salem, "Transcatheter intraarterial therapies: rationale and overview," *Radiology*, vol. 259, no. 3, pp. 641–657, 2011.

[3] F. Giammarile, L. Bodei, C. Chiesa et al., "EANM procedure guideline for the treatment of liver cancer and liver metastases with intra-arterial radioactive compounds," *European Journal of Nuclear Medicine and Molecular Imaging*, vol. 38, no. 7, pp. 1393–1406, 2011.

[4] X.-D. Wang, R.-J. Yang, X.-C. Cao, J. Tan, and B. Li, "Dose delivery estimated by bremsstrahlung imaging and partition model correlated with response following intra-arterial radioembolization with 32p-glass microspheres for the treatment of

[5] H. Ahmadzadehfar, H.-J. Biersack, and S. Ezziddin, "Radioembolization of liver tumors with yttrium-90 microspheres," *Seminars in Nuclear Medicine*, vol. 40, no. 2, pp. 105–121, 2010.

[6] J. S. Welsh, "Beta decay in science and medicine," *American Journal of Clinical Oncology: Cancer Clinical Trials*, vol. 30, no. 4, pp. 437–439, 2007.

[7] H. Ahmadzadehfar, A. Sabet, M. Muckle et al., "^{99m}Tc-MAA/90Y-Bremsstrahlung SPECT/CT after simultaneous Tc-MAA/^{90}Y-microsphere injection for immediate treatment monitoring and further therapy planning for radioembolization," *European Journal of Nuclear Medicine and Molecular Imaging*, vol. 38, no. 7, pp. 1281–1288, 2011.

[8] S. Vinjamuri and S. Ray, "Phosphorus-32: the forgotten radiopharmaceutical?" *Nuclear Medicine Communications*, vol. 29, no. 2, pp. 95–97, 2008.

[9] S. Shen, G. L. DeNardo, A. Yuan, D. A. DeNardo, and S. J. DeNardo, "Planar gamma camera imaging and quantitation of yttrium-90 bremsstrahlung," *Journal of Nuclear Medicine*, vol. 35, no. 8, pp. 1381–1389, 1994.

[10] L. P. Clarke, S. J. Cullom, R. Shaw et al., "Bremsstrahlung imaging using the gamma camera: factors affecting attenuation," *Journal of Nuclear Medicine*, vol. 33, no. 1, pp. 161–166, 1992.

[11] S. Ito, H. Kurosawa, H. Kasahara et al., "90Y bremsstrahlung emission computed tomography using gamma cameras," *Annals of Nuclear Medicine*, vol. 23, no. 3, pp. 257–267, 2009.

[12] A. K. Shukla, S. C. Kheruka, E. Werner et al., "Localization and quanification of incorporated beta emitting radionuclides using bremsstrahlung imaging," *Indian Journal of Nuclear Medicine*, vol. 21, pp. 27–31, 2006.

[13] A. K. Shukla, S. C. Kheruka, M. lassmann et al., "Standardization of organ specific bremsstrahlung imaging using whole body phantom," *Journal of Medical Physics*, vol. 30, no. 1, pp. 1–13, 2005.

[14] E. Rault, S. Vandenberghe, S. Staelens, R. Van Holen, and I. Lemahieu, "Optimization of Y90 bremsstrahlung image reconstruction using multiple energy window subsets," *Journal of Nuclear Medicine*, vol. 49, supplement 1, p. 399P, 2008.

[15] C. Cipriani, G. Atzei, G. Argirò et al., "Gamma camera imaging of osseous metastatic lesions by strontium-89 bremsstrahlung," *European Journal of Nuclear Medicine*, vol. 24, no. 11, pp. 1356–1361, 1997.

[16] S. M. Rhymer, J. A. Parker, and M. R. Palmer, "Detection of ^{90}Y extravasation by bremsstrahlung imaging for patients undergoing ^{90}Y-ibritumomab tiuxetan therapy," *Journal of Nuclear Medicine Technology*, vol. 38, no. 4, pp. 195–198, 2010.

[17] K. T. Sato, R. J. Lewandowski, M. F. Mulcahy et al., "Unresectable chemorefractory liver metastasis: radioembolization with Y90 microspheres-safety," *Radiology*, vol. 247, no. 2, pp. 507–515, 2008.

[18] R. V. P. Mantravadi, D. G. Spigos, and S. M. Karesh, "Work in progress: intra-arterial P-32 chromic phosphate for prevention of postoperative liver metastases in high-risk colorectal cancer patients," *Radiology*, vol. 148, no. 2, pp. 555–559, 1983.

[19] C. Couinaud, "Liver anatomy: portal (and suprahepatic) or biliary segmentation," *Digestive Surgery*, vol. 16, no. 6, pp. 459–467, 1999.

[20] S. Nathan and S. V. Rao, "Radial versus femoral access for percutaneous coronary intervention: implications for vascular complications and bleeding," *Current Cardiology Reports*, vol. 14, pp. 502–509, 2012.

hepatocellular carcinoma," *Journal of Gastrointestinal Surgery*, vol. 14, no. 5, pp. 858–866, 2010.

[21] A. Kennedy, S. Nag, R. Salem et al., "Recommendations for radioembolization of hepatic malignancies using yttrium-90 microsphere brachytherapy: a consensus panel report from the radioembolization brachytherapy oncology consortium," *International Journal of Radiation Oncology Biology Physics*, vol. 68, no. 1, pp. 13–23, 2007.

[22] S. Vandenberghe, Y. D'Asseler, R. van de Walle et al., "Iterative reconstruction algorithms in nuclear medicine," *Computerized Medical Imaging and Graphics*, vol. 25, no. 2, pp. 105–111, 2001.

[23] J. F. Boan, M. Valero, and J. Arbizu, *Improving Treatment Design by Image Fusion Techniques. Liver Embolization with Y-90 Microspheres*, Springer, Berlin, Germany, 2008.

[24] Y. D'Asseler, "Advances in SPECT imaging with respect to radionuclide therapy," *Quarterly Journal of Nuclear Medicine and Molecular Imaging*, vol. 53, no. 3, pp. 343–347, 2009.

[25] B. Petri, R. Nance, J. Hanada, and J. Stevens, "P-32 bremsstrahlung SPECT helps assess intracavitary therapy," *Clinical Nuclear Medicine*, vol. 17, no. 9, pp. 709–710, 1992.

[26] A. J. Sebastian, T. Szyszko, A. Al-Nahhas, K. Nijran, and N. P. Tait, "Evaluation of hepatic angiography procedures and bremsstrahlung imaging in selective internal radiation therapy: a two-year single-center experience," *CardioVascular and Interventional Radiology*, vol. 31, no. 3, pp. 643–649, 2008.

[27] W. D. Kaplan, R. E. Zimmerman, and W. D. Bloomer, "Therapeutic intraperitoneal 32P: a clinical assessment of the dynamics of distribution," *Radiology*, vol. 138, no. 5, pp. 683–688, 1981.

[28] R. Mansberg, N. Sorensen, V. Mansberg, and H. van der Wall, "Yttrium 90 Bremsstrahlung SPECT/CT scan demonstrating areas of tracer/tumour uptake," *European Journal of Nuclear Medicine and Molecular Imaging*, vol. 34, no. 11, p. 1887, 2007.

[29] H. Ahmadzadehfar, M. Muckle, A. Sabet et al., "The significance of bremsstrahlung SPECT/CT after yttrium-90 radioembolization treatment in the prediction of extrahepatic side effects," *European Journal of Nuclear Medicine and Molecular Imaging*, vol. 39, no. 2, pp. 309–315, 2012.

[30] J. A. Siegel, S. Whyte-Ellis, L. S. Zeiger, S. E. Order, and P. E. Wallner, "Bremsstrahlung SPECT imaging and volume quantitation with 32 Phosphorus," *Antibody, Immunoconjugates, and Radiopharmaceuticals*, vol. 7, no. 1, pp. 1–10, 1994.

[31] D. Minarik, K. Sjögreen-Gleisner, O. Linden et al., "90Y bremsstrahlung imaging for absorbed-dose assessment in high-dose radioimmunotherapy," *Journal of Nuclear Medicine*, vol. 51, no. 12, pp. 1974–1978, 2010.

[32] D. Minarik, M. Ljungberg, P. Segars, and K. S. Gleisner, "Evaluation of quantitative planar 90Y bremsstrahlung whole-body imaging," *Physics in Medicine and Biology*, vol. 54, no. 19, pp. 5873–5883, 2009.

[33] H. Nguyen, G. Ghanem, R. Morandini et al., "Tumor type and vascularity: important variables in infusional brachytherapy with colloidal 32P," *International Journal of Radiation Oncology Biology Physics*, vol. 39, no. 2, pp. 481–487, 1997.

[34] E. I. Parsai, K. M. Ayyangar, R. R. Dobelbower, and J. A. Siegel, "Clinical fusion of three-dimensional images using Bremsstrahlung SPECT and CT," *Journal of Nuclear Medicine*, vol. 38, no. 2, pp. 319–324, 1997.

[35] M. Uchiyama, H. Narita, M. Makino et al., "Strontium-89 therapy and imaging with bremsstrahlung in bone metastases," *Clinical Nuclear Medicine*, vol. 22, no. 9, pp. 605–609, 1997.

[36] G. Hines, S. Spencer, J. Markert, S. Shen, and L. Bender, "Confirmation of Phosphorus-32 (P-32) administration for malignant brain tumor treatment using bremsstrahlung imaging with a gamma camera," *Journal of Nuclear Medicine*, vol. 48, supplement 2, p. 447P, 2007.

[37] N. Tehranipour, A. Al-Nahhas, R. Canelo et al., "Concordant F-18 FDG PET and Y-90 Bremsstrahlung scans depict selective delivery of Y-90-microspheres to liver tumors: confirmation with histopathology," *Clinical Nuclear Medicine*, vol. 32, no. 5, pp. 371–374, 2007.

[38] L. Sherman and P. Goodwin, "SPECT Instrumentation: performance, lesion detection and recent innovations," *Seminars in Nuclear Medicine*, vol. 17, pp. 184–199, 1987.

[39] M. Amoui, E. Pirayesh, S. Akhlaghpoor et al., "Correlation between CT/MRI and bremsstrahlung SPECT of32 after radioembolization of hepatic tumors," *Iranian Journal of Radiology*, vol. 7, no. 1, pp. 1–5, 2010.

[40] H. Narita, M. Uchiyama, T. Ooshita et al., "Imaging of strontium-89 uptake with bremsstrahlung using NaI scintillation camera," *Kakuigaku*, vol. 33, no. 11, pp. 1207–1212, 1996.

[41] Y. H. Kao, E. H. Tan, T. K. B. Teo, C. E. Ng, and S. W. Goh, "Imaging discordance between hepatic angiography versus Tc-99m-MAA SPECT/CT: a case series, technical discussion and clinical implications," *Annals of Nuclear Medicine*, vol. 25, no. 9, pp. 669–676, 2011.

14

Central Nervous System Tuberculosis: An Imaging-Focused

Morteza Sanei Taheri,[1] **Mohammad Ali Karimi,**[1] **Hamidreza Haghighatkhah,**[1]
Ramin Pourghorban,[1] **Mohammad Samadian,**[2] **and Hosein Delavar Kasmaei**[3]

[1]*Department of Radiology, Shohada-e-Tajrish Hospital, Shahid Beheshti University of Medical Sciences, Tehran, Iran*
[2]*Department of Neurosurgery, Loghman Hakim Hospital, Shahid Beheshti University of Medical Sciences, Tehran, Iran*
[3]*Department of Neurology, Shohada-e-Tajrish Hospital, Shahid Beheshti University of Medical Sciences, Tehran, Iran*

Correspondence should be addressed to Mohammad Ali Karimi; mkarimidr@yahoo.com

Academic Editor: Paul Sijens

Central nervous system (CNS) tuberculosis is a potentially life threatening condition which is curable if the correct diagnosis is made in the early stages. Its clinical and radiologic manifestations may mimic other infectious and noninfectious neurological conditions. Hence, familiarity with the imaging presentations of various forms of CNS tuberculosis is essential in timely diagnosis, and thereby reducing the morbidity and mortality of this disease. In this review, we describe the imaging characteristics of the different forms of CNS tuberculosis, including meningitis, tuberculoma, miliary tuberculosis, abscess, cerebritis, and encephalopathy.

1. Introduction

With the outbreak of acquired immunodeficiency syndrome (AIDS) and increasing frequency of other immunocompromising conditions in recent decades, tuberculosis has resurged and remained a major worldwide health problem. Although *Mycobacterium tuberculosis* can involve any organ, most commonly the lung, central nervous system (CNS) tuberculosis is the most devastating form of the disease. Approximately 5–10% of all patients with tuberculosis and up to 20% of patients with AIDS-related tuberculosis have CNS involvement [1–3].

CNS tuberculosis usually results from hematogenous spread, while direct spread from intra- or extracranial focus is rare [4]. The clinical and radiologic manifestations of CNS tuberculosis may mimic other infectious and noninfectious neurological conditions, such as brain tumors. Therefore, familiarity of infectious diseases specialists with the imaging presentations of CNS tuberculosis is essential for prompt and accurate diagnosis of this entity. Herein, we describe the different forms of CNS tuberculosis including meningitis, cerebritis, cerebral abscesses, tuberculomas, miliary tuberculosis, and spinal or calvarial involvement [5–7].

2. Tuberculous Meningitis

Meningitis is the most common manifestation of CNS tuberculosis which is most frequently seen in the children and adolescents [8, 9]. Tuberculous meningitis is mostly due to the hematogenous spread of *Mycobacterium tuberculosis*; however, it can also occur secondary to extension and/or rupture of a subpial or subependymal focus (i.e., Rich focus) to the subarachnoid spaces or into the ventricular system [10]. Tuberculous meningitis often has an insidious course with a nonspecific clinical presentation in early stages, especially in children. Therefore, the imaging plays a key role in the timely diagnosis and decreasing the morbidity and mortality.

Enhancing exudate in the basal cisterns is the most common and also a relatively specific manifestation of leptomeningeal tuberculosis on computed tomography (CT) and magnetic resonance (MR) images [11]. The exudate is composed of neutrophils, mononuclear cells, erythrocytes, and

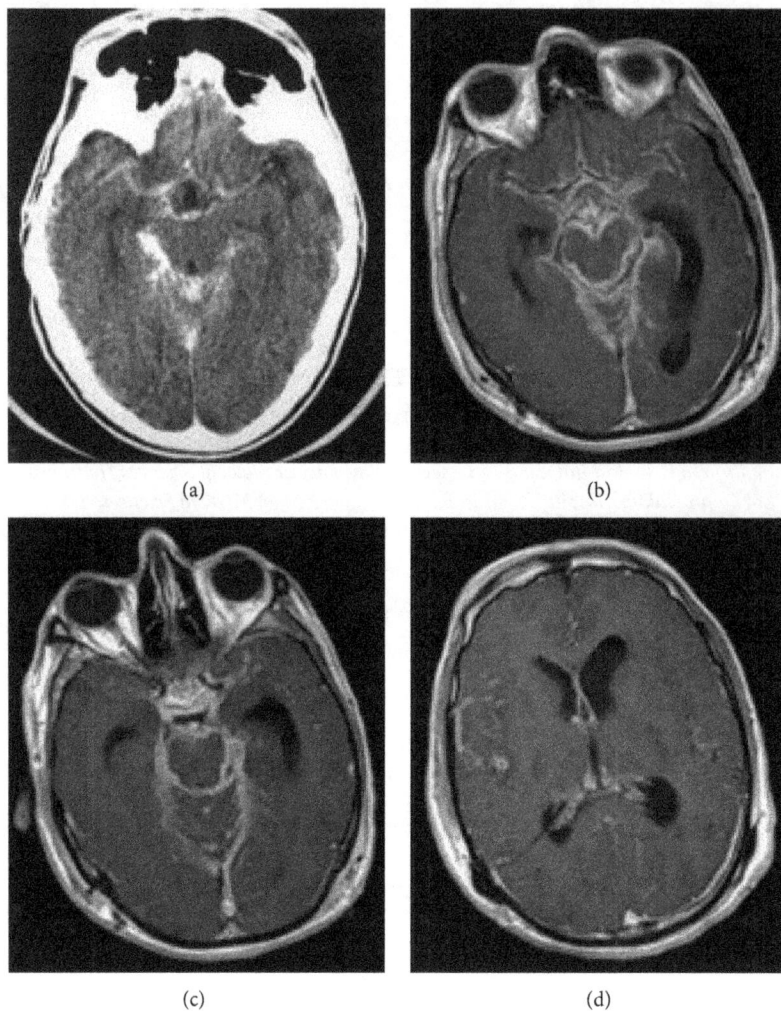

FIGURE 1: Meningeal tuberculosis. (a) Axial postcontrast brain CT shows typical thick enhancement of basilar cisterns. (b) Axial postcontrast T1-weighted MR images in a different patient ((b), (c), and (d)) demonstrate enhancing basilar exudates and leptomeningeal enhancement. A small tuberculoma in right temporal region (d) and hydrocephaly (more severe in left ventricle) and the evidence of prior craniotomy (Burr hole, left pneumoventricle) are also evident.

bacilli in the basal portions of the brain. Meningeal enhancement has been found in up to 90% of cases and is considered to be the most sensitive feature of tubercular meningitis [6, 11, 12]. The subpial exudate is primarily located in the inferomedial surface of the frontal lobes, the anteromedial surface of the temporal lobes, the superior aspect of the cerebellum, and the floor of the third ventricle [13]. Extension to suprasellar, interpeduncular, and pontomesencephalic cisterns may also occur from these primary sites [10]. In most cases, some degree of meningeal involvement is seen within the sulci over the cerebral convexities, the sylvian fissures, and also the ependymal surfaces of the ventricles; the latter usually occurs in the later stages of the disease [1, 14, 15].

On CT images, the obliteration of the basal cisterns by isodense or mildly hyperdense exudates is the most common finding in tuberculous meningitis [1, 6, 13, 16]. The findings are better appreciated on MR imaging than on CT, especially on postcontrast MR images which show the enhancing cisternal exudates and leptomeningeal enhancement (Figure 1) [5].

Parmar et al. demonstrated that postcontrast fluid attenuation inversion recovery (FLAIR) images may have a higher specificity compared to contrast-enhanced T1-weighted images in detection of leptomeningeal enhancement [17]. Magnetization transfer spin echo imaging following contrast injection is superior to the conventional postcontrast imaging in demonstrating meningeal inflammation [7]. In later stages, there may be widening of subarachnoid spaces.

A similar pattern of meningeal enhancement may be seen in other infective meningitis, inflammatory diseases such as rheumatoid arthritis, sarcoidosis, or carcinomatous meningitis [7].

Other radiologic manifestations of tuberculous meningitis may be related to its possible complications, including progressive hydrocephalus, vasculitis, infarction, and cranial neuropathies [6, 7].

Communicating hydrocephalus, which is considered the most common complication of tuberculous meningitis, is usually secondary to the obstruction of cerebrospinal fluid

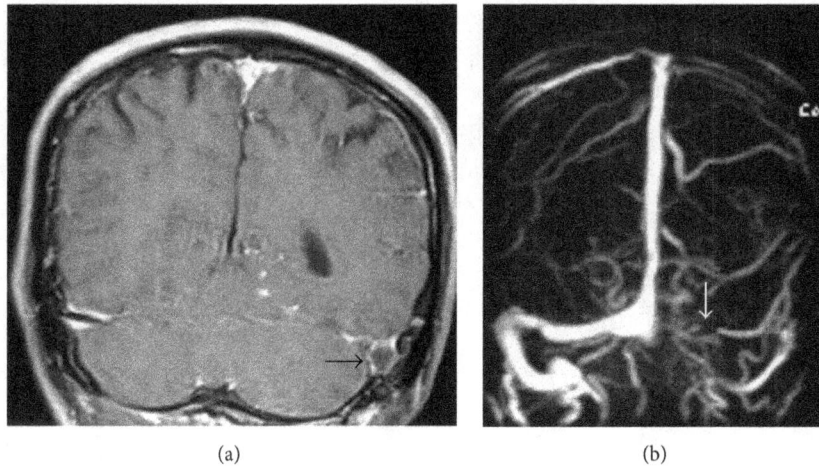

FIGURE 2: Dural venous sinus thrombosis as an only imaging evidence of tuberculous meningitis in a 45-year-old male who presented with headache and cerebrospinal fluid PCR positive for *Mycobacterium tuberculosis*. (a) Coronal postcontrast T1-weighted MR image demonstrates a filing defect within dilated left sigmoid sinus (*black arrow*). (b) MR angiogram reveals nonvisualization of transverse and sigmoid sinuses in left side (*white arrow*).

(CSF) flow in the basal cisterns [1, 4, 6, 7]. In some cases, the hydrocephalus may be noncommunicating, resulting from obstruction due to tuberculoma or rarely tuberculous abscess.

Ischemic infarct is also a common complication, being detected in 20–41% of patients on CT, mostly within the basal ganglia or internal capsule regions and resulting from vascular compression and occlusion of small perforating vessels (necrotizing arteritis) [14, 18, 19], particularly the lenticulostriate and thalamoperforating arteries, vessels which perfuse the so-called medial tuberculosis zone [16]. Tuberculous meningitis may also cause dural venous sinus thrombosis with resultant hemorrhagic infarct. Rarely, tuberculosis may present as isolated dural venous sinus thrombosis without any evidence of meningitis or its complications (Figure 2).

Cranial nerve involvement occurs due to vascular compromise, ischemia, or nerve entrapment in the basal exudates in 17–40% of cases, most commonly affecting the second, third, fourth, and seventh cranial nerves [13, 15]. The affected cranial nerves are best evaluated by MRI, where they may appear thickened, especially in their proximal segments, with high signal intensity on T2-weighted images and marked enhancement on postcontrast images.

3. Parenchymal Tuberculosis

Parenchymal disease may be isolated or associated with tuberculous meningitis. Parenchymal involvement usually presents as tuberculoma. It can also manifest as cerebritis, cerebral abscess, miliary tuberculosis, or tuberculosis encephalopathy.

3.1. Cerebritis and Cerebral Abscess. Parenchymal tuberculosis may occur with or without accompanying meningitis. Tuberculosis cerebritis or abscess may have an appearance similar to that of pyogenic bacterial infection on neuroimaging studies.

Focal tuberculous cerebritis is very rare [5], with hypo- and hypersignal intensities on T1- and T2-weighted images, respectively, and causes small areas of patchy enhancement on postcontrast images.

Tuberculous abscess is rare and is characterized by a central area of liquefaction with pus. It may be solitary or multiple and is frequently multiloculated (Figure 3) [15]. Tuberculous abscess is different from tuberculomas which contain central caseation and liquefaction mimicking pus. The tuberculous abscess is hypodense with peripheral edema and mass effect on CT. On T2-weighted images, central necrotic area has increased signal intensity. Postcontrast images demonstrate ring enhancement that is usually thin and uniform, although it may be irregular and thick (Figure 4), especially in immunocompromised patients [1, 3, 6, 7, 20, 21].

Magnetization transfer (MT) images improve the conspicuity of all CNS tuberculosis lesions [22–27]. On MR spectroscopy, the peak of amino acids, which could be detected in pyogenic abscess, is not usually seen in tuberculous abscess [22, 27].

3.2. Tuberculoma. Tuberculoma is the most common parenchymal lesion in CNS tuberculosis which could be found in any portion of the intracranial space. The lesion may be solitary or multiple and may be seen with or without meningitis. Histologically, the mature tuberculoma is composed of a necrotic caseous center surrounded by a capsule that contains fibroblasts, epithelioid cells, Langhans giant cells, and lymphocytes [28].

On nonenhanced CT scans, tuberculoma may be isodense, hyperdense, or of mixed density. On contrast-enhanced CT, it may present a pattern of ring-like enhancement or, less likely, as an area of nodular or irregular nonhomogeneous enhancement. A central nidus of calcification with surrounding ring-like enhancement, known as the target sign, suggests the diagnosis [19]. Nonenhanced MR studies show a mixed, predominantly low signal intensity lesion with

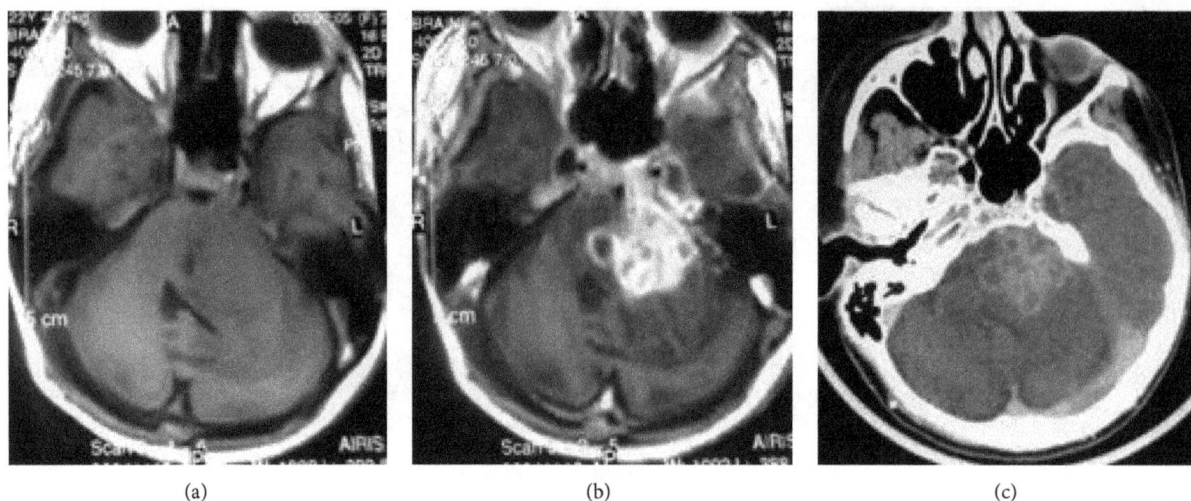

(a)   (b)   (c)

FIGURE 3: Tuberculous abscess mimicking a cerebellopontine angle tumor in a 22-year-old female with miliary pulmonary tuberculosis, right hemiparesis, left facial paresis, and sixth and seventh cranial nerves involvement. Axial T1-weighted image (a) shows a predominantly isosignal lesion in the left hemisphere of cerebellum with extension to CPA and prepontine cistern accompanied by marked peripheral edema and mass effect. Multilobulated enhancement of the lesion is seen in the postcontrast T1-weighted (b) and CT (c) images.

a central zone of high signal intensity and surrounding high signal intensity edema on T2-weighted or FLAIR images [29]. The central high signal intensity zone corresponds to caseating necrosis, and the low signal intensity of the capsule may be related to a layer of collagenous fibrosis with high protein concentration and low water content [29].

Like contrast-enhanced CT, postcontrast MR images usually show a pattern of ring-like enhancement (Figure 5).

Caseating solid granulomas are usually hypointense and strikingly hypointense on T1- and T2-weighted images, respectively. This relative hypointensity is attributed to the granulation tissue and compressed glial tissue in the central core resulting in a greater cellular density than the brain parenchyma. Noncaseating granulomas do not show typical imaging pattern and are usually hypointense to isointense on T1-weighted and hyperintense on T2-weighted images. Homogeneous enhancement is seen after administration of contrast media [7].

Follow-up CT or MR studies are useful in monitoring the response to medical treatment. Paradoxical enlargement of a preexisting tuberculoma or evolution of a new intracranial and spinal tuberculoma in patients receiving adequate treatment may be occasionally seen. However, with continuation of antituberculous therapy, eventual resolution of the tuberculoma usually occurs [29, 30].

Sometimes, healed tuberculomas appear as calcified foci on nonenhanced CT (Figure 6). Similarly, calcification in the basal cisterns has been demonstrated a few years after meningeal tuberculosis [31].

3.3. Miliary Tuberculosis. Miliary tuberculosis is seen mostly in severely immunocompromised patients and is usually associated with meningeal involvement or extracranial primary sites [32]. Since the dissemination is hematogenous,

the lesions are usually located at the corticomedullary junctions. The lesions are tiny (2-3 mm in diameter) scattered lesions that may be invisible on noncontrast MR sequences (Figures 7(a) and 7(b)). In visible lesions, MRI shows small lesions that are hypointense on T2-weighted sequences. These lesions occasionally can be seen as small hypodensities on CT scan [13].

Postcontrast T1-weighted MR images show numerous, round, small, homogeneous, enhancing (usually ring enhancement) lesions (Figure 7(c)) [22]. Invisible lesions that may or may not enhance after intravenous injection of gadolinium can be clearly visible on magnetization transfer spin echo T1-weighted imaging with or without contrast [23].

3.4. Tuberculous Encephalopathy. Tuberculous encephalopathy typically occurs in young children who may present with convulsion, stupor, and coma with no signs of meningeal irritation or focal neurological deficit. Neuroimaging studies show severe cerebral edema, which may be unilateral or bilateral. Myelin loss in the white matter may result in hypodensity on CT images and hyperintensity on T2-weighted MR images [7, 10, 33].

4. Miscellaneous Forms of CNS Tuberculosis

Osseous and nonosseous spinal/spinal cord tuberculosis, subdural/epidural abscess, and calvarial tuberculosis (Figure 8) are other forms of tuberculosis that may involve CNS with direct or indirect pathways.

Tuberculous spinal meningitis presents on MR imaging as a CSF loculation and obliteration of the spinal subarachnoid space, with loss of the outline of the spinal cord in the cervicothoracic spine and matting of the nerve roots in the lumbar region. Contrast-enhanced imaging reveals nodular,

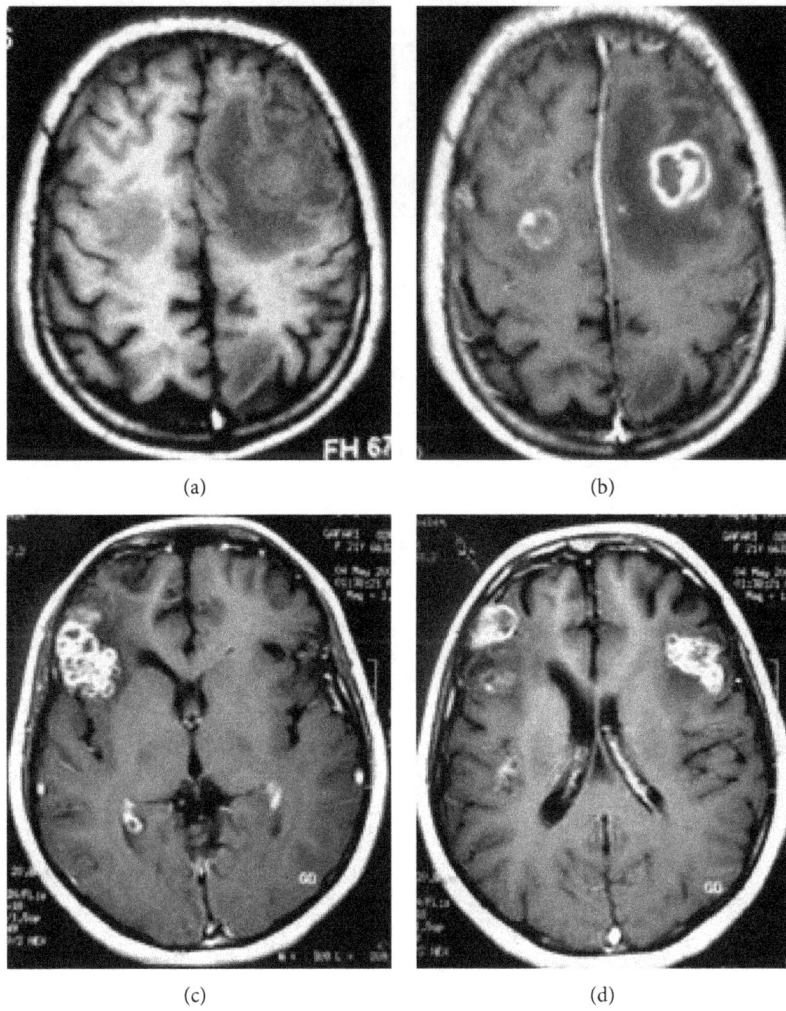

(a)

(b)

(c)

(d)

FIGURE 4: Tuberculous brain abscess. Axial pre- and postcontrast T1-weighted MR images ((a) and (b)) in a 38-year-old male with cognitive and speech disorders show two hypointense lesions in both frontal lobes with peripheral edema, which is severe on left side, and have thick ring-like enhancement (b). (c) and (d) Axial postcontrast T1-weighted MR images in a 22-year-old female with pulmonary miliary tuberculosis and 3-month history of headache, nausea, vomiting, and recent seizure demonstrate bifrontal irregularly enhancing lesions with mild peripheral edema.

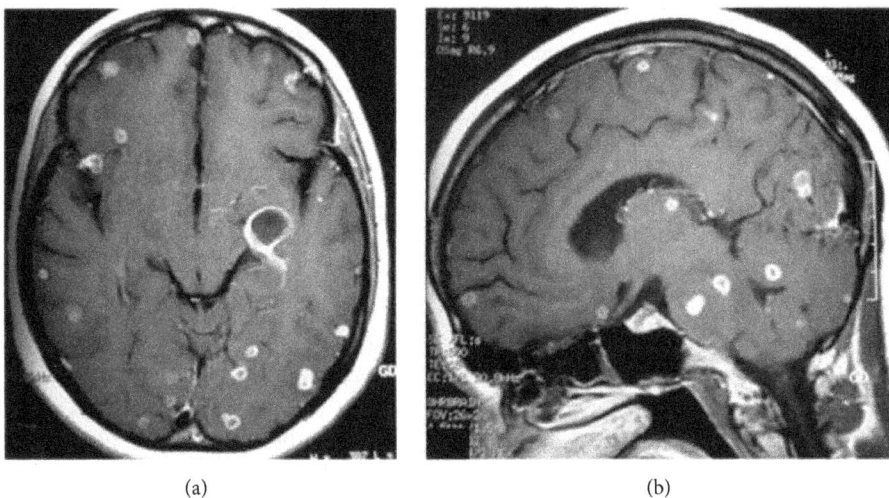

(a)

(b)

FIGURE 5: Multiple supra- and infratentorial tuberculomas in a 27-year-old female with history of pulmonary tuberculosis. Tuberculomas are seen as multiple small ring enhancing lesions without peripheral edema in axial and sagittal postcontrast T1-weighted MR images.

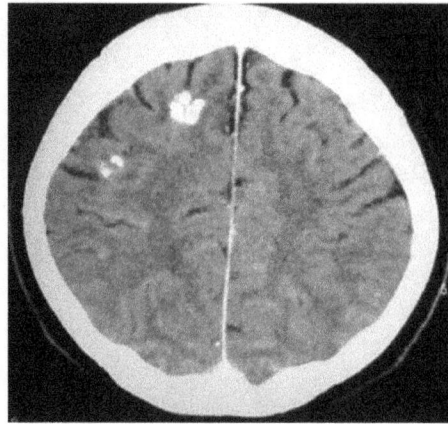

FIGURE 6: Treated tuberculoma. Axial noncontrast CT image shows two calcified lesions in right frontal lobe without edema or mass effect.

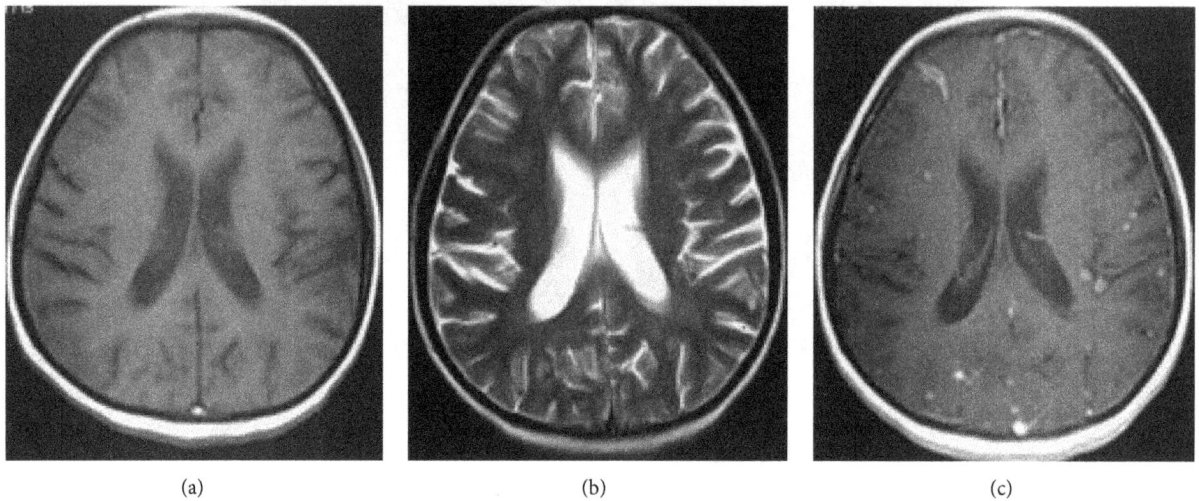

(a)   (b)   (c)

FIGURE 7: Miliary brain tuberculosis in a 20-year-old female with 3-month history of cough, weight loss, newly added generalized headache, dizziness, nausea, and vomiting. There is no obvious abnormality in the T1- (a) and T2-weighted (b) images. Axial postcontrast T1-weighted MR image (c) shows numerous bilateral tiny enhancing nodules scattered throughout the brain parenchyma.

thick, linear intradural enhancement, which may completely fill the subarachnoid spaces [5].

Longstanding arachnoiditis may result in the development of syringomyelia (spinal cord cavitation) that typically demonstrates CSF signal intensity on all MR sequences [5, 29].

Tuberculous spondylitis results from hematogenous spread of infection to the vertebral body via paravertebral venous plexus of Batson. Typical presentation is involvement of multiple vertebral bodies with sparing of intervertebral disc in early stage and disc involvement in later stages. Paraspinal extension and resultant paravertebral abscess (Pott's abscess) as well as subdural/epidural abscess formation with associated spinal cord compression (Figure 9) are other common findings.

Intracranial subdural or epidural abscess formation may or may not be associated with a primary CNS tuberculous focus and have imaging findings identical to that of other

pyogenic abscesses, that is, iso- to hypointensity on T1-weighted images, hyper- or mixed signal intensity on T2-weighted images, and rim enhancement on postcontrast images [29].

5. Conclusion

CNS tuberculosis has various imaging appearances, including meningitis, tuberculoma, miliary tuberculosis, abscess, cerebritis, and encephalopathy. In addition, the radiologic manifestations of this disease are not always typical and sometimes may be mistaken with other lesions such as brain tumors. Familiarity with the various imaging presentations of CNS tuberculosis is of key importance for the radiologists and infectious diseases specialists in timely diagnosis, thereby reducing the morbidity and mortality of this potentially life threatening disease.

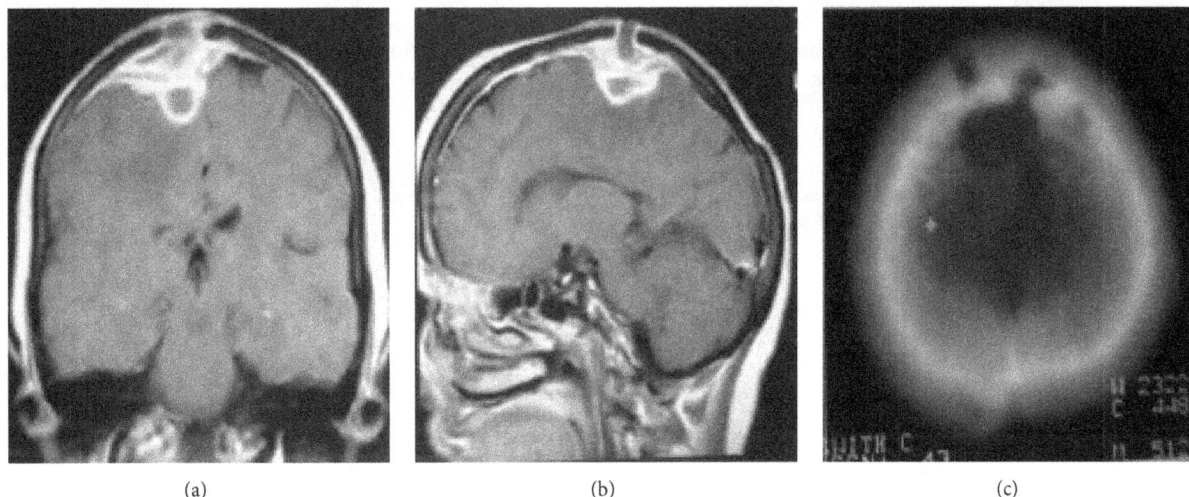

(a)   (b)   (c)

FIGURE 8: Tuberculous abscess with epidural and subdural empyema and calvarial osteomyelitis. Coronal (a) and sagittal (b) postcontrast T1-weighted MR images demonstrate epidural and subdural collections over the bifrontal cerebral convexities (more on the right side) with intraparenchymal and calvarial extension. Peripheral edema and irregular marked enhancement of the lesion as well as dural enhancement are evident. The bony destructive lytic lesions are seen in the bone window CT image (c).

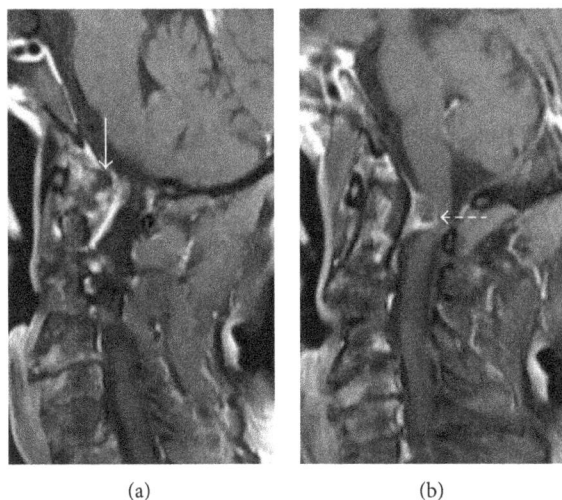

(a)   (b)

FIGURE 9: Postcontrast sagittal T1-weighted MR images reveal atlantoaxial tuberculosis with peripherally enhancing epidural abscess (*arrow*) accompanied by cord compression (*dashed arrow*) in a 62-year-old female who presented with gradual bilateral paralysis.

Conflict of Interests

The authors declare that there is no conflict of interests regarding the publication of this paper.

References

[1] A. Bernaerts, F. M. Vanhoenacker, P. M. Parizel et al., "Tuberculosis of the central nervous system: overview of neuroradiological findings," *European Radiology*, vol. 13, no. 8, pp. 1876–1890, 2003.

[2] J. Berenguer, S. Moreno, F. Laguna et al., "Tuberculous meningitis in patients infected with the human immunodeficiency virus," *The New England Journal of Medicine*, vol. 326, no. 10, pp. 668–672, 1992.

[3] J. E. Vidal, A. C. P. de Oliveira, F. B. Filho et al., "Tuberculous brain abscess in AIDS patients: report of three cases and literature review," *International Journal of Infectious Diseases*, vol. 9, no. 4, pp. 201–207, 2005.

[4] R. B. Rock, M. Olin, C. A. Baker, T. W. Molitor, and P. K. Peterson, "Central nervous system tuberculosis: pathogenesis and clinical aspects," *Clinical Microbiology Reviews*, vol. 21, no. 2, pp. 243–261, 2008.

[5] J. Burrill, C. J. Williams, G. Bain, G. Conder, A. L. Hine, and R. R. Misra, "Tuberculosis: a radiologic review," *Radiographics*, vol. 27, no. 5, pp. 1255–1273, 2007.

[6] G. Bathla, G. Khandelwal, V. G. Maller, and A. Gupta, "Manifestations of cerebral tuberculosis," *Singapore Medical Journal*, vol. 52, no. 2, pp. 124–131, 2011.

[7] V. V. Ahluwalia, G. Dayananda Sagar, T. P. Singh, N. Arora, S. Narayan, and M. M. Singh, "MRI spectrum of CNS tuberculosis," *Journal, Indian Academy of Clinical Medicine*, vol. 14, no. 2, pp. 83–90, 2013.

[8] M. C. Raviglione, D. E. Snider Jr., and A. Kochi, "Global epidemiology of tuberculosis: morbidity and mortality of a worldwide epidemic," *The Journal of the American Medical Association*, vol. 273, no. 3, pp. 220–226, 1995.

[9] S. Andronikou, J. Wilmshurst, M. Hatherill, and R. VanToorn, "Distribution of brain infarction in children with tuberculous meningitis and correlation with outcome score at 6 months," *Pediatric Radiology*, vol. 36, no. 12, pp. 1289–1294, 2006.

[10] D. K. Dastur, D. K. Manghani, and P. M. Udani, "Pathology and pathogenetic mechanisms in neurotuberculosis," *Radiologic Clinics of North America*, vol. 33, no. 4, pp. 733–752, 1995.

[11] S. Andronikou, B. Smith, M. Hatherill, H. Douis, and J. Wilmshurst, "Definitive neuroradiological diagnostic features of tuberculous meningitis in children," *Pediatric Radiology*, vol. 34, no. 11, pp. 876–885, 2004.

[12] G. Uysal, G. Köse, A. Güven, and B. Diren, "Magnetic resonance imaging in diagnosis of childhood central nervous system tuberculosis," *Infection*, vol. 29, no. 3, pp. 148–153, 2001.

[13] A. Arbeláez, E. Medina, F. Restrepo, and M. Castillo, "Cerebral tuberculosis," *Seminars in Roentgenology*, vol. 39, no. 4, pp. 474–481, 2004.

[14] J. R. Jinkins, R. Gupta, and J. Rodriguez-Carbajal, "MR imaging of central nervous system tuberculosis," *Radiologic Clinics of North America*, vol. 33, no. 4, pp. 771–786, 1995.

[15] C. Morgado and N. Ruivo, "Imaging meningo-encephalic tuberculosis," *European Journal of Radiology*, vol. 55, no. 2, pp. 188–192, 2005.

[16] G. V. Shah, "Central nervous system tuberculosis: imaging manifestations," *Neuroimaging Clinics of North America*, vol. 10, no. 2, pp. 355–374, 2000.

[17] H. Parmar, Y.-Y. Sitoh, P. Anand, V. Chua, and F. Hui, "Contrast-enhanced flair imaging in the evaluation of infectious leptomeningeal diseases," *European Journal of Radiology*, vol. 58, no. 1, pp. 89–95, 2006.

[18] D. K. Dastur, V. S. Lalitha, P. M. Udani, and U. Parekh, "The brain and meninges in tuberculous meningitis-gross pathology in 100 cases and pathogenesis.," *Neurology India*, vol. 18, no. 2, pp. 86–100, 1970.

[19] M. L. H. Whiteman, "Neuroimaging of central nervous system tuberculosis in HIV-infected patients," *Neuroimaging Clinics of North America*, vol. 7, no. 2, pp. 199–214, 1997.

[20] P. Sharma, R. K. Garg, R. Verma, M. K. Singh, and R. Shukla, "Incidence, predictors and prognostic value of cranial nerve involvement in patients with tuberculous meningitis: a retrospective evaluation," *European Journal of Internal Medicine*, vol. 22, no. 3, pp. 289–295, 2011.

[21] R. K. Garg, "Tuberculosis of the central nervous system," *Postgraduate Medical Journal*, vol. 75, no. 881, pp. 133–140, 1999.

[22] R. Trivedi, S. Saksena, and R. K. Gupta, "Magnetic resonance imaging in central nervous system tuberculosis," *Indian Journal of Radiology and Imaging*, vol. 19, no. 4, pp. 256–265, 2009.

[23] R. K. Gupta, N. Husain, M. K. Kathuria, S. Datta, R. K. S. Rathore, and M. Husain, "Magnetization transfer MR imaging correlation with histopathology in intracranial tuberculomas," *Clinical Radiology*, vol. 56, no. 8, pp. 656–663, 2001.

[24] S. Saxena, M. Prakash, S. Kumar, and R. K. Gupta, "Comparative evaluation of magnetization transfer contrast and fluid attenuated inversion recovery sequences in brain tuberculoma," *Clinical Radiology*, vol. 60, no. 7, pp. 787–793, 2005.

[25] R. K. Gupta, M. K. Kathuria, and S. Pradhan, "Magnetization transfer MR imaging in CNS tuberculosis," *The American Journal of Neuroradiology*, vol. 20, no. 5, pp. 867–875, 1999.

[26] R. Gupta, "Magnetization transfer MR imaging in central nervous system infections," *Indian Journal of Radiology and Imaging*, vol. 12, no. 1, pp. 51–58, 2002.

[27] R. K. Gupta, D. K. Vatsal, N. Husain et al., "Differentiation of tuberculous from pyogenic brain abscesses with in vivo proton MR spectroscopy and magnetization transfer MR imaging," *American Journal of Neuroradiology*, vol. 22, no. 8, pp. 1503–1509, 2001.

[28] T. K. Kim, K. H. Chang, C. J. Kim, J. M. Goo, M. C. Kook, and M. H. Han, "Intracranial tuberculoma: comparison of MR with pathologic findings," *The American Journal of Neuroradiology*, vol. 16, no. 9, pp. 1903–1908, 1995.

[29] B. D. Ku and S. Yoo, "Extensive meningeal and prenchymal calcified tuberculoma as long-term residual sequelae of tuberculous meningitis," *Neurology India*, vol. 57, no. 4, pp. 521–522, 2009.

[30] B. Afghani and J. M. Lieberman, "Paradoxical enlargement or development of intracranial tuberculomas during therapy: case report and review," *Clinical Infectious Diseases*, vol. 19, no. 6, pp. 1092–1099, 1994.

[31] J. Lorber, "Intracranial calcifications following tuberculous meningitis in," *Acta Radiologica*, vol. 50, no. 1-2, pp. 204–210, 1958.

[32] N. Krishnan, B. D. Robertson, and G. Thwaites, "The mechanisms and consequences of the extra-pulmonary dissemination of *Mycobacterium tuberculosis*," *Tuberculosis*, vol. 90, no. 6, pp. 361–366, 2010.

[33] P. M. Udani and D. K. Dastur, "Tuberculous encephalopathy with and without meningitis clinical features and pathological correlations," *Journal of the Neurological Sciences*, vol. 10, no. 6, pp. 541–561, 1970.

15

Evaluation of Hemodynamics in Focal Steatosis and Focal Spared Lesion of the Liver using Contrast-Enhanced Ultrasonography with Sonazoid

Kazue Shiozawa,[1,2] Manabu Watanabe,[1] Takashi Ikehara,[1] Michio Kogame,[1] Mie Shinohara,[1] Masao Shinohara,[1] Koji Ishii,[1] Yoshinori Igarashi,[1] Hiroyuki Makino,[2] and Yasukiyo Sumino[1]

[1] Division of Gastroenterology and Hepatology, Department of Internal Medicine, Toho University Medical Center, Omori Hospital, 6-11-1 Omorinishi, Ota-ku, Tokyo 143-8541, Japan

[2] Division of Gastroenterology and Hepatology, Department of Internal Medicine, Saiseikai Yokohamashi Tobu Hospital, 3-6-1 Shimosueyoshi, Tsurumi-ku, Yokohama-shi, Kanagawa 230-0012, Japan

Correspondence should be addressed to Manabu Watanabe; manabu62@med.toho-u.ac.jp

Academic Editor: David Maintz

We aim to investigate the hemodynamics in focal steatosis and focal spared lesion of the liver using contrast-enhanced ultrasonography (CEUS) with Sonazoid. The subjects were 47 patients with focal steatosis and focal spared lesion. We evaluated enhancement patterns (hyperenhancement, isoenhancement, and hypoenhancement) in the vascular phase and the presence or absence of a hypoechoic area in the postvascular phase for these lesions using CEUS. Of the 24 patients with focal steatosis, the enhancement pattern was isoenhancement in 19 and hypoenhancement in 5. Hypoechoic areas were noted in the postvascular phase in 3 patients. Of the 23 patients with focal spared lesions, the enhancement pattern was isoenhancement in 18 and hyperenhancement in 5. No hypoechoic areas were noted in the postvascular phase in any patient. The hemodynamics in focal steatosis and focal spared lesions in nondiffuse fatty liver can be observed using low-invasive procedures in real-time by CEUS. It was suggested that differences in the dynamics of enhancement in the vascular phase of CEUS were influenced by the fat deposits in the target lesion, the surrounding liver parenchyma, and the third inflow.

1. Introduction

Nondiffuse fatty liver is considered to develop when the fat accumulation ability of hepatocytes or fat deposition becomes heterogeneous throughout the liver and is classified into the following 4 types: focal steatosis, multifocal steatosis, lobar or segmental steatosis, and focal spared lesion in fatty liver [1]. Based on imaging studies, insulin and nutrient levels in the blood flowing into the corresponding hepatic areas are considered to be causative in the frequent development of focal steatosis and focal spared lesion [2].

Some cases of focal steatosis and focal spared lesion exhibit an oval or mass-like appearance on imaging, and differentiation from liver tumors may be problematic. In this study, we performed contrast-enhanced ultrasonography (CEUS) for focal steatosis and focal spared lesions using Sonazoid (Daiichi Sankyo Pharmaceutical, Tokyo, Japan), in order to diagnose liver mass lesions, and obtained information on the hemodynamics of focal steatosis and focal spared lesions. Herein, we report these data with a review of the literature.

2. Materials and Methods

The subjects were 47 patients in whom liver mass lesions were detected on abdominal ultrasonography during health check-up and underwent CEUS with Sonazoid. The findings of these patients were investigated retrospectively. These were diagnosed with focal steatosis (24 cases) or a focal spared lesion (23 cases) on dynamic computed tomography (CT) and magnetic resonance imaging [3, 4]. At first, the presence or absence of an existing blood vessel within the lesion was evaluated by color doppler ultrasonography (CDUS). Next, CEUS was performed using an Aplio XG (Toshiba Medical Systems, Tokyo, Japan) with a convex probe (PVT-375BT, 3.75 MHz center frequency). The mechanical index (MI) for the acoustic output was set to 0.2, and a single focus point was set at the lower margin of the lesion. An intravenous bolus injection of Sonazoid (0.5 mL) was administered via a left cubital venous line followed by flushing with 10 mL of normal saline. The lesion was evaluated with regard to the following findings: the dynamics of the enhancement in the vascular phase (0–40 seconds), the presence or absence of an existing blood vessel within the lesion in the vascular phase, and the presence or absence of a hypoechoic area in the postvascular phase (after 15 minutes). Digital cine clips of the CEUS images were stored on the hard disk of the scanner and transferred to a high performance personal computer for subsequent analysis. The dynamics of the enhancement in the vascular phase were compared with those in the surrounding liver and classified into the following 3 enhancement patterns: hyperenhancement, isoenhancement and hypoenhancement. The postvascular phase was observed using the advanced dynamic flow (ADF) mode in some cases. Using the ADF mode, Sonazoid bubbles phagocytosed by Kupffer cells were destroyed, with a high MI of 1.0 [5]. Since the presence or absence of hypoechoic areas in the postvascular phase cannot be readily identified, particularly in high-echoic lesions, this procedure is useful for such determination.

All CEUS images were reviewed by two hepatologists, one was with 15 years of experience and other was with 27 years of experience.

2.1. Statistical Analysis. The presence or absence of an existing blood vessel in the lesion and the enhancement pattern (hyperenhancement, isoenhancement, and hypoenhancement) in the vascular phase were compared using Fisher's exact test. Statistical analyses were performed using SPSS version 11.0 (Statistical Package for the Social Sciences) for Windows (Microsoft) and $P < 0.05$ was considered to indicate a statistically significant difference.

This study was approved by the Ethical Review Board of Toho University Medical Center, Omori Hospital.

3. Results

3.1. Focal Steatosis. Of the 24 patients with focal steatosis (Table 1), 13 and 11 were male and female, respectively, and the mean age was 61.8 ± 14.3 years (median: 64.5 years). The mean major axis of the lesion was 20.0 ± 9.5 mm (median: 19.5 mm) and the location was S3 in 1 patient (near the umbilical portion), S4 in 16 (transverse part of the portal vein in 8, near the falciform ligament of the liver (Sappey's vein area) in 6, and the gallbladder bed and adjacent to IVC in 1 each), S5 in 6 (the gallbladder bed in 3, the right lobe surface in 1, and other area of the right lobe in 2), and S8 (right lobe surface) in 1.

The enhancement pattern in the vascular phase of CEUS was isoenhancement in 19 patients and hypoenhancement in 5 (Figure 1). An existing blood vessel was noted in the lesion in the vascular phase in 7 patients. On comparison of the enhancement patterns, the patterns were isoenhancement and hypoenhancement of the lesions in 5 and 2 of the 7 patients with existing blood vessels, respectively, and in 14 and 3 of the lesions of the 17 patients with no existing blood vessels, respectively, showing no significant difference.

A hypoechoic area was noted in the postvascular phase in 3 patients, which was also evident using the ADF mode in these same 3 patients.

3.2. Focal Spared Lesion. Of the 23 patients with focal spared lesions (Table 2), 15 and 8 were male and female, respectively, and the mean age was 52.9 ± 14.1 years (median: 52 years). The mean major axis of the lesion was 22.8 ± 11.8 mm (median: 20 mm), and the location was S3 in 1 patient (near the umbilical portion), S4 in 5 (transverse part of the portal vein in 3, and Sappey's vein area and the gallbladder bed in 1 each), S5 in 7 (the gallbladder bed in 6, and the right lobe surface in 1), S6 in 5 (the right lobe surface in 4, and the right hepatic hilum in 1), S7 (right lobe surface) in 2, and S8 in 3 (the right lobe surface in 1, and other area of the right lobe in 2).

The enhancement pattern in the vascular phase of CEUS was isoenhancement of the lesion in 18 patients and hyperenhancement of the lesion in 5 (Figure 2).

An existing blood vessel was noted in the lesion in the vascular phase in 5 patients. On comparison of the enhancement patterns, the patterns were hyperenhancement and isoenhancement of the lesions in 3 and 2 of the 5 patients with existing blood vessels, respectively, and in 2 and 16 of the lesions of the 18 patients with no existing blood vessels, respectively, showing a significant difference ($P = 0.048$), and existing blood vessels were more often noted in the cases with hyperenhancement.

No hypoechoic areas were noted in the postvascular phase in any patient. Nine patients were observed using the ADF mode, but no hypoechoic areas were noted.

4. Discussion

Fatty liver is caused by the accumulation of triglycerides and other nutrients within hepatocytes and is roughly divided into diffuse and nondiffuse fatty liver. Nondiffuse fatty liver is further classified into 4 types: focal steatosis, multifocal steatosis, lobar or segmental steatosis, and focal spared lesion in the fatty liver [1]. The characteristic hemodynamic profile of the liver is considered to be involved in the maldistribution of fat in the liver parenchyma. The blood supply to the liver is derived from the hepatic artery and portal vein. The portal vein supplies 70% to 80% of the blood, delivering nutrients and other substances derived from the intestine [6]. It has been reported that, in nondiffuse fatty liver, localized fat and nonfat deposition are likely to occur in specific lesions, such as the dorsal S4 lesion of the liver, around the gallbladder and Sappey's vein area [7–9]. Matsui et al. [2, 10] investigated many cases using CT during arterial portography (CTAP)

TABLE 1: Of the 24 lesions with focal steatosis, patients character, location, size, enhancement pattern in the vascular phase of CEUS, presence of existing blood vessel in the CDUS and/or the vascular phase, presence of hypoechoic area in the postvascular phase, and ADF mode of CEUS.

No.	Age	Sex	Location	Size (mm)	Vessels seen on CDUS or/and CEUS	CEUS Vascular	CEUS Postvascular/ADF
1	60	F	S4/Transverse portion	28	+	Iso	−*
2	73	F	S4/Sappey's vein area	25	+	Hypo	−
3	72	M	S5/GB bed	25	+	Iso	−
4	80	M	S4/Transverse portion	36	+	Iso	−
5	45	M	S4/GB bed	8	+	Iso	+
6	49	M	S4/Sappey's vein area	21	+	Iso	−
7	62	M	S4/Sappey's vein area	15	+	Hypo	−
8	76	F	S4/Transverse portion	20		Iso	−
9	85	F	S3/Umbilical portion	7		Iso	−
10	59	M	S4/Transverse portion	18		Hypo	−
11	48	F	S4/Sappey's vein area	12		Iso	−
12	68	F	S4/Transverse portion	14		Iso	−
13	67	F	S4/Adjacent to IVC	40		Iso	−
14	50	M	S5/Right lobe surface	15		Iso	−
15	31	M	S8/Right lobe surface	8		Iso	−
16	66	F	S5/GB bed	30		Iso	−
17	74	M	S4/Transverse portion	8		Iso	−
18	80	F	S4/Transverse portion	27		Iso	−
19	64	M	S4/Sappey's vein area	31		Iso	−
20	45	F	S4/Sappey's vein area	20		Iso	−
21	65	M	S5/GB bed	19		Hypo	−
22	40	M	S5/Other area of the right lobe	15		Iso	−
23	49	F	S5/Other area of the right lobe	8		Iso	+
24	75	M	S4/Transverse portion	30		Hypo	+

GB: gall bladder, Iso: isoenhancement, hypo: hypoenhancement, ADF: advanced dynamic flow.
* −: no hypoechoic area, +: hypoechoic area.

and clarified that the above-described lesions, in which fat deposition/nonfat deposition are likely to occur, exhibit defects of enhancement on CTAP, in the absence of any apparent lesion, that is, the defects correspond to pseudolesions, and the presence of a blood vessel (third inflow) flowing into the liver other than the portal vein is involved in the appearance of the pseudolesions. The third inflow includes the right gastric vein, cystic vein, and Sappey's vein [11]. Since the portal blood flow is important in the transport of dietary fat from the intestine, the concentrations of hormones, such as insulin, and nutrients in the third inflow, could be different from those in the portal blood, and these differences could contribute to the heterogeneous deposition of fat [2].

For focal steatosis and focal spared lesions, hemodynamics has been reported on CEUS using SonoVue (Bracco, Milan, Italy) [12–14]. However, to our knowledge, there has been no report on the use of CEUS using Sonazoid. CEUS using SonoVue can only be used to evaluate the vascular phase. In contrast, the vascular and postvascular phase (Kupffer phase) can be evaluated with CEUS using Sonazoid based upon the characteristic of Sonazoid following phagocytosis by Kupffer cells.

Liu et al. [12] reported the hemodynamics of 25 lesions in 20 patients with focal steatosis by CEUS using SonoVue, in which hypoenhancement and isoenhancement of the lesions were observed in the vascular phase in 44% each and hyperenhancement was observed in 12%. In our study, isoenhancement and hypoenhancement of the lesions were noted in 19 (79%) and 5 (21%) of the 24 patients, and no hyperenhancement was observed in any patient. Considering the findings of Liu et al., it was suggested that focal steatosis tends to present as hypoenhanced or isoenhanced lesions in the vascular phase of CEUS.

Liu et al. also investigated the time required for contrast agent to reach and enter the lesion with focal steatosis [12]. The time to reach the hypoenhanced lesions, which was 1–21 seconds, was delayed compared with the time (1–7 seconds) taken for the surrounding liver parenchyma. They did not mention the reason for this, but, in all likelihood, the staining intensity or speed may have tended to decrease in the hypoenhanced regions compared to that in the surrounding liver parenchyma due to the exclusion/narrowing of blood vessels by the fatty cells; that is, exclusion of the sinusoid by fat droplets [15]. Therefore, hyperenhancement is unlikely to

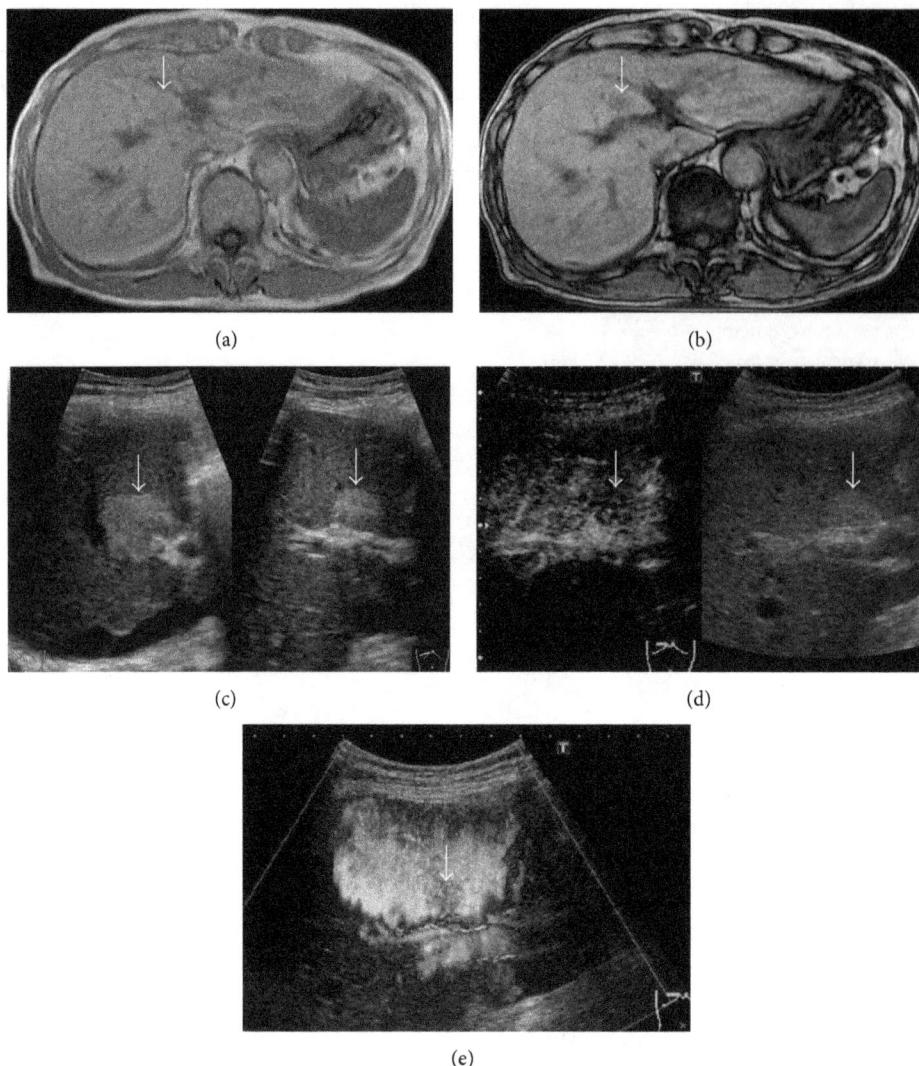

FIGURE 1: A 75-year-old male (case no. 24) with focal steatosis in the S4 (transverse portion). (a) In-phase T1-weighted magnetic resonance image (MRI) scan shows the isointense lesion (arrow) in the S4 (transverse portion). (b) The lesion is hypointense on an out of-phase T1-weighted MRI scan (arrow) and is diagnosed as focal steatosis. (c) Gray-scale ultrasonography (US) (right intercostal axis) shows a hyperechoic lesion (arrow). (d) Left: in the vascular phase (17 seconds) of contrast-enhanced ultrasonography (CEUS) (right subcostal axis), the lesion (arrow) is hypoenhancement compared with the surrounding liver. Right: gray-scale US (monitor mode) (arrow). (e) In the advanced dynamic flow (ADF) mode of the postvascular phase of CEUS (right intercostal axis), the lesion shows a hypoechoic area (arrow).

occur in focal steatosis, and the cause of hyperenhancement in the 12% in the study reported by Liu et al. remains unclear.

Among the 23 patients with focal spared lesions, isoenhancement and hyperenhancement of the lesions were noted in the vascular phase of CEUS in 18 and 5 patients, respectively, and no hypoenhancement was noted in any patient. In the focal steatosis cases described above, enhancement tended to decrease in the focal steatosis lesion, compared with that in the surrounding liver parenchyma, due to the influence of fatty cells. In these focal spared lesions, isoenhancement was noted in most cases, but hyperenhancement was noted in some cases. This may have been due to fatty cell-induced exclusion and narrowing of blood vessels in the surrounding liver parenchyma by fatty cells [16, 17], in

contrast to focal steatosis, and enhancement of the lesion may have appeared to be increased relative to that of the surrounding liver parenchyma. In normal liver parenchyma, arterial blood generally flows in first, followed by perfusion via the portal blood flow. Since ectopic venous circulation other than the portal vein, that is, the third inflow, is involved in focal spared lesions, the third inflow may have entered the focal spared lesion earlier than the portal blood perfusion within the liver parenchyma, resulting in more rapid and stronger enhancement compared with the surrounding liver parenchyma.

Regarding the existing blood vessels and the enhancement pattern in focal steatosis and focal spared lesions, no significant correlation was noted between the presence of an

TABLE 2: Of the 23 lesions with focal spared lesions, patients character, location, size, enhancement pattern in the vascular phase of CEUS, presence of existing blood vessel in the CDUS and/or the vascular phase, presence of hypoechoic area in the postvascular phase, and ADF mode of CEUS.

No.	Age	Sex	Location	Size (mm)	Vessels seen on CDUS or/and CEUS	CEUS	
						Vascular	Postvascular/ADF
1	44	M	S4/GB bed	60.9	+	hyper	−*
2	75	F	S5/GB bed	12	+	Iso	−
3	69	F	S6/Right hepatic hilum	14	+	hyper	−
4	48	M	S5/GB bed	12	+	Iso	−
5	35	F	S4/Sappey's vein area	21	+	hyper	−
6	52	M	S5/GB bed	17		Iso	−
7	45	M	S6/Right lobe surface	19		Iso	−
8	70	M	S7/Right lobe surface	41		Iso	−
9	37	F	S6/Right lobe surface	20		Iso	−
10	62	F	S8/Other area of the right lobe	18		Iso	−
11	52	M	S5/Right lobe surface	12		hyper	−
12	59	M	S8/Right lobe surface	23		hyper	−
13	64	M	S4/Transverse portion	22		Iso	−
14	45	M	S5/GB bed	18		Iso	−
15	24	M	S5/GB bed	20		Iso	−
16	71	F	S8/Other area of the right lobe	15		Iso	−
17	47	F	S3/Umbilical portion	13		Iso	−
18	59	M	S4/Transverse portion	40		Iso	−
19	34	M	S4/Transverse portion	20		Iso	−
20	36	M	S6/Right lobe surface	30		Iso	−
21	60	M	S7/Right lobe surface	35		Iso	−
22	56	M	S6/Right lobe surface	27		Iso	−
23	72	F	S5/GB bed	14		Iso	−

GB: gall bladder, hyper: hyperenhancement, Iso: isoenhancement, ADF: advanced dynamic flow.
* −: no hypoechoic area.

existing blood vessel and the enhancement pattern in focal steatosis. In contrast, in focal spared lesions, existing blood vessels were noted in 3 of the 5 cases with hyperenhancement, showing a significant difference. The presence or absence of an existing blood vessel may influence the enhancement dynamics in focal spared lesions.

In the postvascular phase, hypoechoic areas were noted in 3 of the 24 focal steatosis cases, and these hypoechoic areas were also observed using the ADF mode in each of these cases. In contrast, no hypoechoic areas were noted in any of the 23 cases of focal spared lesion or of the 9 cases observed using the ADF mode. These findings suggest that the phagocytic ability of Kupffer cells is reduced in fat-containing cells compared with normal liver cells.

It was clarified that hemodynamics in lesions can be observed using low-invasive procedures in real-time by CEUS using Sonazoid in comparison with the previous CT angiography. And it was suggested that Kupffer function (phagocytosis) in the lesions could be evaluated by observing the postvascular phase. In addition, hypoechoic areas were noted in some of the focal steatosis cases in the postvascular phase. We require attention for differentiation of these lesions and malignant tumors.

Among the limitations, this study was retrospective in nature, that is, the number of cases was small, the lesions were not diagnosed histologically, and it was unclear whether the existing blood vessel within the lesions represented an artery, vein, or portal vein. It may be necessary to increase the number of cases and perform further evaluations including histopathological investigation.

5. Conclusion

We investigated the hemodynamics in focal steatosis and focal spared lesions in nondiffuse fatty liver by CEUS using Sonazoid. It was suggested that differences in the dynamics of enhancement in the vascular phase of CEUS were influenced by fat deposits in the target lesion and the surrounding liver parenchyma and the third inflow and that the fat deposition-associated phagocytic ability of Kupffer cells is involved with the presence or absence of the hypoechoic area in the postvascular phase.

As for the knowledge provided in this study, it will seem that it is necessary in future in distinguishing a malignant tumor from these lesion.

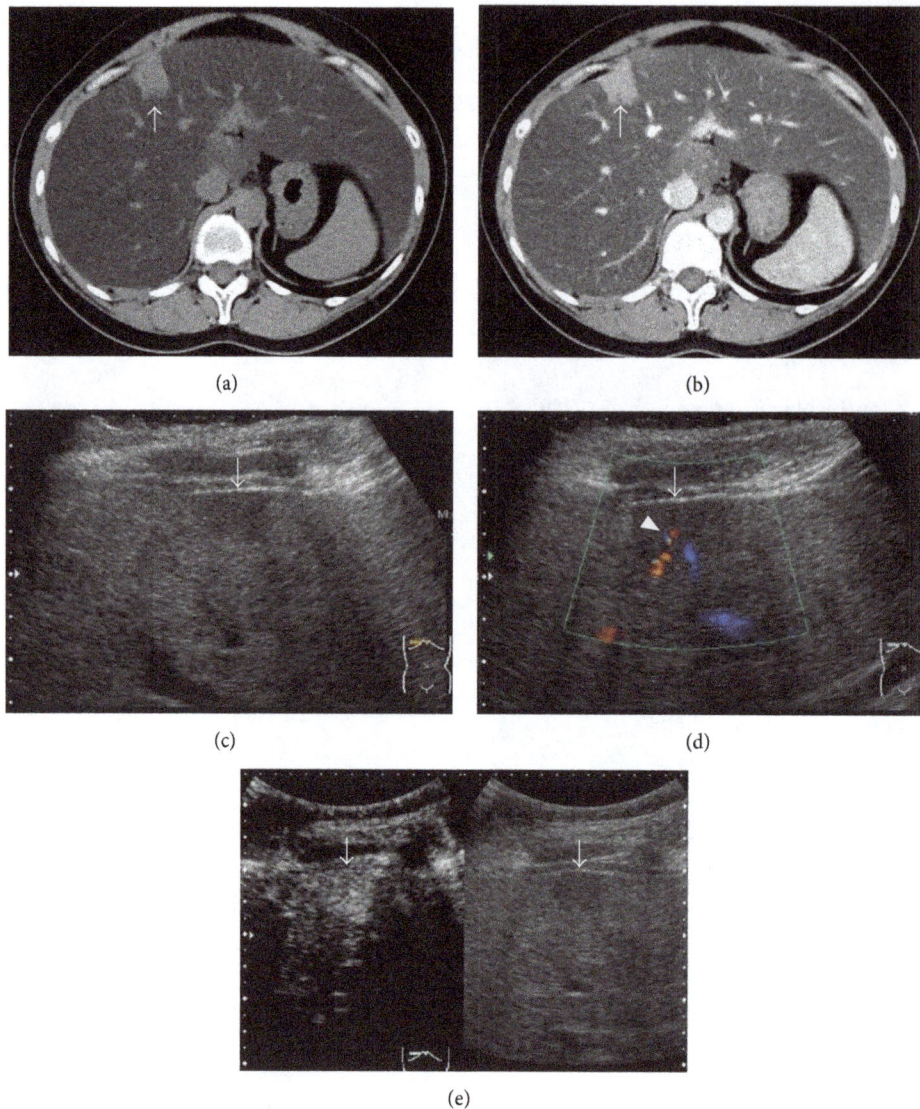

(a)

(b)

(c)

(d)

(e)

FIGURE 2: A 35-year-old female (case No. 5) with focal spared lesion in the S4 (near the falciform ligament of liver so called Sappey's vein area). (a) Unenhanced computed tomography (CT) scan shows a hyperattenuating lesion (arrow) in the S4. (b) Enhanced CT scan shows the lesion (arrow) of hyperattenuation in the portal phase. (c) Gray-scale US (right intercostal axis) shows a hypoechoic lesion (arrow). (d) Color Doppler ultrasonography (CDUS) (right intercostal axis) shows hepato petal flow (arrow head) toward the lesion (arrow). (e) Left: In the vascular phase (13 seconds) of CEUS (right intercostal axis), the lesion (arrow) is hyperenhancement compared with the surrounding liver. Right: Gray-scale US (monitor mode) (arrow).

Abbreviations

CEUS: Contrast-enhanced ultrasonography
CT: Computed tomography
CDUS: Color Doppler ultrasonography
MI: Mechanical index
ADF: Advanced Dynamic Flow
CTAP: CT during arterial portography.

Consent

All procedures followed were in accordance with the ethical standards of the responsible committee on human experimentation (institutional and national) and with the Helsinki Declaration of 1975, as revised in 2008 [5]. Informed consent was obtained from all patients for being included in the study.

Conflict of Interests

There are no financial or other relations that could lead to a conflict of interests.

References

[1] B. W. Dong, M. H. Chen, J. G. Li, B. Wang, and K. Yan, "Further study on sonographic patterns of non-formity fatty liver," *Chinese Journal of Ultrasonography*, vol. 2, pp. 62–63, 1993.

[2] O. Matsui, M. Kadoya, S. Takahashi et al., "Focal sparing of segment IV in fatty livers shown by sonography and CT: correlation with aberrant gastric venous drainage," *The American Journal of Roentgenology*, vol. 164, no. 5, pp. 1137–1140, 1995.

[3] K. W. Kim, M. J. Kim, S. S. Lee et al., "Sparing of fatty infiltration around focal hepatic lesions in patients with hepatic steatosis: sonographic appearance with CT and MRI correlation," *The American Journal of Roentgenology*, vol. 190, no. 4, pp. 1018–1027, 2008.

[4] S. Hirohashi, K. Ueda, H. Uchida et al., "Nondiffuse fatty change of the liver: discerning pseudotumor on MR images enhanced with ferumoxides-initial observations," *Radiology*, vol. 217, no. 2, pp. 415–420, 2000.

[5] S. Yoshikawa, H. Iijima, M. Saito et al., "Crucial role of impaired Kupffer cell phagocytosis on the decreased Sonazoid-enhanced echogenicity in a liver of a nonalchoholic steatohepatitis rat model," *Hepatology Research*, vol. 40, no. 8, pp. 823–831, 2010.

[6] R. C. Sanders, J. D. Dolk, and N. S. Miner, "Liver," in *Exam Preparation for Diagnostic Ultrasound: Abdomen and OG/GYN*, p. 3, Lippincott Williams & Wilkins, Baltimore, Md, USA, 1st edition, 2002.

[7] Y. Kawamori, O. Matsui, S. Takahashi, M. Kadoya, T. Takashima, and S. Miyayama, "Focal hepatic fatty infiltration in the posterior edge of the medial segment associated with aberrant gastric venous drainage: CT, US, and MR findings," *Journal of Computer Assisted Tomography*, vol. 20, no. 3, pp. 356–359, 1996.

[8] O. Matsui, T. Takashima, M. Kadoya et al., "Staining in the liver surrounding gallbladder fossa on hepatic arteriography caused by increased cystic venous drainage," *Gastrointestinal Radiology*, vol. 12, no. 1, pp. 307–312, 1987.

[9] J. Yoshikawa, O. Matsui, T. Takashima et al., "Focal fatty change of the liver adjacent to the falciform ligament: CT and sonographic findings in five surgically confirmed cases," *American Journal of Roentgenology*, vol. 149, no. 3, pp. 491–494, 1987.

[10] O. Matsui, M. Kadoya, J. Yoshikawa et al., "Aberrant gastric venous drainage in cirrhotic livers: imaging findings in focal areas of liver parenchyma," *Radiology*, vol. 197, no. 2, pp. 345–349, 1995.

[11] W. Dahnert, "Third inflow to liver," in *Radiology Review Manual*, W. Dahnert, Ed., p. 675, Lippincott Williams & Wilkins, Philadelphia, Pa, USA, 5th edition, 2003.

[12] L. P. Liu, B. W. Dong, X. L. Yu, D. K. Zhang, C. S. Kang, and X. H. Zhao, "Evaluation of focal fatty infiltration of the liver using color doppler and contrast-enhanced sonography," *Journal of Clinical Ultrasound*, vol. 36, no. 9, pp. 560–566, 2008.

[13] L. P. Liu, B. W. Dong, X. L. Yu, D. K. Zhang, X. Li, and H. Li, "Analysis of focal spared areas in fatty liver using color doppler imaging and contrast-enhanced microvessel display sonography," *Journal of Ultrasound in Medicine*, vol. 27, no. 3, pp. 387–394, 2008.

[14] T. Gabata, O. Matsui, M. Kadoya et al., "Aberrant gastric venous drainage in a focal spared area of segment IV in fatty liver: demonstration with color Doppler sonography," *Radiology*, vol. 203, no. 2, pp. 461–463, 1997.

[15] G. C. Farrell, N. C. Teoh, and R. S. McCuskey, "Hepatic microcirculation in fatty liver disease," *Anatomical Record*, vol. 291, no. 6, pp. 684–692, 2008.

[16] I. Mihmanli, F. Kantarci, M. H. Yilmaz et al., "Effect of diffuse fatty infiltration of the liver on hepatic artery resistance index," *Journal of Clinical Ultrasound*, vol. 33, no. 3, pp. 95–99, 2005.

[17] L. Oguzkurt, T. Yildirim, D. Torun, F. Tercan, O. Kizilkilic, and E. A. Niron, "Hepatic vein Doppler waveform in patients with diffuse fatty infiltration of the liver," *European Journal of Radiology*, vol. 54, no. 2, pp. 253–257, 2005.

16

The Spleen Revisited: An Overview on Magnetic Resonance Imaging

João Palas, António P. Matos, and Miguel Ramalho

Radiology Department, Hospital Garcia de Orta, 2801-951 Almada, Portugal

Correspondence should be addressed to Miguel Ramalho; miguel-ramalho@netcabo.pt

Academic Editor: Andreas H. Mahnken

Despite being well visualized by different cross-sectional imaging techniques, the spleen is many times overlooked during the abdominal examination. The major reason is the low frequency of splenic abnormalities, the majority consisting of incidental findings. There has been a steady increase in the number of performed abdominal magnetic resonance imaging (MRI) studies; therefore, it is important to be familiar to the major MRI characteristics of disease processes involving the spleen, in order to interpret the findings correctly, reaching whenever possible the appropriate diagnosis. The spleen may be involved in several pathologic conditions like congenital diseases, trauma, inflammation, vascular disorders and hematologic disorders, benign and malignant tumors, and other disease processes that focally or diffusely affect the spleen. This paper presents a description and representative MRI images for many of these disorders.

1. Introduction

Splenic disease has always been a challenge to the radiologist. Despite of being well visualized by different cross sectional imaging techniques, the spleen is many times overlooked during the abdominal examination. The major reason is the low frequency of splenic abnormalities, the majority consisting of incidental findings.

There has been a steady increase in the number of performed abdominal magnetic resonance imaging (MRI) studies; therefore, it is important to be familiar to the major MR imaging characteristics of disease processes involving the spleen, in order to interpret the findings correctly, reaching whenever possible the appropriate diagnosis. Nowadays, MRI permits the characterization of the most common splenic lesions, such as cysts, small hemangiomas, and hamartomas, and improvement in the detection of malignant diseases such as lymphoma and metastases [1].

The spleen may be involved by several pathologic conditions including congenital diseases, trauma, inflammation, vascular disorders and hematologic disorders, benign and malignant tumors, and other disease processes that focally or diffusely affects the spleen. This article presents a description and representative MRI images for many of these disorders.

2. The Normal Spleen

The spleen is located in the left hypogastric quadrant of the abdomen and is fixed in its intraperitoneal position beneath the 9th to 11th intercostal spaces by the splenorenal, splenocolic, splenogastric, and phrenicosplenic ligaments. The configuration of the spleen is variable (typically coffee bean shaped), as well as the size, which is related with the patient's morphological type and age [2]. The organ's convex face lies adjacent to the diaphragm. The concave side of the spleen has contact with the stomach, left kidney, and colon flexure. The splenic hilum is found within this concavity and acts as an entry and exit route for the arterial, venous, and lymphatic vessels and nerves. The spleen is divided into two compartments, namely, the red and white pulp, separated by the marginal zone. The white pulp is made up of T- and B-lymphocytes and is located centrally, while the red pulp is composed of rich plexuses of tortuous venous sinuses [3].

On T1-weighted MR images, the normal signal intensity of the spleen is lower than that of hepatic tissue. Conversely, on T2-weighted images, the spleen shows higher signal intensity, appearing brighter than the liver [4] (Figure 1). The distinctive microscopic anatomy of the spleen may be reflected on diffusion-weighted images (DWI) and ADC

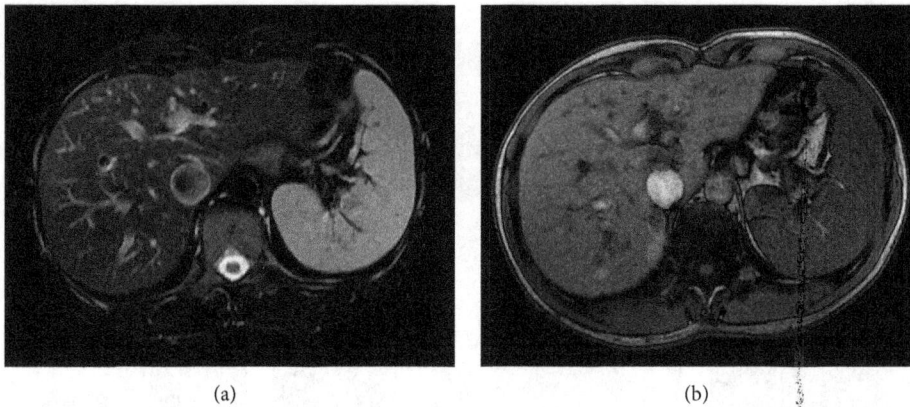

(a)   (b)

FIGURE 1: The normal spleen. Axial T2wi FSE with fat suppression (a) and axial T1wi out-of-phase GRE (b). The spleen shows the typical coffee bean configuration. On T1wi (b), the normal signal intensity of the spleen is lower than that of hepatic tissue. Conversely, on T2wi, the spleen shows higher signal intensity.

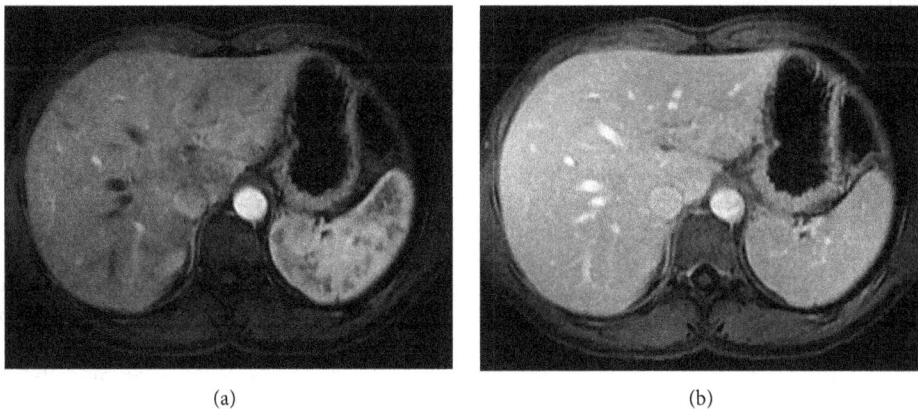

(a)   (b)

FIGURE 2: Pattern of enhancement of the normal spleen. Postcontrast axial T1wi 3D-GRE with fat suppression in the arterial (a) and venous (b) phase. The spleen shows a heterogeneous pattern enhancement immediately after contrast material administration (a), secondary to differences in flow between the red and white pulps, becoming homogeneous in venous (b) and interstitial phases.

maps. Prior studies have shown significant differences in the mean ADCs between the spleen and other abdominal organs [5, 6].

The spleen demonstrates a heterogeneous serpentine or arciform pattern enhancement immediately after contrast material administration, secondary to differences in flow between the red and white pulps, becoming homogeneous in venous and interstitial phases [4] (Figure 2). Any heterogeneity after this period is considered pathologic [7, 8].

3. Congenital Diseases and Normal Variants

The congenital absence of spleen is known as asplenia and the presence of one or more spleens is known as polysplenia. Both are very rare and usually associated with other congenital abnormalities.

The accessory spleens may be found in 10% of the population [9], more frequently in women, usually with less than 4 cm in size and located near the splenic hilum or near the pancreatic tail (Figure 3). More than two accessory spleens occur in less than 5%. The presence of accessory splenules may arise within the substance of solid organs, notably the pancreas [10]. The presence of a well-marginated rounded mass located within 3 cm of the distal tail of the pancreas with signal intensity features of the spleen on all MR sequences suggests the diagnosis of intrapancreatic accessory spleen (IPAS) [11]. However, other entities may mimic the signal intensity and postgadolinium enhancement features of IPAS. Therefore, DWI and SPIO-enhanced MRI can be used to characterize the lesion and to establish the definite diagnosis [3].

Splenosis develops when splenic tissue is seeded within the abdomen or pelvis (Figure 4) following trauma [12].

The "upside-down spleen" is a normal variant due to an abnormal splenic rotation where the hilum is superiorly located and the convex border is medial and adjacent to the left kidney [13] (Figure 5).

All these normal variants and congenital abnormalities are usually easy to recognize.

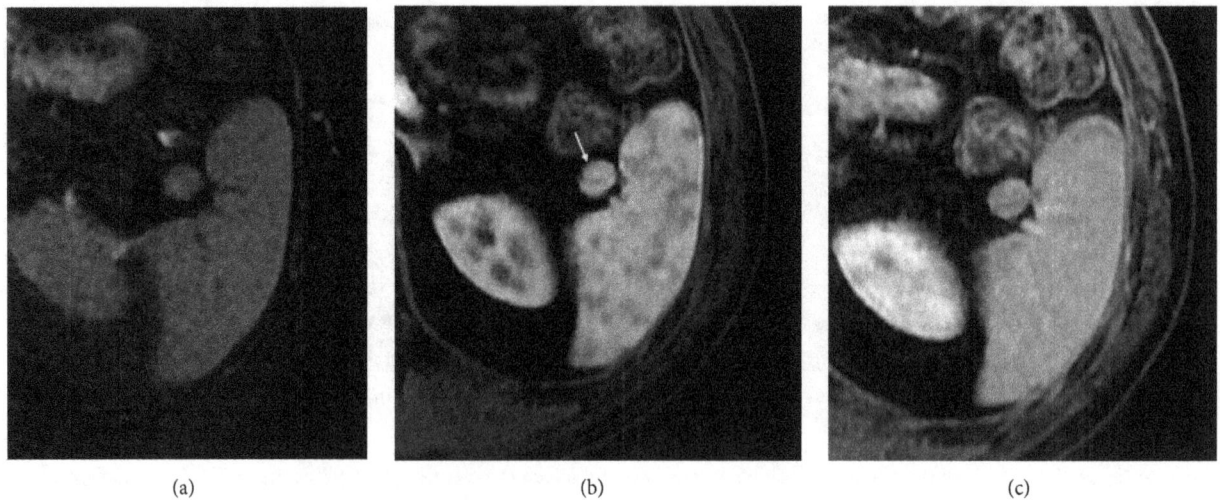

FIGURE 3: Accessory spleen. Axial T2wi FSE with fat suppression (a) and postcontrast axial 3D-GRE T1wi with fat suppression images at the arterial (b) and venous (c) phases. An accessory spleen is shown near the splenic hilum. Note the similar signal intensity and dynamic behavior comparable with the splenic parenchyma.

4. Inflammatory/Infectious Diseases

4.1. Abscesses. Splenic abscess is an uncommon lesion with high mortality rates, because of delayed detection and treatment [14, 15]. The frequency of splenic abscess has recently increased due to the higher number of immunocompromised patients, as those with hematologic disorders (e.g., leukemia), those with recreational intravenous drug abuse, and those with acquired immunodeficiency syndrome (AIDS). These lesions may be single or multiple [7].

Splenic abscesses are hypointense on T1-weighted images and have a moderate to high signal intensity on T2-weighted images, with irregular and undefined margins [8, 16]. Gas might be seen within the abscess as signal voids in the antidependent position and might be recognized by the presence of susceptibility artifact on T1-weighted in-phase and out-of-phase GRE sequences which appear greater on sequences with higher TE the sequence with higher TE (usually in-phase images). Following intravenous contrast administration, peripheral enhancement may be seen, although it is less often intense compared to liver abscess, perhaps due to the fairly bright enhancement of the normal splenic parenchyma in the arterial phase [8, 16] (Figure 6).

Candidiasis is the opportunistic infection that most frequently affects the liver and the spleen in immunocompromised patients. MRI is superior to CT for the detection and characterization of splenic microabscesses (<1 cm), most commonly secondary to candidiasis and appear as multiple hyperintense lesions in T2-weighted images with peripheral ring enhancement on gadolinium-enhanced images [7, 8] (Figure 7).

4.2. Histoplasmosis. Although it might be seen in patients with competent immune systems, the prevalence of histoplasmosis is greater in immunocompromised patients. MR imaging demonstrates the acute and subacute phases of this disease as scattered hypointense lesions on both T1- and T2-weighted images. Old granulomas can be calcified, causing with the characteristic signal intensity changes with blooming artifacts on MR images [8].

4.3. Sarcoidosis. Sarcoidosis is a granulomatous systemic disease of unknown etiology that may involve several organs and not infrequently the spleen. Of patients with systemic sarcoidosis, 24 to 59% have biopsy-documented splenic sarcoidosis [17].

Nodular sarcoidosis has been reported to demonstrate low signal intensity in all MR sequences. The lesions are most conspicuous on T2-weighted fat-suppressed or early phase contrast-enhanced images. Sarcoid lesions enhance minimally on delayed images (Figure 8).

5. Vascular Lesions

5.1. Infarct. Splenic infarcts may result from venous or arterial blood supply interruption. The vascular occlusions can be the result of a tromboembolic process caused by any type of hemolytic anemia, endocartitis or chronic valvular diseases, Gaucher disease, portal hypertension, or vascular collagen diseases [8, 18].

The typical MR appearance of a splenic infarct is a triangular wedge-shaped area, at the periphery of the spleen, with varying signal intensity according to the age of the infarct. It shows no enhancement after gadolinium injection and it is better depicted in late vascular phases, when the spleen is homogeneously enhanced [7, 8] (Figure 9).

5.2. Hematoma. Splenic hematoma is usually secondary to trauma [18]. Like splenic infarcts, the MR appearance is variable, depending on the age of the lesion. On acute (1 to 2 days) and early subacute phase (2 to 7 days) hematomas show

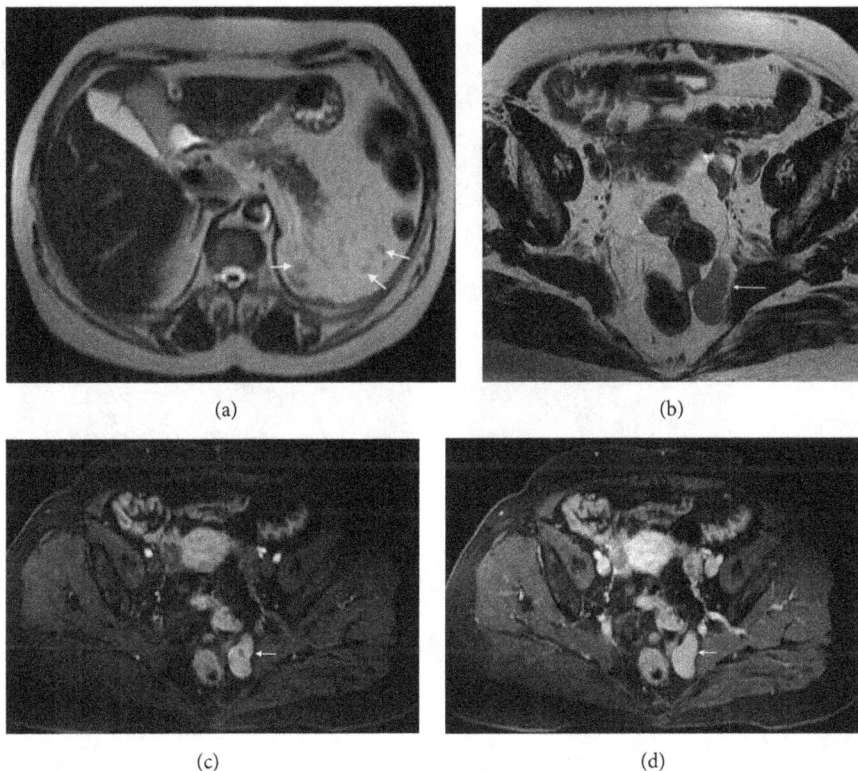

(a)   (b)

(c)   (d)

FIGURE 4: Pelvic splenosis. Axial (a) T2wi SSFSE, axial (b) T2 wi FSE and postcontrast axial T1wi 3D-GRE with fat suppression in the arterial (c) and venous (d) phase. This patient with history of splenectomy following a car accident underwent pelvic MRI to clarify pelvic masses depicted in previous CT. There are multiple nodular masses in the left hypochondrium (arrows, (a)) consistent with splenosis. There are also multiple well-defined nodules in the pelvis demonstrating high signal intensity on T2wi (arrow, (b)), with heterogeneous enhancement immediately after contrast material administration (c), becoming homogeneous in the venous (d) phase, consistent with splenosis.

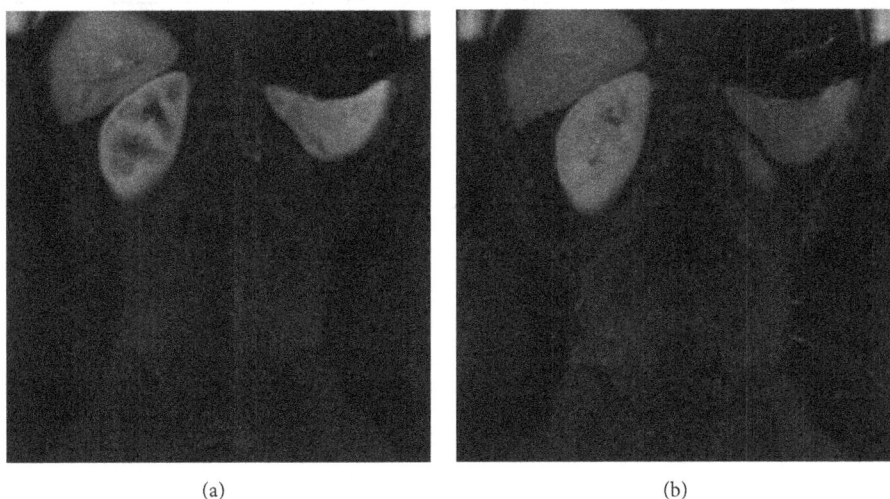

(a)   (b)

FIGURE 5: Upside-down spleen. Coronal postcontrast 3D-GRE T1wi with fat suppression at the arterial (a) and venous (b) phases. An abnormal splenic rotation is seen. The hilum is superiorly located and the convex border is adjacent to the left kidney.

low signal intensity on T2-weighted images and intermediate and increasingly higher signal intensity on T1-weighted images, respectively. On late subacute phase (7 to 14–28 days), hematomas show hyperintensity on both T1- and T2-weighted images (Figure 10). After 3 weeks (chronic), the hematoma may have a cystic appearance, regarded as a hyperintensity lesion on T2-weighted sequences with low signal intensity on T1-weighted images [18]. Older hematomas appear hypointense on both T1- and T2-weighted images, due to its fibrotic component.

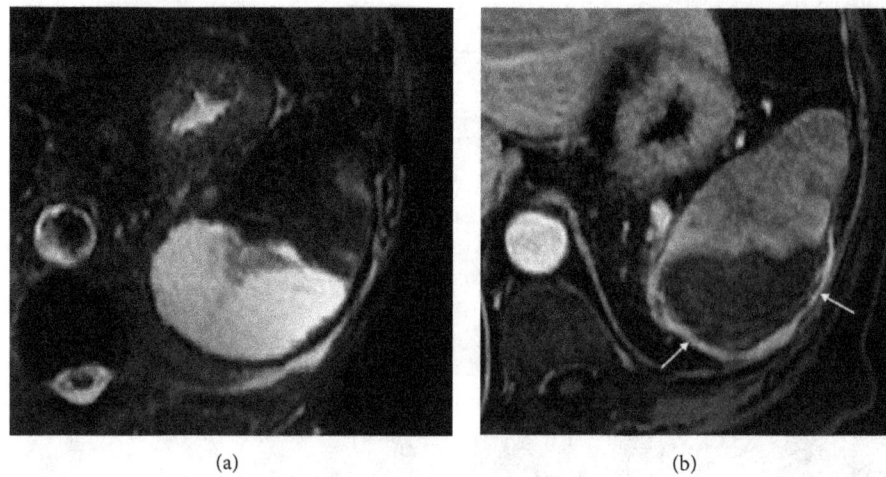

(a)

(b)

FIGURE 6: Splenic abscess. Axial T2wi SSFSE with fat suppression (a) and postcontrast axial T1wi 3D-GRE with fat suppression in the venous (b) phase. A large subcapsular splenic abscess is depicted. This lesion is marked hyperintense on T2wi and hypointense on T1wi with irregular margin. Note the faint enhancement of the splenic capsule (arrows, (b)).

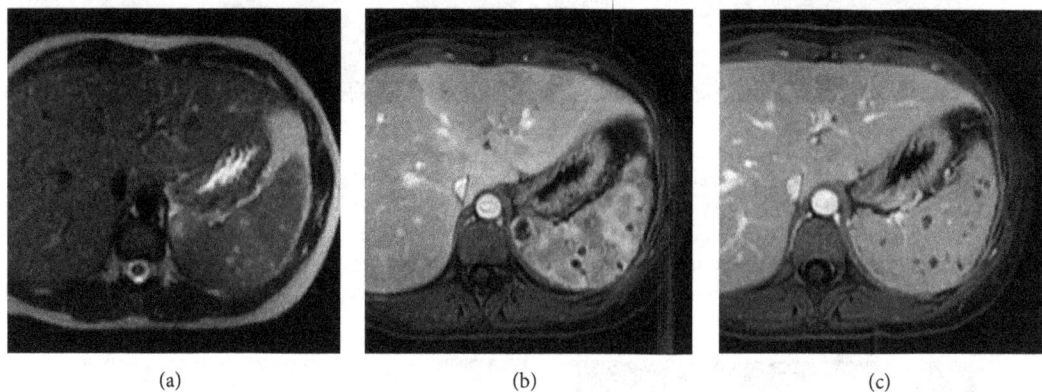

(a)   (b)   (c)

FIGURE 7: Microabscesses in an HIV patient with candidiasis. Axial T2wi SSFSE (a) and postcontrast axial 3D-GRE T1wi with fat suppression at the arterial (b) and venous (c) phases images. Multiple ill-defined T2w hyperintense lesions (a) with peripheral ring enhancement on gadolinium-enhanced images ((b) and (c)) are depicted, consistent with abscesses.

6. Benign Tumors

6.1. Cysts. Cysts are the most common benign focal splenic masses. They may be separated into epithelial or true cysts (approximately 25% of splenic cysts), which are lined with epithelium, and pseudocysts that can be posttraumatic or secondary to pancreatitis, in which the wall is fibrotic and lacks a true cellular lining (account for approximately 75% of splenic cysts) [1, 19].

Posttraumatic pseudocysts are thought to represent the final stage in evolution of a splenic hematoma, although some have suggested that they might also be secondary to infarct or infection [16, 18]. Pancreatic pseudocysts arising in the tail of the pancreas may involve the spleen by extending either beneath the splenic capsule or into the proper splenic parenchyma. Patients usually have a history of acute pancreatitis [16].

MRI shows the characteristic findings of a cyst, that is, a well-defined round mass, with thin or imperceptible wall, homogeneous hypointense on T1-weighted images, and hyperintense on T2-weighted images, with no enhancement on postcontrast images [18] (Figure 11).

It is often impossible to distinguish between true and false cysts; the clinical presentation and patient history may help to narrow the differential diagnoses. Cyst wall trabeculation or peripheral septations are much more commonly found in true cysts [7].

6.2. Hydatid Cyst (Echinococcus granulosus). Usually involves the liver or lungs but occasionally may also involve the spleen. Splenic hydatid cysts are very rare even in endemic regions (less than 2%) [19]. On MRI these cysts share imaging characteristics to those located in the liver. They are hyperintense on T2-weighted images and hypointense on T1-weighted images. They can be either unilocular or contain daughter cysts, distributed peripherally or throughout the lesion, giving a multilocular appearance. A "serpent" or

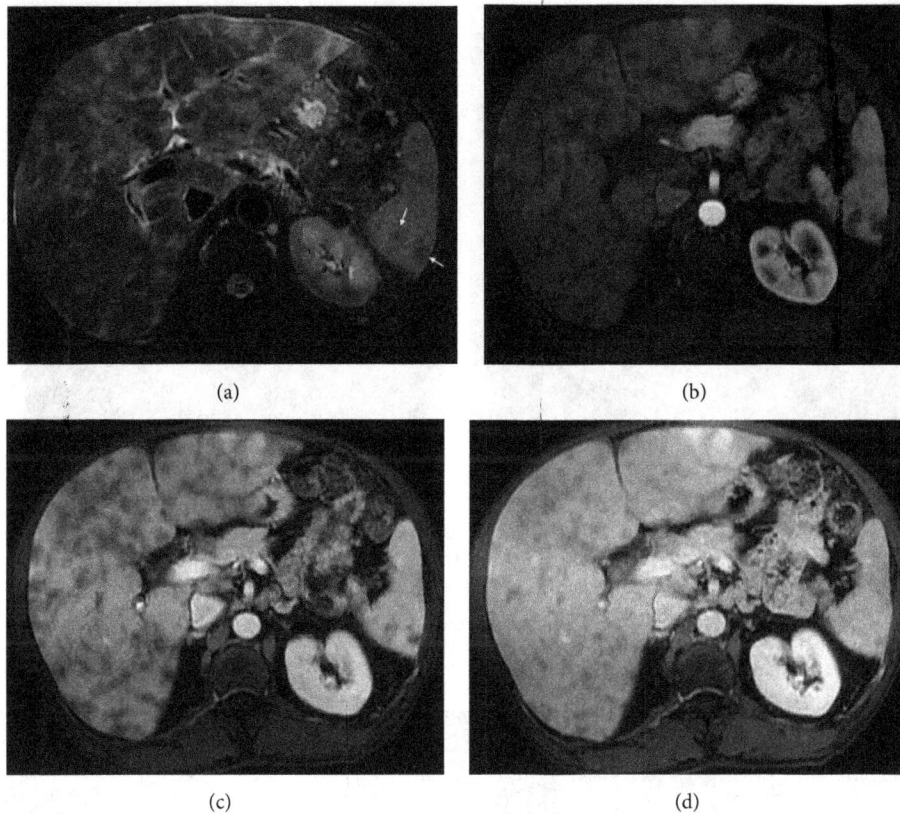

FIGURE 8: Sarcoidosis. Axial T2wi FSE with fat suppression (a) and postcontrast axial T1wi 3D-GRE with fat suppression in the arterial (b), venous (c) and interstitial phases (d). Low signal intensity nodules are depicted in the spleen on the T2wi sequences (arrows, (a)). The lesions are most conspicuous on fat-suppressed T2wi or early phase (b) contrast-enhanced images. Note the progressive enhancement of the sarcoid lesions on venous (c) and delayed images (d).

"snake" sign is occasionally noted representing collapsed parasitic membranes within the cyst. Continuous and irregular, 4- to 5-mm-thick, low signal intensity rim surrounding the cyst corresponding to the dense fibrous capsule encasing the parasitic membranes is frequently seen. Typically, no enhancement is noted following IV contrast administration [18, 20] (Figure 12).

6.3. *Hemangiomas*. Splenic hemangiomas are the most common benign solid tumor of the spleen. Their frequency in large autopsy series is 0.03%–14%, and they are more frequently found in males (1.4 versus 1.0) [19, 21]. These lesions are believed to be congenital in origin, arising from sinusoidal epithelium. Most of them are less than 2 cm in diameter; however, once large they may spontaneously rupture, causing intra-abdominal hemorrhage. Histologically, they are composed of endothelial-lined blood-filled spaces of varying size and can be characterized by the size of these spaces as capillary or cavernous lesions [16].

Diffuse hemangiomatosis of the spleen is a rare benign vascular condition occurring as a manifestation of systemic angiomatosis (associations with Klippel-Trénaunay-Weber, Turner, Kasabach-Merritt-like, and Beckwith-Wiedemann syndromes have been reported) or, less commonly, confined to the spleen [8].

Most hemangiomas are well-defined homogeneous, hypo- to isointense on T1-weighted images and most commonly hyperintense on T2-weighted images compared with splenic parenchyma [21] (Figure 13). On dynamic contrast-enhanced studies, they usually show peripheral enhancement with centripetal, delayed progression (see Figure 13). Uncommonly, similarly to liver hemangiomas, these lesions may undergo sclerosis and late phase images are important to suggest the correct diagnosis. The typical nodular peripheral enhancement of hepatic hemangiomas is uncommonly seen in splenic hemangiomas [22].

6.4. *Hamartomas*. Hamartoma is an infrequently benign, usually asymptomatic tumor of the spleen, with an autopsy incidence of 0.13% and no gender predilection. Approximately, one-sixth of hamartomas are found in children (<16 years). They are nonneoplastic tumors composed of a mixture of normal elements of splenic red and white pulp components [19, 23]. They are considered to be congenital in origin, but some theories associate it with previous trauma.

Hamartomas are a sharply defined, rounded, single solid lesion that sometimes may be multiple (Figure 14). On MRI, they are usually isointense on T1-weighted images and heterogeneously hyperintense on T2-weighted images [22]. After intravenous gadolinium administration, there is

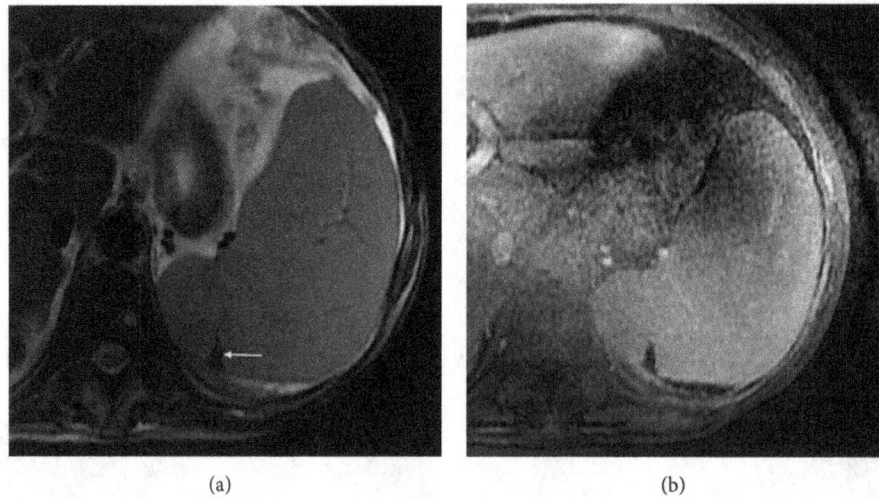

(a)   (b)

FIGURE 9: Splenic infarct. Axial T2wi FSE (a) and axial postcontrast fat-suppressed 3D-GRE T1wi at the venous (b) phase. A small triangular wedge-shaped area at the periphery of the spleen is noted (arrow, (a)), with hypointensity signal on both T1 and T2wi, with no enhancement on postcontrast images.

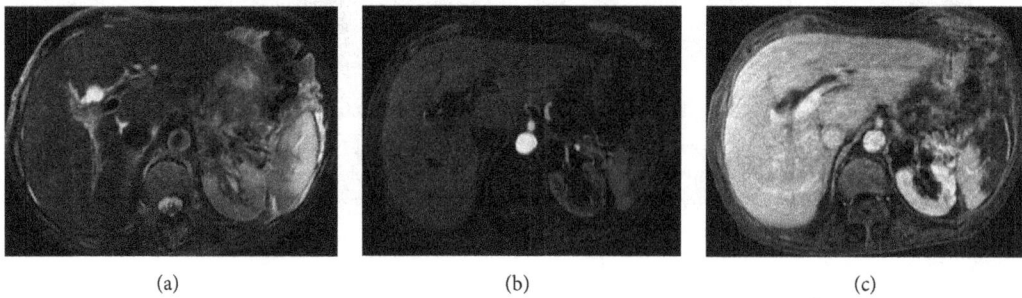

(a)   (b)   (c)

FIGURE 10: Hematoma. Axial (a) T2wi SSFSE and postcontrast axial T1wi 3D-GRE with fat suppression in the arterial (b) and interstitial (c) phases. A chronic hematoma is depicted with a cystic appearance, regarded as a lesion with moderate hyperintensity on T2wi sequences (a) and hypointensity on T1wi with no perceptible enhancement ((b), (c)).

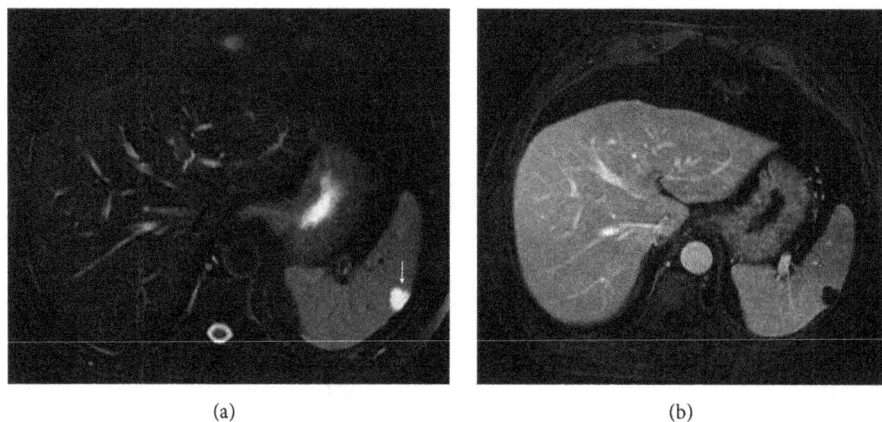

(a)   (b)

FIGURE 11: Splenic cyst. Axial T2wi FSE with fat suppression (a) and postcontrast axial 3D-GRE T1wi with fat suppression at the interstitial (b) phase. Note the thin-walled and well-defined nodule, homogeneously hyperintense on T2wi (a), with no enhancement on post contrast image, characteristic of cysts.

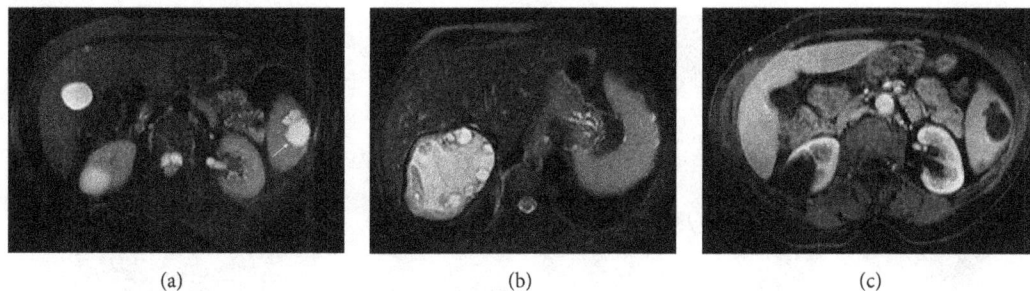

FIGURE 12: Hydatid cyst. Axial T2wi SSFSE with fat suppression ((a) and (b)) and axial postcontrast T1wi 3D-GRE with fat suppression in the venous (c) phase. A classic hydatid cyst is visualized in the liver (b). A concomitant splenic hydatid cyst is depicted as a multilocular lesion with moderate hyperintensity on T2wi (arrow, (a)) and hypointensity on T1wi (c). A fibrotic thickened continuous low signal intensity rim surrounding the cyst is seen on T2wi ((a), (b)). No enhancement is noted following IV contrast administration (c).

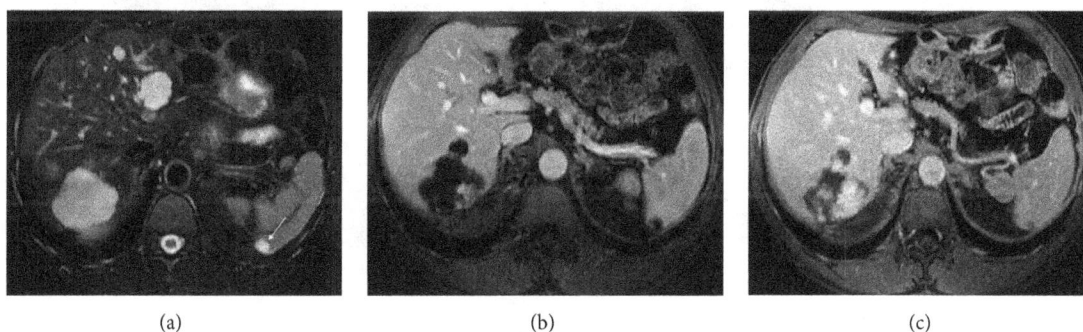

FIGURE 13: Splenic hemangioma. Axial T2wi FSE with fat suppression (a) and postcontrast axial 3D-GRE T1wi with fat suppression at the arterial (b) and interstitial (c) phases. The hemangioma is depicted as a well-defined, homogeneous, and hyperintense lesion on T2wi (arrow, (a)), with a peripheral enhancement with centripetal and delayed progression, on postcontrast images ((b) and (c)). Note the hepatic hemangiomas on the same imaging plane.

usually diffuse heterogeneous enhancement, which may be useful in distinguishing this lesion from the typical peripheral enhancement noted in hemangiomas (see Figure 14). Prolonged enhancement may be appreciated, which has been attributed to stagnant contrast material within the sinusoids of the red pulp of splenic tissue. Persistent areas of hypointensity may also be seen and correspond to areas of necrosis within the lesion [7, 16, 21].

6.5. Littoral Cell Angioma. Littoral cell angioma is a relatively new clinicopathological entity of a rare benign tumor of the spleen that develops from the lining cells of the red-pulp sinuses, the so-called "littoral cells", giving rise to littoral cell angioma [24]. It has no malignant histological features and has a benign clinical course.

Lesions are of variable size and commonly multinodular. They are composed of anastomosing vascular channels with irregular lumina featuring cyst-like spaces and lined by tall endothelial cells.

On MRI, lesions are inhomogeneously hyperintense on T2-weighted images, with signal intensity similar to that of hemangiomas and slightly hypointense on unenhanced T1-weighted images. Littoral cell angiomas may show low signal intensity on all sequences due to hemosiderin accumulation within neoplastic littoral cells [25]. Dynamic postcontrast

T1-weighted images depict delayed contrast enhancement, suggestive of a vascular lesion with contrast media pooling (Figure 15).

6.6. Lymphangioma. Lymphangioma is a rare vascular benign lesion filled with lymph instead of red blood cells as seen in hemangioma [18]. Usually diagnosed in childhood, it may appear as solitary or multiple splenic lesions or as a diffuse involvement replacing most of the splenic parenchyma, known as lymphangiomatosis [16].

Cystic lymphangioma is the most frequent type and is characterized by a honeycomb of large and small thin-walled cysts containing lymph-like clear fluid. On MRI, lymphangiomas usually present as well-defined multilocular cystic lesions, with thin septations and hyperintensity on T2-weighted sequences. However, some of the cysts may be hyperintense on T1-weighted images, due to protein or hemorrhagic content [1, 16, 19].

7. Malignant Tumors

7.1. Lymphoma. Lymphoma is the most common splenic malignancy. Both Hodgkin's and non-Hodgkin's lymphoma may present in the spleen as the primary site (less than 1%) or as part of systemic involvement [1].

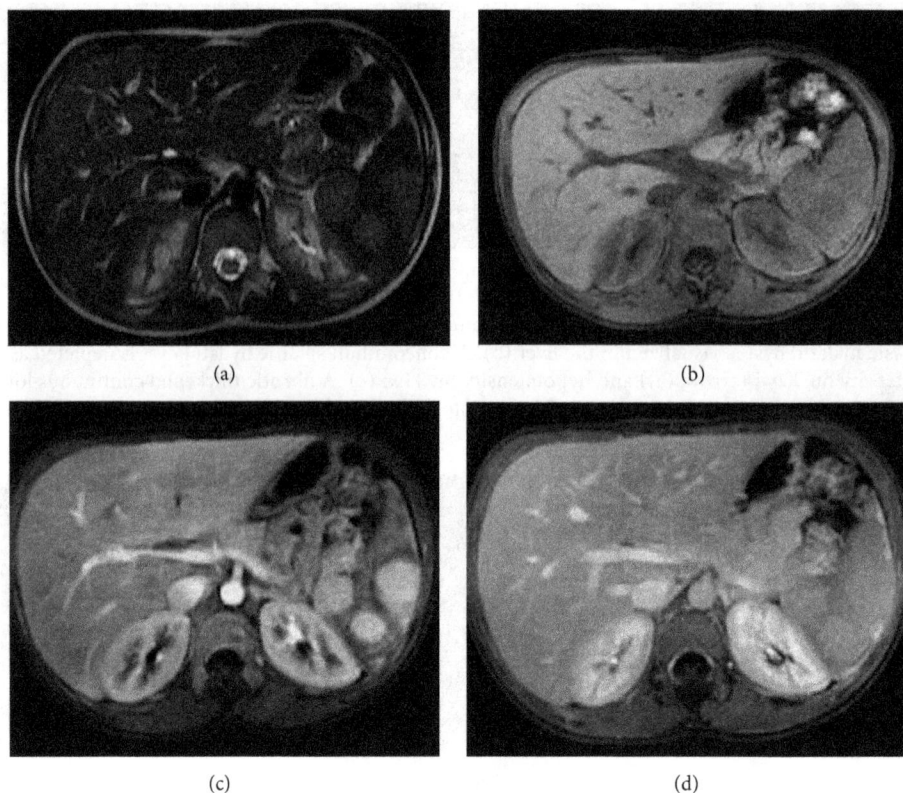

FIGURE 14: Splenic hamartoma. Axial T2wi SSFSE (a), pre- (b) and postcontrast axial T1w 3D-GRE with fat suppression in the arterial (c) and venous (d) phase. Multiple rounded lesions are seen on T2wi (a) and T1wi (b). These lesions demonstrate hyperenhancing characteristics on the arterial phase (c) progressing to isointensity on the venous phase (d).

Splenic involvement in lymphoma may produce homogeneous enlargement (the most common finding, although it may be absent in up to 30% of patients), multiple small (or miliary) nodules, a single solitary mass, or a combination of these appearances [16, 19].

Immediate postcontrast MRI images surpass CT in their evaluation; nevertheless, the role of MRI has not been established yet.

Lymphomatous nodules are typically isointense to splenic parenchyma on T1- and T2-weighted images, although they may present some hypointensity on T2-weighted images, which may help to distinguish from metastatic lesions (Figure 16). Lymphomatous lesions are usually hypovascular with lower signal intensity relative to normal spleen on postcontrast images, thereby increasing conspicuity [16, 23].

7.2. *Metastasis.* Although the spleen is the most vascular organ in the body, it is an infrequent site for metastatic disease. Metastatic involvement of the spleen is somewhat uncommon, occurring in up to 7% of patients with widespread malignancy. According to most series, splenic metastases are mainly due to melanoma and breast cancers and in a less percentage from cancers of the lung, colon, stomach, ovary, endometrium, and prostate [7, 18].

Splenic metastatic lesions may be solitary, multiple, or diffuse and differ in number and size from a few millimeters to several centimeters. At MR imaging, metastases typically appear as hyperintense masses on T2-weighted images and hypo- to isointense masses on T1-weighted images with inhomogeneous contrast enhancement, usually with peripheral ring-like pattern [19, 23, 26] (Figure 17). Central tumor necrosis is seen as regions of hyperintensity on T2-weighted images [27]. The presence of blood products from hemorrhage or other paramagnetic substances, such as melanin from melanocytic melanomas, may result in high signal intensity on T1-weighted images [18].

7.3. *Perisplenic Neoplasms Infiltrating the Spleen.* Implants on the serosal surface of the spleen are seen in patients with peritoneal carcinomatosis, commonly from ovarian or gastrointestinal primary neoplasms. These implants may cause indentation and scalloping of the surface of the spleen. Direct tumor invasion of the spleen is uncommon, but can be seen in tumors originating from the pancreas, stomach, colon or left kidney, and retroperitoneum (Figure 18) [28].

7.4. *Angiosarcoma.* Angiosarcoma is exceedingly rare, yet it is the most common primary malignant nonlymphoid tumor of the spleen [29]. These tumors are highly aggressive (nearly 80% of patients die 6 months after the diagnosis) and usually manifest as widespread metastatic disease or splenic rupture [7, 8, 16]. Association with thoratrast has been reported.

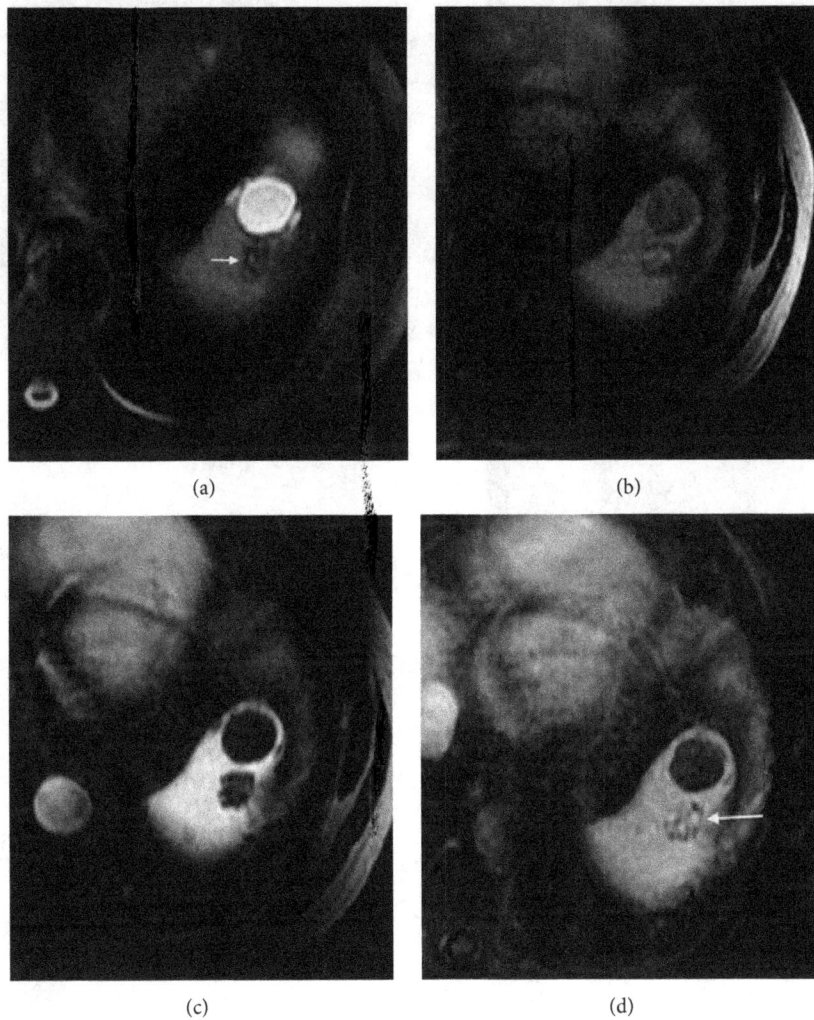

FIGURE 15: Littoral cell angioma. Axial T2wi FSE with fat suppression (a), pre- (b) and postcontrast axial 3D-GRE T1wi with fat suppression at the venous phase (c) and after 10 minutes of contrast injection (d). A hypointense nodular lesion is depicted on T2wi (arrow, (a)), with areas of magnetic susceptibility artifact, and hypovascular nodules that show subtle peripheral enhancement with progressive slow centripetal accumulation of contrast (arrow, (d)). This mass was thought to represent a sclerosed splenic hemangioma. This heterogeneous splenic appearance is also possible with angiosarcoma and in cases of splenic hemangiomatosis. Note the anteriorly adjacent splenic cyst.

Angiosarcoma typically appears as multiple nodular heterogeneous masses, with variable signal intensity on T1-weighted and T2-weighted images, due to the presence of hemorrhage with different ages, siderotic nodules, and areas of necrosis. Following the intravenous administration of gadolinium, the lesion demonstrates heterogeneous enhancement. MRI seems to be more precise than CT in the overall assessment and staging of this type of tumor and is of particular value for timely diagnosis [30].

There are other extremely rare primary malignant splenic tumors including malignant fibrous histiocytoma, leiomyosarcoma, fibrosarcoma, malignant teratoma, and Kaposi sarcoma, all of which are with nonspecific appearance.

8. Diffuse Diseases

8.1. Splenomegaly. Splenomegaly is a radiologic and clinical sign, classically described when the craniocaudal splenic length is more than 12 cm (Figure 19). This may result from congestion (portal hypertension, splenic vein occlusion, or thrombosis), infiltrative disease (Gaucher disease or histiocytosis), hematologic disorders (polycythemia vera, myelofibrosis), inflammatory's/infectious diseases (HIV, mononucleosis, amyloidosis, Feltys syndrome, or mycobacterial infection), cysts, or tumors (leukemia, lymphoma, or metastases) [7, 10, 23].

8.2. Siderotic Nodules. Foci of hemosiderin deposition are seen in about 9%–12% of patients with portal hypertension and are the so-called Gamma-Gandy bodies (Figure 20). These foci of hemosiderin have low signal intensity on all pulse sequences and exhibit "blooming" artifact on gradient echo sequences, secondary to iron deposition [8, 23].

8.3. Gaucher Disease. Gaucher disease is an autosomal recessive lysosomal disorder secondary to lack of the enzyme

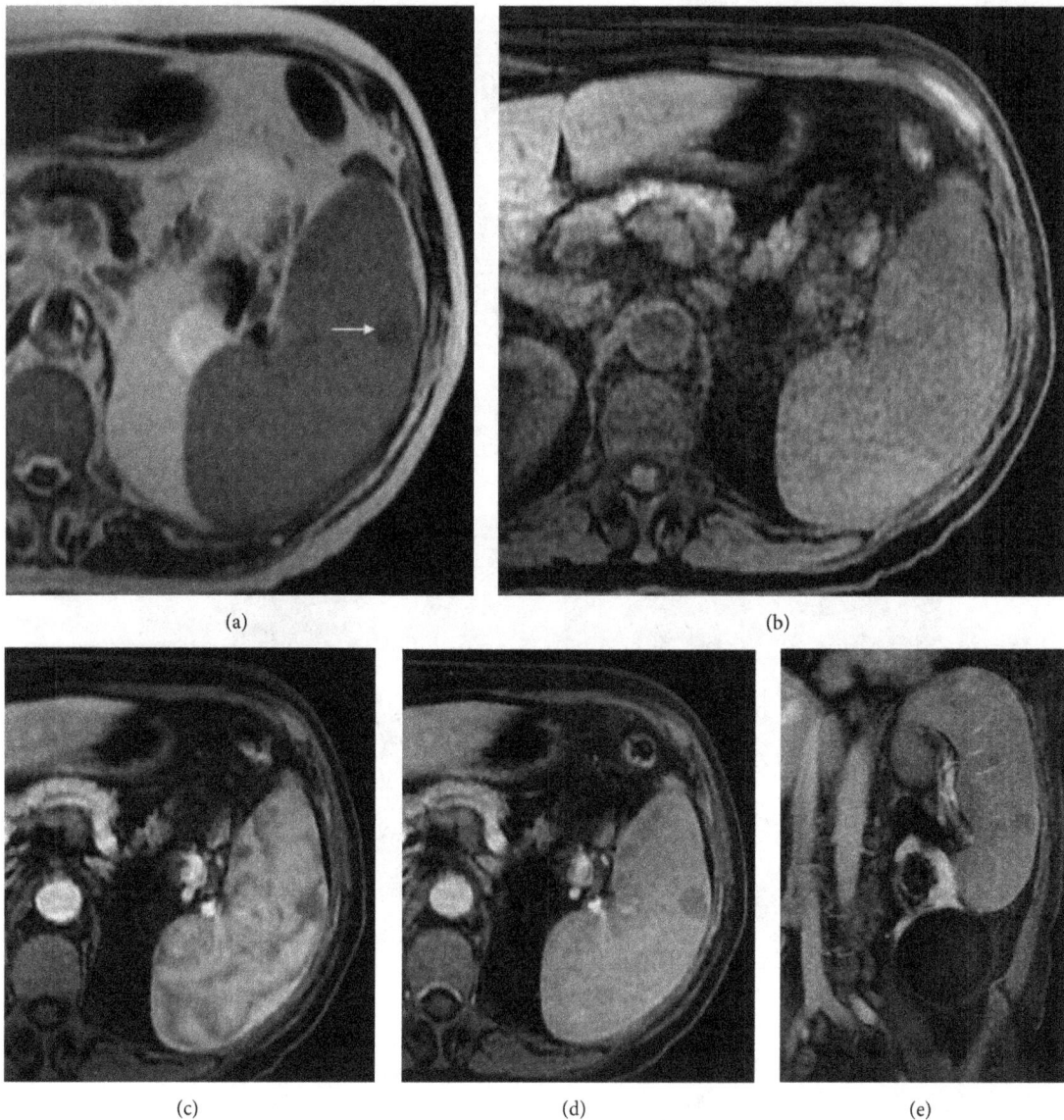

(a)

(b)

(c)   (d)   (e)

FIGURE 16: Lymphoma. Axial T2wi SSFSE (a), axial pre- (b) and postcontrast T1wi 3D-GRE with fat suppression in the arterial (c) and venous (d) phase. Coronal fat-suppressed T1wi 3D-GRE in the interstitial phase (e). The spleen is enlarged. Lymphomatous nodules are isointense to splenic parenchyma on T1wi (b) and T2wi (a). One nodule is moderately hypointense T2wi (arrow, (a)). This feature aids in distinction against metastatic lesions, which are commonly hyperintense. Lymphomatous lesions demonstrate hypovascular nature with lower signal intensity relative to normal spleen on postcontrast images ((c), (d) (e)), thereby increasing conspicuity.

glucocerebrosidase, leading to the accumulation of gluco-cerebrosides in the cells of the reticuloendothelial system, causing hepatosplenomegaly. Splenic infarcts and fibrosis associated with Gaucher disease may exhibit a multifocal pattern [8].

8.4. Hemosiderosis and Sickle Cell Disease. Hemosiderosis, with splenic involvement, shows diffuse diminished signal intensity of the organ on both T1- and T2-weighted images relative to musculature as a result of hemosiderin deposition [1] (Figure 21).

Sickle cell disease is common in the Afro-descendent population with a prevalence of 0.2% (homozygous form)

and 8%–10% (heterozygous form). The spleen is the most commonly organ involved. In patients with sickle cell disease, the spleen appears as a nearly signal void area due to iron deposition from blood transfusion. Autosplenectomy is often found in patients with homozygous sickle cell disease [7, 8] (Figure 22).

8.5. Extramedullary Hematopoiesis. Extramedullary hemato-poiesis is a compensatory response to failure of the bone marrow cells. A focal mass-like involvement of the liver and spleen, which are the main affected organs, may be present. On MRI, the appearance of the nodular lesions depends on the evolution of the hematopoiesis. Active lesions

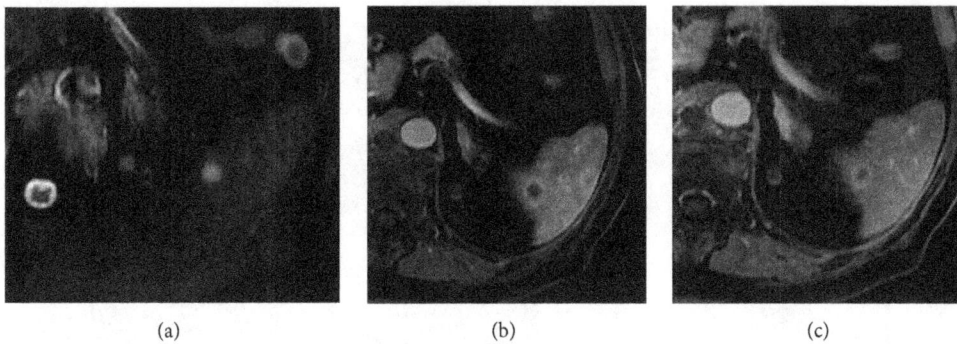

FIGURE 17: Splenic metastasis on a patient with a small-cell lung carcinoma. Axial T2wi SSFSE (a) and postcontrast axial 3D-GRE T1wi with fat suppression at the arterial (b) and venous (c) phases. Note the nodular lesion depicted as a hyperintense nodule on T2wi with peripheral ring-like enhancement.

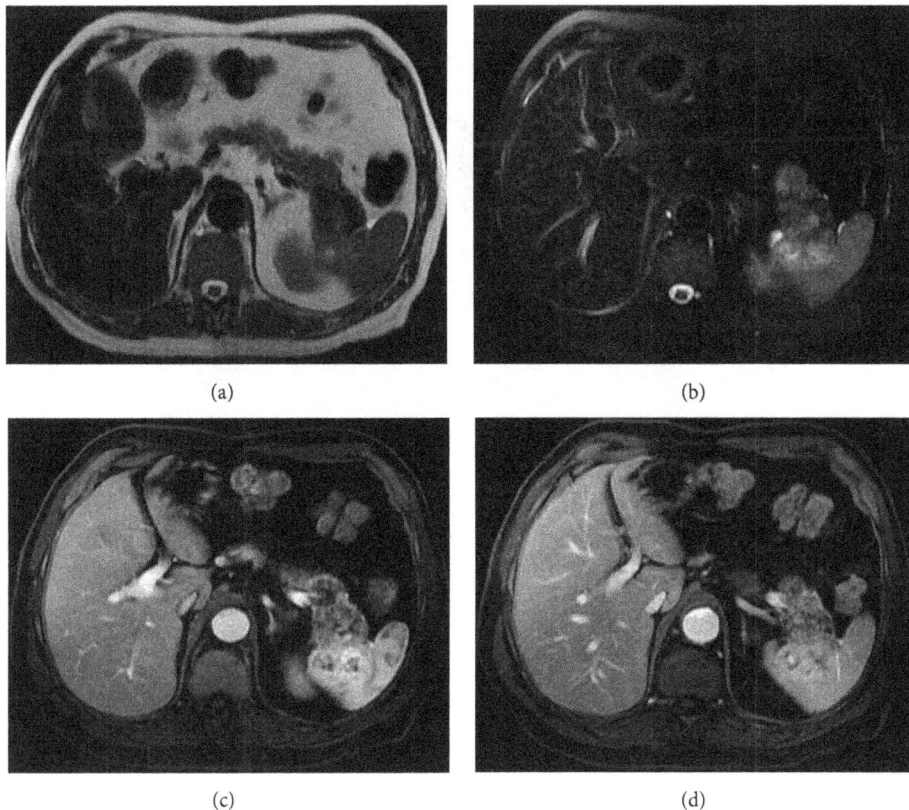

FIGURE 18: Pancreatic tail clear cell renal cell carcinoma metastases with infiltration of the spleen through the splenic hilum. Axial T2wi SSFSE without (a) and with (b) fat suppression and axial postcontrast T1wi 3D-GRE with fat suppression in the arterial (c) and venous (d) phase. A large heterogeneous mass is seen in the pancreatic tail infiltrating the spleen.

reveal intermediate signal intensity on T1-weighted images, high signal intensity on T2-weighted images, and moderate enhancement after administration of intravenous gadolinium. Older lesions are hypointense on T1- and T2-weighted images and do not show any enhancement. These lesions usually demonstrate low signal intensity on in-phase T1-weighted GRE images compared with that on out-of phase images due to the presence of iron [8].

9. Conclusion

Focal and diffuse lesions of the spleen are uncommon and usually discovered incidentally on cross-sectional imaging studies. Due to the widespread of MRI there has been an increase in the detection of diseases involving the spleen. By virtue of its excellent contrast resolution and the possibility of tissue characterization through the use of different sequences,

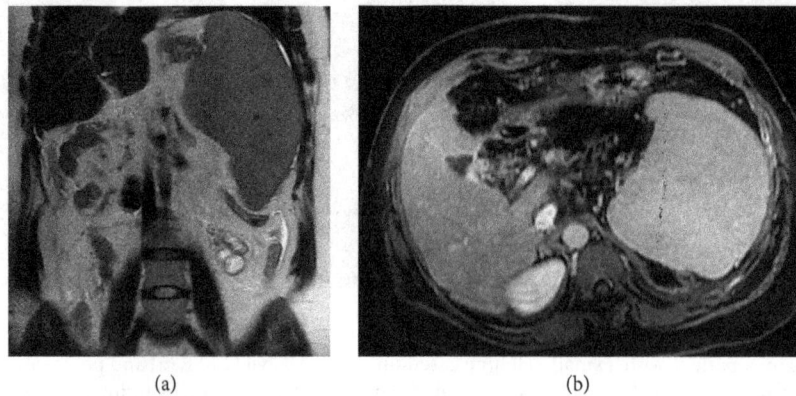

FIGURE 19: Splenomegaly. Coronal T2wi SSFSE (a) and postcontrast axial T1wi 3D-GRE with fat suppression in the interstitial phase (b). A homogeneous splenomegaly resulting from congestion (portal hypertension) is easily seen.

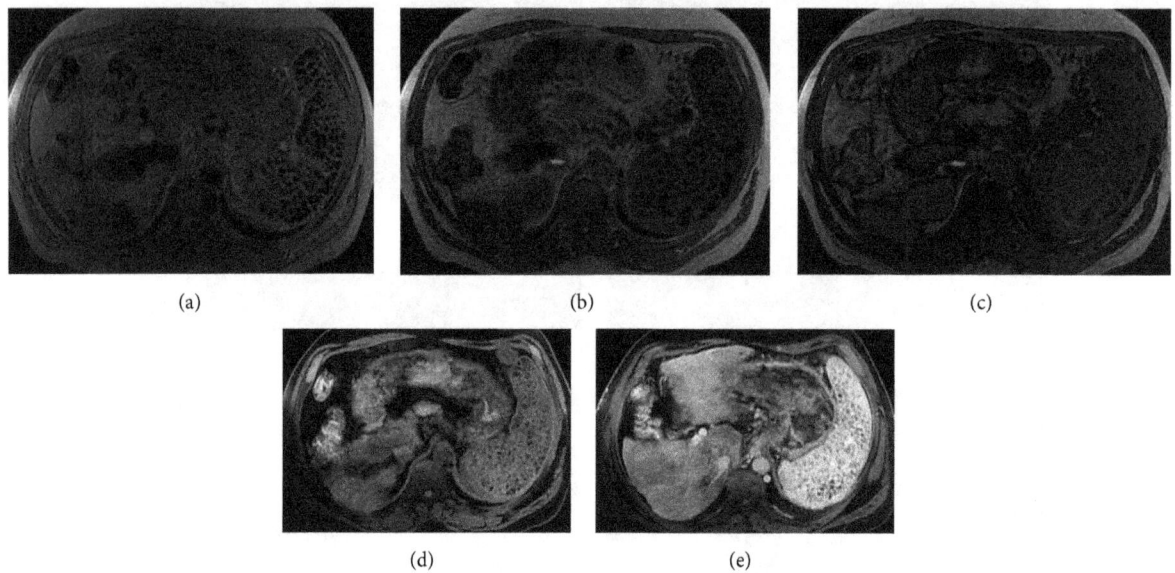

FIGURE 20: Siderotic splenic nodules (Gamma-Gandy bodies). Axial T2* (a), axial 2D-GRE T1w in-phase (b) and out-of-phase (c), and pre (d) and postcontrast axial 3D-GRE T1wi with fat suppression at the arterial phase (e). Note the splenomegaly with multiple foci of hemosiderin with low signal intensity on all pulse sequences and exhibiting the "blooming" artifact on in-phase (longer TE) GRE sequences, secondary to iron deposition. No enhancement is depicted.

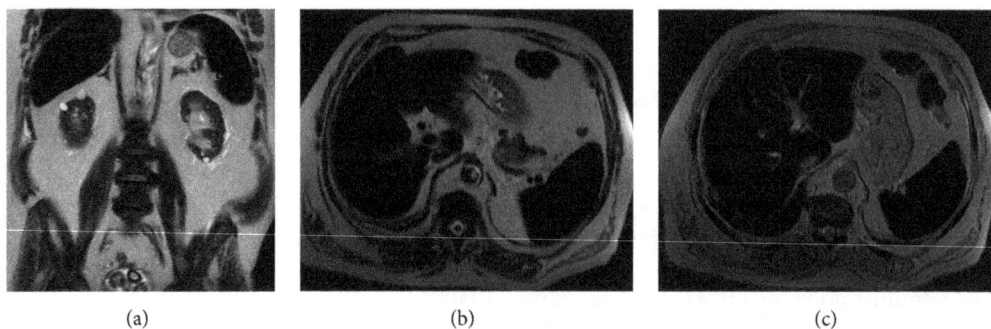

FIGURE 21: Paroxysmal nocturnal hemoglobinuria. Coronal (a) and axial (b) T2wi SSFSE and axial T2* (c) images. This patient with paroxysmal nocturnal hemoglobinuria shows diffuse diminished signal intensity of the liver and spleen on T2wi as a result of hemosiderin deposition. Notice the iron accumulation on the renal cortex (a).

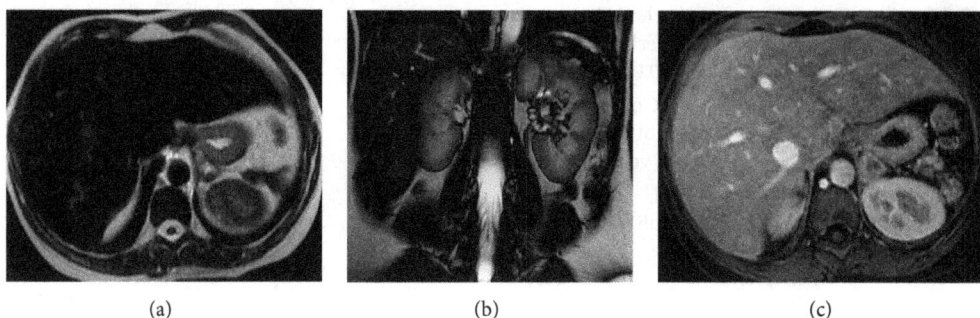

(a)   (b)   (c)

FIGURE 22: Autosplenectomy is found in a patient with homozygous sickle cell disease. Axial T2wi SSFSE (a), coronal SSFP (b), and postcontrast axial 3D-GRE T1wi with fat suppression at the arterial phase (c). Note the small remnant of spleen and the diffuse diminished signal intensity of the hepatic parenchyma on both T1wi and T2wi as a result of iron deposition.

MRI provides an excellent tool for the evaluation and characterization of various splenic lesions.

Awareness of the MRI appearance of the most common splenic disease processes is important for the radiologist to interpret the findings correctly, reaching whenever possible the appropriate diagnosis.

Disclosure

This paper was presented in part at the 25th European Congress of Radiology, 2013.

Conflict of Interests

The authors declare that there is no conflict of interests regarding the publication of this paper.

References

[1] A. Luna, R. Ribes, P. Caro, L. Luna, E. Aumente, and P. R. Ros, "MRI of focal splenic lesions without and with dynamic gadolinium enhancement," *American Journal of Roentgenology*, vol. 186, no. 6, pp. 1533–1547, 2006.

[2] T. Benter, L. Klühs, and U. Teichgräber, "Sonography of the spleen," *Journal of Ultrasound in Medicine*, vol. 30, pp. 1281–1293, 2011.

[3] K. M. Jang, S. H. Kim, S. J. Lee, M. J. Park, M. H. Lee, and D. Choi, "Differentiation of an intrapancreatic accessory spleen from a small (<3-cm) solid pancreatic tumor: value of diffusion-weighted MR imaging," *Radiology*, vol. 266, pp. 159–167, 2013.

[4] R. C. Semelka, J. P. Shoenut, P. H. Lawrence, H. M. Greenberg, T. P. Madden, and M. A. Kroeker, "Spleen: dynamic enhancement patterns on gradient-echo MR images enhanced with gadopentetate dimeglumine," *Radiology*, vol. 185, no. 2, pp. 479–482, 1992.

[5] T. Yoshikawa, H. Kawamitsu, D. G. Mitchell et al., "ADC measurement of abdominal organs and lesions using parallel imaging technique," *American Journal of Roentgenology*, vol. 187, no. 6, pp. 1521–1530, 2006.

[6] A. B. Rosenkrantz, M. Oei, J. S. Babb, B. E. Niver, and B. Taouli, "Diffusion-weighted imaging of the abdomen at 3.0 Tesla: image quality and apparent diffusion coefficient reproducibility compared with 1.5 Tesla," *Journal of Magnetic Resonance Imaging*, vol. 33, no. 1, pp. 128–135, 2011.

[7] L. S. Rabushka, A. Kawashima, and E. K. Fishman, "Imaging of the spleen: CT with supplemental MR examination," *Radiographics*, vol. 14, no. 2, pp. 307–332, 1994.

[8] K. M. Elsayes, V. R. Narra, G. Mukundan, J. S. Lewis Jr., C. O. Menias, and J. P. Heiken, "MR imaging of the spleen: spectrum of abnormalities," *Radiographics*, vol. 25, no. 4, pp. 967–982, 2005.

[9] G. Gayer, R. Zissin, S. Apter, E. Atar, O. Portnoy, and Y. Itzchak, "CT findings in congenital anomalies of the spleen," *British Journal of Radiology*, vol. 74, no. 884, pp. 767–772, 2001.

[10] H. M. Karakaş, N. Tunçbilek, and O. O. Okten, "Splenic abnormalities: an overview on sectional images," *Diagnostic and Interventional Radiology*, vol. 11, pp. 152–158, 2005.

[11] V. Herédia, E. Altun, F. Bilaj, M. Ramalho, B. W. Hyslop, and R. C. Semelka, "Gadolinium- and superparamagnetic-iron-oxide-enhanced MR findings of intrapancreatic accessory spleen in five patients," *Magnetic Resonance Imaging*, vol. 26, no. 9, pp. 1273–1278, 2008.

[12] S. Merran, P. Karila-Cohen, and V. Servois, "CT anatomy of the normal spleen: variants and pitfalls," *Journal de Radiologie*, vol. 88, no. 4, pp. 549–558, 2007.

[13] J. L. Westcott and E. L. Krufky, "The upside-down spleen," *Radiology*, vol. 105, no. 3, pp. 517–521, 1972.

[14] S. Paris, S. M. Weiss, W. H. Ayers Jr., and L. E. Clarke, "Splenic abscess," *American Surgeon*, vol. 60, no. 5, pp. 358–361, 1994.

[15] K. Y. Liu, Y. M. Shyr, C. H. Su, C. W. Wu, L. Y. Lee, and W. Y. Lui, "Splenic abscess—a changing trend in treatment," *South African Journal of Surgery*, vol. 38, no. 3, pp. 55–57, 2000.

[16] D. M. Warshauer and H. L. Hall, "Solitary splenic lesions," *Seminars in Ultrasound, CT and MRI*, vol. 27, no. 5, pp. 370–388, 2006.

[17] T. Sekine, Y. Amano, F. Hidaka et al., "Hepatosplenic and muscular sarcoidosis: characterization with MR imaging," *Magnetic Resonance in Medical Sciences*, vol. 11, pp. 83–89, 2012.

[18] M. Urrutia, P. J. Mergo, L. H. Ros, G. M. Torres, and P. R. Ros, "Cystic masses of the spleen: radiologic- pathologic correlation," *Radiographics*, vol. 16, no. 1, pp. 107–129, 1996.

[19] A. Giovagnoni, C. Giorgi, and G. Goteri, "Tumours of the spleen," *Cancer Imaging*, vol. 5, no. 1, pp. 73–77, 2005.

[20] M. Yuksel, G. Demirpolat, A. Sever, S. Bakaris, E. Bulbuloglu, and N. Elmas, "Hydatid disease involving some rare locations in the body: a pictorial essay," *Korean Journal of Radiology*, vol. 8, no. 6, pp. 531–540, 2007.

[21] M. Ramani, C. Reinhold, R. C. Semelka et al., "Splenic heman-
     giomas and hamartomas: MR imaging characteristics of 28
     lesions," *Radiology*, vol. 202, no. 1, pp. 166–172, 1997.

[22] R. M. Abbott, A. D. Levy, N. S. Aguilera, L. Gorospe, and
     W. M. Thompson, "Primary vascular neoplasms of the spleen:
     radiologic-pathologic correlation," *Radiographics*, vol. 24, no. 4,
     pp. 1137–1163, 2004.

[23] A. Kamaya, S. Weinstein, and T. S. Desser, "Multiple lesions
     of the spleen: differential diagnosis of cystic and solid lesions,"
     Seminars in Ultrasound, CT and MRI, vol. 27, no. 5, pp. 389–403,
     2006.

[24] S. Falk, H. J. Stutte, and G. Frizzera, "Littoral cell angioma: a
     novel splenic vascular lesion demonstrating histiocytic differ-
     entiation," *American Journal of Surgical Pathology*, vol. 15, no.
     11, pp. 1023–1033, 1991.

[25] A. D. Levy, R. M. Abbott, and S. L. Abbondanzo, "Littoral
     cell angioma of the spleen: CT features with clinicopathologic
     comparison," *Radiology*, vol. 230, no. 2, pp. 485–490, 2004.

[26] V. M. Runge and N. M. Williams, "Dynamic contrast-enhanced
     magnetic resonance imaging in a model of splenic metastasis,"
     Investigative Radiology, vol. 33, no. 1, pp. 45–50, 1998.

[27] P. F. Hahn, R. Weissleder, D. D. Stark, S. Saini, G. Elizondo, and
     J. T. Ferrucci, "MR imaging of focal splenic tumors," *American
     Journal of Roentgenology*, vol. 150, no. 4, pp. 823–827, 1988.

[28] R. K. Kaza, S. Azar, M. M. Al-Hawary, and I. R. Francis,
     "Primary and secondary neoplasms of the spleen," *Cancer
     Imaging*, vol. 10, no. 1, pp. 173–182, 2010.

[29] S. Falk, J. Krishnan, and J. M. Meis, "Primary angiosarcoma
     of the spleen: a clinicopathologic study of 40 cases," *American
     Journal of Surgical Pathology*, vol. 17, no. 10, pp. 959–970, 1993.

[30] W. M. Thompson, A. D. Levy, N. S. Aguilera, L. Gorospe,
     and R. M. Abbott, "Angiosarcoma of the spleen: imaging
     characteristics in 12 patients," *Radiology*, vol. 235, no. 1, pp. 106–
     115, 2005.

17

Knowledge on Irradiation, Medical Imaging Prescriptions, and Clinical Imaging Referral Guidelines among Physicians in a Sub-Saharan African Country (Cameroon)

Boniface Moifo,[1,2] **Ulrich Tene,**[1] **Jean Roger Moulion Tapouh,**[1,3] **Odette Samba Ngano,**[4] **Justine Tchemtchoua Youta,**[1] **Augustin Simo,**[5] **and Joseph Gonsu Fotsin**[1]

[1]Department of Radiology and Radiation Oncology, Faculty of Medicine and Biomedical Sciences, The University of Yaoundé I, Yaoundé, Cameroon
[2]Radiology Department, Yaoundé Gynaecology, Obstetrics and Pediatrics Hospital (YGOPH), P.O. Box 4362, Yaoundé, Cameroon
[3]Radiology Department, Yaoundé University Teaching Hospital, Yaoundé, Cameroon
[4]Department of Radiation Oncology, Yaoundé General Hospital, Yaoundé, Cameroon
[5]National Radiation Protection Agency (NRPA), Yaoundé, Cameroon

Correspondence should be addressed to Boniface Moifo; bmoifo@yahoo.fr

Academic Editor: Paul Sijens

Background. Clinical imaging guidelines (CIGs) are suitable tools to enhance justification of imaging procedures. *Objective.* To assess physicians' knowledge on irradiation, their self-perception of imaging prescriptions, and the use of CIGs. *Materials and Methods.* A questionnaire of 21 items was self-administered between July and August 2016 to 155 referring physicians working in seven university-affiliated hospitals in Yaoundé and Douala (Cameroon). This pretested questionnaire based on imaging referral practices, the use and the need of CIGs, knowledge on radiation doses of 11 specific radiologic procedures, and knowledge of injurious effects of radiation was completed in the presence of the investigator. Scores were allocated for each question. *Results.* 155 questionnaires were completed out of 180 administered (86.1%). Participants were 90 (58%) females, 63 (40.64%) specialists, 53 (34.20%) residents/interns, and 39 (25.16%) general practitioners. The average professional experience was 7.4 years (1–25 years). The mean knowledge score was 11.5/59 with no influence of sex, years of experience, and professional category. CIGs users' score was better than nonusers (means 14.2 versus 10.6; $p < 0.01$). 80% of physicians (124/155) underrated radiation doses of routine imaging exams. Seventy-eight (50.3%) participants have knowledge on CIGs and half of them made use of them. "Impact on diagnosis" was the highest justification criteria follow by "impact on treatment decision." Unjustified requests were mainly for "patient expectation or will" or for "research motivations." 96% of interviewees believed that making available national CIGs will improve justification. *Conclusion.* Most physicians did not have appropriate awareness about radiation doses for routine imaging procedures. A small number of physicians have knowledge on CIGs but they believe that making available CIGs will improve justification of imaging procedures. Continuous trainings on radiation protection and implementation of national CIGs are therefore recommended.

1. Introduction

The medical use of ionizing radiation is becoming the most significant man-made source of exposure for the population in the western world and also in developing countries [1, 2]. In a community-based level, to reduce the burden of medical imaging radiation, we need to apply the two cornerstones of radiation protection of patient which are justification and optimization of exposures. This concerns all the steps of the imaging process starting from the elaboration of the request forms by referring physicians to the validation, realization, and interpretation of the imaging examinations. The last two are those that deserve the quality of the imaging procedure and are on the responsibility of radiographers and radiologists. The referring physician has the responsibility to prescribe the best imaging procedure for the patient clinical condition, giving the clinical and administrative data useful for the validation of that choice. Many countries develop or adopt clinical imaging guidelines (CIGs) to support the physicians' prescription of the most suitable imaging procedure for the patient clinical condition [3–5]. These CIGs are justification based tools expressing for a given clinical setting possible imaging procedures and for each imaging procedure the level of indication, the level of scientific proof (reliability and accuracy), the level of irradiation, and some comments (procedure for substitution, etc.). Hence, referring clinicians must be aware of the level of patients' doses and the possible harmful effects of this exposure in order to justify irradiating medical imaging procedure.

In Cameroon, there are evidences of the lack of completeness of imaging request forms [6, 7]. Many studies on radiation protection established the poor knowledge of medical professionals on standards and principles of radiation protection [6, 8, 9]. This is enhanced by the lack of training on radiation protection and the absence of "guide for better use of medical imaging procedure" [10]. Various studies from different parts of the world have demonstrated general lack of knowledge on radiation doses and their adverse potential in the absence of referral guidelines among referring physicians [2, 11–19]. This situation in many developing countries is unlikely to be as much as this [11, 20]. The level of awareness concerning radiation doses of a given imaging exam influences clinician behaviors [21]. If they do not have enough information related to radiation doses and safety, their actions will not be safe and will result in adverse effects.

As part of a project to improve best clinical practices, with a view of clinicians' awareness on radiation risk and justification of the request of medical imaging procedures, we conducted a survey to investigate the radiation dose knowledge and use of CIGs among physicians in relation to their referral practice in a pool of seven first reference hospitals in Cameroon.

2. Materials and Methods

This cross-sectional study was conducted in seven university-affiliated hospitals in Yaoundé and Douala in Cameroon from July to August 2016. Confidentiality and anonymity were maintained according to the regulations mandated by Research Ethics Committee of Faculty of Medicine and Biomedical Sciences of University of Yaoundé I, in accordance with the Declaration of Helsinki.

2.1. Target. Recruitment was done by convenience sampling of all physicians who were consulting during this period on a voluntary basis. The participants were informed that the results would be used only for a scientific study.

2.2. Questionnaire. A self-administered questionnaire was filled by the physician in the presence of the investigator who collected it immediately. This questionnaire was based on a model used by Borgen and Stranden in Norway in 2014 [12]. The questions concerned reasons for referring for imaging procedures, knowledge and use of clinical imaging referral guidelines (CIGs), knowledge on radiation doses of 11 most prescribed medical imaging procedures, knowledge on stochastic and deterministic effects of radiation, the need of training on ionizing radiation, and the need of CIGs. We removed questions for which the answers were not yet available in our milieu like those on the source of radiation or had other items for the better understanding of national specificities such as past training on justification or radioprotection and the facilities support of CIGs. Age, gender, professional category, place of degree graduation, and years of professional experience of the respondents were also registered.

2.3. Statistical Analysis. We constructed a total radiation knowledge score ranging from 0 to 59 following the quotation used by Borgen and Stranden in Norway [12]. For the imaging procedures, a correct answer was coded 3 points, each yielding a maximum of 33 points. Knowing the existence of adverse effects of radiation was coded 2 points; the value of a radiation dose of two chest X-ray incidences and international unit of the effective radiation dose were coded 4 points each. Knowing the terms stochastic and deterministic was coded 4 points, and correct categorization of the six detrimental effects correctly was coded 2 points each, resulting in a maximum of 16 points. Missing data gave 0 points, and a total radiation knowledge score was noted for all participants.

Data were analyzed using the Statistical Package for the Social Sciences for windows (SPSS 19.0) to determine descriptive statistics including frequency distribution, mean, standard deviation, and percentages. Level of knowledge, attitude, and practices were calculated as a percentage of correct answers in each section. Levels less than 50% were considered poor knowledge. For comparison, we used ANOVA test or Student's t-test and Chi square test of Pearson or Fischer for means and frequencies, respectively, between professional category, level of experience, and services when it was suitable.

3. Results

3.1. Demographics. Of the 180 participants solicited, 155 questionnaires (86.1%) were completed. Twenty-five participants did not consent to participate to the survey. The mean age (range) of participants was 34.8 (23–56) years with female predominance (58%). The average experience of all physicians including postgraduation years was 7.4 years (1–25 years). The main hospital unit of interviewed physicians was Internal Medicine (68/155). Sixty-three respondents (40.7%) were specialists. Table 1 shows the distribution of general characteristics of respondents according to their professional category.

3.2. Global Knowledge Score of Respondents on Irradiation. The mean total knowledge score was 11.5/59 (11.3 for men and 11.7 for women). Gathering respondents into groups based on clinical experience of more than or less than 10 years, the means scores were 11.6 and 11.0, respectively. Table 2 shows

TABLE 1: General characteristics of respondents according to their professional category.

General characteristics	Interne/residents $n = 53$	General practitioners $n = 39$	Specialists $n = 63$	p value
Mean age in years (SD*)	30.6 (3.78)	31.6 (4.8)	40.2 (6.3)	**<0.01**
Sex, n = M/F (%)	17/36 (**40.7**)	12/27 (34.2)	36/27 (25.1)	**<0.01**
Mean years of experience (SD*)	4.2 (2.7)	4.4 (3.6)	**7.4** (5.8)	**<0.01**
Place of training degree: national/abroad (% of abroad)	46/7 (13.2)	29/10 (25.6)	44/19 (30.2)	**0.09**
Hospital working units of respondents, n (% in the professional category)				
Internal medicine, $n = 68$	24 (45.3)	17 (43.5)	27 (42.9)	
Surgery, $n = 32$	9 (17)	4 (10.3)	19 (30.2)	
Gynecology, $n = 22$	9 (17)	4 (10.3)	9 (14.3)	**<0.01**
Pediatric, $n = 20$	10 (18.9)	3 (7.7)	7 (11.1)	
Emergency, $n = 13$	1 (1.9)	11 (28.2)	1 (0.6)	

*Standard deviation.

TABLE 2: Global knowledge of physicians with regard to their general characteristics.

General characteristics	Global knowledge score		p value
	Mean	SD*	
Sex: male/female	11.7/11.3	7.0/6.7	0.68
Place of degree training: national/abroad	12.0/11.0	6.9/6.5	0.08
Years of experience: <10 years/≥10 years	11.6/11.0	7.0/6.5	0.66
Resident or interne physician	12.0	7.5	
Specialist physician	11.5	6.9	0.18
General practitioners	10.3	5.6	
Physician in emergency unit	13.0	9.5	
Physician in internal medicine unit	11.7	7.3	
Physician in surgery unit	11.1	6.1	0.84
Physician in gynecology unit	11.2	4.8	
Physician in pediatric unit	10.3	6.8	

*Standard deviation.

the mean global knowledge score of physicians with regard to sex, years of experience, site of training, and their working units. Differences between these groups were not statistically significant.

3.3. Knowledge on Irradiation during Some Imaging Procedures. All the respondents recognized that ionizing radiation has dissimilar injurious effects on patients; 95.5% of them had mistaken the effective radiation international dose unit (millisievert). None of them were able to give the approximate dose of a frontal chest X-ray exam (≈0.05 mSv) which is the most prescribed X-ray procedure.

More than 85% of the physicians undervalued radiation doses (in terms of number of chest X-ray doses) of routine imaging procedures: 85.8 to 86.5% underrated the doses of lumbar, abdominal, and thoracic CT scans, while 88.4 to 98.7% underrated the doses of intravenous pyelography, barium enema, lumbar spine, and pelvic X-rays. Magnetic resonance imaging (MRI) and ultrasound were considered as radiating procedures, respectively, by 83% and 28% of respondents.

TABLE 3: Respondents ($n = 25$) matching responses with deterministic and stochastic harmful effects of X-rays.

Type of effects	Stochastics, n (%)	Deterministic, n (%)
Infertility	9 (36)	16 (64)
Leukemia	12 (48)	13 (52)
Genetic abnormality	13 (52)	12 (48)
Fetal malformation	14 (56)	11 (44)
Radiation-induced cancer	16 (64)	9 (36)

Only 25 (16.1%) out of 106 clinicians knowing that X-rays had harmful effects declared that they were familiar with deterministic and stochastic terms. When sorting six harmful effects of X-rays as either stochastic or deterministic, these 25 clinicians' mean score (correct answers) was 48% (Table 3).

3.4. Physicians' Perception on Their Prescriptions of Medical Imaging Procedures and the Use and Need of Clinical Referral Imaging Guidelines. Regarding the use of clinical

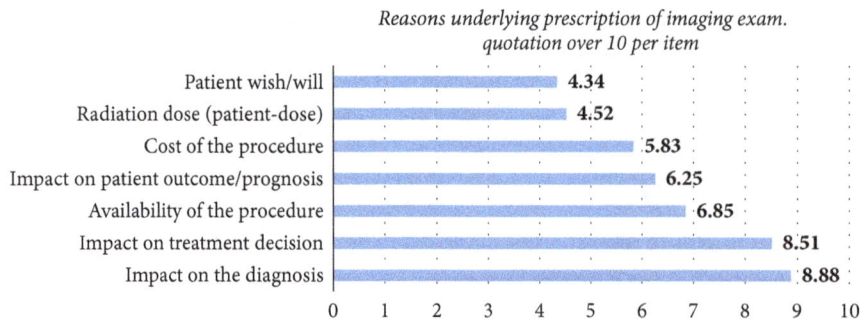

Reasons underlying prescription of imaging exam.
quotation over 10 per item

FIGURE 1: Weighting of physicians' reasons for the prescription of imaging procedure.

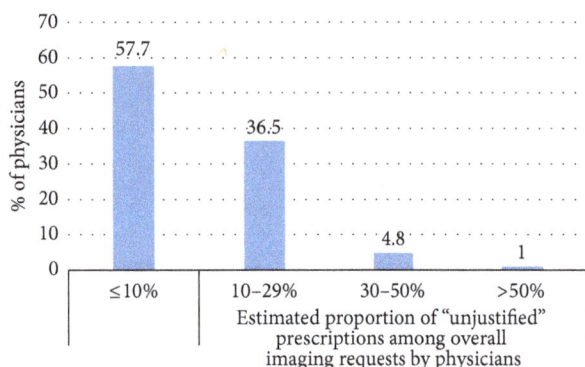

FIGURE 2: Proportion of imaging prescriptions considered by physicians unlikely to affect treatment/diagnosis.

referral guidelines for imaging, we found that 78 (50.3%) respondents have knowledge on referral guidelines and only a half of them (36) had made use of it. Overall, there was no statistically significant difference concerning the use of guidelines ($p > 0.05$) among clinicians in different categories, experience, place of training, and hospital units of work. 72.9% of participants reported that they never had training on radiation protection since their graduation. Seventy-six physicians (49%) defined clinical imaging referral guidelines (CIGs) as a tool for limitation of dose, while 23.2% defined them as a tool for justification.

Among the reasons underlying the request of an imaging exam (Figure 1), "impact on the diagnosis" was the highest weighted, with a mean score of 8.8/10 (median: 9). The importance of "patient's wish" was the lowest (mean: 4.3/10; median: 4), followed by considerations on "radiation dose to patient" (mean: 4.52/10; median: 4). The choice of a given imaging technique when prescribing was sustained by the basic knowledge acquired during medical training for 60% or by their personal experience for 20% of respondents.

Despite the fact that "impact on diagnosis or treatment" was the main reason for the request of imaging procedures, nearly two-thirds (67.1%) of physicians declared that they sometime requested for imaging that would not likely have an effect on treatment/diagnosis. The proportion of these requests represented less than 10% of overall prescriptions for 57.7% of the physicians (Figure 2). The main reason for these

prescriptions was the "patient expectation or will" weighted 3.9 on 8 (median: 4) followed by "research motivations" with 2.5 (median: 2) as shown in Figure 3.

Concerning physicians' self-perception on the need of training on radiation protection, 71% of respondents agreed to have had a training on justification and 27% on radiation protection. Nearly two-thirds (67.7%) of physicians claimed to have been sensitized on patient irradiation in diagnostic imaging. There is a wish for 95.5% of physicians to dispose national clinical imaging guidelines. All participants thought that making available CIGs will improve their knowledge and then their behavior regarding prescriptions of imaging procedures. The most suitable CIGs support preferred by our respondents was a didactic version for computer, smartphone, or tablet (32.2%) followed by smart software version (23.2%).

3.5. Knowledge on Irradiation in Relation with Imaging Requests and Use of CIGs. Total knowledge score on irradiation was better in respondents using CIGs than those who did not use CIGs (average score: 14.2 versus 10.6, $p < 0.01$). However, this knowledge score was similar: (1) among respondents who had training on justification ($n = 110$) compared to those who did not have training ($n = 45$) (average score: 11.6 versus 11.1, $p = 0.67$) and (2) among respondents who had training in radiation protection ($n = 42$) compared to those who did not have training ($n = 113$) (average score: 12.7 versus 11.0, $p = 0.15$) and (3) for physicians who admitted ($n = 100$) to sometimes prescribe imaging tests unlikely to affect treatment/diagnosis compared to those who denied ($n = 55$) (average score: 11.7 versus 10.9, $p = 0.46$).

4. Discussion

4.1. Strength and Limitations. This is a first ever study from Cameroon among referring clinicians on their attitude and knowledge concerning radiation exposure of patients during common radiology investigations and their familiarity to the irradiation doses and exposure dose unit and self-assessment of their medical imaging requests. However, the use of questionnaires has inherent limitations, as some answers reflect respondents' subjective opinions. In the present study, respondents' self-report on their own practice should be interpreted with care. The immediate filling of

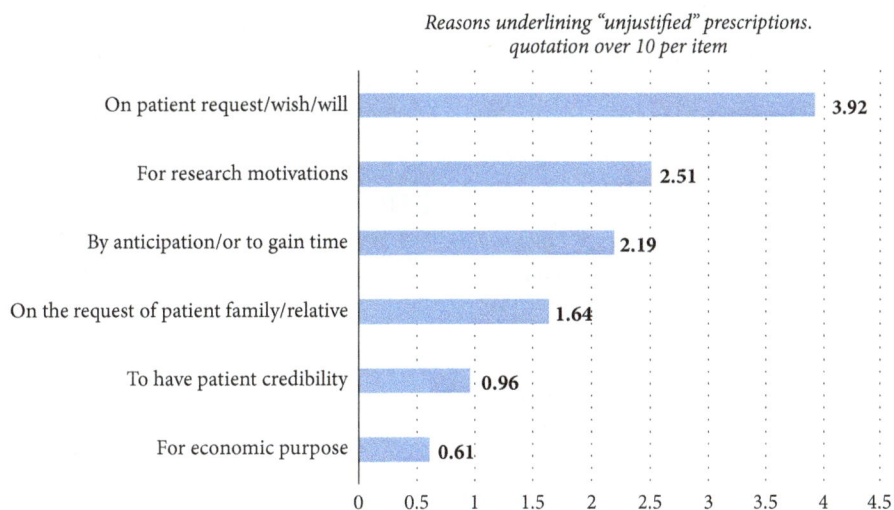

FIGURE 3: Physicians' reasons for prescriptions of imaging procedures unlikely to affect treatment/diagnosis.

the questionnaire in the presence of the investigator avoided responses after consultation of documents. The anonymity of the questionnaire raised complexity related to judgment of an individual respondent. The quotation points of open questions and those related to the practice allowed having less subjective responses and the possibility of appraising practical attitudes. Nevertheless, national generalization of results of this study should be raised carefully due to the impossibility of randomly choosing clinicians. But up to 86% respondents seen in their office is a nonnegligible participation rate. The predominance of specialists reflects the normal distribution of the medical professional population at the university-affiliated hospitals in the country.

4.2. Global Radiation Knowledge Score of Respondents. Our study had shown that, in Cameroon, clinicians had poor knowledge on radiation with a worse mean score less than 20% (11.5/59) [12, 14–20, 22–28]. All the three professional respondent groups possessed the same very low knowledge on radiation. Even though in agreement with previous reports, it was noteworthy that only 23% of the clinicians had used clinical imaging referral guidelines (CIGs), which is in the range of the level of use in other studies (10–40%) [20, 29]. Two main reasons of this, as worldwide demonstrated, are the absence of diffused national CIGs and the insufficiency of training on justification as it was reported in other studies in the same settings [7, 10]. This could corroborate some findings of our study. Firstly, the general knowledge was worse in clinicians who said they did not use referral guidelines. Secondly, neither the self-reported participations to specific training on justification (71% of clinicians) nor those on radiation protection (27%) significantly modified their knowledge on irradiation. Lastly, the poor general knowledge of doctors seems not to be link to the high rate of imaging prescriptions unlikely to have an effect on therapeutic decision.

4.3. Specific Knowledge on Irradiation during Imaging Procedures. Like in other countries in Africa and in the world,

this study confirmed the underestimation of irradiation dose of the most prescribed imaging exams by doctors in Cameroon [12, 20, 23, 30–32]. Despite the fact that they had poor knowledge on irradiation, all of them recognized the dissimilar injurious effect of ionizing radiation of some imaging modalities. This reveals their superficial knowledge on the topic, probably acquired during medical training.

In fact, critical findings obtained during this study sustained this superficial knowledge. For all the imaging procedures evaluated in this study, none of the participants were able to have 50% of the correct range of patient-dose for common imaging procedures. The proportion (for all procedures) of respondents with false answers in this study was the highest one ever obtained in a developing country to the best of our knowledge, with a global tendency of all participants (like elsewhere) to the underestimation [12, 20, 23, 29, 30]. Surprisingly, we found a high proportion (up to 80%) of clinicians thinking that MRI is an ionizing exam [12, 13, 31]. Some authors like Moifo et al. attributed this to the new integration of MRI in our country [10]. But this high proportion compared to other studies conducted in developing countries suggests that things are becoming worse, maybe due to the rarity of this modality (just three medical centers having MRI machine for about 25 million inhabitants). This statement cannot be transposed to ultrasound procedures which are widespread in Cameroon but 28% of respondents considered it as an ionizing technic with a radiation dose up to 1-10-folds higher than one chest X-ay (modal class). We think that this could be due to very superficial knowledge on radiation issue doubled by the insufficiency of training on radiation protection. For instance, they ould not be able to estimate the radiation dose of a complex imaging technic if they could not state correctly the international radiation unit (95.5% of wrong answers) or if they were not able to state properly (no good answer) the radiation dose of a single chest X-ray.

Concerning adverse effect of imaging radiation, physicians are not comfortable with the terms stochastic and deterministic, and only 48% were able to dissociate stochastic from deterministic harmful effects of radiation. And even this could be due to the 50% probability to randomly choose between deterministic or stochastic on this question. It could be different if we had formulated the question a little bit different with an open answer. Nevertheless, this confirms the approximate knowledge of the respondents.

4.4. Self-Perception of Imaging Prescriptions and Use and Need of Referral Guidelines. The imaging referral practices of respondents reflect clearly their level of awareness concerning clinical imaging issue [21]. For instance, the poor level of knowledge concerning patient-dose during imaging procedure is confirmed by the poor consideration to "radiation dose" as criteria influencing the choice of a given imaging procedure. The level of irradiation should contribute to the justification of an imaging procedure alongside with the impact on diagnosis and the therapeutic decision [3–5]. Furthermore, this study reveals a very high proportion of clinicians erquesting for imaging tests whose results are unlikely to affect patients' treatment/diagnosis, like in some developing countries [20, 31] but in greater proportion than in developed countries [12, 29]. But in our settings, respondents argue their choice by facing the burden of patients environment (family, friend, or other relatives), helping them to grant some time for elaborating diagnostic or for building some notion by making research. All these reasons could be avoided if they have in disposition a tool helping them like CIGs for better prescription of imaging examinations. Instead, we found that only half of the physicians knew the existence of CIGs and less than one-quarter had ever used it. Similar proportions have been described in developed and developing countries [20, 29]. It had been shown that incorporating the imaging guideline tools in the process of justification of imaging referral reduces significantly the proportion of useless examinations in imaging diagnostics [2]. When we ask for the type of facility tools the respondents may like to possess in light of making it easier to use the guidelines, the choice focused on didactic version for computer, smartphone, or tablet followed by smart software version. This means that the better way to spread CIGs in our environment should integrate ITC (information technology and communication).

5. Conclusion

The level of awareness of clinicians in Cameroon of irradiation during imaging procedure is very low and superficial and this affects the quality of their imaging prescriptions. This is enhanced by the lack of training on radiation protection and clinical imaging referral guidelines (CIGs). Improving justification of imaging request may pass through recurrent training on radiation protection to both undergraduates and postgraduates clinicians and by adopting national CIGs, followed by the vulgarization of these national CIGs through ITC.

Conflicts of Interest

The authors declare that there are no conflicts of interest regarding the publication of this paper.

Acknowledgments

Thanks are due to all the referring physicians who kindly accepted to participate in this survey. IAEA and NRPA for workshops in radiation protection through the Projects RAF/9/053/9012/03 (Optimization in Pediatric Imaging) and RAF/9/053/9011/01 (Implementing and Use of Clinical Imaging Guidelines for Africa) are acknowledged. The authors wish to thank Dr. Teingueng Ouogue Francisse for proofreading and English typesetting of this manuscript.

References

[1] F. O. Ujah, N. B. Akaagerger, E. H. Agba, and J. T. Iortile, "A comparative study of patients radiation levels with standard diagnostic reference levels in federal medical center and bishop murray hospitals in makurdi," *Archives of Applied Science Research*, vol. 4, no. 2, pp. 800–802, 2012.

[2] United Nations, Ed., *Sources and effects of ionizing radiation: United Nations Scientific Committee on the Effects of Atomic Radiation: UNSCEAR 2008 Report to the General Assembly, with Scientific Annexes*, United Nations, New York, NY, USA, 2010.

[3] ACR Appropriateness Criteria®, American College of Radiology, July 2014.

[4] European Commission, "Radiation Protection N° 178: Referral Guidelines for Medical Imaging Availability and Use in the European Union," 2014, https://ec.europa.eu/energy/sites/ener/files/documents/178.pdf.

[5] Guide du bon Usage des Examens d'Imagerie Médicale, Société Française de Radiologie, Paris, france, (Editions SFR), 2005, http://gbu.radiologie.fr/.

[6] B. Moifo, M. Ndeh Kamgnie, F. Ninying Fuh, and O. F. Zeh, "Pertinence des indications d'examens d'imagerie médicale à Yaoundé—Cameroun," *Health Sciences and Diseases*, vol. 14, no. 4, pp. 1–8, 2013.

[7] B. Moifo, K. M. Ndeh, F. N. Fuh, J. Tambe, H. Tebere, and F. J. Gonsu, "Assessment of the completeness of medical imaging request forms in a sub-Saharan African setting," *Medecine et Sante Tropicales*, vol. 24, no. 4, pp. 392–396, 2014.

[8] P. Ongolo-Zogo, M. B. Nguehouo, J. Yomi, and S. Nko'o Amven, "Knowledge in radiation protection: a survey of professionals in medical imaging, radiation therapy and nuclear medicine units in yaounde," *Radioprotection*, vol. 48, no. 1, pp. 39–49, 2013.

[9] P. Ongolo-Zogo, C. Mpeke Mokubangele, B. Moifo, and J. Gonsu Fotsin, "Evaluating pediatric patient dose during computed tomography in two university teaching hospitals in Yaoundé—Cameroun," *Radioprotection*, vol. 47, no. 4, pp. 533–542, 2012.

[10] B. Moifo, A. L. Edzimbi, H. Tebere, J. Tambe, R. N. Samba, and J. G. Fotsin, "Referring physicians' knowledge on justification of medical exposure in diagnostic imaging in a sub-saharan African country, Cameroon," *Open Journal of Radiology*, vol. 4, no. 1, pp. 60–68, 2014.

[11] K. Ghazikhanlou Sani, M. Jafari, M. Mohammadi, M. Mojiri, and A. Rahimi, "Iranian physicians' knowledge about radiation dose, received by patients in diagnostic radiology," *Iranian Journal of Radiation Research*, vol. 6, no. 4, pp. 207–211, 2009.

[12] L. Borgen and E. Stranden, "Radiation knowledge and perception of referral practice among radiologists and radiographers compared with referring clinicians," *Insights into Imaging*, vol. 5, no. 5, pp. 635–640, 2014.

[13] A. Ahidjo, I. Garba, Z. Mustapha, and A. M. Abubakar, "Referring doctors knowledge about radiation doses in patients undergoing common radiological examinations," *Journal of Medicine and Medical Sciences*, vol. 3, no. 4, pp. 222–225, 2012.

[14] K. E. Thomas, J. E. Parnell-Parmley, S. Haidar et al., "Assessment of radiation dose awareness among pediatricians," *Pediatric Radiology*, vol. 36, no. 8, pp. 823–832, 2006.

[15] S. Shiralkar, A. Rennie, M. Snow, R. B. Galland, M. H. Lewis, and K. Gower-Thomas, "Doctors' knowledge of radiation exposure: questionnaire study," *British Medical Journal*, vol. 327, no. 7411, pp. 371–372, 2003.

[16] A. D. Quinn, C. G. Taylor, T. Sabharwal, and T. Sikdar, "Radiation protection awareness in non-radiologists," *British Journal of Radiology*, vol. 70, pp. 102–106, 1997.

[17] C. I. Lee, A. H. Haims, E. P. Monico, J. A. Brink, and H. P. Forman, "Diagnostic CT scans: assessment of patient, physician, and radiologist awareness of radiation dose and possible risks," *Radiology*, vol. 231, no. 2, pp. 393–398, 2004.

[18] K. Jacob, G. Vivian, and J. R. Steel, "X-ray dose training: are we exposed to enough?" *Clinical Radiology*, vol. 59, no. 10, pp. 928–934, 2004.

[19] A. Arslanoglu, S. Bilgin, Z. Kubal, M. N. Ceyhan, M. N. Ilhan, and I. Maral, "Doctors' and intern doctors' knowledge about patients ionizing radiation exposure doses during common radiological examinations," *Diagnostic and Interventional Radiology*, vol. 13, no. 2, pp. 53–55, 2007.

[20] P. Singh, S. Aggarwal, A. M. S. Kapoor, R. Kaur, and A. Kaur, "A prospective study assessing clinicians attitude and knowledge on radiation exposure to patients during radiological investigations," *Journal of Natural Science, Biology and Medicine*, vol. 6, no. 2, pp. 398–401, 2015.

[21] M. Prabhat, S. Sudhakar, B. Kumar, and P. Ramaraju, "Attitude and perception (KAP) of dental undergraduates interns on radiographic protectiona questionnaire based cross-sectional study," *Journal of Advanced Oral Research*, vol. 2, pp. 45–50, 2011.

[22] D. J. Brenner and H. Hricak, "Radiation exposure from medical imaging: time to regulate?" *Journal of the American Medical Association*, vol. 304, no. 2, pp. 208-209, 2010.

[23] J. A. Soye and A. Paterson, "A survey of awareness of radiation dose among health professionals in Northern Ireland," *British Journal of Radiology*, vol. 81, no. 969, pp. 725–729, 2008.

[24] H. E. Rice, D. P. Frush, M. J. Harker, D. Farmer, and J. H. Waldhausen, "Peer assessment of pediatric surgeons for potential risks of radiation exposure from computed tomography scans," *Journal of Pediatric Surgery*, vol. 42, no. 7, pp. 1157–1164, 2007.

[25] J. P. Renston, A. F. Connors Jr., and A. F. Dimarco, "Survey of physicians' attitudes about risks and benefits of chest computed tomography," *Southern Medical Journal*, vol. 89, no. 11, pp. 1067–1073, 1996.

[26] C. M. Heyer, S. Peters, and S. Lemburg, "Awareness of radiation exposure of thoracic CT scans and conventional radiographs: what do non-radiologists know?" *Fortschr Röntgenstr*, vol. 179, no. 3, pp. 261–267, 2007.

[27] A. Finestone, T. Schlesinger, H. Amir, E. Richter, and C. Milgrom, "Do physicians correctly estimate radiation risks from medical imaging?" *Archives of Environmental Health*, vol. 58, no. 1, pp. 59–61, 2003.

[28] M. J. Correia, A. Hellies, M. G. Andreassi, B. Ghelarducci, and E. Picano, "Lack of radiological awareness among physicians working in a tertiary-care cardiological centre," *International Journal of Cardiology*, vol. 103, no. 3, pp. 307–311, 2005.

[29] L. Borgen, E. Stranden, and A. Espeland, "Clinicians' justification of imaging: do radiation issues play a role?" *Insights Imaging*, vol. 1, no. 3, pp. 193–200, 2010.

[30] R. F. Abdellah, S. A. Attia, A. M. Fouad, and A. W. Abdel-Halim, "Assessment of physicians' knowledge, attitude and practices of radiation safety at suez canal university hospital, egypt," *Open Journal of Radiology*, vol. 5, no. 4, pp. 250–258, 2015.

[31] H. Mohammad, J. T. Iortile, I. Garba, and M. A. Suwaid, "Knowledge of radiation and it effects among Doctors in Makurdi, North Central Nigeria," *International Research Journal of Basic and Clinical Studies*, vol. 1, no. 7, pp. 103–106, 2013.

[32] J. Newton, D. Knight, and G. Woolhead, "General practitioners and clinical guidelines: a survey of knowledge, use and beliefs," *British Journal of General Practice*, vol. 46, no. 410, pp. 513–517, 1996.

18

An Objective Study of Anatomic Shifts in Intracranial Hypotension using Four Anatomic Planes

Shamar J. Young [iD],[1] **Ronald G. Quisling,**[2] **Sharatchandra Bidari,**[2] **and Tina S. Sanghvi**[1]

[1]*Department of Radiology, University of Minnesota, 420 Delaware St SE, Minneapolis, MN 55455, USA*
[2]*Department of Diagnostic Radiology, University of Florida, 1600 SW Archer Rd, Gainesville, FL 32610, USA*

Correspondence should be addressed to Shamar J. Young; youn1862@umn.edu

Academic Editor: Stefan O. R. Pfleiderer

Purpose. Intracranial hypotension (IH) often remains undetected using current MR diagnostic criteria. This project aims to demonstrate that central incisural herniation is highly effective in helping to make this diagnosis. *Materials and Methods.* Magnetic resonance imaging (MRI) was analyzed in 200 normal and 81 clinically known IH patients. MRI reference lines approximating the plane of the incisura, the plane of the diaphragma sella, the plane of the foramen magnum, and the plane of the visual pathway were utilized to measure the position of selected brain structures relative to these reference lines. *Results.* All IH patients had highly statistically significant ($p < 0.0001$) measurable evidence of downward central incisural herniation when compared to normal controls. The first of the important observations was a downward shift of the mammillary bodies, which shortened the midsagittal width of the interpeduncular fossa cistern. A concurrent downward shift and deformity of the tuber cinereum accompanied the mammillary body shift. The second essential observation was an abnormal clockwise rotation of the long axis of the visual pathway. A severity grading system is proposed based on the extent of these shifts as well as secondary shifts of the brain stem, splenium, and cerebellar tonsils. *Conclusion.* This study objectively delineates the anatomic shifts of brain structures adjacent to the incisura and foramen magnum. This methodology is sufficient to recognize the features of IH and to stratify the spectrum of IH findings into a functional grading system for quantifying the results of interventional therapy.

1. Introduction

While much has been learned about intracranial hypotension (IH) in the last several years, for a variety of reasons, an initial misdiagnosis still remains common [1, 2]. In part, the diagnostic challenge stems from the myriad of reported presenting clinical symptoms. Although the complaint of headache is most common [3], nausea/vomiting [4], cranial neuropathies [5–9], radiculopathies [10], Parkinsonism [11], quadriplegia [12], and even coma [13–17] have also been described. To complicate matters further, the originally described diagnostic finding of low opening cerebral spinal fluid (CSF) pressure has also come into question. Normal CSF pressures have been seen in patients with well documented symptoms of IH, suggesting a wide range for normal baseline CSF pressures as well as significant variation in the pressure decline required to yield symptoms between individuals [18, 19].

Thus CSF volume, rather than the actual CSF pressure, is likely the pathophysiological variable at play [18, 20].

Unfortunately, the clinically experienced diagnostic dilemmas are matched by similar limitations in imaging. Reported magnetic resonance imaging (MRI) features of IH have lacked measureable criteria to provide an objective basis for diagnosis. Similarly, no published criteria exist to grade the extent or severity of IH nor to document interval progression/improvement following treatment. The MRI findings of IH are primarily the result of CSF volume loss and compensatory mechanisms according to the Monroe-Kellie doctrine [5]. Loss of CSF results in loss of sufficient buoyant force to prevent the brain from descending downward. Compensatory subdural effusions can develop, which in some cases also causes rupture of subdural bridging veins transforming subdural hygromas into subdural hematomas and thereby adding additional downward herniation force

[19]. In the absence of unilateral subdural hematomas, most cases of IH produce central incisural herniation, rather than the more common asymmetric, or paracentral downward transtentorial herniation typically associated with asymmetric supratentorial mass effect.

Prior reported imaging indicators of IH include subdural fluid collections, pachymeningeal enhancement, engorgement of venous structures, pituitary hyperemia, and "sagging" of the brain [10, 21]. Although these findings may be present in patients with IH, none occur with sufficient frequency to qualify as essential diagnostic criteria. For example, pachymeningeal enhancement is the most well recognized imaging finding of IH, reported in up to 83% of patients [22–30]; however, lack of enhancement does not preclude diagnosis. Messori et al. found subdural fluid collections in less than half of their IH patient population [20]. Brainstem "slumping," an MRI sign considered specific for IH [28, 31–33], has only been reported in approximately 51% of cases [34]. Thus, in the absence of these reported findings there has been no means of differentiating normal from abnormal in a substantial number of patients. Furthermore, lack of a severity grading scale precludes a means of documenting treatment effectiveness.

The goals for this retrospective review were twofold. This study tests the hypothesis that central incisural herniation is present in IH and can be quantitatively described. This hypothesis is tested by measuring interval distances between relevant brain structures and fixed anatomically based planes of reference both at the tentorial hiatus and at the foramen magnum in both normal and IH patient populations. Secondly, the study aims to stratify IH patients based upon the extent of the brain displacement to create a grading system which can objectively evaluate posttreatment effects.

2. Material and Methods

2.1. Definition of Planes of Reference and Description of Distances Measured

2.1.1. Description of the Specific Measurements Relative to the Plane of the Incisura Ventral to the Mesencephalon. The plane of the incisura, formed by interconnecting the Galenic venous confluence point (which includes the internal cerebral veins, the mesencephalic veins, and the basal veins of Rosenthal) with the base of the dorsum sella (Figure 1), provides the best estimate of the actual tentorial free margins forming the tentorial hiatus. The incisura includes all CSF spaces within the tentorial hiatus as well as the midbrain. Supratentorial structures adjacent to the plane of the incisura but ventral to the midbrain include the tuber cinereum and the mammillary bodies. Apposed structures immediately below the plane of the incisura include the belly of the pons. The interpeduncular fossa crosses the plane of the incisura. Its apex, which is open, is estimated by the distance between the caudal mammillary body surface superiorly and the belly of the pons inferiorly. The base of the interpeduncular fossa is the undersurface of the central midbrain. The normal relationship between these supra- and infratentorial structures

and their measurements including the mammillary-pontine distance, height of the interpeduncular cistern at the plane of the cecum, and the ratio of these measurements are illustrated in Figure 1. Objective measurable evidence of downward central incisural herniation is the reduction of the distance between the mammillary bodies and the belly of the pons and the downward displacement of the mammillary bodies toward, then crossing the plane of the incisura. The measurement of the distance from the incisural line to the mammillary bodies is illustrated in Figure 1. Additionally, as central incisural herniation proceeds and the mammillary bodies descend below the plane of the incisura, the normal rectangular configuration of the interpeduncular fossa as seen on the sagittal projection compresses anteriorly forming more of a triangle. This change in interpeduncular shape is an easily discernable finding and is also illustrated in Figure 1.

2.1.2. Description of the Specific Measurements Relative to the Plane of the Incisura Dorsal to the Mesencephalon. The splenium of the corpus callosum is located superior to the plane of the incisura. The distance between the caudal surface of the splenium and the plane of the incisura has been measured and is illustrated in Figure 1.

2.1.3. Description of the Specific Measurements Relative to the Position of the Mesencephalon. The mesencephalon crosses the plane of the incisura with roughly half above and half below. The iter reference point corresponds to the porus of the cerebral aqueduct. The distance between the iter and the plane of the incisura estimates the normal position of the mesencephalon and was measured as illustrated in Figure 1. Reduction in this distance is a measure of downward displacement.

2.1.4. Description of the Specific Measurements Relative to the Plane of the Long Axis of the Visual Pathway. The second anatomic displacement related to downward central incisural herniation is a clockwise rotation of the visual pathway relative to the plane of the long axis of the visual pathway. The tuberculum-venous confluence reference line provides a means of evaluating the spatial orientation of the visual pathway relative to the central skull base as delineated by the plane of the diaphragm sella. The line is formed by the interconnection between the same Galenic venous confluence mentioned in creation of the plane of the incisura and the tuberculum sella. This is an artificial reference line rather than an anatomic line, but does parallel the normal ascending oblique orientation of the optic chiasm, as shown in Figure 2. This plane of reference can then be used to detect the clockwise rotation of the visual pathway axis in the context of central incisural herniation. This angle was measured and is illustrated in Figure 1.

2.1.5. Description of the Specific Measurements of the Optic Chiasm Position Relative to the Plane of the Diaphragm Sella. The third anatomic displacement related to downward central incisural herniation is downward displacement of the optic chiasm relative to the entrance of the sella that is estimated by the plane of the tuberculum sella, the plane

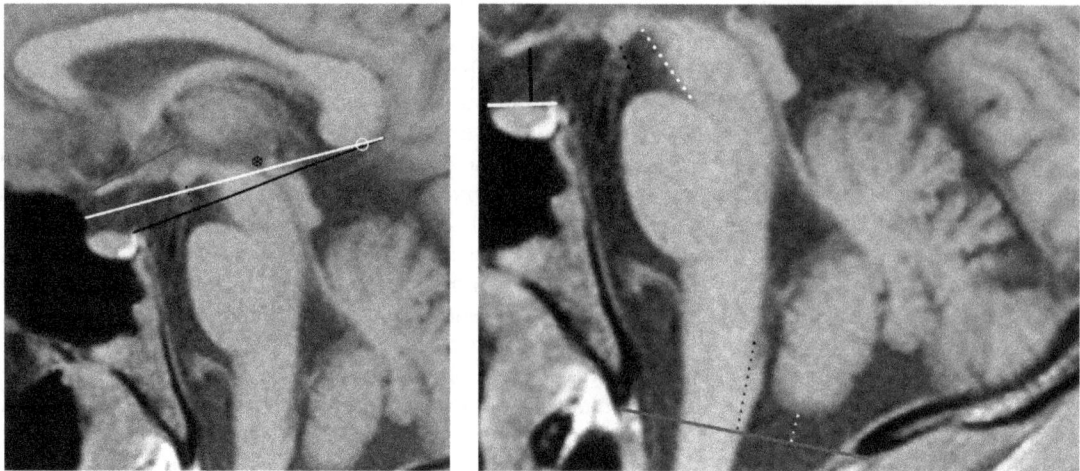

(a) Anatomic reference planes and measured distanced intervals for supratentorial structures adjacent to the tentorial hiatus (incisura). The supratentorial reference planes are noted as follows: the *plane of the incisura* (approximated by the black line), the *tuberculum-venous confluence line* (approximated by the white line), and the *long axis of the visual pathway* (approximated by the gray reference line). The measured distances are shown by the mammillary body to incisura line distance (triangles measured interval), the splenium of the corpus callosum to incisura line distance (white circle), and the iter (point) to tuberculum-venous confluence line distance (black snowflake) demonstrated in a normal patient

(b) Anatomic reference planes and measured distanced intervals for additional supra- and infratentorial structures. This sagittal midline MRI image of the posterior fossa demonstrates additional measurements. The first of these is the measured interval (black line) between the undersurface of the optic chiasm and the plane of the diaphragm sella (white line). The interpeduncular fossa distances are also demonstrated with the mammillary body-pontine distance (black dotted line) representing the apex; the base (width of the floor of the tegmentum portion of the midbrain) is shown as well (white dotted line). The ratio is calculated from the apex to base relationship. The plane of the foramen magnum (gray line) is defined by the interconnection of the opisthion with the basion points of the skull. Since the decussation of the pyramids cannot be determined reliably on sagittal MRI, the distance between the obex and the foramen magnum line (black triangle line) was used as an alternative distance interval in order to assess caudal brain stem displacement. The distance from the caudal aspect of the cerebellar tonsil to the foramen magnum line is shown (white triangle line)

FIGURE 1: Incisural and foramen magnum related anatomic planes of reference and their MRI equivalent reference lines. *Technical note.* A symbol (rather than a line) has been used in the figures, when a measured distance is close to or equal to zero.

that establishes the position of the diaphragm sella and also delineates the intracranial surface of the central skull base. This reference line represents the interconnection of the tuberculum sella anteriorly with the diaphragm sella insertion point posteriorly. Note, the tuberculum sella is also the anterior point for diaphragm sella insertion. This distance was measured and is illustrated in Figure 1.

2.1.6. Description of the Specific Measurements Relative to the Plane of the Foramen Magnum. The plane of the foramen magnum is created by interconnecting the basion with the opisthion points of the osseous foramen magnum. The decussation of the pyramids, which defines the cervicomedullary junction, is estimated by drawing a vertical line across the medulla from the obex of the caudal fourth ventricle. This methodology has been shown to fall within a few millimeters of the pyramidal decussation [35]. The position of the normal cervicomedullary junction is defined by the distance between the cervicomedullary junction and the plane of the foramen magnum. The position of the caudal poles of the tonsils is defined by the interval between the tonsils and the plane of the foramen magnum. Both the distance of the plane of the foramen magnum to the caudal tip of the cerebellar tonsil and

the distance from the plane of the foramen magnum to the obex were obtained as illustrated in Figure 1. These anatomic relationships between the cervicomedullary junction and the cerebellar tonsils relative to the plane of the foramen magnum allow independent assessment of secondary displacement of the brainstem versus the caudal poles of the cerebellar tonsils in the context of central incisural herniation. These changes can sometimes be confused with Chiari malformations.

2.1.7. Additional Imaging Features Associated with IH. All patients, including both normal and IH categories, were evaluated for a presence of the venous engorgement, dural venous sinus distension (as positive if the borders of the dominant transverse sinus were convex rather than concave), presence of subdural hygromas/hematomas, and pituitary enlargement.

2.2. Study Description. After institutional review board approval was obtained, a retrospective review of the electronic medical records (EMR) and picture archiving and communication system (PACS) was performed of patients undergoing brain MRIs from 3/2004 to 9/2012. Inclusion into the IH group required clinical and radiographic evidence of IH that

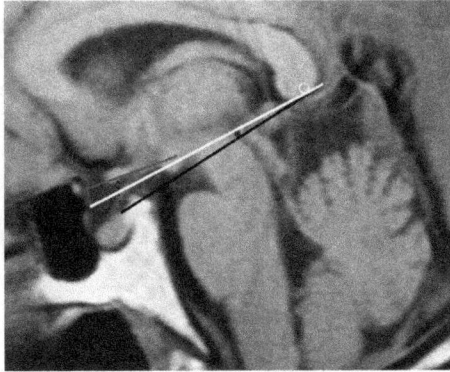

(a) Grade 1 or early (minimal) central incisural herniation. Findings include caudal shift of the mammillary bodies from their normal position located above the *tuberculum-venous confluence line* (white reference line) to a position interposed between the *tuberculum-venous confluence line* (white reference line) and *the incisural line* (black reference line). Concurrently, the interval between the optic chiasm and the plane of the diaphragm sella (black triangle line) is shortened beyond normal range. Additionally, the long axis of the chiasm/visual tract (gray line) rotates from a positive upward angle relative the tuberculum-venous confluence line (white line) into an orientation which is either parallel or at a slightly negative angle. The splenium of the corpus callosum (white circle) to incisura line (black reference line) distance is essentially zero

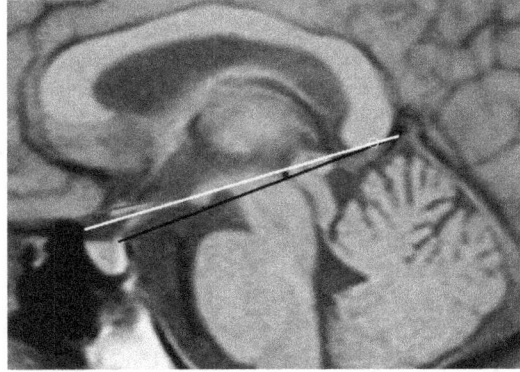

(b) Grade 2 or moderate central incisural herniation. Findings include progressive caudal shift of the mammillary bodies from their grade 1 position just below the tuberculum-venous confluence line (white reference line) to a position at the incisural line (black reference line). The distance interval between the mammillary body and the belly of the pons is now noticeably diminished and its shape is altered from a quadrangular to a triangular appearance. The optic chiasm/diaphragm sella interval continues to decrease. The tuber cinereum changes from a straight line into a caudal sagging shape. The long axis of the chiasm/visual tracts is now oriented at a negative angle (gray reference line), another characteristic sign of advanced central incisural herniation, relative to the tuberculum-venous confluence line (white reference line). The iter (black snowflake) and splenial (white circle) positions, formerly supratentorial, now approach the incisural line (black reference line)

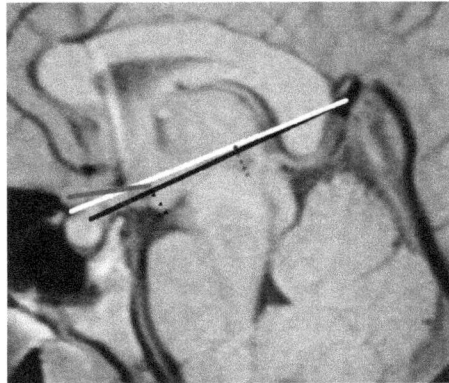

(c) Grade 3 advanced central incisural herniation. Findings include progressive caudal shift of the mammillary bodies from their grade 2 position at or minimally below the incisural line (black reference line) to an infratentorial position (black triangle distance). The interval distance between the mammillary body and the belly of the pons is now significantly diminished and the interpeduncular fossa is clearly triangular in shape. The optic chiasm has nearly reached the entrance of the sella. The long axis of the chiasm/visual tracts (gray reference line) is now at a significantly negative angle relative to the tuberculum-venous confluence line (white reference line). The iter position and the splenium have crossed beyond the incisural line into the posterior fossa. The iter to tuberculum-venous confluence line is depicted by the black snowflake line. The splenium to incisural line is depicted by the white circle line. The tuber cinereum clearly sags inferiorly and begins to buckle over the dorsum sella (another characteristic sign of advanced central incisural herniation). The interpeduncular fossa is close to being completely effaced as the mammillary bodies approach the belly of the pons

FIGURE 2: Grading downward central incisural herniation. *Technical note*. A symbol (rather than a line) has been used in the figures when a measured distance is close to or equal to zero.

met the international classification of headache disorders 3rd edition criteria for IH. A list was obtained from our clinical colleagues and a search of the radiology report database was performed for "intracranial hypotension." This produced a group of patients with both clinical and MRI findings of IH. If findings of IH were found on MRI only and the patient was not on the list provided by our clinical colleagues, the EMR was searched to determine whether patients did indeed meet HIS-3 criteria for IH. Those that did were also included. Exclusionary criteria included hydrocephalus, acute global brain swelling, and pseudotumor cerebri as seen on MRI, all of which can also produce central incisural herniation.

The normal and IH patient cohorts were retrospectively reviewed independently by two attending neuroradiologists (RQ and TS). The control group consisted of patients imaged during the same time period without clinical symptomatology of IH and who were felt, after review by the same two neuroradiologists, to have normal brain MRIs. All distance measurements were obtained using midline, T1-weighted, sagittal-projection, MRI sequences using 3 mm slice thicknesses. Measurements were given a positive value when the structure of interest was located above the reference line and a negative number if below. The mean ages of normal and IH patients were compared using a t-test. Fishers exact test was used to compare the proportions of males and females in the two groups. All analyses were completed in SAS 9.3. Means and standard deviations for normal ($n = 200$) and all IH patients ($n = 81$) as well as for IH patients with grades 1, 2, and 3 were calculated. For each response variable, the means of normal and IH patients were compared, controlling for sex and the potential interaction in sex and normal/IH patients.

A simple grading system for downward central incisural herniation was created by assessing the mammillary bodies' relationship to the incisural line. Grade 1 displacement is defined as mammillary body position above the incisural line. In grade 2 they reach the incisural line and in grade 3 they descend below the incisural line. These grades are illustrated in Figures 2 and 3.

3. Results

A total of 81 consecutive patients with IH and 200 normal patients were examined. The mean age of 40.4 years (range 13–81 years) for IH patients was not significantly different than the mean age of 39.9 years (range 0–94 years) for normal patients ($p > 0.05$). The normal group consisted of 45% (90) women and 55% (110) men, which differed significantly from the IH cohort which had 74% (60) women and 26% (21) men ($p = 0.02$).

A total of ten interval measurements were made examining the changes related to the visual pathway, the incisura, and the foramen magnum. For each, the mean and standard deviations for each measurement in both the normative group and the IH groups (including grade 1 (early), grade 2 (moderate), and grade 3 (advanced)) are presented in Table 1. With the exception of the distance from the mammillary body tip to the incisura line the difference in normal and IH groups did not differ significantly for females and males. Table 2 provides the p values for these variables between the

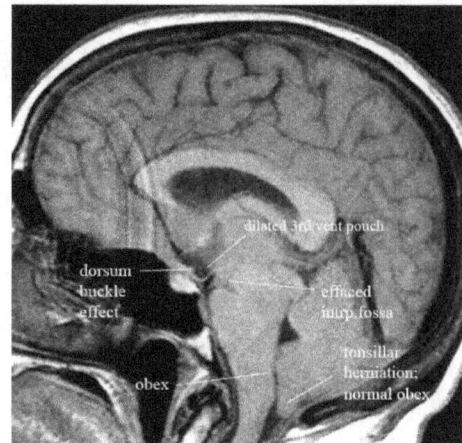

FIGURE 3: Very advanced grade 3 central incisural herniation. Imaging features of the most advanced state are presented in this figure. Notice that in this most advanced state of central incisural herniation the mammillary bodies have reached the belly of the pons completely effacing the interpeduncular fossa. The tuber cinereum typically buckles over the dorsum sella (a second characteristic sign of central incisural herniation), which creates a pocket of CSF within the lower third ventricle. The suprasellar space is effaced as the optic chiasm position reaches the entrance to the sella. The long axis of the chiasm/visual tracts is oriented at a significantly negative angle relative to the *tuberculum-venous confluence line*. The iter and the splenium have crossed the *incisural line* well into the posterior fossa. The obex position is low and the cerebellar tonsils are also herniated beyond normal range.

normative group and displacements in the IH grades. The p values for the distance from the mammillary body tip to the incisura line are also provided in Table 2 for both males and females as the interaction between the sexes was significant. Comparison between all IH patients and the normative group is not included but resulted in p values < 0.0001 in all cases.

Although the complete data can be found in Tables 1 and 2, some of the most important results are highlighted here. The normal visual pathway angle is initially positive, 7.42 degrees; however, downward central incisural herniation causes a progressive clockwise radial shift measuring −0.68 degrees (IH grade 1), diminishing to −1.19 degrees (IH grade 2) and finally to −9.71 degrees (IH grade 3). The mammillopontine distance progressively decreases, as evidenced by mean measurements of 7.07 mm (normal), 5.32 mm (grade 1), 4.60 mm (grade 2), and 3.79 mm (grade 3). The mammillary body tip to incisura line also progressively decreases from 3.4 mm (normal) to 2.26 mm (IH grade 1), 0 mm (IH grade 2), and −3.8 mm (IH grade 3).

The presence of the classical findings of IH was also investigated. Subdural hygromas/hematomas were seen in 48%, 41%, and 39% of grade 1, grade 2, and grade 3 IH patients, respectively. Dural thickening/enhancement was seen in 63%, 53%, and 50% of grade 1, grade 2, and grade 3 IH patients, respectively. Pituitary enlargement was seen in 22%, 29%, and 39% of grade 1, grade 2, and grade 3 IH patients, respectively, while venous distension was seen in 26%, 35%, and 36% of grade 1, grade 2, and grade 3 patients, respectively.

TABLE 1: Average measurements of recorded distances, comparing normal with grades of IH.

Variable	Normal	All IH	Grade 1	Grade 2	Grade 3
Distance from mammillary body tip to incisura line	3.39 (1.90)	−0.98 (3.47)	2.26 (1.19)	0 (0)	−3.80 (3.05)
Distance from the diaphragm sella to the optic chiasm	5.16 (1.60)	2.07 (1.62)	3.53 (1.37)	1.8 (1.19)	1.12 (1.12)
Angle of the optic chiasm	7.42* (3.93)	−4.95* (10.2)	−0.68* (7.63)	−1.19* (5.41)	−9.71* (11.5)
Height of the interpeduncular cistern at the plane of the cecum	12.76 (1.84)	11.03 (2.24)	11.61 (1.79)	11.51 (1.67)	10.39 (2.61)
Mammillopontine distance	7.07 (1.33)	4.47 (1.70)	5.32 (1.58)	4.6 (1.53)	3.79 (1.61)
Ratio of interpeduncular cistern	0.56 (0.11)	0.40 (0.14)	0.46 (0.11)	0.40 (0.12)	0.36 (0.15)
Distance from iter to tuberculum-venous confluence line	0.20 (1.93)	−2.51 (4.28)	−0.62 (2.78)	−1.16 (3.12)	−4.67 (4.82)
Distance from splenium of the corpus callosum to the incisura line	0.99 (1.57)	−0.73 (2.72)	0.52 (1.91)	0.06 (1.83)	−2.01 (3.02)
Distance from caudal pole of tonsils to plane of the foramen magnum	1.98 (2.45)	−2.20 (5.80)	−3.31 (7.88)	−1.55 (3.48)	−1.71 (4.91)
Distance from obex to plane of foramen magnum	8.36 (2.95)	5.30 (4.4)	4.98 (5.73)	5.27 (3.48)	5.52 (3.93)

All measurements without * are in mm with standard deviations provided in (). * demarks measurements in degrees.

TABLE 2: p values of Table 2 measurements.

Variable	Nrl-1	Nrl-2	Nrl-3	1-2	1–3	2-3
Distance from mammillary body tip to incisura line	0.04 (0.10)	<0.0001 (<0.0001)	<0.0001 (<0.0001)	0.05 (0.002)	<0.0001 (<0.0001)	<0.0001 (<0.0001)
Distance from the diaphragm sella to the optic chiasm	<0.0001	<0.0001	<0.0001	0.0007	<0.0001	0.28
Angle of the optic chiasm	<0.0001	<0.0001	<0.0001	0.93	<0.0001	<0.0001
Height of the interpeduncular cistern at the plane of the cecum	0.007	0.02	<0.0001	0.89	0.04	0.10
Mammillopontine distance	<0.0001	<0.0001	<0.0001	0.07	0.0006	0.24
Ratio of interpeduncular cistern	<0.0001	<0.0001	<0.0001	0.08	0.009	0.59
Distance from iter to tuberculum-venous confluence line	0.11	0.11	<0.0001	0.76	<0.0001	<0.0001
Distance from splenium of the corpus callosum to the incisura line	0.32	0.07	<0.0001	0.40	<0.0001	0.0001
Distance from caudal pole of tonsils to plane of the foramen magnum	<0.0001	0.0003	<0.0001	0.23	0.12	0.86
Distance from obex to plane of foramen magnum	<0.0001	0.0008	0.0008	0.96	0.50	0.60

Table providing p values. Nrl = normal patient cohort, 1 = grade 1 IH patients, 2 = grade 2 IH patients, and 3 = grade 3 IH patients.

None of these abnormalities were seen in the normal patient cohort.

4. Discussion

IH remains a difficult clinical diagnosis, made more difficult because although CSF pressure measurements often fall objectively into the normal range, they are relatively low in symptomatic patients [18, 19]. Evidence of central incisural downward herniation was evident in every case of symptomatic IH. Thus, understanding the primary structural shifts related to IH versus those which occur secondarily is essential.

The need to provide objective measures for the detection of IH has been addressed by a couple authors previously. Pannullo et al. investigated the position of the cerebellar tonsils relative to the foramen magnum and the position of the iter relative to the incsiural line in 7 patients with IH, comparing them to normative data from Reich et al. [24, 36]. They found that downward displacement of the tonsils and/or iter was present in 6 of 7 patients [24]. Messori et al. described 4 different anatomical measurements (the position of the cerebellar tonsils, fourth ventricle, and infundibular recess as well as the angle between the bicommissural line and a line tangential to the floor of the fourth ventricle) in 8 patients with IH, comparing them to 89 normal controls [20]. A subsequent analysis revealed that the cerebellar tonsils, fourth ventricle, and infundibular recess measurements were statistically different between the IH and normal controls. However, the number of patients with IH reviewed was low (less than 10) in each of these papers and they reviewed less anatomic measurements than this study has.

This paper objectively demonstrates several interesting findings in terms of anatomic pathophysiology in IH patients. Progressive clockwise rotation of the visual (optic tract) axis occurs as the lateral geniculate bodies of the thalami progressively descend downward with increasing severity of IH, as defined by our proposed grading system. Detection of this rotational displacement is achieved by comparing the long axis of the visual pathway to the tuberculum-venous confluence reference line. In abnormal IH patients it switches to a negative radial orientation, an important diagnostic feature of central incisural herniation, especially in early stages of IH when findings can otherwise easily be missed. Additionally and concurrent with rotatory visual pathway shift, there is depression of the optic chiasm relative to the diaphragma sella line. In advanced IH the optic chiasm actually reaches the entrance to the sella.

Central incisural herniation affects the mammillary bodies and the tuber cinereum differently. The downward displacement of the mammillary bodies begins from its normal position above both the tuberculum-venous confluence line and the incisural line. Caudal displacement of the mammillary bodies is stratified into grades of severity based upon which reference lines are crossed. In grade 1 displacement mammillary body position is below the tuberculum-venous confluence line but above the incisural line. In grade 2, the mamillary bodies reach the incisural line and in grade 3

they descend below the incisural line (see Figures 2(a)–2(c)). The mammillopontine distance was also studied by Shah et al. 2013 who found cutoff values of 5.5 mm or less for the mammillopontine distance (and 50° or less for the pontomesencephalic angle) to be both sensitive and specific in strengthening the MRI diagnosis of intracranial hypotension. Our results are very similar as the mammillopontine distance average seen in grade 1 is 5.32 mm with a standard deviation of 1.58 mm (Table 1), with decreasing values as the grade progresses [37].

This study brings to light two additional MRI signs not previously reported: the closure of the interpeduncular fossa and buckling of the tuber cinereum over the dorsum. The deformity of the interpeduncular fossa was measured by calculating a ratio of the decreasing apex width versus the unchanging base width. In practical terms this translates into shift from a rectangular shape of the interpeduncular fossa to a triangular shape (see Figures 2(b) and 2(c)). In the most advanced state of incisural herniation, the interpeduncular fossa is completely effaced (see Figure 3). The caudal sag and buckling of the tuber cinereum are illustrated in Figures 1, 2(b), and 2(c). Recognizable caudal shift of the rostral brain stem was measured by downward shift of the iter relative to the incisural line. Caudal displacement of the splenium was recognized in the same manner. Both were caudally displaced only in the more advanced cases of IH. Again, Shah et al. also found no statistically significant difference in the lateral ventricular angle, also referred to as the "corpus callosal angle," between control subjects and patients with intracranial hypotension [37].

Evidence of concurrent caudal brain stem displacement was based on evidence that the cervicomedullary junction (using the obex as a landmark) approached or passed the foramen magnum line. The posterior fossa structures were among the most stable in our analysis and thus are not a useful finding in either diagnosis or grading IH severity.

The commonly quoted hallmarks of IH including pituitary engorgement, subdural hygroma/hematoma, pachymeningeal enhancement, and venous distension were distributed sporadically across this data set. When present, these findings are certainly helpful in diagnosing IH. However, they were evident in roughly the same proportion across all three severity grades and therefore fail as a means of stratification. They also were not present with sufficient incidence to be considered an essential IH diagnostic finding. The fact that subdural hygroma/hematoma and pachymeningeal enhancement did not increase in prevalence with increasing grade may suggest that these patients have slowly developed severe IH rather than suffering acute onset or that the variation of compensatory mechanisms and factors leading to the presentation of the secondary factors is greater than previously noted. However, further investigation into this area is needed.

The stratification of the data in the IH group into mild, moderate, and advanced, corresponding to IH grades 1, 2, and 3, was born from a need to evaluate the consequence of IH therapy using objective reproducible criteria. The movement of structures relative to these anatomically based reference planes provides such criteria.

TABLE 3: Suggested cutoff distances for the proposed grades.

Variable	Suggested cutoff values
Distance from mammillary body tip to incisura line	1.25
Distance from the diaphragm sella to the optic chiasm	3.65
Angle of the optic chiasm	1.7*
Height of the interpeduncular cistern at the plane of the cecum	11.85
Mammillopontine distance	5.75
Ratio of interpeduncular cistern	0.49
Distance from iter to tuberculum-venous confluence line	−1.15
Distance from splenium of the corpus callosum to the incisura line	0.2
Distance from caudal pole of tonsils to plane of the foramen magnum	−0.1
Distance from obex to plane of foramen magnum	6.85

All suggested values are in mm except for those denoted by ∗ which are in degrees.

Table 3 gives our recommended values for each measurement which could be considered abnormal; however, upon review of the measurement data and grading system, two key structural relationships are recommended to diagnose IH. When the mammillary bodies descend to or beyond the level of the incisural line, the patient has substantial caudal migration and is considered grade 2 (if at the line) or grade 3 (if below the line). In this setting, no further assessment is necessary to confirm significant central incisural herniation. However, if the patient's mammillary bodies remain above the incisural line but below the tuberculum-venous confluence line and the patient has symptoms compatible with IH measuring the angle of the visual pathway is the next step. If the long axis visual pathway angle is more than 1 positive degree compared to the tuberculum-venous confluence line, it falls within normal limits. If the visual angle parallels or is less (i.e., negative angle), then findings are indicative of early IH-related central incisural herniation and proactive spinal imaging or testing may be considered.

This study has several limitations, including its retrospective nature. The grading system which is introduced primarily to provide an objective method of following posttreatment changes is not correlated with patient symptoms, an area of anticipated future research for this group. The grading system will also need validation. The reproducibility of the lines was also not tested directly in this study. The lines were utilized by multiple members of the research group; however differences were not scientifically addressed and this is yet another area of interest for further investigation by this group. Another weakness is the inability to reliably correlate MRI findings with onset of symptoms, as some believe that symptoms and MRI findings may become more profound over time. Lastly while it is the practice at our institution to image all patients with suspected IH by MRI given the IHS-III diagnostic clinical guidelines, this study may have missed potential IH patients. In particular, those patients with very mild symptoms and those not meeting HIS-III criteria may have been missed.

In conclusion, this study reveals that IH is always accompanied by central incisural herniation and changes to the visual pathway. Supratentorial structures ventral to the mesencephalon are most susceptible to central incisural shift.

The study of this movement allowed a grading system to be suggested, allowing patients to be objectively followed after therapy. We also suggest an objective means for diagnosing subtle cases of IH. Intracranial changes previously reported in the literature, especially associated with venous congestion in the pituitary gland and dura, were not consistent findings and therefore are considered adjunctive findings, although helpful when present.

Conflicts of Interest

The authors have no pertinent conflicts to disclose.

References

[1] G. Hoseman, "cited by Bell WE," in *Nachwirkengen der Lumbalanasthesie und ihre Benampfung. Verhandl. deutsch. path. Gesellsch. Chir*, vol. 38, p. 17, 1909.

[2] W. I. Schievink, "Misdiagnosis of spontaneous intracranial hypotension," *JAMA Neurology*, vol. 60, no. 12, pp. 1713–1718, 2003.

[3] W. I. Schievink, V. M. Morreale, J. L. D. Atkinson, F. B. Meyer, D. G. Piepgras, and M. J. Ebersold, "Surgical treatment of spontaneous spinal cerebrospinal fluid leaks," *Journal of Neurosurgery*, vol. 88, no. 2, pp. 243–246, 1998.

[4] J. Zwicker and C. Lum, "A treatable mimic of Chiari malformation with syringomyelia," *The Canadian Journal of Neurological Sciences Le Journal Canadien Des Sciences Neurologiques*, vol. 36, no. 4, pp. 480–482, 2009.

[5] P. Berlit, E. Berg-Dammer, and D. Kuehne, "Abducens nerve palsy in spontaneous intracranial hypotension," *Neurology*, vol. 44, no. 8, p. 1552, 1994.

[6] J. C. Horton and R. A. Fishman, "Neurovisual findings in the syndrome of spontaneous intracranial hypotension from dural cerebrospinal fluid leak," *Ophthalmology*, vol. 101, no. 2, pp. 244–251, 1994.

[7] G. T. A. Warner, "Spontaneous intracranial hypotension causing a partial third cranial nerve palsy: A novel observation," *Cephalalgia*, vol. 22, no. 10, pp. 822–823, 2002.

[8] E. Ferrante, A. Savino, A. Brioschi, R. Marazzi, MF. Donato, and M. Riva, "Transient oculomotor cranial nerves palsy in spontaneous intracranial hypotension," *J Neurosurg Sci*, vol. 42, no. 3, pp. 177–179, 1998.

[9] K. M. Brady-McCreery, S. Speidel, M. A. W. Hussein, and D. K. Coats, "Spontaneous intracranial hypotension with unique strabismus due to third and fourth cranial neuropathies," *Binocular Vision & Strabismus Quarterly*, vol. 17, no. 1, pp. 43–48, 2002.

[10] W. I. Schievink, "Spontaneous spinal cerebrospinal fluid leaks and intracranial hypotension," *Journal of the American Medical Association*, vol. 295, no. 19, pp. 2286–2296, 2006.

[11] A. S.-Ï. Pakiam, L. Christine, and A. E. Lang, "Intracranial hypotension with parkinsonism, ataxia, and bulbar weakness," *JAMA Neurology*, vol. 56, no. 7, pp. 869–872, 1999.

[12] W. I. Schievink and M. M. Maya, "Quadriplegia and cerebellar hemorrhage in spontaneous intracranial hypotension," *Neurology*, vol. 66, no. 11, pp. 1777-1778, 2006.

[13] C. E. Beck, N. W. Rizk, L. T. Kiger, D. Spencer, L. Hill, and J. R. Adler, "Intracranial hypotension presenting with severe encephalopathy," *Journal of Neurosurgery*, vol. 89, no. 3, pp. 470–473, 1998.

[14] R. W. Evans and B. Mokri, "Spontaneous intracranial hypotension resulting in coma," *Headache: The Journal of Head and Face Pain*, vol. 42, no. 2, pp. 159-160, 2002.

[15] E. Ferrante, I. Arpino, A. Citterio, and A. Savino, "Coma resulting from spontaneous intracranial hypotension treated with the epidural blood patch in the Trendelenburg position premedicated with acetazolamide," *Clinical Neurology and Neurosurgery*, vol. 111, no. 8, pp. 699–702, 2009.

[16] J. L. Kashmere, M. J. Jacka, D. Emery, and D. W. Gross, "Reversible coma: A rare presentation of spontaneous intracranial hypotension," *Canadian Journal of Neurological Sciences*, vol. 31, no. 4, pp. 565–568, 2004.

[17] S. Kremer, L. Taillandier, E. Schmitt et al., "Atypical clinical presentation of intracranial hypotension: Coma [1]," *Journal of Neurology*, vol. 252, no. 11, pp. 1399-1400, 2005.

[18] B. Mokri, S. F. Hunter, J. L. D. Atkinson, and D. G. Piepgras, "Orthostatic headaches caused by CSF leak but with normal CSF pressures," *Neurology*, vol. 51, no. 3, pp. 786–790, 1998.

[19] M. Paldino, A. Y. Mogilner, and M. S. Tenner, "Intracranial hypotension syndrome: a comprehensive review," *Neurosurgical Focus*, vol. 15, no. 6, pp. 1–8, 2003.

[20] A. Messori, B. F. Simonetti, L. Regnicolo, P. Di Bella, F. Logullo, and U. Salvolini, "Spontaneous intracranial hypotension: The value of brain measurements in diagnosis by MRI," *Neuroradiology*, vol. 43, no. 6, pp. 453–461, 2001.

[21] L. Spelle, A. Boulin, C. Tainturier, A. Visot, P. Graveleau, and L. Pierot, "Neuroimaging features of spontaneous intracranial hypotension," *Neuroradiology*, vol. 43, no. 8, pp. 622–627, 2001.

[22] A. Franzini, G. Messina, V. Nazzi et al., "Spontaneous intracranial hypotension syndrome: A novel speculative physiopathological hypothesis and a novel patch method in a series of 28 consecutive patients - Clinical article," *Journal of Neurosurgery*, vol. 112, no. 2, pp. 300–306, 2009.

[23] T. C. Brightbill, R. S. Goodwin, and R. G. Ford, "Magnetic resonance imaging of intracranial hypotension syndrome with pathophysiological correlation," *Headache: The Journal of Head and Face Pain*, vol. 40, no. 4, pp. 292–299, 2000.

[24] S. C. Pannullo, J. B. Reich, G. Krol, M. D. F. Deck, and J. B. Posner, "MRI changes in intracranial hypotension," *Neurology*, vol. 43, no. 5, pp. 919–926, 1993.

[25] L. Spelle, A. Boulin, L. Pierot, P. Graveleau, and C. Tainturier, "Spontaneous intracranial hypotension: MRI and radionuclide cisternography findings [5]," *Journal of Neurology, Neurosurgery & Psychiatry*, vol. 62, no. 3, pp. 291-292, 1997.

[26] O. C. Bruera, L. Bonamico, J. A. Giglio, V. Sinay, J. A. Leston, and M. D. L. Figuerola, "Intracranial hypotension: The nonspecific nature of MRI findings," *Headache: The Journal of Head and Face Pain*, vol. 40, no. 10, pp. 848–852, 2000.

[27] R. L. Mittl and D. M. Yousem, "Frequency of unexplained meningeal enhancement in the brain after lumbar puncture," *American Journal of Neuroradiology*, vol. 15, no. 4, pp. 633–638, 1994.

[28] B. Mokri, D. G. Piepgras, and G. M. Miller, "Syndrome of orthostatic headaches and diffuse pachymeningeal gadolinium enhancement," *Mayo Clinic Proceedings*, vol. 72, no. 5, pp. 400–413, 1997.

[29] K. L. Schoffer, T. J. Benstead, and I. Grant, "Spontaneous intracranial hypotension in the absence of magnetic resonance imaging abnormalities," *Canadian Journal of Neurological Sciences*, vol. 29, no. 3, pp. 253–257, 2002.

[30] W. I. Schievink and J. Tourje, "Intracranial hypotension without meningeal enhancement on magnetic resonance imaging: case report," *Journal of Neurosurgery*, vol. 92, no. 3, pp. 475–477, 2000.

[31] W. I. Schievink, F. B. Meyer, J. L. D. Atkinson, and B. Mokri, "Spontaneous spinal cerebrospinal fluid leaks and intracranial hypotension," *Journal of Neurosurgery*, vol. 84, no. 4, pp. 598–605, 1996.

[32] W. I. Schievink, "Spontaneous spinal cerebrospinal fluid leaks: a review.," *Neurosurgical focus [electronic resource].*, vol. 9, no. 1, p. e8, 2000.

[33] R. A. Fishman and W. P. Dillon, "Dural enhancement and cerebral displacement secondary to intracranial hypotension," *Neurology*, vol. 43, no. 3, pp. 609–611, 1993.

[34] W. I. Schievink, M. M. Maya, C. Louy, F. G. Moser, and J. Tourje, "Diagnostic criteria for spontaneous spinal CFS leaks and intracranial hypotension," *American Journal of Neuroradiology*, vol. 29, no. 5, pp. 853–856, 2008.

[35] R. G. Quisling, S. G. Quisling, and J. Parker Mickle, "Obex/nucleus gracilis position: Its role as a marker for the cervicomedullary junction," *Pediatric Neurosurgery*, vol. 19, no. 3, pp. 143–150, 1993.

[36] J. B. Reich, J. Sierra, M. D. F. Deck, and F. Plum, "MRI description and clinical correlation of dynamic upward and downward transtentorial and foramen magnum brain herniation," *Annals of Neurology*, vol. 33, pp. 795–799, 1993.

[37] L. M. Shah, L. A. McLean, M. E. Heilbrun, and K. L. Salzman, "Intracranial hypotension: Improved MRI detection with diagnostic intracranial angles," *American Journal of Roentgenology*, vol. 200, no. 2, pp. 400–407, 2013.

19

Automated Determination of Arterial Input Function for Dynamic Susceptibility Contrast MRI from Regions around Arteries using Independent Component Analysis

Sharon Chen,[1] Yu-Chang Tyan,[1,2,3,4] Jui-Jen Lai,[5] and Chin-Ching Chang[5]

[1]Department of Medical Imaging and Radiological Sciences, Kaohsiung Medical University, Kaohsiung 807, Taiwan
[2]Center for Infectious Disease and Cancer Research, Kaohsiung Medical University, Kaohsiung 807, Taiwan
[3]Graduate Institute of Medicine, College of Medicine, Kaohsiung Medical University, Kaohsiung 807, Taiwan
[4]Institute of Medical Science and Technology, National Sun Yat-sen University, Kaohsiung, Taiwan
[5]Department of Medical Imaging, Kaohsiung Medical University Hospital, Kaohsiung 807, Taiwan

Correspondence should be addressed to Sharon Chen; sharchen@kmu.edu.tw

Academic Editor: Weili Lin

Purpose. Quantitative cerebral blood flow (CBF) measurement using dynamic susceptibility contrast- (DSC-) MRI requires accurate estimation of the arterial input function (AIF). The present work utilized the independent component analysis (ICA) method to determine the AIF in the regions adjacent to the middle cerebral artery (MCA) by the alleviated confounding of partial volume effect. *Materials and Methods*. A series of spin-echo EPI MR scans were performed in 10 normal subjects. All subjects received 0.2 mmol/kg Gd-DTPA contrast agent. AIFs were calculated by two methods: (1) the region of interest (ROI) selected manually and (2) weighted average of each component selected by ICA (weighted-ICA). The singular value decomposition (SVD) method was then employed to deconvolve the AIF from the tissue concentration time curve to obtain quantitative CBF values. *Results*. The CBF values calculated by the weighted-ICA method were 41.1 ± 4.9 and 22.1 ± 2.3 mL/100 g/min for cortical gray matter (GM) and deep white matter (WM) regions, respectively. The CBF values obtained based on the manual ROIs were 53.6 ± 12.0 and 27.9 ± 5.9 mL/100 g/min for the same two regions, respectively. *Conclusion*. The weighted-ICA method allowed semiautomatic and straightforward extraction of the ROI adjacent to MCA. Through eliminating the partial volume effect to minimum, the CBF thus determined may reflect more accurate physical characteristics of the T2* signal changes induced by the contrast agent.

1. Introduction

Perfusion is a fundamental physiological characteristic of brain tissues that can be measured by MRI techniques. One of the MRI methods commonly applied in clinical settings for measuring cerebral blood flow (CBF) is the dynamic susceptibility contrast MRI (DSC-MRI) [1, 2]. The DSC-MRI, an exogenous contrast technique, allows rapid measurements of MRI signal change when the paramagnetic bolus agent passes through the brain tissue. DSC-MRI with high SNR has led to widespread clinical applications such as initial investigation of stroke and tumor imaging [2, 3].

High concentrations of lanthanide contrast agents (e.g., Gd-DTPA) produce significant T2 and T2* relaxation and

cause the signal to drop by about 50% when the blood-brain barrier is intact. Vilringer et al. [4] presented a first-order model to explain the local magnetic inhomogeneity across vessels due to the induced susceptibility difference. They found that inhomogeneity occurs mainly in the regions of tissue around vessels and the magnitude of variability is inversely proportional to the square of the distance from the center of the vessel. In contrast to T1 signal enhancement, which has a short range of interaction, the T2 susceptibility effect extends beyond the vascular space, affecting much of the surrounding brain tissue [5]. Duhamel et al. [6] found that the arterial input function (AIF) determined from regions within arteries, instead of around arteries, could result in uncertainty in the estimated mean transit time (MTT).

One can conclude from these experiments that it is more accurate to measure AIF from regions around the artery.

AIF plays an important role in the quantification of CBF for perfusion measurements. CBF can be obtained by deconvolving AIF from the measured concentration time curve of tissue with dilution theory equation [7, 8]. How and where the AIF was determined has been one of the key aspects in calculating perfusion parameters. While obtaining the local AIF for each imaging voxel is difficult, a surrogate AIF is usually derived from one of the major arteries, for example, the middle cerebral artery (MCA) [5, 6]. Practically, the AIF is commonly determined by manual selection of regions of interest (ROIs) surrounding large arteries [5, 9]. Compared with that derived from regions within large vessels, AIF derived from tissues adjacent to vessels avoids flow artifacts and possible signal saturations while examining T2 changes resulting from the contrast agent passage. In addition, it provides more accurate CBF quantification since the relaxivity constant embedded in the concentration time curves of the AIF would be closer to that of the tissue. Next to the understanding of AIF characteristics, postprocessing of signal extraction is very important. Van Osch et al. [10, 11] have recently used calibration curves incorporated with partial volume correction algorithm by selecting manually a region covering the tissue around the internal carotid artery, which showed improved reproducibility of AIF determination. However, in their study, AIF was obtained from blood signals and the vessel was required to be parallel to the main magnetic field because the phase shift is linear along with the cross session of the vessel. On the other hand, partial volume correction factor is also a way to eliminate the partial volume effect by scaling the tail of concentration time curve of artery and vein [12, 13]. For AIF determination by automatic method of ROI selection, several research groups [14, 15] proposed methods by setting criteria related to the characteristics of the dynamic signal/concentration time curves, such as full width at half maximum (FWHM), the maximum concentration (MC), time-to-peak (TTP), and arrival time (AT). Although the processes were automatic, these methods were limited by the lack of biophysical meanings for criterion selected because the MRI signal was combined with both T1 and T2 effects, which could vary with different imaging systems, protocols, and patients or subjects.

Manual ROI technique and criterion ROI method are subjective and cumbersome in resolving the confounding signal which is mixed with various tissue components around vessels. Therefore, there has been thriving use of numerical method to automatically segment the ROI. The statistical methods that examine the difference in signal characteristics are appropriate for solving the problem of signal mixture. Martel et al. [16, 17] applied factor analysis (FA) technique combined with principle component analysis (PCA) to remove much of the random noise contamination when extracting the vessel factor image with the signal intensity curve for 107 patients with acute stroke. However, additional assumptions with *a priori* knowledge were needed to yield factors with physiological significance. Murase et al. [18] presented the fuzzy *c*-means (FCM) method for determining AIF within the mask around the internal carotid artery.

This method was complex in mask decision and had difficulty defining the number of clusters. Moreover, determining the fuzzy rules of the cluster was subjective and difficult.

A blind source separation method such as independent component analysis (ICA), which decomposes the mixture signals into basic components, can be employed to extract the signal of interest. ICA is a model-free multivariate statistical method that has been employed to identify pixels that have a common underlying time-response behaviors involving the spatially independent cortical activation areas in functional MRI (fMRI) [19–25]. It had also been used as a segmentation technique to visualize the different hemodynamic compartments [26, 27] and to remove the confounding signals from large vessels to improve images with significantly less artifacts [28]. The present work proposed using ICA to define regions around the artery and to determine an accurate AIF from the regions. AIFs were also obtained from ROIs that were drawn manually and from the regions within arteries as determined by ICA. CBFs were then calculated by these AIFs for comparison. The resultant CBF from ICA-based method got closer values 41.1 ± 4.9 mL/100 g/min and 22.1 ± 2.3 mL/100 g/min for gray matter and white matter, compared to the standard values of nuclear medicine, 43.1 mL/100 g/min and 21.3 mL/100 g/min, respectively [29].

2. Materials and Methods

2.1. Simulation Experiment. The purpose of simulation experiment is to evaluate the performance of image segmentation by ICA. Three squared blocks (each with 81 pixels) representing the artery (in red), artery-surrounding tissue (in green), and tissue (in blue), respectively, are shown in Figure 1(a). The signals mimicking the contrast agent effect on vessel and parenchyma are calculated from Kiselev's approach [30]. In his approach, he utilized Pade approximation to bridge the deviance between theoretically known limits with the account for the results of the Monte Carlo simulation [5]. The deviance caused by the effect of contrast agent is due to the local field inhomogeneity around the vessel and capillary. The force of inhomogeneous field around the vessel is the susceptibility difference between inside and outside vessel, which is the static dephasing regime (SDR) effect. Another force causing the field inhomogeneity around capillary is due to the proton diffusing out toward the tissue, which is called the diffusional narrowing regime (DNR) effect.

In our simulation, we simply assumed the signal of artery-surrounding tissue is affected only by the SDR effect and that of tissue is affected by the combination of the DNR and SDR effects. The input bolus of artery was given as

$$C_a(t) = \frac{C_{\max}(t/t_0)}{\exp(-t/t_0 + 1)}, \tag{1}$$

where $C_{\max} = 3$ mM and $t_0 = 7$ ms [30]. The concentration of contrast agent in blood in the studied tissue was obtained through the calculation of dilution theory (mean transit time was assumed as 2.6 s). The inhomogeneity of field around vessels was related to several factors, such as magnetic field ($B_0 = 1.5$ T), pulse sequence (Gradient Echo with TE = 45 ms),

(a)

(b)

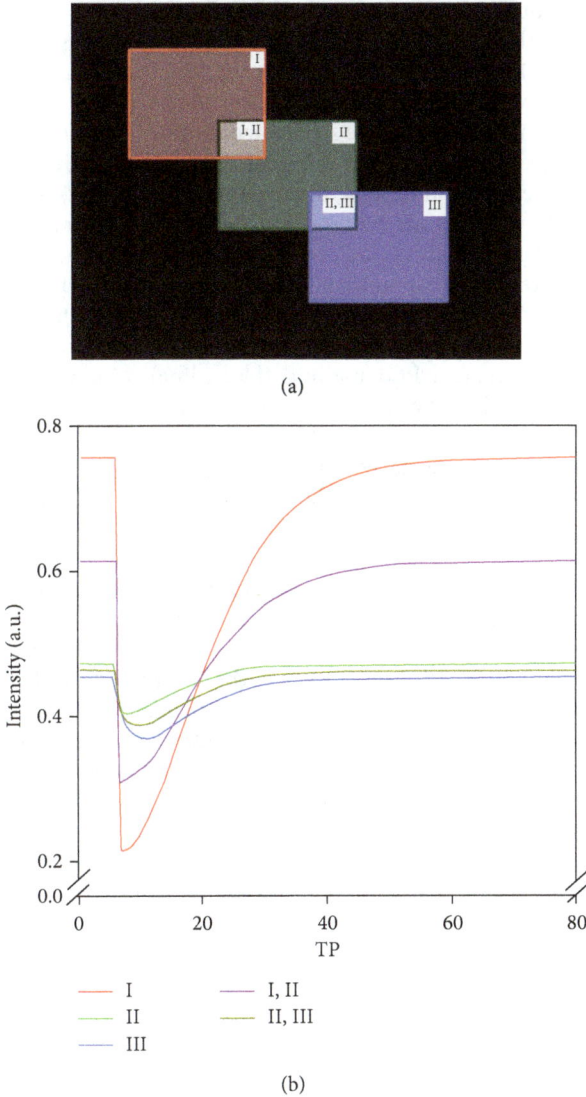

FIGURE 1: (a) The physiological signals for artery (I), surrounding tissue (II), and tissue (III) are simulated in three blocks (in red, green, and blue, resp.). The partial volume fractions between (I, II) and (II, III) were 0.5. (b) The generated raw signals were calculated from Kiselev's approach [30].

blood volume fraction ($\zeta_a = 0.005$; $\zeta_v = 0.01$; $\zeta_c = 0.02$), vessel radius ($\rho_a = \rho_v = 100\,\mu m$; $\rho_c = 3.5\,\mu m$), the magnetic susceptibility of venous blood ($\chi_0 = 0.038$ ppm), the baseline relaxation rate ($R_{2a_0} = 6.21\,1/s$; $R_{2v_0} = 13.43\,1/s$), and the relaxivity [30]. The relaxivity was estimated from the known parameters following the asymptotic forms in [30].

The noise-free signal time curves for the three components (I, II, and III) were converted from the simulated concentration time curves and shown in Figure 1(b). The partial volume fraction in the overlapped areas (I&II and II&III) was set to be 0.5. Various levels of noise were added to generate contrast-to-noise ratios (CNRs) ranged from 30 to 70 for the arterial signal time curve. Images of 80 time points with 1.5 s per time point were simulated for each CNR. Using ICA, 10 components were extracted and three of them were

selected for each of the three signal sources. The IC maps were transferred into z-value maps, and the first 50 voxels with maximum z-values were selected. The performance of segmentation was evaluated with percent detected voxels in the ROIs with and without partial volume averaging.

2.2. MRI Acquisition. Eight healthy volunteers (4 males and 4 females), 30–45 years old (average = 35.5 years), participated in this study with informed consent. All experiments were performed at Chang Gung Memorial Hospital with protocols approved by the institutional review board.

A single-shot spin-echo EPI sequence was employed to perform the perfusion imaging on a 1.5 T MR scanner (Magnetom Vision, Siemens, Erlangen, Germany) with the following parameters: TR/TE = 1,500/60 ms, flip angle = 90°, field of view = $218 \times 218\,mm^2$, matrix size = 64×64, and slice thickness = 6 mm. Seven image slices with 60 time points per slice were obtained for each subject. The images of the first three time point images were discarded as dummy scans. In each perfusion measurement, the contrast agent Gd-DTPA (0.2 mmol/kg b.w., Magnevist, Schering, Berlin, Germany) was injected in the left antecubital vein using an MR-compatible injector (Spectris, Medrad Inc., Indianola, PA). The injection rate was set to be 5 mL/s and the volume of the dose was 25 mL. The time point (TP) of injection was at 7th TP of scan. Two volunteers were excluded from the evaluation due to significant motions during the DSC-MRI scan.

2.3. Data Processing. AIF was selected using both the manual and ICA methods. For the manual method, a region (about 30 pixels) around the MCA was singled out as the candidate of AIF calculation. As for the ICA method, the data process is described as follows.

ICA decomposed the input data into their constituent sources, according to statistical independence [31, 32]. In this technique, an unmixed matrix ($W_{q \times p}$) is employed to project data into its own reconstructed source ($N_{q \times v}$) in the q direction where data distribution is non-Gaussian:

$$M_{q_0 \times v} \approx N_{q \times v} = W_{q \times p} X_{p \times v}, \tag{2}$$

where $M_{q_0 \times v}$ is the source matrix with q_0 sources and spatial size v; $X_{p \times v}$ is the observed data matrix with p time series; $W_{q \times p}$ is the unmixed matrix with $q \times p$ matrix size; $N_{q \times v}$ is the component matrix which is employed to approach the original component source (M), where $q \leq q_0$.

Forty constitutional IC maps (covering 99% of the eigenvalues) were generated based on tissue characteristics with which tissue had its temporal performance in the independent spatial domain. Of all IC maps, two maps of interest, namely, the artery (ICA-a) and the tissue around the artery (ICA-s), were selected according to their hemodynamic characteristics; that is, artery has early, narrow, and high peak features of responsive concentration. In order to decide a global AIF, the selected IC map was transferred into z-value maps, and the first 50 voxels of maximum z-value were used as the ROI of AIF calculation. The z-value is defined as $z_i = (x_i - \text{mean}_{IC})/\text{Std}_{IC}$, where x_i is the voxel value of an IC image; "mean$_{IC}$" and "Std$_{IC}$" are the average and standard deviation over an IC map [32]. Therefore, the time course per voxel in the ROI was weighted by the z-value of the IC map to generate an AIF. This weighted time course embodied the tissue's response to contrast agent and facilitated deciding a more purified region with respect to the representation of tissue. That is because, in ICA calculation, the temporal behaviors of voxels having the same tissue properties were grouped into a component map because it contributed the same value to the location of anatomy. Taking this advantage, ICA selected voxels with higher weighting to calculate AIF and removed the partial volume effect. The weighted-AIF can be defined by

$$AIF = \sum_i^n Q_i \times S_i \quad n = \text{voxels in VOI}, \qquad (3)$$

where S_i is the signal intensity time curve of the ith voxel in the ROI selected after z-value thresholding and region clustering in each ICA map of interest. Q_i is the weighting matrix of the ith voxel whose value is the normalized value from the IC map, and herein AIF is termed as AIF$_{(ICA-w)}$.

Before calculating CBF, the MR signal intensity was transferred into the concentration of contrast agent [5, 30] by the following equation:

$$C(t) = \frac{-K}{TE} \ln \left(\frac{S(t)}{S_0} \right), \qquad (4)$$

where K is the relaxivity, which is related to the tissue type and magnetic field. For 1.5 T magnetic field, K is about 7.62 m/M/s; $S(t)$ is the signal intensity at time t; and S_0 is the baseline intensity before the contrast arrival. Afterward, the concentration time curve of candidate AIFs was fitted using the data period of 7th–25th time points with a gamma-variate function to determine the TTP, arrival time, FWHM, and peak height as the indicators of AIF for comparison of two AIFs. Later, the concentration of candidate AIFs was employed to calculate CBF using the SVD deconvolution method with adaptive thresholds [33].

3. Results

In the simulation experiment, the performance of signal segmentation with ICA as a function of CNR was presented in Figure 2. The three IC component maps (which selected at most 50 pixels for each ROI) corresponding to each of the three signal sources were demonstrated in Figures 2(a)–2(e) for different CNR levels. The alleviation of partial volume effect (in I&II and II&III areas) was observed as CNR increase. The segmentation performance at various CNR was summarized in Figure 2(f). Comparing to surrounding tissue, the localization of signal for artery and tissue was fully achieved. The partial volume effect affected the signal decomposition, especially for regions containing boundary at low CNR condition. However, the segmentation of surrounding tissue was quite accurate, even at low CNR level (>90% accuracy).

Figure 3 shows the resultant segmentations at three regions for one clinical dataset: a region drawn manually by the manual ROI method and two regions segmented by the ICA method. It was found that ICA yielded better segmented boundaries along the MCA compared with the manual ROI, especially at the regions where the partial volume effect prevailed. In addition, the AIF concentration time curves for all subjects obtained from different methods were presented in Figure 4. As can be seen, the dynamic curve of the selected ROI showed its own tissue characteristic. The artery curve (solid dark gray line) had greater amplitude than the others and there was a clear recirculation after the first bolus passage. The surrounding tissue curve (solid light gray line) showed a lower peak than both the artery curve and the curve obtained from the manual ROI method (black line). Moreover, the manual ROI curve showed an intermediate characteristic between the above two. Although characteristics of AIF vary among subjects in onset time, peak height, FWHM and TTP, a consistent tendency among three AIFs determined by the different tissue location was consistent across subjects.

The results of AIF concentration time curves fitted with gamma-variate function for all eight subjects were listed in Table 1. The table showed the statistics of paired t-test between (a) manual ROI (Manu-roi) and the artery ROI with the weighted-ICA method (ICA-aw); (b) manual ROI (Manu-roi) and the surrounding tissue ROI with the weighted-ICA method (ICA-sw); and (c) artery ROI (ICA-aw) and the surrounding tissue ROI (ICA-sw) with the weighted-ICA method. Significant differences in peak height were found in various tissues, with the highest value in the artery and the lowest value in the surrounding tissue. A similar significant pattern was observed in arrival time, with the fastest for the artery and the slowest for the surrounding tissue. In addition, the TTP for the manual ROI was found to be longer than that for the other two methods while the FWHM for the surrounding tissue is smaller than that for the other two methods.

Table 2 showed the CBF values of gray and white matters and their ratios, obtained using AIFs calculated from the ROI selected by three methods. CBF values obtained from the AIF$_w$ of surrounding tissue were significantly smaller than those obtained from the other two datasets. The CBF values calculated by the weighted-ICA method (ICA-sw) were 41.1 ± 4.9 and 22.1 ± 2.3 mL/100 g/min for cortical gray matter (GM) and deep white matter (WM) regions, respectively. The CBF values obtained from the manual ROIs were 53.6 ± 12.0 and 27.9 ± 5.9 mL/100 g/min for the same two regions, respectively. The CBF values and GM/WM ratios obtained from both methods (ICA and manual ROI) were in good agreement with those found in the literature [9].

4. Discussion

The partial volume effect is a common problem in the segmentation of the AIF location. It is almost impossible to select a region surrounding the arteries without partial volume confounding. However, the data-driven method provides a subjective approach to selecting the region of interest with characteristic information that can be used to avoid the partial volume effect. As the method used in

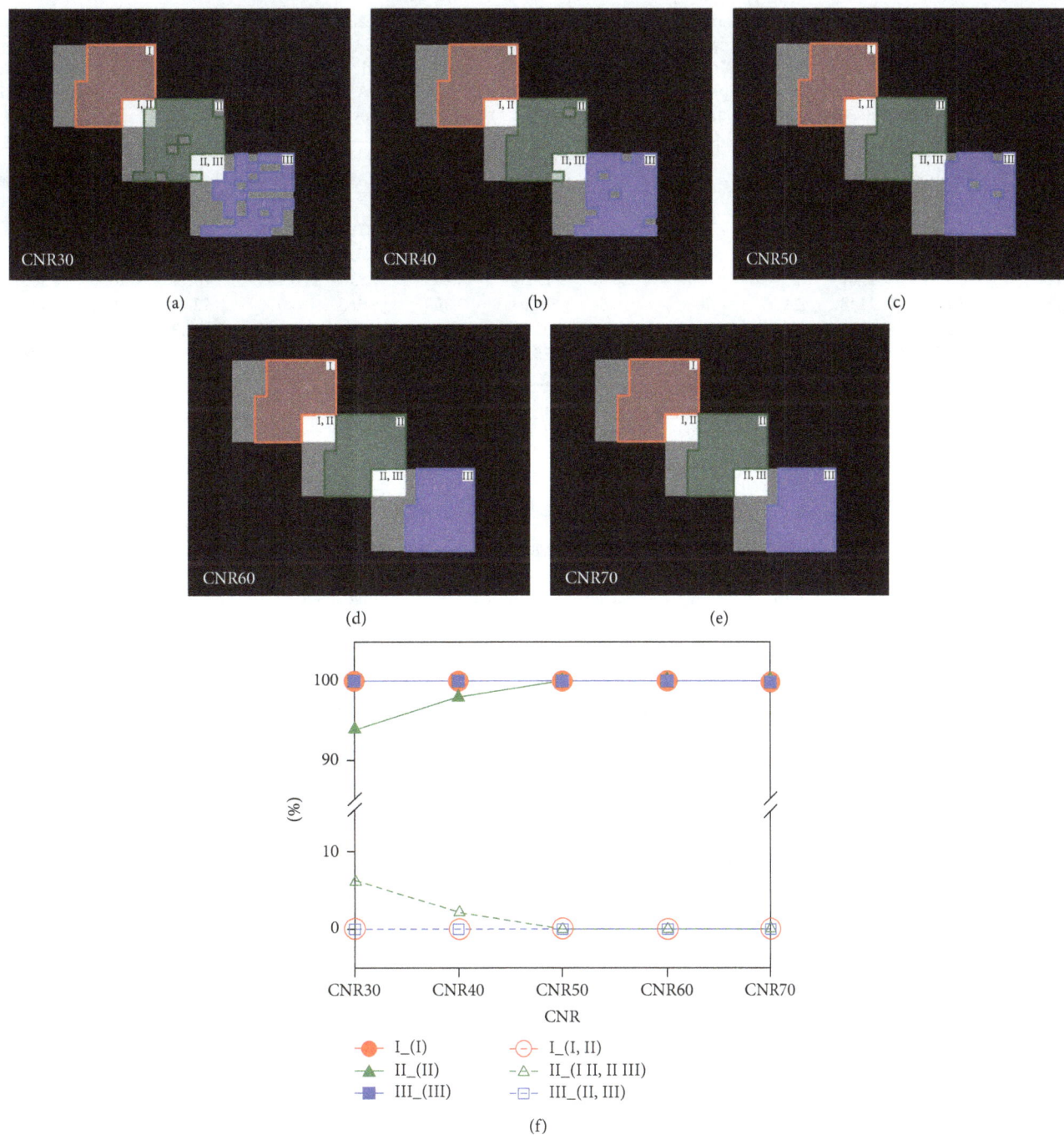

FIGURE 2: The performance of signal segmentation for three ROIs after ICA. The spatial segmentation of ROIs was listed in (a)–(e) along different CNRs. The area symbols for artery, surrounding tissue, and tissue are denoted as I, II, and III, respectively. The performance in signal segmentation is summarized in (f). The solid line denotes the true rate of selected region located in the ROI and the dash line is the false rate outside ROI.

this present study, ICA is a helpful tool and its applications are emerging in decades [31, 32]. Kao et al. [27] employed ICA aided by Bayesian estimation to segment the artery and to refine tissue classification. Other methods, for example, Murase et al. [18], utilized a fuzzy clustering method to identify the voxels belonging to the tissue around the artery after manually outlining the region. Even though the partial

volume information is unknown from *a priori* knowledge, the relative fraction of the partial volume can be assessed by ICA processing. For the performance as shown in our simulation (in Figure 2), a good segmenting control was achieved in the region around the artery by weighting IC values. Then, the region possessing high source characteristics can be extracted by fraction thresholding of the partial volume. In a similar

TABLE 1: Comparisons of time-to-peak (TTP), arrival time (the first time point above the mean time response), FWHM, and peak high after gamma fitting in 8 subjects as determined by manual ROI (Manu-roi) and ICA in artery (ICA-aw) and surrounding tissue (ICA-sw). Below the table, there is statistic comparison with paired t-test for manual and weighted-ICA ROI. Significant difference between Manu-roi and ICA-aw ROI is found in TTP, onset time, and peak high and that between Manu-roi and ICA-sw ROI is found in TTP, onset time, FWHM, and peak. For ICA-aw and ICA-sw, there are significant differences in onset time, FWHM, and peak high.

	TTP (sec)			Onset time (sec)			FWHM (sec)			Peak high (#/mL)		
	Manu-roi	ICA-aw	ICA-sw	Manu-roi	ICA-aw	ICA-sw	Manu-roi	ICA-aw	ICA-sw	Manu-roi	ICA-aw	ICA-sw
#1 (36 y, m)	26.70	25.89	26.07	21.12	19.64	21.89	7.650	7.305	5.775	546.6	1423	324.4
#2 (33 y, m)	29.36	27.66	27.98	20.94	20.55	21.68	9.615	8.295	7.365	528.4	1020	456.5
#3 (32 y, m)	28.20	27.20	27.27	21.09	20.01	22.67	9.450	9.375	7.005	421.6	1077	337.3
#4 (46 y, m)	26.58	27.81	27.50	21.42	20.97	22.37	6.495	7.830	6.885	401.4	960.2	305.9
#5 (35 y, f)	24.74	24.18	24.03	18.68	18.60	19.08	9.060	8.655	6.090	427.8	792.2	508.3
#6 (35 y, f)	22.69	22.16	21.71	18.24	17.48	17.67	6.960	7.515	5.865	438.0	671.2	463.1
#7 (38 y, f)	30.50	29.41	29.58	22.85	22.88	25.73	12.53	9.240	4.920	422.3	903.7	309.9
#8 (29 y, f)	27.25	26.42	26.37	20.15	19.00	22.37	11.12	9.855	4.380	361.2	1033	411.1
Mean	27.00	26.34[a]	26.31[a]	20.56	19.89[a]	21.68[a,b]	9.110	8.509	6.036[a,b]	443.4	985.0	389.6[a,b]
Std[c]	2.487	2.281	2.456	1.503	1.642	2.427	2.060	0.931	1.036	62.78	222.6	79.98

[a]Significantly ($P < 0.05$, paired t-test) higher than Manu-roi.
[b]Significantly ($P < 0.05$, paired t-test) higher than ICA-aw.
[c]Standard deviation.

TABLE 2: rCBFs are calculated by the AIFs determined by the manual ROI (Manu-roi) and ICA-based ROI (weighted-ICA) method in gray and white matter regions. The paired t-test is employed to test the difference between the manual and ICA-based method in the artery (GM_a and WM_a) and surrounding tissue (GM_s and WM_s) and between the artery and surrounding tissue in the ICA-based method in gray and white matter regions.

rCBF (mL/100 g/min)	Manu-roi			ICA-aw			ICA-sw		
	GM_m	WM_m	$(G/W)_m$	GM_a	WM_a	$(G/W)_a$	GM_s	WM_s	$(G/W)_s$
#1 (36 y, m)	66.98	38.35	1.746	56.13	35.17	1.596	41.94	24.83	1.689
#2 (33 y, m)	54.22	28.22	1.921	54.25	30.78	1.762	40.83	21.98	1.857
#3 (32 y, m)	42.26	24.05	1.757	48.00	30.60	1.569	35.02	21.14	1.656
#4 (46 y, m)	45.79	29.57	1.549	40.33	30.16	1.337	38.70	24.55	1.576
#5 (35 y, f)	64.09	28.75	2.229	60.73	28.78	2.110	46.52	23.68	1.964
#6 (35 y, f)	49.08	21.95	2.236	48.09	22.13	2.173	46.75	21.17	2.208
#7 (38 y, f)	37.33	20.13	1.855	41.74	24.73	1.688	34.05	17.71	1.922
#8 (29 y, f)	69.27	32.20	2.151	66.52	34.73	1.915	45.10	21.55	2.093
Mean	53.63	27.90	1.931	51.97	29.64	1.769[a]	41.11[a,b]	22.08[a,b]	1.871[a,b]
Std[c]	12.01	5.879	0.253	9.118	4.476	0.2839	4.935	2.309	0.221

GM = gray matter; WM = white matter; G/W = the ratio of gray matter and white matter.
[a]Significantly ($P < 0.05$, paired t-test) higher than ROI_m in GM, WM, and G/W.
[b]Significantly ($P < 0.05$, paired t-test) higher than A_{wic} in GM, WM, and G/W.
[c]Standard deviation.

outcome also with respect to the clinical case in Figure 3, the regions selected from different locations were capable of determining a candidate AIF. The manual ROI method was more prone to the partial volume effect than the ICA when examining the surrounding tissue. It led to substantial uncertainty and required professional training to select an ROI for AIF determination.

As for ICA's specificity, ICA utilizes the spatial independence of constituent sources attributed to each voxel to decompose signals. These constituent sources include vessel components, tissue components, motion artificial components, and noise components induced by the contrast agent. For sources with more negentropy property (non-Gaussian), the ICA generates component maps with higher discrimination of the source signal [26, 27]. From the component maps, the source map of interest (i.e., vessel or tissue) is

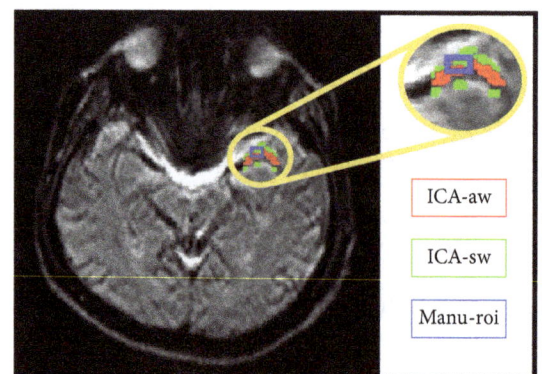

FIGURE 3: Regions selected by the manual ROI and ICA method (blue: manual selection; red and green: artery and its surrounding tissue selected by weighted-ICA).

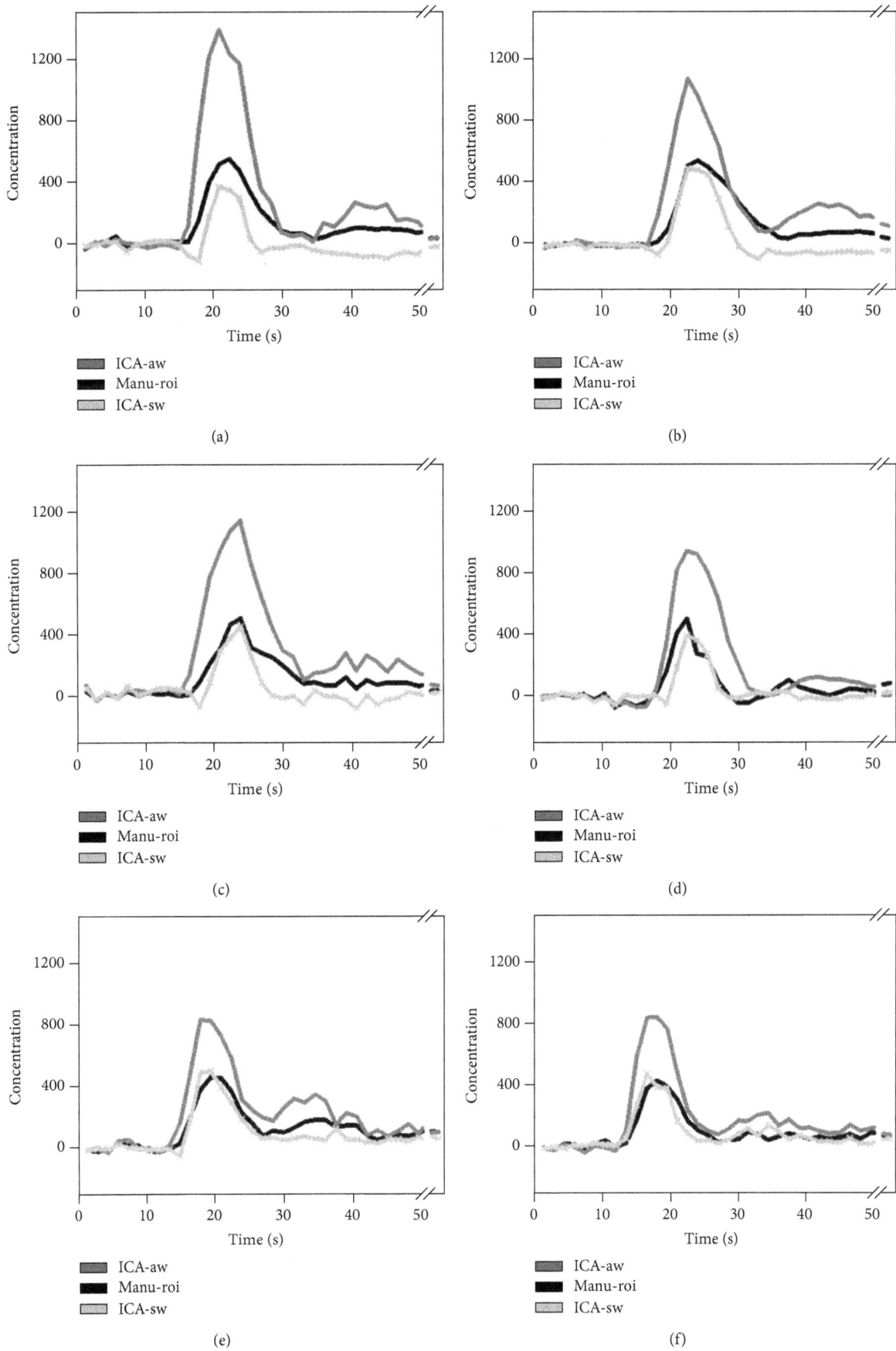

FIGURE 4: Continued.

(g)

(h)

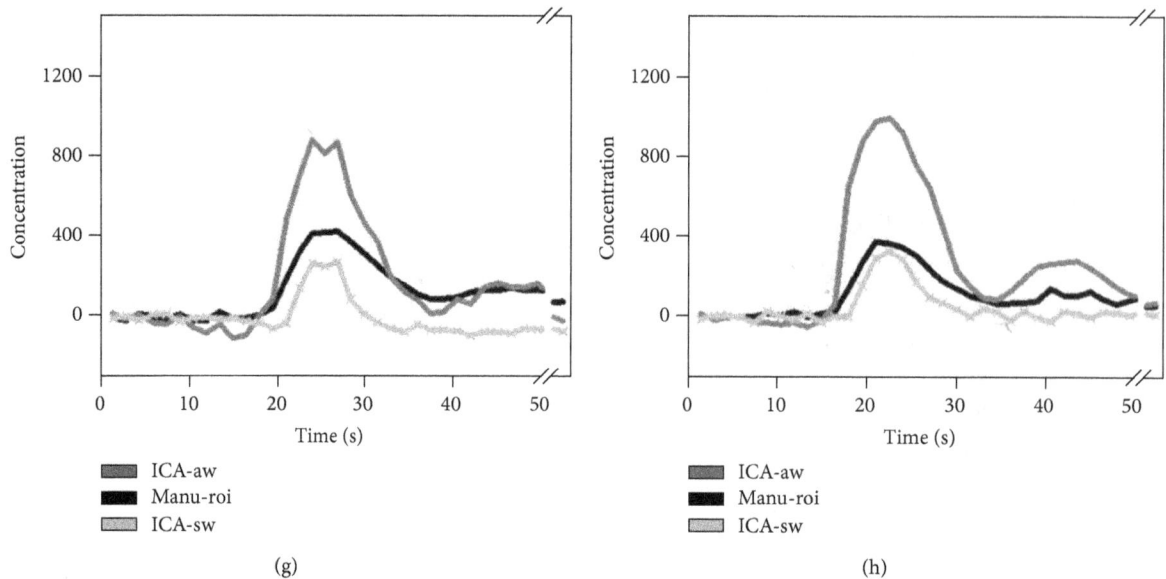

FIGURE 4: Different AIFs were determined for eight subjects in (a)–(h). (1) The artery with weighted-ICA (solid dark gray line); (2) the average with manual ROI (solid black line); and (3) the surrounding tissue with weighted-ICA (solid light gray line). This figure also shows the result.

selected. Furthermore, the area confounded with higher partial volume effect can be removed by z-thresholding and weighting processing for the map of interest. ICA provides a good segmentation tool for locating the area of signal specificity as demonstrated in the simulation experiment and MRI perfusion data. Although ICA provides a better signal decomposition for tissue characteristics, its resultant constitution was normalized based on the hypothesis of statistic independence. This essential hypothesis restricted its application on the calculation of absolute partial volume in each brain tissue. However, if the density of brain parenchyma is involved in the treatment of disease, especially for the assessment of medication, an absolute estimation of tissue characteristics is worth further studies.

Except for the processor of data analysis, the signal we acquired can represent that the meaningful perfusion signal is not acquired easily because generally the signal is caused due to the tissue susceptibility and hemodynamic response. Therefore, according to the theoretical derivation of DSC-MR perfusion application, AIF derived from the region within the artery may not be a good choice because the relaxivities of arterial and tissue water differ. Previous studies assumed the same relaxivities for blood and tissue, which resulted in the overestimation of CBF in a nonlinear relation with the concentration in blood [30, 34]. Kiselev et al. suggested that the relaxivity of tissue should consider the contribution of both the static dephasing regime (SDR) and diffusional narrowing regime (DNR) effects [34–36]. The relaxation effect of Gd-DTPA in brain tissue was found to be several-fold larger than that in bulk blood [36]. Consequently, using AIF obtained from blood signals would introduce significant errors in quantifying CBF in brain tissue, unless the relaxivity of tissue could be independently measured. Besides the location at which the AIF needed to be determined, several properties of AIF were also in addition assessed for the

comparison of CBF calculated among tissue in our present work. In Table 1, the manual ROI method was found to produce AIFs with different TTP, arrival time, FWHM, and peak height. These feature indexes revealed some biophysical properties of the contrast agent-affected compartments in the artery, surrounding tissue, and the region between them. The within-subject variation was mainly caused by the partial volume of tissue and blood. In addition, for the manual ROI method, the uncertainty of ROI selection (i.e., operating at different time sessions or by different operators) could lead to more variable results. This circumstance should be avoided in the application of study and clinical practice.

In addition, a notion worth considering in the deconvolution process was that both the various shapes of the AIF and the thresholding in SVD processing could result in different CBF values. This effect was demonstrated by computer simulation using AIFs with various heights and areas (see Figure 5). In conclusion, using the nonideal AIFs will induce a large error in CBF estimation (Table 3). Next to the calculation of CBF, in this study, we also considered the averaged-AIF as the reference base. Although the comparison of averaged-AIF and weighted-AIF showed no significant difference to each other, it provided cross-checking of the intracorrelation evaluation (not shown averaged result). The top 50 voxels with highest z-value were highly consistent with each other and provided a partial volume free in the region.

In conclusion, quantitative CBF measurement involves a complex combination between tissue physiology, hemodynamic physics, data acquisition technique, and data analysis [37]. In the present work, we focused on the exploration of data mining, especially for the avoidance of partial volume effect. The benefits of this work were contributed for a more precise calculation of CBF: (1) ICA provides a semiautomatic tool for selecting the component of interest; (2) ICA decomposes the signal by reducing the partial volume effect; (3)

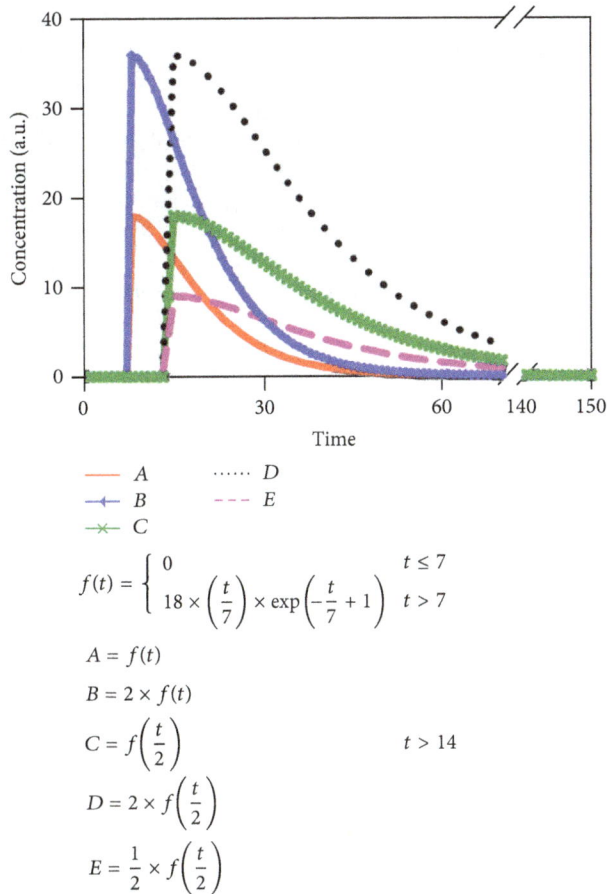

$$f(t) = \begin{cases} 0 & t \le 7 \\ 18 \times \left(\dfrac{t}{7}\right) \times \exp\left(-\dfrac{t}{7} + 1\right) & t > 7 \end{cases}$$

$$A = f(t)$$

$$B = 2 \times f(t)$$

$$C = f\left(\frac{t}{2}\right) \qquad\qquad t > 14$$

$$D = 2 \times f\left(\frac{t}{2}\right)$$

$$E = \frac{1}{2} \times f\left(\frac{t}{2}\right)$$

FIGURE 5: Various AIFs (A–E) are employed to test the deconvolution calculation for flow in dilution theory. "A" (red line) is the ideal AIF defined in the paper [38] and the ideal flow is 80 mL/100 g·min. The thresholding value is the cut-off value in adaptive SVD calculation [33]. B–E curves are the nonideal AIFs simulated.

TABLE 3: Estimated flow obtained from calculation of Figure 5.

	Estimated flow	Area under curve	Thresholding (%)
A	76.40	262.43	13.64
B	38.20	524.86	27.27
C	84.73	523.18	25.82
D	42.36	1046.36	51.64
E	168.91	262.43	12.95

Note: the signal-to-noise ratio is 27.7 for A.

the determination of AIF in the tissue around the artery is necessary for CBF quantification.

Competing Interests

The authors declare that they have no competing interests.

Acknowledgments

This study was supported in part by two grants, NSC-98-2314-B-037-034-MY3 from the National Science Council and KMU-Q099023, KMU-TP104A14, and KMU-M105006 from Kaohsiung Medical University Research Foundation (KMU-M102001), Taiwan. Thanks are due to Chang Gung Memorial Hospital, Lin-Kou, Taiwan, for the data acquisition.

References

[1] B. R. Rosen, J. W. Belliveau, J. M. Vevea, and T. J. Brady, "Perfusion imaging with NMR contrast agents," *Magnetic Resonance in Medicine*, vol. 14, no. 2, pp. 249–265, 1990.

[2] F. Calamante, D. G. Gadian, and A. Connelly, "Quantification of perfusion using bolus tracking magnetic resonance imaging in stroke: assumptions, limitations, and potential implications for clinical use," *Stroke*, vol. 33, no. 4, pp. 1146–1151, 2002.

[3] T. Sugahara, Y. Korogi, M. Kochi, Y. Ushio, and M. Takahashi, "Perfusion-sensitive MR imaging of gliomas: comparison between gradient-echo and spin-echo echo-planar imaging techniques," *American Journal of Neuroradiology*, vol. 22, no. 7, pp. 1306–1315, 2001.

[4] A. Vilringer, B. R. Rosen, J. W. Belliveau et al., "Dynamic imaging with lanthanide chelates in normal brain: contrast due to magnetic susceptibility effects," *Magnetic Resonance in Medicine*, vol. 6, no. 2, pp. 164–174, 1988.

[5] J. L. Boxerman, L. M. Hamberg, B. R. Rosen, and R. M. Weisskoff, "MR contrast due to intravascular magnetic susceptibility perturbations," *Magnetic Resonance in Medicine*, vol. 34, no. 4, pp. 555–566, 1995.

[6] G. Duhamel, G. Schlaug, and D. C. Alsop, "Measurement of arterial input functions for dynamic susceptibility contrast magnetic resonance imaging using echoplanar images: comparison of physical simulations with in vivo results," *Magnetic Resonance in Medicine*, vol. 55, no. 3, pp. 514–523, 2006.

[7] A. G. Sorensen, "What is the meaning of quantitative CBF?" *American Journal of Neuroradiology*, vol. 22, no. 2, pp. 235–236, 2001.

[8] N. A. Thacker, M. L. J. Scott, and A. Jackson, "Can dynamic susceptibility contrast magnetic resonance imaging perfusion data be analyzed using a model based on directional flow?" *Journal of Magnetic Resonance Imaging*, vol. 17, no. 2, pp. 241–255, 2003.

[9] L. Ostergaard, D. F. Smith, P. Vestergaard-Poulsen et al., "Absolute cerebral blood flow and blood volume measured by magnetic resonance imaging bolus tracking: comparison with positron emission tomography values," *Journal of Cerebral Blood Flow & Metabolism*, vol. 18, no. 4, pp. 425–432, 1998.

[10] M. J. P. Van Osch, E.-J. P. A. Vonken, C. J. G. Bakker, and M. A. Viergever, "Correcting partial volume artifacts of the arterial input function in quantitative cerebral perfusion MRI," *Magnetic Resonance in Medicine*, vol. 45, no. 3, pp. 477–485, 2001.

[11] M. J. P. van Osch, E.-J. P. A. Vonken, M. A. Viergever, J. van der Grond, and C. J. G. Bakker, "Measuring the arterial input function with gradient echo sequences," *Magnetic Resonance in Medicine*, vol. 49, no. 6, pp. 1067–1076, 2003.

[12] A. Bjørnerud and K. E. Emblem, "A fully automated method for quantitative cerebral hemodynamic analysis using DSC-MRI," *Journal of Cerebral Blood Flow and Metabolism*, vol. 30, no. 5, pp. 1066–1078, 2010.

[13] L. Knutsson, E. Lindgren, A. Ahlgren et al., "Reduction of arterial partial volume effects for improved absolute quantification of DSC-MRI perfusion estimates: comparison between

tail scaling and prebolus administration," *Journal of Magnetic Resonance Imaging*, vol. 41, no. 4, pp. 903–908, 2015.

[14] K. A. Rempp, G. Brix, F. Wenz, C. R. Becker, F. Gückel, and W. J. Lorenz, "Quantification of regional cerebral blood flow and volume with dynamic susceptibility contrast-enhanced MR imaging," *Radiology*, vol. 193, no. 3, pp. 637–641, 1994.

[15] X. Li, J. Tian, E. Li, X. Wang, J. Dai, and L. Ai, "Adaptive total linear least square method for quantification of mean transit time in brain perfusion MRI," *Magnetic Resonance Imaging*, vol. 21, no. 5, pp. 503–510, 2003.

[16] A. L. Martel, A. R. Moody, S. J. Allder, G. S. Delay, and P. S. Morgan, "Extracting parametric images from dynamic contrast-enhanced MRI studies of the brain using factor analysis," *Medical Image Analysis*, vol. 5, no. 1, pp. 29–39, 2001.

[17] A. L. Martel, D. Fraser, G. S. Delay, P. S. Morgan, and A. R. Moody, "Separating arterial and venous components from 3D dynamic contrast-enhanced MRI studies using factor analysis," *Magnetic Resonance in Medicine*, vol. 49, no. 5, pp. 928–933, 2003.

[18] K. Murase, K. Kikuchi, H. Miki, T. Shimizu, and J. Ikezoe, "Determination of arterial input function using fuzzy clustering for quantification of cerebral blood flow with dynamic susceptibility contrast-enhanced MR imaging," *Journal of Magnetic Resonance Imaging*, vol. 13, no. 5, pp. 797–806, 2001.

[19] M. J. McKeown, S. Makeig, G. G. Brown et al., "Analysis of fMRI data by blind separation into independent spatial components," *Human Brain Mapping*, vol. 6, no. 3, pp. 160–188, 1998.

[20] M. J. McKeown and T. J. Sejnowski, "Independent component analysis of fMRI data: examining the assumptions," *Human Brain Mapping*, vol. 6, no. 5-6, pp. 368–372, 1998.

[21] S. Dodel, J. M. Herrmann, and T. Geisel, "Localization of brain activity—blind separation for fMRI data," *Neurocomputing*, vol. 32-33, pp. 701–708, 2000.

[22] V. D. Calhoun, T. Adali, G. D. Pearlson, and J. J. Pekar, "A method for making group inferences from functional MRI data using independent component analysis," *Human Brain Mapping*, vol. 14, no. 3, pp. 140–151, 2001.

[23] E. Formisano, F. Esposito, N. Kriegeskorte, G. Tedeschi, F. Di Salle, and R. Goebel, "Spatial independent component analysis of functional magnetic resonance imaging time-series: characterization of the cortical components," *Neurocomputing*, vol. 49, pp. 241–254, 2002.

[24] F. Esposito, E. Seifritz, E. Formisano et al., "Real-time independent component analysis of fMRI time-series," *NeuroImage*, vol. 20, no. 4, pp. 2209–2224, 2003.

[25] V. Kiviniemi, J.-H. Kantola, J. Jauhiainen, A. Hyvärinen, and O. Tervonen, "Independent component analysis of nondeterministic fMRI signal sources," *Neuroimage*, vol. 19, no. 2, pp. 253–260, 2003.

[26] F. Calamante, M. Mørup, and L. K. Hansen, "Defining a local arterial input function for perfusion MRI using independent component analysis," *Magnetic Resonance in Medicine*, vol. 52, no. 4, pp. 789–797, 2004.

[27] Y.-H. Kao, W.-Y. Guo, Y.-T. Wu et al., "Hemodynamic segmentation of MR brain perfusion images using independent component analysis, thresholding, and Bayesian estimation," *Magnetic Resonance in Medicine*, vol. 49, no. 5, pp. 885–894, 2003.

[28] T. J. Carroll, V. M. Haughton, H. A. Rowley, and D. Cordes, "Confounding effect of large vessels on MR perfusion images analyzed with independent component analysis," *American Journal of Neuroradiology*, vol. 23, no. 6, pp. 1007–1012, 2002.

[29] K. L. Leenders, D. Perani, A. A. Lammertsma et al., "Cerebral blood flow, blood volume and oxygen utilization: normal values and effect of age," *Brain*, vol. 113, no. 1, pp. 27–47, 1990.

[30] V. G. Kiselev, "On the theoretical basis of perfusion measurements by dynamic susceptibility contrast MRI," *Magnetic Resonance in Medicine*, vol. 46, no. 6, pp. 1113–1122, 2001.

[31] A. Hyvarinen, J. Karhunen, and E. Oja, *Independent Component Analysis*, John Wiley & Sons, New York, NY, USA, 2001.

[32] A. Hyvärinen and E. Oja, "A fast fixed-point algorithm for independent component analysis," *Neural Computation*, vol. 9, no. 7, pp. 1483–1492, 1997.

[33] H.-L. Liu, Y. Pu, Y. Liu et al., "Cerebral blood flow measurement by dynamic contrast MRI using singular value decomposition with an adaptive threshold," *Magnetic Resonance in Medicine*, vol. 42, no. 1, pp. 167–172, 1999.

[34] V. G. Kiselev, "Transverse relaxation effect of MRI contrast agents: a crucial issue for quantitative measurements of cerebral perfusion," *Journal of Magnetic Resonance Imaging*, vol. 22, no. 6, pp. 693–696, 2005.

[35] D. A. Yablonskiy and E. M. Haacke, "Theory of NMR signal behavior in magnetically inhomogeneous tissues: the static dephasing regime," *Magnetic Resonance in Medicine*, vol. 32, no. 6, pp. 749–763, 1994.

[36] B. F. Kjølby, L. Østergaard, and V. G. Kiselev, "Theoretical model of intravascular paramagnetic tracers effect on tissue relaxation," *Magnetic Resonance in Medicine*, vol. 56, no. 1, pp. 187–197, 2006.

[37] F. Calamante, "Arterial input function in perfusion MRI: a comprehensive review," *Progress in Nuclear Magnetic Resonance Spectroscopy*, vol. 74, pp. 1–32, 2013.

[38] B. R. Rosen, J. W. Belliveau, and D. Chien, "Perfusion imaging by nuclear magnetic resonance," *Magnetic Resonance Quarterly*, vol. 5, no. 4, pp. 263–281, 1989.

20

Impact of the Ceiling-Mounted Radiation Shielding Position on the Physician's Dose from Scatter Radiation during Interventional Procedures

Lucie Sukupova ⓘ**,**[1] **Ondrej Hlavacek,**[2] **and Daniel Vedlich**[2]

[1]*Department of the Director, Institute for Clinical and Experimental Medicine, Videnska 1958/9, 140 21 Prague 4, Czech Republic*
[2]*Radiodiagnostic and Interventional Radiology Department, Institute for Clinical and Experimental Medicine, Videnska 1958/9, 140 21 Prague 4, Czech Republic*

Correspondence should be addressed to Lucie Sukupova; lucie.sukupova@gmail.com

Academic Editor: Andreas H. Mahnken

The effect of the ceiling-mounted radiation shielding on the amount of the scatter radiation was assessed under conditions simulating obese patients for clinically relevant exposure parameters. Measurements were performed in different projections and with different positions of the ceiling-mounted shielding: without shielding; shielding closest to the patient; and shielding closest to the physician performing the procedure. The protection provided by the shielding was assessed for cardiology when the femoral access is used and for radiology when the physician performs the procedure in the abdominal area. The results show that the use of the ceiling-mounted shielding can decrease the dose from the scatter radiation by 95% at the position of the performing physician. In cardiology, the impact is more pronounced when the left oblique projection is used. In radiology, a large decrease was observed for right oblique projections, compared to cardiology. The ceiling-mounted shielding should be placed as close to the physician as possible. The idea of creating the largest radiation shadow by placing the radiation shielding as close to the patient as possible does not provide as effective radiation protection of the operator as it might be thought.

1. Introduction

It is widely accepted that low dose exposures can increase cancer risk, and as a consequence the scatter radiation produced by patients during fluoroscopy guided procedures may present a risk for performing physicians [1]. Physicians performing interventional procedures in close proximity to patients are exposed to potentially low levels of scattered dose for long time period [2], making radiation protection of the interventional staff an important issue [3, 4]. There are practical ways of reducing occupational doses to interventional staff, including the use of protective shielding. Protective shielding may be personal—aprons, thyroid shields, and glasses—or could be part of the X-ray system and its accessories as ceiling-mounted shielding, table shielding with vertical extension, disposable pads, or shielding placed over patients [5–10]. Doses to both staff and patients can also be reduced through the use of modified angiography system setups (frame rate, X-ray field size, spectral filtration, projection, etc.). These are described in [5] and will not be discussed here.

In some situations, shielding placed correctly can significantly improve the radiation protection of the staff; Fetterly et al. [11] reviewed effects of different types shielding and its influence on protection from scatter radiation. Fetterly et al. were dealing with the positioning of the lower, middle, and upper body shielding and its influence on protection from scatter radiation. The authors measured doses by simulating procedures performed on angiography systems but only in the posteroanterior (PA) projection, which is not commonly used in cardiology, and sometimes radiology procedures. Physicians use projections including left anterior oblique (LAO) and right anterior oblique (RAO), often tilted in the cranial (CR) or caudal (CD) directions. In the LAO projection, the X–ray beam is entering the patient from the right hand side, and in the CR projection the X-ray beam is entering from the lower part of the patient's body towards the head direction.

In this study, the influence of the ceiling-mounted shielding and its positioning on the occupational doses of performing physicians due to the scatter radiation from different projections under conditions simulating the exposures during interventional procedures was investigated.

2. Materials and Methods

Two angiography systems, each equipped with a ceiling-mounted radiation shielding, were chosen for this study. The first, Artis Q (installed in 2016, Siemens, Erlangen, Germany) has a 25 cm flat panel detector and is used for cardiac procedures. The cine mode Coro_CARE (dose saving mode) was chosen for measurement, each cine acquisition running for 4 s with the frame rate 15 fr/s, as used clinically. The exposure parameters were set automatically by the use of the automatic dose rate control (ADRC), which is used on both angiography systems. The exposure parameters were as follows: 86–96 kVp, 340–780 mA, pulse width 5.2–9.0 ms, 0.0 mm Cu additional filtration, and small and large focus.

The second system, Artis Zee (installed in 2012, Siemens, Erlangen, Germany), with a flat panel detector of 48 cm diagonally is used for interventional radiology. On Artis Zee, the mode for abdominal procedures (biliary tract dilation, nephrostomy) was chosen for measurement, with each cine acquisition running for 4 s with the frame rate 7.5 fr/s (this is intentionally higher for better measurement accuracy: 1 single frame or 1 fr/s is used routinely). The exposure parameters chosen by the ADRC were as follows: 81–115 kVp, 478–668 mA, pulse width 36–39 ms, 0.0 mm Cu additional filtration, and large focus.

The attenuation of the patient was simulated by the anthropomorphic Alderson male adult RANDO phantom, the torso with head, but without arms and legs. Due to the relatively small size of the RANDO phantom (much smaller than our average patient of 85 kg), higher attenuation was simulated by adding the PMMA slabs to the RANDO phantom. For the cardiology system, 4 cm of the PMMA was placed above the phantom and 2 cm under the phantom. The RANDO phantom with added PMMA slabs simulates a patient weighting between 85 and 90 kg, which corresponds more closely to our patient group. For the radiology system, an additional 2 cm of the PMMA was placed both right and left side of the RANDO phantom to simulate larger patients. Larger patients produce more scatter radiation, because they require more radiation to be used (a patient with the PA diameter of 29 cm requires about 200% more radiation than a patient with the diameter of 24 cm [12]) and hence produce much more scatter [12].

The amount of scatter radiation was measured by the Radcal 9095 system (Radcal Corporation, Monrovia, California, USA) with the cylindrical 1800 cc ionization chamber 10X6-1800 (the active volume 1 800 cm^3). Correction for energy dependence [13] and angle dependence [14] is negligible. The measurements were performed in the dose accumulation mode. The geometry was as follows: the patient table with the RANDO phantom placed 90 cm above the floor, source

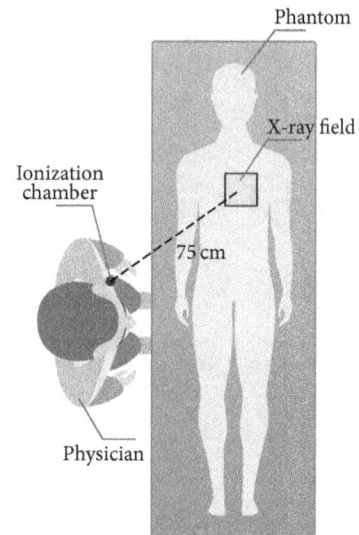

FIGURE 1: The geometry of measurement on the angiography system for cardiology.

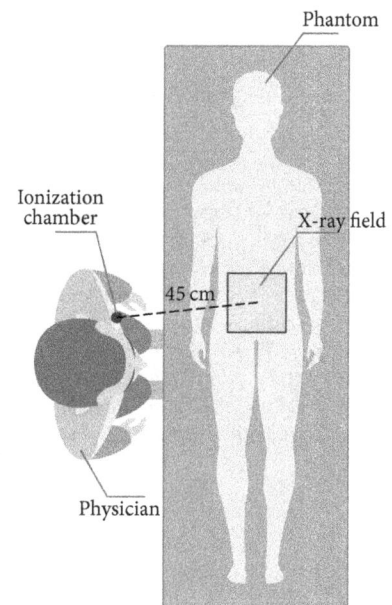

FIGURE 2: The geometry of measurement on the angiography system for radiology.

to table distance of 60 cm, and source to detector distance of 110 cm. The centre of the ionization chamber was placed 135 cm above the floor which corresponds to the chest of the performing physician. The distance of the centre of the ionization chamber from the X-ray field was different for cardiology and radiology and is shown in Figures 1 and 2.

The radiation shielding tested was the ceiling-mounted shielding for the upper body with equivalent of 0.5 mm Pb (OT54001, Mavig, Germany) together with a panel curtain 0.5 mm Pb equivalent (OT94001, Mavig, Germany) which provides a patient contour cutout. At all the measurements, a table-mounted (undertable) shield for the lower body with equivalent of 0.5 mm Pb was also used, but only in one position.

For the cardiology system, the heart of the RANDO phantom was irradiated. The ionization chamber was placed 75 cm from the centre of the X-ray field, which corresponds to the chest of the physician when femoral access is used (illustrated in Figure 1). The X-ray field size at 60 cm from the X-ray tube (at the interventional reference point distance) was 10 cm × 10 cm.

For the radiology system, a lower abdominal area of the RANDO phantom was irradiated. The ionization chamber was placed 45 cm from the centre of the X-ray field, which corresponds to the chest of the physician (illustrated in Figure 2). The X-ray field size at 60 cm from the X-ray tube (at the interventional reference point distance) was 18 cm × 18 cm.

The amount of the scatter radiation was measured for the position of the physician standing at the right hand side of the patient at the physician's left chest side for three positions of the ceiling-mounted shielding:

(a) Without the shielding

(b) With the shielding placed closest to the patient (the dose measured relatively far behind the shielding)

(c) With the shielding placed closest to the physician (the dose measured just behind the shielding).

All the three positions are illustrated in Figure 3 for cardiology and in Figure 4 for radiology. Unfortunately, in some projections, for example, steep RAO projections, the measurements in positions B and C were the same, because the position of the ionization chamber and the radiation shielding was complicated due to the presence of the flat panel detector.

3. Results and Discussion

3.1. Results. For cardiology, the doses from the scatter radiation per 10-frame acquisition were measured for 22 different projections that are routinely used in cardiology. Each measurement was performed twice. The results are given in Table 1. Digits in bold do not differ significantly at 0.05 level of significance. For some projections, the doses with their standard deviations are shown in Figures 5 and 6.

For radiology, the doses from the scatter radiation were measured for 9 different projections that are routinely used. Doses are included in Table 2. All doses were taken for a 10-frame acquisition. For some projections, the values are the same for shielding placed close to the patient as for shielding placed close to the physician due to the complicated geometry (obstruction caused by the position of the flat panel detector or X-ray tube). In these cases, there are only two values in the cell.

The dose to the phantom for each projection was driven by the ADRC. It is known that the dose for steep projections is higher [15–17]. Therefore, the doses from the scatter radiation for each projection were normalized to the P_{KA} values that

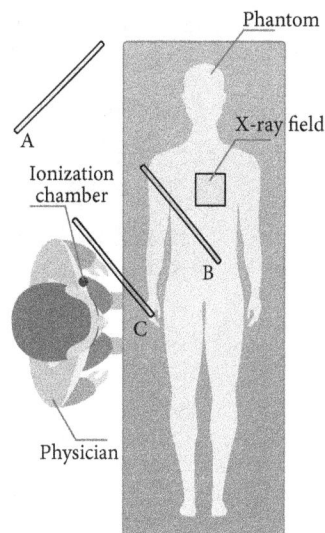

FIGURE 3: Different positions of the ceiling-mounted shielding for cardiology.

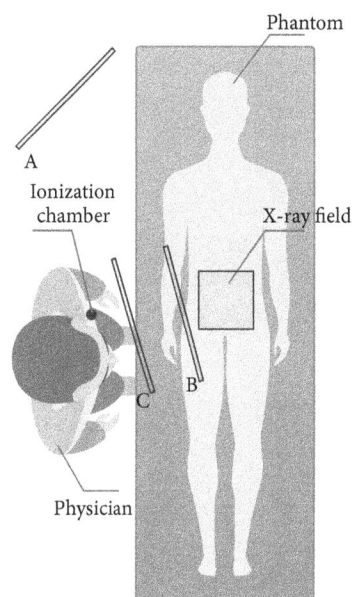

FIGURE 4: Different positions of the ceiling-mounted shielding for radiology.

were gained during the measurement from the KAP-meter (with uncertainty 5%) and are shown in Table 3 for cardiology.

In the same way, as for cardiology, the doses from the scatter radiation for each projection were normalized to the P_{KA} values and are shown in Table 4.

3.2. Discussion. In cardiology, the doses to the physician from the scatter radiation are the highest from LAO projections. In these projections the X-ray tube is on the right side of the patient, therefore close to the physician when the right side radial or femoral access is used. The dose from the scatter radiation can go up to 2.8 μGy per 10 fr when the

TABLE 1: Doses (μGy) from scatter radiation per 10 frames in cardiology for different projections (in each cell, dose without the use of shielding, with shielding placed close to the patient, and with shielding placed close to the physician. Digits in bold do not differ significantly at 0.05.).

	RAO			0°	LAO		
	90°	60°	30°		30°	60°	90°
CD							
30°			0.77/0.17/0.08	0.69/0.12/0.06	2.76/0.28/0.12		
15°		0.18/**0.07/0.03**	0.27/0.10/0.04	0.54/0.21/0.03	1.73/0.73/0.06	2.36/**0.10/0.05**	
0°	0.30/**0.05/0.03**	0.19/**0.05/0.04**	0.19/0.08/0.03	0.59/0.44/0.02	1.20/0.74/0.05	2.27/0.09/0.04	2.40/**0.08/0.04**
CR							
15°		0.22/**0.06/0.03**	0.45/0.28/0.06	0.76/0.47/0.09	2.59/0.46/0.07		
30°			0.74/0.38/0.13	0.83/0.60/0.11	4.51/0.97/0.29		

TABLE 2: Doses (μGy) from scatter radiation per 10 fr in radiology for different projections (in each cell, dose without the use of shielding, with shielding placed close to the patient, and with shielding placed close to the physician. Hyphens mean that the values could not be measured because the dose rate was too high. When there are only two values in the cell, the measurements with shielding placed close to the patient and with shielding placed close to the physician were the same. All the values differ significantly at 0.05.).

	RAO		0°	LAO	
	90°	30°		30°	90°
CD					
20°		28.38/1.43		---/4.45/3.55	
0°	10.72/2.67	34.68/1.55	48.35/4.64/0.89	137.31/15.97/2.32	---/5.02
CR					
20°		44.35/2.92/2.01		119.69/6.55/4.22	

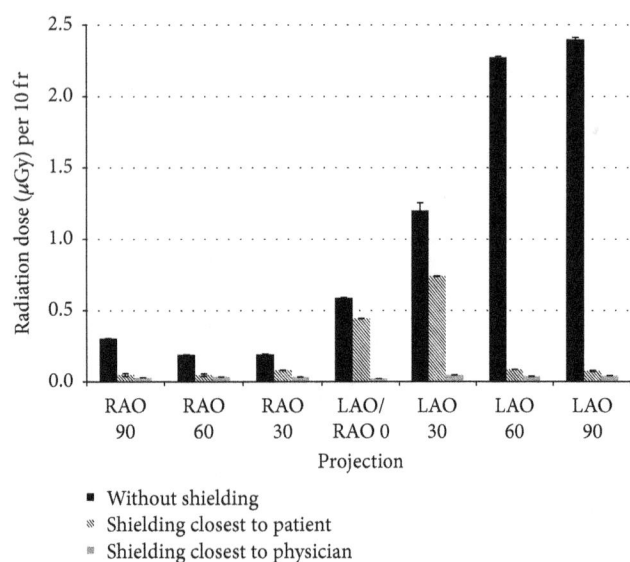

FIGURE 5: Doses from the scatter radiation in cardiology for RAO 90° to LAO 90°, CD/CR 0°.

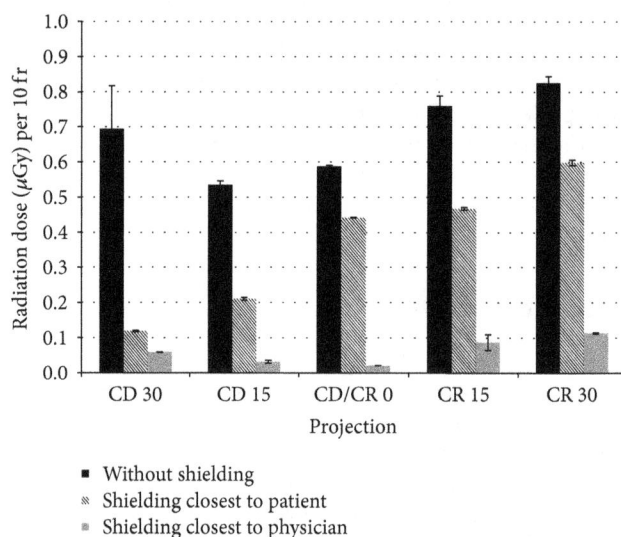

FIGURE 6: Doses from the scatter radiation in cardiology for LAO/RAO 0°, CD 30° to CR 30°.

ceiling-mounted shielding is not used (Table 1). However, the dose from scatter radiation appears to be lowered by more than 95% when the ceiling-mounted shielding is used. If the shielding is placed as close to the physician as possible (as opposed to placing the shielding as close to the patient as possible), there is another decrease of the dose by 50% in LAO projections. This decrease with the positioning of the shielding was not observed for RAO projections. With regards to LAO/RAO 0°, CD/CR projections, the use of the shielding can lower the dose by 30–80% when placed as close to the patient as possible and by another 20–80% when placed as close to the physician as possible.

Doses from scatter radiation for the position of the shielding closest to the patient and closest to the physician were not significantly different at the level 0.05 for some projections (these values are in bold in Table 1), which may

TABLE 3: Dose from scatter radiation normalized to P_{KA} (μGy/μGy $*$ m^2) for cardiology (in each cell dose without the use of shielding, with shielding placed close to the patient and with shielding placed close to the physician).

| | RAO | | | 0° | LAO | | |
	90°	60°	30°		30°	60°	90°
CD							
30°			0.010/0.002/0.001	0.016/0.003/0.001	0.037/0.004/0.002		
15°		0.005/0.002/0.001	0.007/0.003/0.001	0.019/0.007/0.001	0.040/0.017/0.001	0.081/0.003/0.003	
0°	0.011/0.002/0.001	0.006/0.001/0.001	0.007/0.003/0.001	0.022/0.016/0.001	0.037/0.023/0.001	0.086/0.003/0.001	0.086/0.003/0.002
CR							
15°		0.007/0.002/0.001	0.009/0.006/0.001	0.026/0.016/0.003	0.052/0.009/0.001		
30°			0.007/0.003/0.001	0.016/0.012/0.002	0.043/0.009/0.003		

TABLE 4: Dose from scatter radiation normalized to P_{KA} (μGy/μGy $*$ m^2) for radiology (in each cell dose without the use of shielding, with shielding placed close to the patient, and with shielding placed close to the physician. When there are only two values in the cell, the measurements with shielding placed close to the patient and with shielding placed close to the physician were the same).

| | RAO | | 0° | LAO | |
	90°	30°		30°	90°
CD					
20°		0.021/0.001		----/0.003/0.003	
0°	0.008/0.002	0.026/0.001	0.044/0.004/0.001	0.107/0.012/0.002	----/0.004
CR					
20°		0.034/0.002/0.002		0.090/0.005/0.003	

be caused by the fact that only two measurements in each position were performed.

The highest dose from all projections was measured for LAO 30°, CR 30° projection, when the X-ray tube is close to the physician. In this projection, the dose to the physician can by lowered by 94% when the shielding is placed as close to the physician as possible.

In radiology, the doses to the physician from the scatter radiation are also the highest from LAO projections, when the X-ray tube is on the right side of the patient. In LAO projections, the dose can be as high as almost 140 μGy per 10 fr. The dose could be even higher, for example, for LAO 90°, but the value could not be measured due to the high dose rate. The dose from the scatter radiation can be lowered by 98% when the ceiling-mounted shielding is used. This large decrease was observed for RAO projections too, whereas, in cardiology, the large decreases were seen for LAO projections only. If the shielding is placed as close to the physician as possible compared to placing the shielding as close to the patient as possible, there is another decrease of the dose by 85% in LAO projections. For some projections (LAO 30°, CD 20°; LAO 90°, CR/CD 0°), the dose from the scatter radiation without the use of the shielding could not be measured due to the high dose rate.

The dependence of the dose on the shielding positioning is smaller for some steeper projections in radiology, for example, LAO 30°, CD/CR 20°, because the freedom in the positioning is limited by the small space between the X-ray tube and the physician or the detector and the physician.

The doses from scatter radiation are approximately 35–180 times higher for radiology than for cardiology, depending on the projection. The physician-interventional radiologist usually stands much closer to the exposed area of the patient (the abdominal area in our case), so his dose from scatter radiation is much higher. As the doses from scatter radiation are much higher for radiologists, the eye lens of radiologists may be at higher risk of cataracts making the wearing of glasses with Pb equivalent particularly important for radiologists.

The use of the ceiling-mounted shielding is crucial at LAO projections when the performing physician is standing at the right hand side of the patient. The amount of the scatter radiation for the physician in LAO projections is more than 10 times higher than in the RAO projections.

The physician's dose depends on the P_{KA} value used in the projection, as mentioned above, so the dose from scatter radiation in the steeper projection is higher. The doses from scatter radiation normalized to P_{KA} were determined and are included in Tables 3 and 4.

The values in Tables 3 and 4 show that doses from scatter radiation normalized to P_{KA} are higher for radiology than for cardiology. There may be a number of reasons why. In the case of abdomen imaging, which was simulated here, the physician stands closer to the source of scatter radiation. Other causes might be the larger X-ray fields that are used (10 cm for cardiology versus 18 cm for radiology) and also as more attenuating areas are investigated (the heart in lungs versus the abdominal area), more scatter radiation may be produced.

The results were compared with results from the study of Kuon et al. [17] on invasive cardiology. There was good agreement between their and our results. The physician receives the lowest dose from scatter radiation in RAO 20–30° projections. On the other hand, he receives the highest dose from LAO 60–70°, CD 0–20° projections. The normalized values of scatter dose to P_{KA} were of the same order for their and our study, for example, LAO/RAO 0°, CR/CD 0° 0.023 versus 0.022 $\mu Gy/\mu Gy * m^2$, RAO 90°, CD/CR 0° 0.017 versus 0.011 $\mu Gy/\mu Gy * m^2$, LAO 90°, CR/CD 0° 0.062 versus 0.086 $\mu Gy/\mu Gy * m^2$, and LAO 60°, CD 10–20° 0.072 versus 0.081 $\mu Gy/\mu Gy * m^2$.

The results correspond with results from the study of Fetterly et al. [11], where the authors showed that in the LAO/RAO 0°, CR/CD 0° projection the upper body shielding placed closer to the femoral access, and therefore to the operator, provides better radiation protection than the shielding placed 20 cm farther from the operator and closer to the patient.

If the ceiling-mounted shielding is placed closer to the patient, a larger solid angle is shielded but with lower efficiency. On the other hand, if the shielding is placed close to the operator, a smaller solid angle is shielded but with higher efficiency. This should be taken into account when more people are present in the catheterization laboratory.

This study has its limitations. The measurements were performed for one main operator with changed positions of the upper body shielding, but one position of the lower body shielding. The situation would be different when there are two or more operators or other staff in the catheterization laboratory.

Another limitation is that the operator's position may be different for procedures performed from different access, for example, the patient's left side in cardiology, typical in electrophysiology, when pacemakers are implanted. Similarly in radiology, different approaches will be used when the procedure is performed from the jugular vein access or for procedures outside of the abdominal area, for example, limbs.

The measurements were performed for one size of the phantom and one size of the X-ray field. The results would be different for patients of different sizes and also for different sizes of X-ray field. For smaller patients and smaller fields, less scatter would be expected.

4. Conclusion

The use of radiation shielding has a significant impact on the amount of scatter radiation at the position of the performing physician, so the use of radiation shielding should be recommended in all projections.

The dose of the physician performing interventional procedures may be reduced significantly, when the ceiling-mounted shielding is used correctly during the procedures. The influence of the position of the ceiling-mounted radiation shielding on the physician's dose is more pronounced for LAO projections and also for LAO projections tilted in the CD/CR direction. For cardiology, the position of the ceiling-mounted shielding in RAO projections does not affect the dose from the scatter radiation as significantly as it does for LAO projections. However, this is not the case for radiology, where the position of the shielding affects the dose from the scatter radiation in all projections performed on the abdominal area.

In summary, the ceiling-mounted shielding should be used wherever possible, placed as close to the physician as possible. This approach should be applied only to situations, when there is only one operator in the catheterization laboratory where upper and lower body shielding is used. The situation would be different, when there are more people in a catheterization room. The idea of creating the largest radiation shadow by placing the radiation shielding as close to the patient as possible might be used in these situations but we were not dealing with this aspect in our study.

Conflicts of Interest

The authors declare that there are no conflicts of interest regarding the publication of this article.

Acknowledgments

This work is supported by Ministry of Health, Czech Republic, conceptual development of research organization ("Institute for Clinical and Experimental Medicine (IKEM), IN 00023001").

References

[1] M. P. Little, R. Wakeford, E. J. Tawn, S. D. Bouffler, and A. B. De Gonzalez, "Risks associated with low doses and low dose rates of ionizing radiation: why linearity may be (almost) the best we can do," *Radiology*, vol. 251, no. 1, pp. 6–12, 2009.

[2] Y. Kong, L. Gao, W. Zhuo, and A. Qian, "A survey on radiation exposure of primary operators from interventional X-ray procedures," *Radiation Measurements*, vol. 55, pp. 43–45, 2013.

[3] B. A. Schueler, "Operator shielding: How and why," *Techniques in Vascular and Interventional Radiology*, vol. 13, no. 3, pp. 167–171, 2010.

[4] K. P. Kim, D. L. Miller, A. B. De Gonzalez et al., "Occupational radiation doses to operators performing fluoroscopically-guided procedures," *Health Physics Journal*, vol. 103, no. 1, pp. 80–99, 2012.

[5] H. Heidbuchel, F. H. M. Wittkampf, E. Vano et al., "Practical ways to reduce radiation dose for patients and staff during device implantations and electrophysiological procedures," *Europace*, vol. 16, no. 7, pp. 946–964, 2014.

[6] A. Musallam, I. Volis, S. Dadaev et al., "A randomized study comparing the use of a pelvic lead shield during trans-radial interventions: threefold decrease in radiation to the operator but double exposure to the patient," *Catheterization and Cardiovascular Interventions*, vol. 85, no. 7, pp. 1164–1170, 2015.

[7] A. Ertel, J. Nadelson, A. R. Shroff, R. Sweis, D. Ferrera, and M. I. Vidovich, "Radiation dose reduction during radial cardiac catheterization: evaluation of a dedicated radial angiography absorption shielding drape," *ISRN Cardiology*, vol. 2012, Article ID 769167, 5 pages, 2012.

[8] J. P. Gonzales, C. Moran, and J. E. Silberzweig, "Reduction of operator radiation dose by an extended lower body shield," *Journal of Vascular and Interventional Radiology*, vol. 25, no. 3, pp. 462–468, 2014.

[9] D. L. Miller, E. Vañó, G. Bartal et al., "Occupational radiation protection in interventional radiology: a joint guideline of the cardiovascular and interventional radiology society of Europe

and the society of interventional radiology," *CardioVascular and Interventional Radiology*, vol. 33, no. 2, pp. 230–239, 2010.

[10] H. W. Lange and H. Von Boetticher, "Reduction of operator radiation dose by a pelvic lead shield during cardiac catheterization by radial access: comparison with femoral access," *JACC: Cardiovascular Interventions*, vol. 5, no. 4, pp. 445–449, 2012.

[11] K. A. Fetterly, D. J. Magnuson, G. M. Tannahill, M. D. Hindal, and V. Mathew, "Effective use of radiation shields to minimize operator dose during invasive cardiology procedures," *JACC: Cardiovascular Interventions*, vol. 4, no. 10, pp. 1133–1139, 2011.

[12] B. A. Schueler, T. J. Vrieze, H. Bjarnason, and A. W. Stanson, "An investigation of operator exposure in interventional radiology," *RadioGraphics*, vol. 26, no. 5, pp. 1533–1540, 2006.

[13] Radcal Corporation. RC. Low dose rate radiation applications. Specification sheet,.

[14] D. R. Dance, S. Christofides, A. D. A. Maidment, I. D. McLean, and K. H. Ng, *Diagnostic Radiology Physics. A Handbook for Teachers and Students*, International Atomic Energy Agency, 2014.

[15] S. Agarwal, A. Parashar, N. S. Bajaj et al., "Relationship of beam angulation and radiation exposure in the cardiac catheterization laboratory," *JACC: Cardiovascular Interventions*, vol. 7, no. 5, pp. 558–566, 2014.

[16] A. Varghese, R. S. Livingstone, L. Varghese et al., "Radiation doses and estimated risk from angiographic projections during coronary angiography performed using novel flat detector," *Journal of Applied Clinical Medical Physics*, vol. 17, no. 3, pp. 433–441, 2016.

[17] E. Kuon, C. Glaser, and J. B. Dahm, "Effective techniques for reduction of radiation dosage to patients undergoing invasive cardiac procedures," *British Journal of Radiology*, vol. 76, no. 906, pp. 406–413, 2003.

21

MRI-Based Quantification of Magnetic Susceptibility in Gel Phantoms: Assessment of Measurement and Calculation Accuracy

Emma Olsson (ID), **Ronnie Wirestam** (ID), **and Emelie Lind**

Department of Medical Radiation Physics, Lund University, Skåne University Hospital Lund, 22185 Lund, Sweden

Correspondence should be addressed to Ronnie Wirestam; ronnie.wirestam@med.lu.se

Academic Editor: Paul Sijens

The local magnetic field inside and around an object in a magnetic resonance imaging unit depends on the magnetic susceptibility of the object being magnetized, in combination with its geometry/orientation. Magnetic susceptibility can thus be exploited as a source of tissue contrast, and susceptibility imaging may also become a useful tool in contrast agent quantification and for assessment of venous oxygen saturation levels. In this study, the accuracy of an established procedure for quantitative susceptibility mapping (QSM) was investigated. Three gel phantoms were constructed with cylinders of varying susceptibility and geometry. Experimental results were compared with simulated and analytically calculated data. An expected linear relationship between estimated susceptibility and concentration of contrast agent was observed. Less accurate QSM-based susceptibility values were observed for cylindrical objects at angles, relative to the main magnetic field, that were close to or larger than the magic angle. Results generally improved for large objects/high spatial resolution and large volume coverage. For simulated phase maps, accurate susceptibility quantification by QSM was achieved also for more challenging geometries. The investigated QSM algorithm was generally robust to changes in measurement and calculation parameters, but experimental phase data of sufficient quality may be difficult to obtain in certain geometries.

1. Introduction

An object in an external magnetic field will become magnetized to a degree that is determined by the magnetic susceptibility of the object. The local magnetic field inside and in the surroundings of the object will thus depend on the magnetic susceptibility in combination with the geometry/orientation of the object being magnetized. In susceptibility-weighted magnetic resonance imaging (SWI), the local magnetic field distribution is explored to enhance image contrast and to improve the visibility of various structures on the basis of their magnetic susceptibility [1]. Additionally, quantitative susceptibility mapping (QSM) has developed into a promising method for calculating arbitrary magnetic susceptibility distributions from measured magnetic resonance imaging (MRI) phase data [2–4]. A more complete understanding of the phase behaviour in vivo may also require biophysical considerations of microstructural tissue anisotropy and magnetic susceptibility anisotropy [5].

In vivo, the magnetic susceptibility differs among tissue types and tissue regions, and it can thus be exploited as a source of contrast in MRI. For example, in reference to the cerebrospinal fluid (CSF), i.e., when the CSF magnetic susceptibility is set to 0 ppm, the globus pallidus, which is part of the basal ganglia, has a magnetic susceptibility of 0.105 ppm while white matter has a lower susceptibility of -0.030 ppm [6]. In addition to the effects of normal ageing [7], a number of conditions and processes can alter the magnetic susceptibility of tissue. For example, iron accumulation in inflamed myelin cells, as in a multiple sclerosis (MS) plaque, increases the susceptibility of the myelin [8]. Iron accumulation is also seen in other neurodegenerative diseases, for example, Alzheimer's and Parkinson's diseases [9]. The magnetic susceptibility is also dependent on the oxygen saturation level of blood, and the susceptibility increases with increasing levels of deoxyhemoglobin. Hence, venous blood will show a higher susceptibility than arterial blood, and quantification of magnetic susceptibility can thus be useful in estimations of oxygen extraction fraction (OEF) [10] and cerebral metabolic rate of oxygen ($CMRO_2$) [11]. The change in susceptibility with deoxygenation can also be manifested, for example, in extravasated blood from an intracranial haemorrhage [12]. Quantitative measurements of the susceptibility could also be potentially useful to determine the concentration of an external MRI contrast agent (CA). Relaxivity-based CA quantification, which is the currently most common approach, is associated with several methodological complications in, for example, perfusion and permeability measurements using dynamic contrast-enhanced MRI (DCE-MRI) and dynamic susceptibility contrast MRI (DSC-MRI) [13]. Hence, more accurate CA concentration quantification in vivo would indeed be beneficial, and a few examples of dynamic contrast-enhanced QSM studies have been presented [14–16].

In QSM applications, quantification of magnetic susceptibility in absolute terms is becoming increasingly important, and extensive validation is thus warranted. A number of QSM reconstruction tools exist, and the process of systematically characterizing differences in accuracy between algorithms has recently been initiated by other groups [17–19]. In experimental evaluations, phantoms have the advantage of offering well-defined contents and geometries and constitute an important, though not complete, part of the validation process, and the present investigation serves as a supplement to previous investigations related to the accuracy of phase and susceptibility quantification [e.g., [20–25]]. In the present study, previously described in preliminary terms by Olsson (unpublished report) [26], the QSM approach was evaluated in gel phantoms with inserted cylinders containing known concentrations of gadolinium CA, to establish whether the QSM method can deliver accurate results with respect to quantitative magnetic susceptibility values in absolute terms. Measured phase values and the corresponding magnetic susceptibility estimates, calculated by an established QSM algorithm, were compared to values based on theoretical relationships. Various phantom designs and simulated susceptibility distributions, as well as different parameters and settings in the measurements and in the susceptibility calculation, were investigated in order to establish optimal settings and important sources of error in the attempts to produce accurate magnetic susceptibility maps.

2. Theory

2.1. The Dipole Field and the Magic Angle. A magnetic moment with magnitude m, pointing in the z direction, produces a magnetic flux density component B_z:

$$B_z \propto \frac{m}{d^3} \left(3\cos^2\Theta - 1 \right), \tag{1}$$

where d is the distance from m and Θ is the angle relative to the z-axis. The angle at which the factor $(3\cos^2\Theta - 1)$ equals zero is called the magic angle (i.e., approximately $\pm 54.7°$ or $180°\pm 54.7°$). At the magic angle positions, the magnetic flux density component B_z will be zero independently of the magnitude of the magnetic moment.

2.2. Phase Shift and Magnetic Field. Variations in the local magnetic field with position r lead to differences in MRI resonance frequency and to subsequent phase-shift variations, and the MRI phase evolution $\phi(r)$ is given by

$$\phi(r) = \omega(r) \cdot TE = \gamma \cdot B(r) \cdot TE, \tag{2}$$

where TE is the echo time. In order for the measured phase images to be useful, unwrapping and filtering of background field variations are required. The unwrapping can be accomplished by a region growing algorithm which identifies phase gradients that correspond to a difference by a multiple of 2π and subsequent addition or subtraction of 2π [27]. Filtering is needed because the unwrapped image usually contains a remaining background phase gradient over the entire image. This phase does not arise from the susceptibility distribution inside the object but from, for example, imperfect shimming or susceptibility sources outside the imaging volume. *Projection onto Dipole Fields* (PDF) [28, 29] is one method for background field removal that compares magnetic fields generated from magnetic dipoles inside and outside a region of interest. Other examples of filtering methods are *Laplacian Boundary Value* (LBV) [30] and *Regularization Enabled Sophisticated Harmonic Artefact Reduction for Phase data* (RESHARP) [31].

2.3. Cylindrical Objects. The internal (in) and external (ex) magnetic field alterations ΔB, caused by an infinitely long cylinder, are given by the following analytical expressions:

$$\Delta B_{in} = \frac{\Delta\chi}{6} \left(3\cos^2\theta - 1 \right) B_0 \tag{3}$$

$$\Delta B_{ex} = \frac{\Delta\chi}{2} \frac{a^2}{\rho^2} \sin^2\theta \cos 2\varphi B_0 \tag{4}$$

where $\Delta\chi$ is the difference in susceptibility between the inside and the outside of the cylinder, a is the radius of the cylinder, θ is the angle between the direction of the B_0 field and the cylinder axis, and ρ and φ are the cylindrical coordinates describing a point at distance ρ and at an angle φ relative to a point at the centre of the cylinder.

2.4. Magnetic Susceptibility and Magnetic Field. For more complicated geometries or shapes, the local field change caused by the introduction of an object in the external magnetic field can be described more generally [32, 33] and is often formulated as a convolution (denoted "⊗") of the arbitrary susceptibility distribution with a dipole field kernel; i.e., the corresponding phase is given by

$$\Delta\phi(r) = \gamma \cdot TE \cdot \frac{3\cos^2\theta - 1}{4\pi r^3} \otimes \chi(r) \tag{5}$$

where r and θ are spherical coordinates and χ denotes the magnetic susceptibility. The main idea of QSM is to extract the susceptibility distribution according to (5), using the information of the local magnetic field from the measured phase images. However, problems arise because the dipole kernel is zero at the magic angle. A convolution in real space represents a multiplication in k-space, and extracting the susceptibility distribution from (5) by deconvolution would therefore imply a division by zero at some coordinates in k-space which would, in principle, affect every point of the $\chi(r)$ solution in real space.

Morphology Enabled Dipole Inversion (MEDI) [29, 34–36] is a QSM reconstruction method, designed to solve the ill-posed inverse problem of resolving $\chi(r)$ according to (5). In the MEDI approach, the problem is formulated so that the difference between an estimated field map and the measured field map should be of the order of the noise level ε. This can be written as

$$\left\| W \left(\delta - FT^{-1} \left(D \cdot FT \left(\chi \right) \right) \right) \right\|_2 \leq \varepsilon \qquad (6)$$

where W is a weighting matrix, δ is the measured field, and D is the representation of the dipole field in k-space. "FT" and "FT^{-1}" denote the forward and inverse Fourier transform, respectively. Additionally, MEDI uses the fact that changes in susceptibility follow the morphological boundaries and that the susceptibility map therefore should have gradients in the same locations as the magnitude image [35].

In brief, the inverse problem is solved through an iterative process. An initial guess is made for the susceptibility distribution. Convolving this with the dipole kernel gives an estimated field map. The estimated field map is compared to the measured field map, i.e., the phase image, and the difference, the error, is used to update the initial guess. The updated susceptibility distribution is then used as input when this procedure is repeated. Iterations are made until the result fulfils the requirements. A regularization parameter λ determines how much magnitude versus phase image information is prioritized. The Lagrange multiplier method is used to reformulate the problem in (6) as a minimization of a cost function [35].

3. Materials and Methods

3.1. Phantom Design. In order to evaluate the QSM method with respect to phase measurement as well as mathematical reconstruction, three different phantoms were constructed. Thin-walled plastic cylinders were filled with a paramagnetic gadolinium (Gd) contrast agent solution (Dotarem, Guerbet, France). The employed plastic material and the low thickness of the cylinder walls (of the order of 100 μm) imply that the susceptibility effects created by the cylinders should be negligible. The cylinders were sealed and glued onto the inside of a larger container. The container with cylinders was subsequently filled with agarose gel doped with a small amount of nickel in the form of nickel(II)nitrate hexahydrate, $Ni(NO_3)_2 \cdot 6H_2O$. The gel was designed according to a locally developed preparation routine using, in this study, 1% agarose and 0.24 mM Ni^{2+} [37]. The susceptibility of the gel was calculated using Wiedemann's additivity law for the susceptibility of mixtures, i.e., $\chi = p_1\chi_1 + p_2\chi_2 + \cdots p_n\chi_n$, where p_n is the concentration of substance n [38].

The purpose of the contrast agent was to obtain a controlled increase of the susceptibility inside the cylinders to achieve a difference in susceptibility between the cylinders

TABLE 1: Reference magnetic susceptibility values of the different components of the phantoms.

χ(**water**)	-9.022 ppm
χ_{mol}(**Ni(NO$_3$)$_2$ · 6H$_2$O**)	54 ppm/M
χ_{mol}(**Gd**)	326 ppm/M in reference to water
χ(**gel**)	-9.017 ppm
χ(**0.5 mM Gd**)	-8.859 ppm

TABLE 2: Imaging parameters in the standard protocol used for QSM phase measurements.

Sequence	3D Multi-TE Gradient Echo
Number of echoes	11
Echo spacing, ΔTE	6.78 ms
Flip angle	20°
Band width	150 Hz/pixel
Field of view, FOV	24 cm
Slice thickness	2 mm
Number of averages	1
Matrix size	256 x 240

and the background, resembling different compartments in the human body (including cases of injected external contrast agent, for example, for the purpose of perfusion imaging). Table 1 shows the theoretical absolute values used for the susceptibility of water and nickel, as well as the most commonly reported value of the molar susceptibility for gadolinium (used as a reference value in this study [39]). The calculated susceptibility values for the gel and the 0.5 mM gadolinium solution are also included.

(i) In the first phantom design, cylinders with 5 mm diameter, filled with 0.5 mM Gd solution, were positioned at five different angles relative to the main magnetic field (approximately 0, 30, 55, 75, and 90°). The actual angles were measured in the resulting images.

(ii) The second phantom design consisted of 5 mm diameter cylinders in parallel, with varying concentrations of Gd contrast agent, i.e., [0, 0.2, 0.4, 0.6, 0.8, 1, 2, 4, 6, 8, 10] mM.

(iii) In the third phantom, cylinders in parallel, containing 0.5 mM Gd solution with diameters of [2, 2.6, 4.7, 5, 7.4, 9, 10.8] mm, were used.

3.2. Measurements. Measurements were carried out at room temperature on a 3T MRI unit (Magnetom Trio, Siemens Healthcare GmbH, Erlangen, Germany) using an imaging protocol described in Table 2. The parameters were selected according to the recommendations for QSM of human brain given by the *Cornell MRI Research Lab* [40]. A multi-TE gradient echo sequence was used, because a single TE acquisition is regarded not to be sufficient for deriving the magnetic field from the phase, due to an offset in the magnetic field depending on the conductivity of the material. The phase shifts reported below correspond to the difference in phase between two subsequent TEs, i.e., to a time period ΔTE (*cf.* Table 2), and are based on multiecho data [34, 39, 41]. In the evaluation process, this protocol was subsequently altered to accomplish measurements with isotropic voxels, different spatial resolutions, and shorter TE. The different parameter changes are described more in detail below.

Spatial Resolution. Measurements were performed with varying spatial resolution (altered matrix size and fixed volume of interest). A FOV of 205×205 mm^2 and an excited slab of 32 mm were used. The matrix sizes used were 64×64, 128×128, 256×256, and 512×512, corresponding to isotropic voxels with sides 3.2, 1.6, 0.8, and 0.4 mm, respectively.

Volume Coverage. Measurements in which only the number of slices was varied were carried out, implying varied volume of interest. The voxel size was 0.8×0.8×0.8 mm^3 and the number of slices was 40, 60, 104, and 144. The phantom with different diameters was used, placed with the cylinders perpendicular to the main magnetic field.

3.3. Image Processing and QSM Calculation.
For postprocessing of the measured images, a MEDI MATLAB code package for QSM, from *Cornell MRI Research Lab* [40], was employed. Magnitude and phase images, one set for each TE, were obtained from the MRI experiments. The phase images were unwrapped [27] and subsequently filtered with the PDF approach [28, 29]. The phase images were also masked before they were supplied to the MEDI algorithm, using a threshold approach based on information from the magnitude image, to define the object region to be included in the susceptibility calculation.

3.4. Variations in Postprocessing and QSM Calculation Procedures

Filtering Method. Different methods for phase background removal were compared, i.e., "Projection onto Dipole Fields (PDF)" [28, 29], "Laplacian Boundary Value (LBV)" [30], and "Regularization Enabled Sophisticated Harmonic Artefact Reduction for Phase data, (RESHARP)" [31].

Variation of λ. The susceptibility images were calculated using λ settings 1, 10, 100, 1000, 10 000, and 50 000.

Zero Padding. Zero padding, to potentially reduce artefacts, was performed in the spatial domain by padding the matrix symmetrically with 200 zeros in all three dimensions.

3.5. Simulation.
A simulated set of phase images was constructed by creating a template based on the magnitude images that distinguishes between cylinders and gel. Artificial susceptibility images were then constructed by assigning the theoretical values (*cf.* Table 1) of the susceptibility for agarose gel and gadolinium solution to the respective pixels. From the artificial susceptibility images, a set of simulated phase images was calculated using (5). This set of simulated phase images was then used as input to the MEDI algorithm and simulated

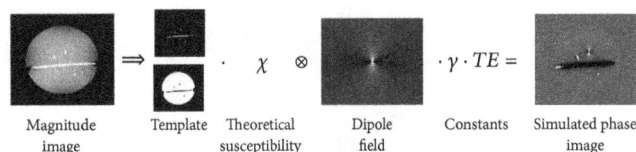

FIGURE 1: Illustration of the construction of a simulated phase image.

QSM maps were obtained. The construction of the simulated phase image is illustrated in Figure 1.

3.6. Image Analysis.
Experimental as well as simulated phase and QSM images were evaluated by measuring the value of interest (mean and standard deviation) in ROIs placed in the cylinders. In the output data from the MEDI software, the background gel region was assigned values which were very close to zero (*cf.* Figure 2), and the background gel thus served as a zero reference (with known susceptibility according to Table 1). Experimental values were compared with the corresponding theoretical and/or simulated values. The calculations of theoretical phase, displayed for the phantom with 0.5 mM Gd cylinders of varying angles and for the phantom with varying Gd contrast agent concentrations, were based on (3) under the assumption that the respective magnetic susceptibility differences $\Delta\chi$ were known, based on the reference values in Table 1. Conversely, (3) can be used to calculate an unknown magnetic susceptibility difference, based on measured phase, and such calculated $\Delta\chi$ estimates, based on measured phase and the infinite-cylinder approximation of (3), are also, for completeness, included in the results.

4. Results

4.1. Cylinder Angle. Figure 2 shows (a) a phase image and (b) a corresponding susceptibility image of the phantom with cylinders of varying angles relative to the B_0 field. So-called blooming effects in the phase image, related to the properties of a dipole field, are seen around cylinders not oriented parallel to the main magnetic field. Some unwanted residues of this blooming effect can be seen in the susceptibility image. In Figure 2(c), analytically calculated phase values, based on the infinite-cylinder approximation (see (3)) and the assumption of known reference values of magnetic susceptibility (Table 1), are compared with the measured phase data for cylinders at different angles. Figure 2(d) shows the expected magnetic susceptibility values (based on the reference values in Table 1), as well as the corresponding results based on experimental phase data, i.e., employing the infinite-cylinder approximation (see (3)) as well as the QSM algorithm. The phase inside the cylinders corresponded well with the theoretical values, and, accordingly, the infinite-cylinder approximation yielded quite reasonable susceptibility estimates based on experimental phase data. However, the QSM calculation returned susceptibility values that deviated

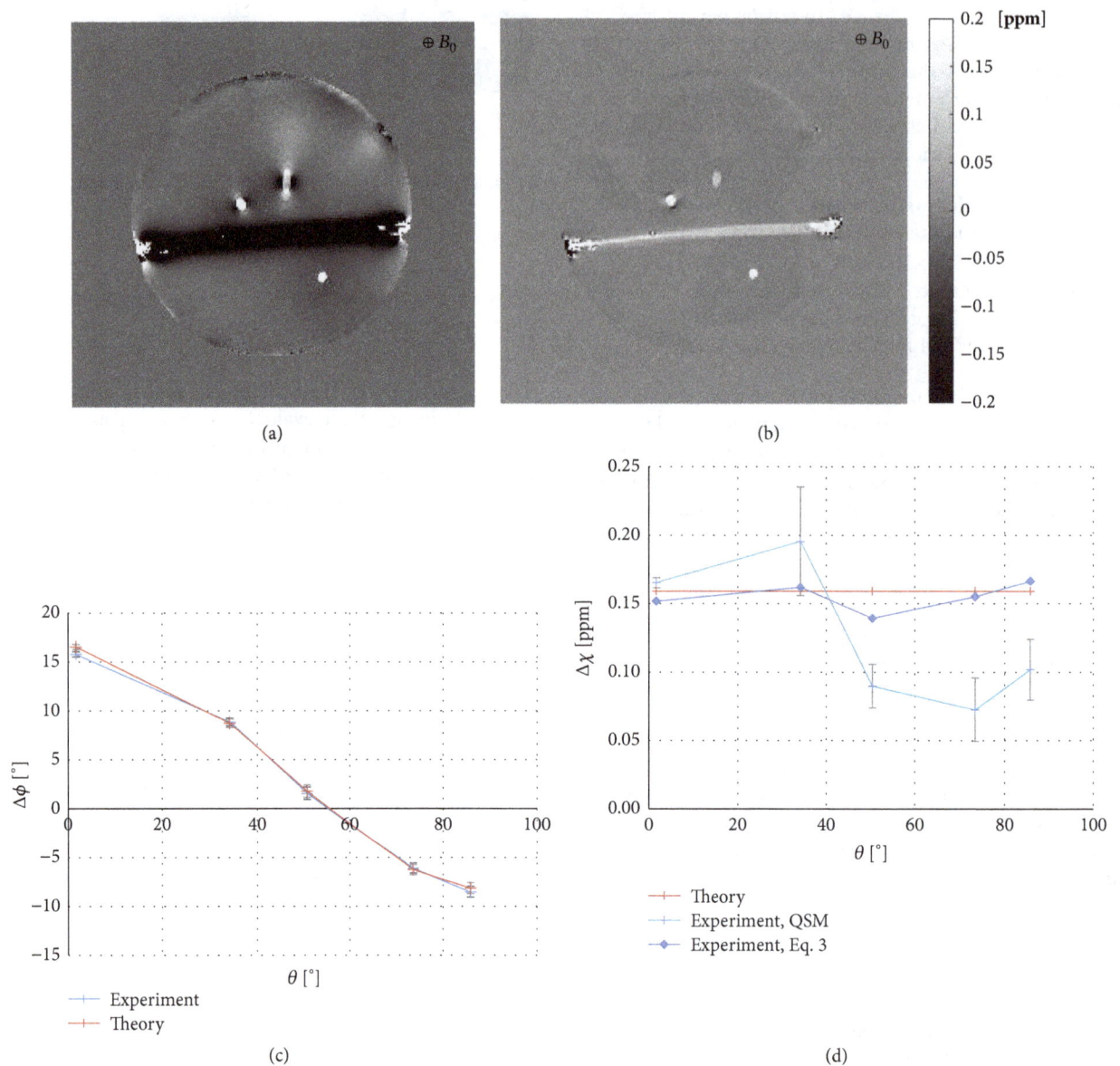

FIGURE 2: (a) Phase image and (b) the corresponding calculated susceptibility image of the phantom with varying angles of the cylinders (slice 17 of 48). The graphs in (c) and (d) show theoretical as well as experimental phase and susceptibility in the cylinders as a function of the angle relative to the main magnetic field. (c) Analytically calculated phase values (based on the infinite-cylinder approximation and the reference values in Table 1) and the corresponding measured phase values. (d) Expected theoretical magnetic susceptibility values (based on the reference values in Table 1) as well as the estimates based on experimental phase data, i.e., employing the infinite-cylinder approximation as well as the QSM algorithm. Error bars correspond to the standard deviation within the region of interest for the experimental QSM data.

considerably from the expected values, for angles larger than the magic angle.

4.2. Concentration of Gadolinium Solution.
An expected linear dependence, for both phase and susceptibility, on the concentration of gadolinium was observed (Figure 3). The QSM algorithm yielded a measured slope of 390 ppm/M, which was slightly higher than the corresponding experimental slope based on the infinite-cylinder approximation (382 ppm/M) (Figure 3(b)). Insufficient phase unwrapping was observed at high concentrations, and, for the phase results, this was compensated for manually by simply adding 2π to

the extracted numerical values. It was, however, not possible to evaluate the QSM output for concentrations above 4 mM.

4.3. Cylinder Diameter.
QSM-based susceptibility estimates for the seven cylinders of various diameters, at parallel and perpendicular orientations, are presented in Figure 4.

4.4. Variation of Measurement Parameters

Spatial Resolution. The phantom with different diameters was measured, with the cylinders oriented perpendicular to the main magnetic field, at different spatial resolutions.

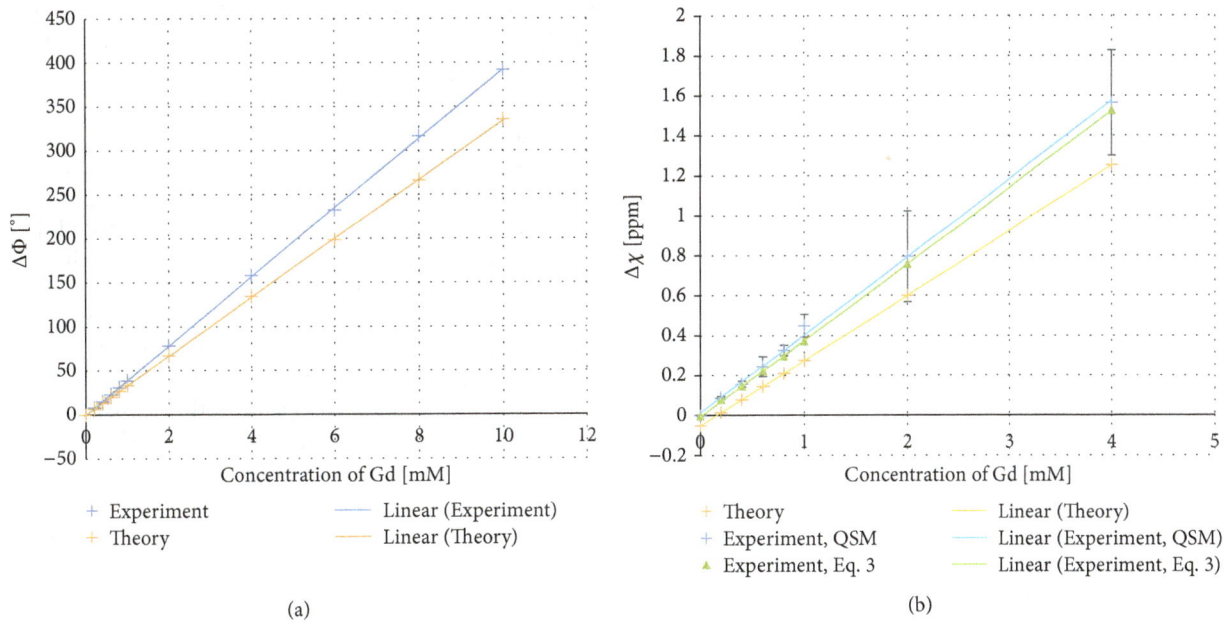

FIGURE 3: Phase and magnetic susceptibility as a function of the concentration of gadolinium contrast agent. (a) Analytically calculated phase (based on the infinite-cylinder approximation and the reference values in Table 1) and measured phase. (b) Expected theoretical magnetic susceptibility values (based on the reference values in Table 1) as well as the estimates based on experimental phase data, i.e., employing the infinite-cylinder approximation as well as the QSM algorithm. For the three highest concentrations in (a), the phase was manually unwrapped. Error bars correspond to the standard deviation within the region of interest for the experimental QSM data.

The susceptibilities in the 5 mm and 10.8 mm cylinders are presented as a function of pixel size in Figure 5.

Volume Coverage. Figure 6 shows the result of measuring with different volume coverage. The same slice thickness (0.8 mm) was used for each acquisition.

4.5. Variations in Postprocessing and QSM Calculation Procedures

Filtering Methods. Susceptibility estimates obtained using phase data filtered with three different methods for background field removal (PDF, LBV, and RESHARP) as well as without any filtering are presented in Figure 7.

Variation of λ. Although clear differences in QSM image quality were observed for different λ settings, the numerical susceptibility values inside cylinders did not vary substantially (approximately ± 0.01 ppm from the measured mean value) when λ varied between 1 and 50000.

Zero Padding. The zero padding did not have any observable effect on the estimated absolute susceptibility values for the phantom with cylinders in various angles relative to the main magnetic field.

4.6. Simulations.
Simulated phase images and the corresponding artificial susceptibility maps, calculated from simulated phase data using the MEDI algorithm, are shown in Figures 8(a)–8(d). Simulated phase images appeared visually similar to corresponding measured phase images, but, in the simulated QSM images (i.e., calculated from simulated phase maps), no susceptibility dependence on the angle of the cylinder axis relative to the B_0 field was observed (see Figure 8(e)). In the phantom with varying cylinder diameters, the simulated phase images resulted in susceptibility values that were in much better agreement with theory than the susceptibility values based on measured phase (see Figure 8(f)). These findings can be compared to results from measured data in Figures 2(d) and 4.

4.7. Phase Profiles.
A profile was positioned through the 5 mm cylinder in measured and simulated phase images of the phantom with cylinders of varying diameters. Profiles were plotted both in-plane and along the slice direction as illustrated in Figures 9(a) and 9(b); i.e., the measurements were identical, except for the use of different slice directions. The results are presented in Figures 9(c)–9(f). Special attention was paid to the amplitude of the peaks at the cylinder edges; no marked difference in peak amplitude was seen between measured and simulated phase for the in-plane profile. However, with the phase profile in the slice direction, the simulated peak phase value was considerably higher than the measured phase.

5. Discussion

Cylindrical objects were used in this investigation due to their geometrical resemblance with blood vessels. Also, the distinct angular dependence of the phase in a cylinder (*cf.* Figure 2(a))

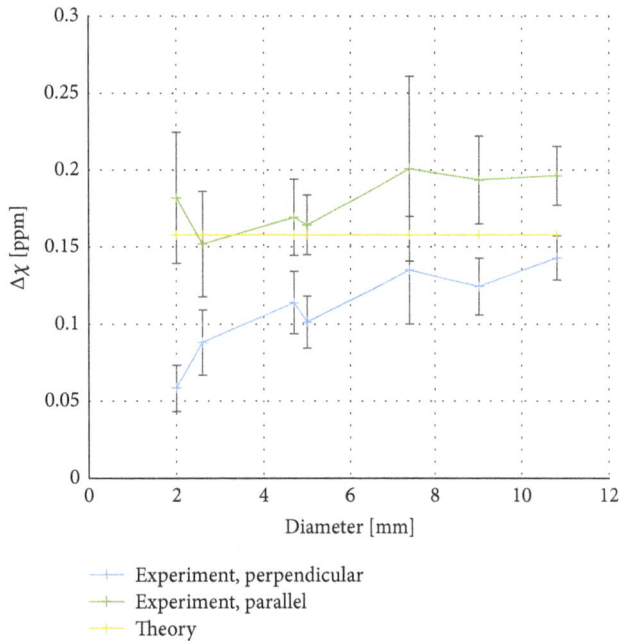

FIGURE 4: Measured susceptibility estimated from the QSM algorithm as a function of cylinder diameter. Results for cylinders parallel and perpendicular to the main magnetic field are compared with the theoretical value. Error bars correspond to the standard deviation within the region of interest for the experimental data.

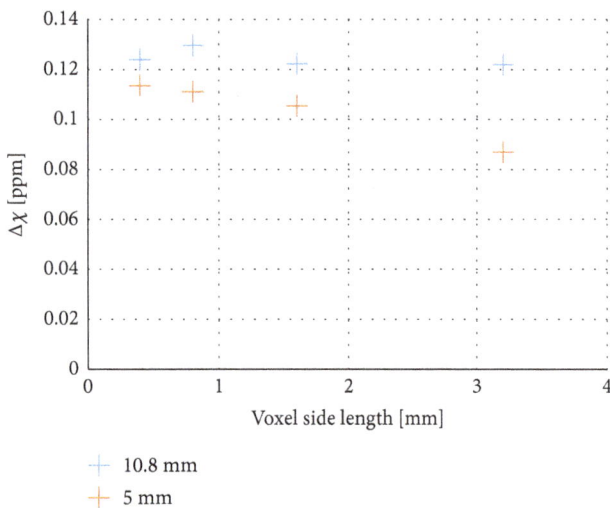

FIGURE 5: Measured susceptibility estimates from the QSM algorithm in the centres of the 10.8 mm and 5 mm diameter perpendicularly oriented cylinders, for different isotropic spatial resolutions.

made it reasonable to assume that cylinders could be a challenge for the QSM algorithm. Another advantage with the use of cylinders is the availability of theoretical relationships between the local magnetic field change and the magnetic susceptibility, as seen in (3) and (4). In the interpretation of the current results, it should, however, be remembered that cylinders show rather limited resemblance with most *in vivo* structures of relevance to clinical investigations. The initial presumption that cylindrical objects could be problematic

for the QSM algorithm seemed, at first, to be valid based on the observation of the measured and theoretical data of the phase and susceptibility inside the cylinders at different angles relative to the main magnetic field (Figure 2(d)). The simulated data, however, indicated that the QSM algorithm did, in fact, generate magnetic susceptibility values that were very close to theory, even for angles larger than the magic angle (*cf.* Figure 8(e)). Furthermore, the simulated data did not show any dependence of estimated susceptibility on the diameter of the phantom (*cf.* Figure 8(f)).

From the measurements on cylinders filled with solutions of varying gadolinium concentrations, it was concluded that the estimated susceptibility varied linearly with the concentration of contrast agent, with an estimated slope of approximately 390 ppm/M using the QSM algorithm and 382 ppm/M using the infinite-cylinder approximation; i.e., the QSM algorithm generated a slightly higher slope than the infinite-cylinder approximation, based on the same experimental phase data. Our current estimates are in good agreement with previous findings for gadoterate meglumine (Dotarem), by Fruytier et al. [42], but higher than the reference (Magnevist) Gd molar susceptibility value of 326 ppm/M [39].

For the 0.5 mM gadolinium solution, also used in the other phantom designs, the susceptibility value was slightly higher than the reference value, in accordance with the results shown in Figure 3(b), as discussed above. Comparing the results of Figures 2(d) and 4 with Figure 3(b) indicates that the deviation of the slope from the reference value (in Figure 3(b)) corresponds well to the slight apparent overestimation of the susceptibility for cylinders approximately parallel to the main magnetic field. Since the phase shift (in Figure 3(a)) and the susceptibility estimates based on the infinite-cylinder approximation (in Figure 3(b)) were also higher than expected from the molar susceptibility reference value, it seems reasonable to conclude that the overestimation was not, at least not entirely, related to the QSM-based susceptibility calculation. The result from the use of simulated phase data confirmed that the problem of estimating the true susceptibility values for different angulations relative to the main magnetic field was not inherent to the MEDI algorithm.

The choice of the regularization parameter λ has previously been shown to influence the quantitative accuracy of the QSM method [35]. However, in the present study, the value of λ seemed to influence primarily the image quality, but the absolute susceptibility estimates did not vary substantially. The fact that the results were not much affected by the choice of λ also suggests that the observed error arises from some other step in the procedure. Hence, three different filtering methods were applied to see if the problems were caused in the background phase removal procedure. Although the results for different filtering methods were not identical, no filtering method returned a systematically more accurate result than the others. An attempt was also made to calculate the susceptibility without filtering. This resulted in images of poor quality, but the angular dependence of the susceptibility estimates remained.

As shown, the phase was measured correctly inside the cylinders but measured and simulated phase data did not

(a)

(b)

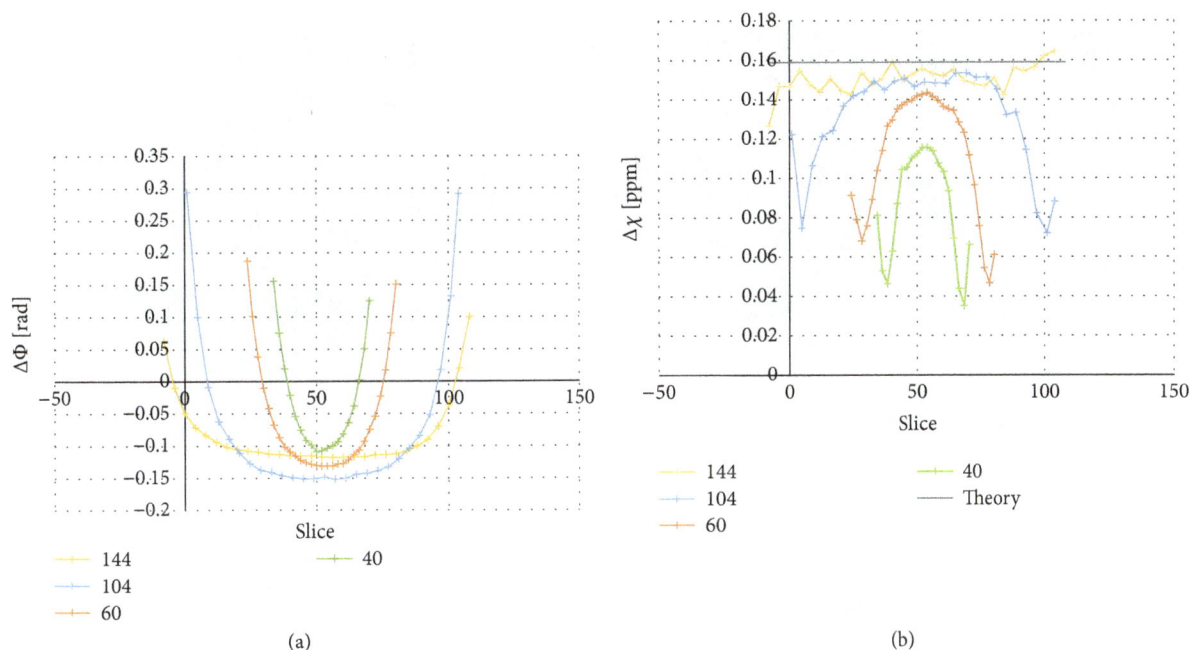

FIGURE 6: The diagrams show (a) the phase and (b) the QSM-based susceptibility, measured in the largest cylinder of the phantom with different diameters for a varying number of slices: 40 slices correspond to an object coverage of 32 mm, 60 slices correspond to 48 mm, 104 slices correspond to 83.2 mm, and 144 slices correspond to 115.2 mm.

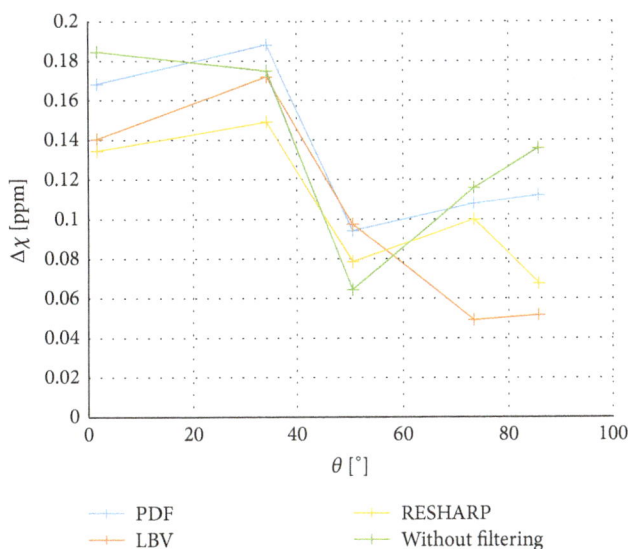

FIGURE 7: QSM-based magnetic susceptibility in cylinders oriented at different angles relative to the main magnetic field, calculated using three different filtering methods (PDF, LBV, and RESHARP) as well as without filtering.

generate the same output from the QSM algorithm. Hence, a reasonable conclusion was that measured phase must differ from simulated phase *outside* the cylinder. The comparison of profiles originating from measured and simulated phase showed that the difference in phase between measurement and simulation occurred just outside the cylinder, and the underestimation was more pronounced when phase was

recorded along the slice direction. Partial volume effects may have been of importance in this context [43], considering the high spatial phase gradient in this region, and it is not entirely straightforward to predict the exact manifestation of the loss of phase information, occurring in the complex sum of voxel components, in a given imaging situation. Depending on the particular MRI unit and imaging protocol, potential effects of applied deapodization filters might also be relevant to consider in this context. Since the magnetization of the cylinder affects the phase not only inside the cylinder but also in the area surrounding the cylinder, the background phase in the vicinity of the cylinder will influence the result of the QSM susceptibility calculation. Hence, if the phase was not correctly measured in the background region, close to the cylinder, this constitutes a plausible explanation to why QSM calculations failed to return accurate values for the magnetic susceptibility. This explanation is also in accordance with the fact that the infinite-cylinder approximation (see (3)) yielded more reasonable magnetic susceptibility estimates than the QSM algorithm.

In this context, it is also relevant to note that the phantom with parallel cylinders of varying diameters was scanned at two different orientations relative to the main magnetic field (0° and 90°), while keeping the slice orientation orthogonal to the cylinders in each acquisition, i.e., with the measurement of the phase being consistent in terms of slice orientation relative cylinder axis. Comparing the QSM susceptibility results in Figure 4 (for 5 mm diameter) with those in Figure 2(d) from the phantom with cylinders of varying angles (for 0° and 90°) shows that the parallel as well as the perpendicular cylinder orientation yielded very similar QSM susceptibility values between the two separate phantoms

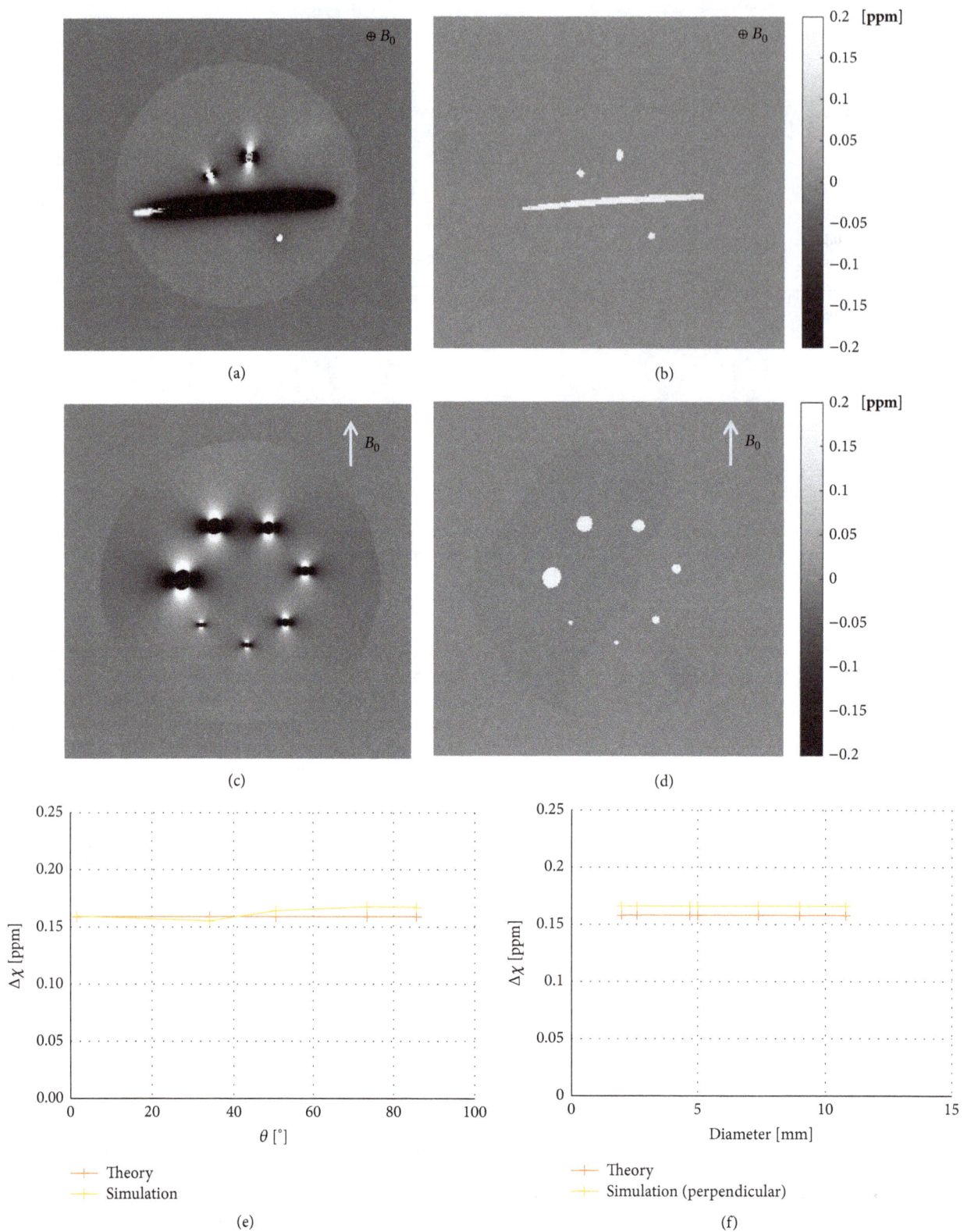

FIGURE 8: (a) Simulated phase image and (b) the corresponding susceptibility image calculated with MEDI for the phantom with cylinders at different angles (slice 17 of 48). (c) Simulated phase image and (d) the corresponding susceptibility image for the phantom with varying diameters (slice 40 of 80). Images were simulated without added noise for a matrix size of 512×512. (d) Susceptibility registered in cylinders with different angles in simulated images. (e) Calculated susceptibility using simulated phase data, for varying cylinder diameter, compared with the theoretical susceptibility. Simulated cylinders corresponded to 0.5 mM Gd, and the assigned values of magnetic susceptibility in the simulated phantom are given in Table 1.

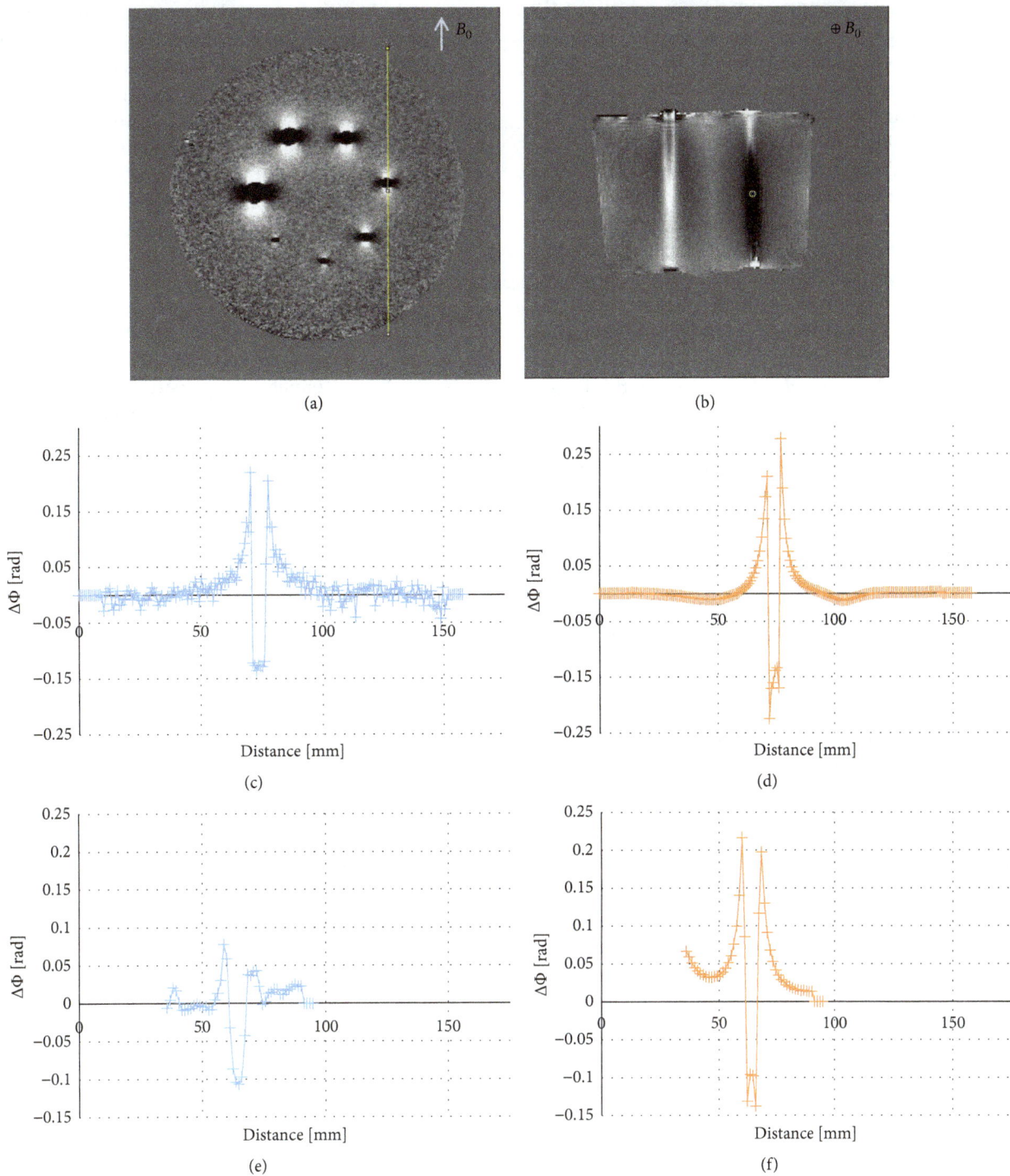

FIGURE 9: Top row: Positioning of a profile through the 5 mm cylinder perpendicular to the main magnetic field (a) in-plane and (b) along the slice direction. Note: the measurements were identical, except for the use of different slice directions. Middle row: values along the profile (when placed perpendicular to the slice direction) through the 5 mm cylinder in a slice in the middle of the volume showing (c) measured and (d) simulated phase. Bottom row: slice direction phase profile through the 5 mm cylinder; comparison between (e) measured phase and (f) simulated phase.

(i.e., 0.16-0.17 ppm in the parallel case and 0.10 ppm in the perpendicular case).

Slice spacing, slice thickness, and volume coverage are also important issues in QSM [44]. In our study, a larger volume coverage of the object resulted in susceptibility values closer to the theoretical value and in susceptibility images with a more uniform slice direction profile, in accordance with previous recommendations for an extended spatial coverage in QSM of deep grey matter [45]. Preliminary attempts to remove slices at the edges of the phase image stack, after the PDF but before the MEDI QSM reconstruction, also resulted in images with less artefacts and a more uniform slice direction profile (data not shown), and this suggests that phase values along the slice direction or at the edges of the imaged volume are influenced by factors which are still unknown (e.g., residual slice aliasing effects, etc.).

Furthermore, the spatial resolution seemed to be of some importance for the accuracy of the estimated susceptibility since the estimated susceptibility values appeared to vary between different voxel sizes. For the smallest cylinders (diameters of 2 mm and 2.6 mm) some degree of partial volume effects can be expected, since the voxel size used was $1\times1\times2$ mm^3, but even for the larger cylinders the estimates differed from the expected values. Figure 5 indicates that there is no dependence on the voxel size for the largest cylinder (10.8 mm in diameter), but for the 5 mm cylinder a higher resolution resulted in a value closer to theory. This implies, not surprisingly, that sufficient spatial resolution is needed to obtain optimal results. At a certain point, the combination of object size and spatial resolution gives sufficiently good measurement conditions, and the systematic error is minimal. For a smaller object, a higher resolution is obviously required to reach that point. However, to establish a clear relationship between image resolution and estimated susceptibility values, more data points would be needed.

Finally, it should be noted that even if experimental phase data were to be accurate, the QSM results would still, in practice, be relative. The assignment of zero phase in the phase maps would imply zero susceptibility, which is normally not the true value for the compartment in question, and, furthermore, the QSM algorithm will typically shift the values of the output data so that the mean value of the volume is close to zero. In the phantoms, the true background susceptibility value is known and thus the expected phase within the cylindrical object can be calculated. In the human body, we do not normally have any such information. Hence, some reference region with known susceptibility is required in order to obtain the correct absolute level of susceptibility within the dataset. CSF has been proposed for such reference purposes, but such an approach is far from straightforward [46].

6. Conclusions

The MEDI algorithm was demonstrated to be quite stable for QSM calculations. The choice of parameters and settings, for example, the regularization parameter λ, the zero padding, and the choice of filtering method seemed not to have a large impact on the quantitative results. Most importantly, when applied to simulated phase maps, MEDI returned accurate susceptibility quantification also for challenging geometries. For experimental phase data, the QSM algorithm did result in a linear relationship between susceptibility and concentration of contrast agent, but correct susceptibility was not obtained for cylindrical objects at an angle close to or larger than the

magic angle. The error seemed to originate from the phase measurement rather than from imperfections in the QSM susceptibility calculation. In our MRI installation, deviation from theory was observed primarily along the slice direction, in the phantom background (i.e., gel) region of the measured phase images. The QSM-based susceptibility results seemed to be somewhat more accurate for large objects and/or good spatial resolution, large volume coverage of the object, and with the slice direction applied along the long axis of the object of interest.

Disclosure

This study has previously been described in preliminary terms by Olsson (unpublished report) [26]. The current research article contains extended data analysis, additional results, and a correspondingly expanded discussion compared with [26].

Conflicts of Interest

The authors declare that there are no conflicts of interest regarding the publication of this paper.

Acknowledgments

This study was supported by the Swedish Research Council [2017-00995], the Swedish Cancer Society [2015/567], and the Crafoord Foundation in Lund [20150753].

References

[1] S. Liu, S. Buch, Y. Chen et al., "Susceptibility-weighted imaging: current status and future directions," *NMR in Biomedicine*, vol. 30, no. 4, Article ID e3552, 2017.

[2] L. Li and J. S. Leigh, "Quantifying arbitrary magnetic susceptibility distributions with MR," *Magnetic Resonance in Medicine*, vol. 51, no. 5, pp. 1077–1082, 2004.

[3] K. Shmueli, J. A. de Zwart, P. van Gelderen, T.-Q. Li, S. J. Dodd, and J. H. Duyn, "Magnetic susceptibility mapping of brain tissue in vivo using MRI phase data," *Magnetic Resonance in Medicine*, vol. 62, no. 6, pp. 1510–1522, 2009.

[4] S. Wharton, A. Schäfer, and R. Bowtell, "Susceptibility mapping in the human brain using threshold-based k-space division," *Magnetic Resonance in Medicine*, vol. 63, no. 5, pp. 1292–1304, 2010.

[5] D. A. Yablonskiy and A. L. Sukstanskii, "Effects of biological tissue structural anisotropy and anisotropy of magnetic susceptibility on the gradient echo MRI signal phase: theoretical background," *NMR in Biomedicine*, vol. 30, no. 4, Article ID e3655, 2017.

[6] I. A. L. Lim, A. V. Faria, X. Li et al., "Human brain atlas for automated region of interest selection in quantitative susceptibility mapping: Application to determine iron content in deep gray matter structures," *NeuroImage*, vol. 82, pp. 449–469, 2013.

[7] Y. Zhang, H. Wei, M. J. Cronin, N. He, F. Yan, and C. Liu, "Longitudinal atlas for normative human brain development and aging over the lifespan using quantitative susceptibility mapping," *NeuroImage*, vol. 171, pp. 176–189, 2018.

[8] C. Stüber, D. Pitt, and Y. Wang, "Iron in multiple sclerosis and its noninvasive imaging with quantitative susceptibility mapping," *International Journal of Molecular Sciences*, vol. 17, no. 1, article 100, 2016.

[9] J. Stankiewicz, S. S. Panter, M. Neema, A. Arora, C. E. Batt, and R. Bakshi, "Iron in chronic brain disorders: imaging and neurotherapeutic implications," *Neurotherapeutics*, vol. 4, no. 3, pp. 371–386, 2007.

[10] K. Kudo, T. Liu, T. Murakami et al., "Oxygen extraction fraction measurement using quantitative susceptibility mapping: Comparison with positron emission tomography," *Journal of Cerebral Blood Flow & Metabolism*, vol. 36, no. 8, pp. 1424–1433, 2016.

[11] J. Zhang, T. Liu, A. Gupta, P. Spincemaille, T. D. Nguyen, and Y. Wang, "Quantitative mapping of cerebral metabolic rate of oxygen ($CMRO_2$) using quantitative susceptibility mapping (QSM)," *Magnetic Resonance in Medicine*, vol. 74, no. 4, pp. 945–952, 2015.

[12] J. H. Duyn and J. Schenck, "Contributions to magnetic susceptibility of brain tissue," *NMR in Biomedicine*, vol. 30, no. 4, p. e3546, 2017.

[13] R. Wirestam, "Using contrast agents to obtain maps of regional perfusion and capillary wall permeability," *Imaging in Medicine*, vol. 4, no. 4, pp. 423–442, 2012.

[14] D. Bonekamp, P. B. Barker, R. Leigh, P. C. M. Van Zijl, and X. Li, "Susceptibility-based analysis of dynamic gadolinium bolus perfusion MRI," *Magnetic Resonance in Medicine*, vol. 73, no. 2, pp. 544–554, 2015.

[15] B. Xu, P. Spincemaille, T. Liu et al., "Quantification of cerebral perfusion using dynamic quantitative susceptibility mapping," *Magnetic Resonance in Medicine*, vol. 73, no. 4, pp. 1540–1548, 2015.

[16] X. L. Xie, A. T. Layton, N. Wang et al., "Dynamic contrast-enhanced quantitative susceptibility mapping with ultrashort echo time MRI for evaluating renal function," *American Journal of Physiology-Renal Physiology*, vol. 310, no. 2, pp. F174–F182, 2016.

[17] C. Langkammer, F. Schweser, K. Shmueli et al., "Quantitative susceptibility mapping: Report from the 2016 reconstruction challenge," *Magnetic Resonance in Medicine*, vol. 79, no. 3, pp. 1661–1673, 2018.

[18] L. Bao, X. Li, C. Cai, Z. Chen, and P. C. M. Van Zijl, "Quantitative susceptibility mapping using structural feature based collaborative reconstruction (SFCR) in the human brain," *IEEE Transactions on Medical Imaging*, vol. 35, no. 9, pp. 2040–2050, 2016.

[19] Y. Wang and T. Liu, "Quantitative susceptibility mapping (QSM): decoding MRI data for a tissue magnetic biomarker," *Magnetic Resonance in Medicine*, vol. 73, no. 1, pp. 82–101, 2015.

[20] D. Zhou, J. Cho, J. Zhang, P. Spincemaille, and Y. Wang, "Susceptibility underestimation in a high-susceptibility phantom: Dependence on imaging resolution, magnitude contrast, and other parameters," *Magnetic Resonance in Medicine*, vol. 78, no. 3, pp. 1080–1086, 2017.

[21] M. C. Langham, J. F. Magland, C. L. Epstein, T. F. Floyd, and F. W. Wehrli, "Accuracy and precision of MR blood oximetry based on the long paramagnetic cylinder approximation of large vessels," *Magnetic Resonance in Medicine*, vol. 62, no. 2, pp. 333–340, 2009.

[22] M. J. Cronin, N. Wang, K. S. Decker, H. Wei, W.-Z. Zhu, and C. Liu, "Exploring the origins of echo-time-dependent quantitative susceptibility mapping (QSM) measurements in healthy tissue and cerebral microbleeds," *NeuroImage*, vol. 149, pp. 98–113, 2017.

[23] C.-Y. Hsieh, Y.-C. N. Cheng, J. Neelavalli, E. M. Haacke, and R. J. Stafford, "An improved method for susceptibility and radius quantification of cylindrical objects from MRI," *Magnetic Resonance Imaging*, vol. 33, no. 4, pp. 420–436, 2015.

[24] H. Xie, Y.-C. N. Cheng, P. Kokeny et al., "A quantitative study of susceptibility and additional frequency shift of three common materials in MRI," *Magnetic Resonance in Medicine*, vol. 76, no. 4, pp. 1263–1269, 2016.

[25] J. Li, S. Chang, T. Liu et al., "Reducing the object orientation dependence of susceptibility effects in gradient echo MRI through quantitative susceptibility mapping," *Magnetic Resonance in Medicine*, vol. 68, no. 5, pp. 1563–1569, 2012.

[26] E. Olsson, *MRI-Based Quantification of Magnetic Susceptibility: Assessment of Measurement And Calculation Accuracy (Unpublished MSc Dissertation)*, Lund University, Lund, 2016.

[27] R. Cusack and N. Papadakis, "New robust 3-D phase unwrapping algorithms: application to magnetic field mapping and undistorting echoplanar images," *NeuroImage*, vol. 16, no. 3, pp. 754–764, 2002.

[28] T. Liu, I. Khalidov, L. de Rochefort et al., "A novel background field removal method for MRI using projection onto dipole fields (PDF)," *NMR in Biomedicine*, vol. 24, no. 9, pp. 1129–1136, 2011.

[29] L. de Rochefort, T. Liu, B. Kressler et al., "Quantitative susceptibility map reconstruction from MR phase data using bayesian regularization: validation and application to brain imaging," *Magnetic Resonance in Medicine*, vol. 63, no. 1, pp. 194–206, 2010.

[30] D. Zhou, T. Liu, P. Spincemaille, and Y. Wang, "Background field removal by solving the Laplacian boundary value problem," *NMR in Biomedicine*, vol. 27, no. 3, pp. 312–319, 2014.

[31] H. Sun and A. H. Wilman, "Background field removal using spherical mean value filtering and Tikhonov regularization," *Magnetic Resonance in Medicine*, vol. 71, no. 3, pp. 1151–1157, 2014.

[32] R. Salomir, B. D. De Senneville, and C. T. W. Moonen, "A fast calculation method for magnetic field inhomogeneity due to an arbitrary distribution of bulk susceptibility," *Concepts in Magnetic Resonance B*, vol. 19, no. 1, pp. 26–34, 2003.

[33] J. P. Marques and R. Bowtell, "Application of a Fourier-based method for rapid calculation of field inhomogeneity due to spatial variation of magnetic susceptibility," *Concepts in Magnetic Resonance*, vol. 25, no. 1, pp. 65–78, 2005.

[34] T. Liu, C. Wisnieff, M. Lou, W. Chen, P. Spincemaille, and Y. Wang, "Nonlinear formulation of the magnetic field to source relationship for robust quantitative susceptibility mapping," *Magnetic Resonance in Medicine*, vol. 69, no. 2, pp. 467–476, 2013.

[35] J. Liu, T. Liu, L. de Rochefort et al., "Morphology enabled dipole inversion for quantitative susceptibility mapping using structural consistency between the magnitude image and the susceptibility map," *NeuroImage*, vol. 59, no. 3, pp. 2560–2568, 2012.

[36] T. Liu, J. Liu, L. De Rochefort et al., "Morphology enabled dipole inversion (MEDI) from a single-angle acquisition: Comparison with COSMOS in human brain imaging," *Magnetic Resonance in Medicine*, vol. 66, no. 3, pp. 777–783, 2011.

[37] J. O. Christoffersson, L. E. Olsson, and S. Sjöberg, "Nickel-doped agarose gel phantoms in MR imaging," *Acta Radiologica*, vol. 32, no. 5, pp. 426–431, 1991.

[38] J. A. Pople, W. G. Schneider, and H. J. Bernstein, *High-Resolution Nuclear Magnetic Resonance*, McGraw-Hill Book Company, Inc, New York, NY, USA, 1959.

[39] L. De Rochefort, R. Brown, M. R. Prince, and Y. Wang, "Quantitative MR susceptibility mapping using piece-wise constant regularized inversion of the magnetic field," *Magnetic Resonance in Medicine*, vol. 60, no. 4, pp. 1003–1009, 2008.

[40] Cornell MRI Research Lab, 2018, http://weill.cornell.edu/mri/pages/qsm.html.

[41] B. Kressler, L. de Rochefort, T. Liu, P. Spincemaille, Q. Jiang, and Y. Wang, "Nonlinear regularization for per voxel estimation of magnetic susceptibility distributions from MRI field maps," *IEEE Transactions on Medical Imaging*, vol. 29, no. 2, pp. 273–281, 2010.

[42] A.-C. Fruytier, J. Magat, F. Colliez, B. Jordan, G. Cron, and B. Gallez, "Dynamic contrast-enhanced MRI in mice at high field: Estimation of the arterial input function can be achieved by phase imaging," *Magnetic Resonance in Medicine*, vol. 71, no. 2, pp. 544–550, 2014.

[43] P. G. Ward, A. P. Fan, P. Raniga et al., "Improved quantification of cerebral vein oxygenation using partial volume correction," *Frontiers in Neuroscience*, vol. 11, p. 89, 2017.

[44] A. Karsa, E. Biondetti, S. Punwani, and K. Shmueli, "The effect of large slice thickness and spacing and low coverage on the accuracy of susceptibility mapping," in *Proceedings of the 24th Annual Meeting of the International Society for Magnetic Resonance in Medicine (ISMRM)*, p. 1555, Singapore, 2016.

[45] A. M. Elkady, H. Sun, and A. H. Wilman, "Importance of extended spatial coverage for quantitative susceptibility mapping of iron-rich deep gray matter," *Magnetic Resonance Imaging*, vol. 34, no. 4, pp. 574–578, 2016.

[46] E. Lind, L. Knutsson, R. Kämpe, F. Ståhlberg, and R. Wirestam, "Assessment of MRI contrast agent concentration by quantitative susceptibility mapping (QSM): application to estimation of cerebral blood volume during steady state," *Magnetic Resonance Materials in Physics, Biology and Medicine*, vol. 30, no. 6, pp. 555–566, 2017.

22

Morphologic and Clinical Outcome of Intracranial Aneurysms after Treatment using Flow Diverter Devices

Anna-Katharina Breu,[1] Till-Karsten Hauser,[1] Florian H. Ebner,[2] Felix Bischof,[3] Ulrike Ernemann,[1] and Achim Seeger[1]

[1]Department of Diagnostic and Interventional Neuroradiology, Eberhard Karls University, Hoppe-Seyler-Street 3, 72076 Tübingen, Germany
[2]Department of Neurosurgery, Eberhard Karls University, Hoppe-Seyler-Street 3, 72076 Tübingen, Germany
[3]Department of Neurology, Eberhard Karls University, Hoppe-Seyler-Street 3, 72076 Tübingen, Germany

Correspondence should be addressed to Achim Seeger; achim.seeger@gmx.de

Academic Editor: Henrique M. Lederman

Flow diverters (FDs) are designed for the endovascular treatment of complex intracranial aneurysm configurations. From February 2009 to March 2013 28 patients (22 females, 6 males) were treated with FD; mean age was 57 years. Data, including aneurysm features, clinical presentation, history of previous bleeding, treatment, and follow-up results, are presented. Early postinterventional neurological deficits (transient: $n = 3$/enduring: $n = 1$) appeared in 4/28 patients (14%), and early improvement of neurological symptoms was observed in 7 patients with previous restriction of cranial nerve function. The overall occlusion rate was 20/26 (77%; 59% after 3 months). 77% achieved best results according to O'Kelly-Marotta score grade D with no contrast material filling (70% of those after 3 months). In 4/6 patients who did not achieve grade D, proximal and/or distal stent overlapping ≥ 5 mm was not guaranteed sufficiently. During follow-up we did not detect any aneurysm recurrence or haemorrhage. In-stent stenosis emerged as the most frequent complication (4/27; 15%) followed by 2 cases of vascular obliteration (AICA/VA). In conclusion endovascular reconstruction using a FD represents a modern and effective treatment in those aneurysms that are not suitable for conventional interventional or surgical treatment. The appearance of severe complications was rare.

1. Introduction

Low porosity stents (flow diverter, FD) play an important role in the effective endovascular treatment of intracranial aneurysms [1–3]. This device is designed for complex aneurysm configurations, fusiform, or wide-necked aneurysms, especially in cases where conventional coiling is not feasible and in locations where clipping is not a treatment option. Even remnants of aneurysms after surgical or endovascular treatment and dissected vessels in selected cases represent an indication for flow diverting treatment [4, 5]. The FD features two main work mechanisms: flow redirection and tissue overgrowth. The high-structural-profile implant bridges the aneurysm neck and reduces the blood flow into

the aneurysm sac because of increased impedance created by the mesh of the implant with high pore density, yet providing blood flow through adjacent perforators and side branches. Flow stasis and formation of a stable aneurysmal thrombus are promoted by reduction of blood circulation within the aneurysm. In addition the FD provides a scaffold for neoendothelialization across the aneurysm neck, which leads to the exclusion of the aneurysm sac from the blood flow in the parent artery and facilitates a sufficient aneurysm occlusion [6]. Indeed questions remain regarding the long-term safety, radiological findings, and clinical outcome. The Flow Diversion in Intracranial Aneurysm Treatment (FIAT) [7] and the Large Aneurysm Randomized Trial: Flow Diversion Versus Traditional GDC Based Endovascular Therapy (LARGE) [8]

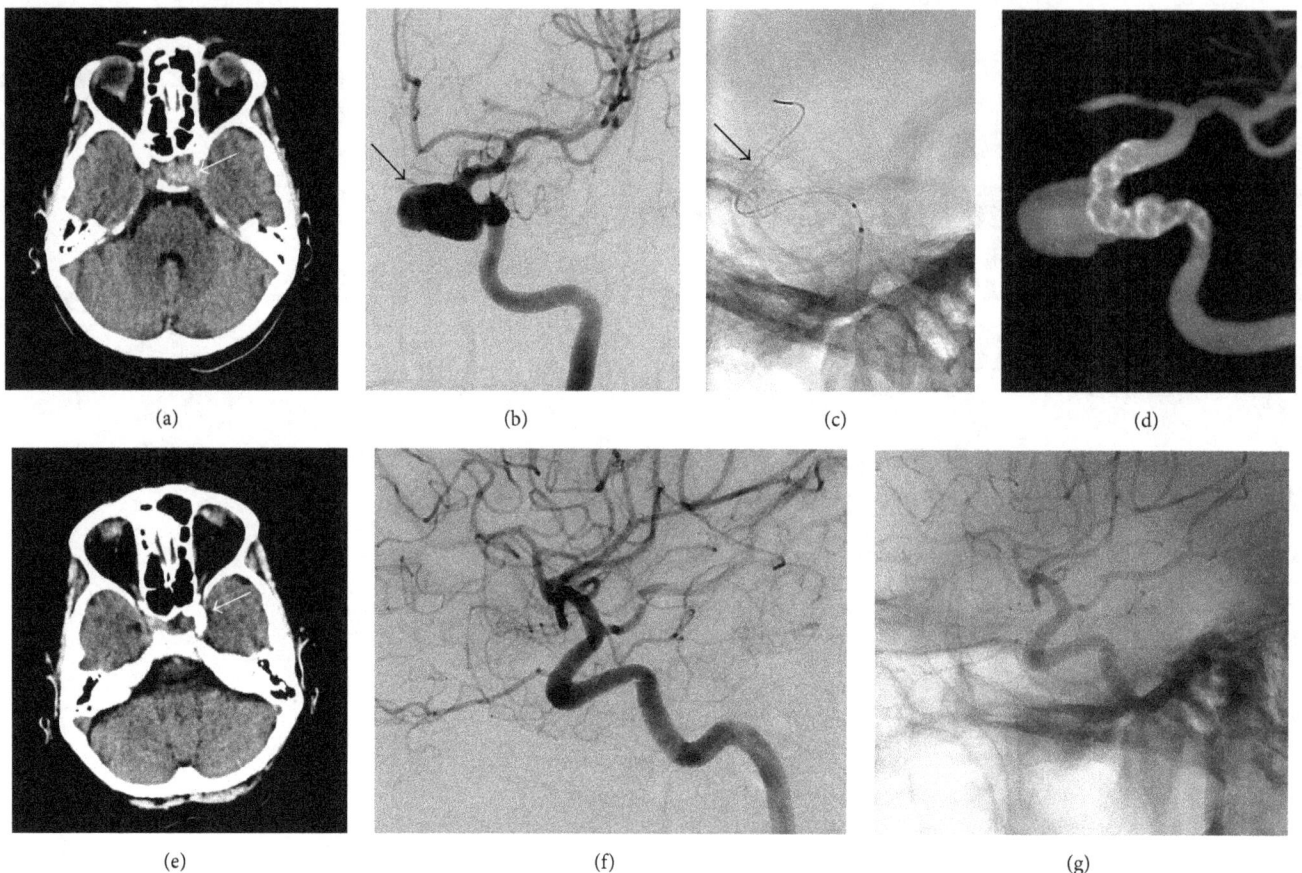

FIGURE 1: Cranial nerve palsy (patient number 1). 55-year-old woman presented with left oculomotor palsy. Cranial CT (a) showed hyperdense mass in the ophthalmic segment of the left carotid artery. Wide-necked intracranial aneurysm was proved by digital subtraction angiography (DSA, b) and the patient was treated using a flow diverter (c, d). In follow-up, clinical symptoms improved; the mass (e) and DSA confirmed no filling of the aneurysm sack (f, g).

are two of the ongoing randomized trials comparing flow diversion with best standard treatment. Interest in the future of flow diversion seems to be rapidly growing. Regarding aneurysm occlusion and vessel remodeling, the early follow-up results are encouraging, but long-term data are needed to assess efficacy and safety. This paper presents a systematic retrospective analysis of the technical findings concerning FD treatment as well as occlusion rate and clinical outcome in mid-term follow-up from 3 months to 3 years.

2. Materials and Methods

From February 2009 to November 2013, 28 patients (22 females, 6 males) were treated with FD; median age was 57 years (range: 8–83 years). A supplementary table providing all patients' clinical symptoms, aneurysm size, and location as well as treatment effects is provided (see supplementary materials in Supplementary Material available online at http://dx.doi.org/10.1155/2016/2187275). Clinical and radiological data were collected retrospectively and the maximum time of follow-up was 3 years.

2.1. Clinical Data. We treated 7 of 28 patients (25%) with FD who had ruptured aneurysms with previous SAH (Hunt

& Hess II = 2, III = 1, V = 2; two without specification); 2/7 patients were treated in the acute period after SAH. We retreated one patient, who had a delayed aneurysm rupture 3 months after FD implantation in another centre due to insufficient aneurysm thrombosis.

12/28 patients (43%) had cranial nerve palsy due to compression by the aneurysm (e.g., patient number 1, see Figure 1). Five patients had unilateral visual loss, four (14%) had affection of the oculomotor nerve, one patient (4%) had affection of the abducens nerve, and two patients (7%) had affection of the fifth and ninth cranial nerve. One patient (4%) had four episodes of transient ischemic attacks. In this case it was assumed that the aneurysm was the origin of recurrent embolisms. Besides those patients with previous aneurysmal bleeding, the aneurysm was found incidentally in asymptomatic patients by neuroradiology examinations in 4/28 patients (14%, see Figure 2); four patients (14%) had unspecific symptoms like headache or dizziness. One patient presented with symptoms indicative of frontal lobe dysfunction caused by a giant aneurysm in the supraophthalmic ICA. Table 1 summarizes the clinical data.

The aneurysm size was classified as small (<10 mm; $n = 15$), large (10–20 mm; $n = 11$), and giant (>20 mm; $n = 2$). In 39% (11/28 patients), the diameter of the neck was

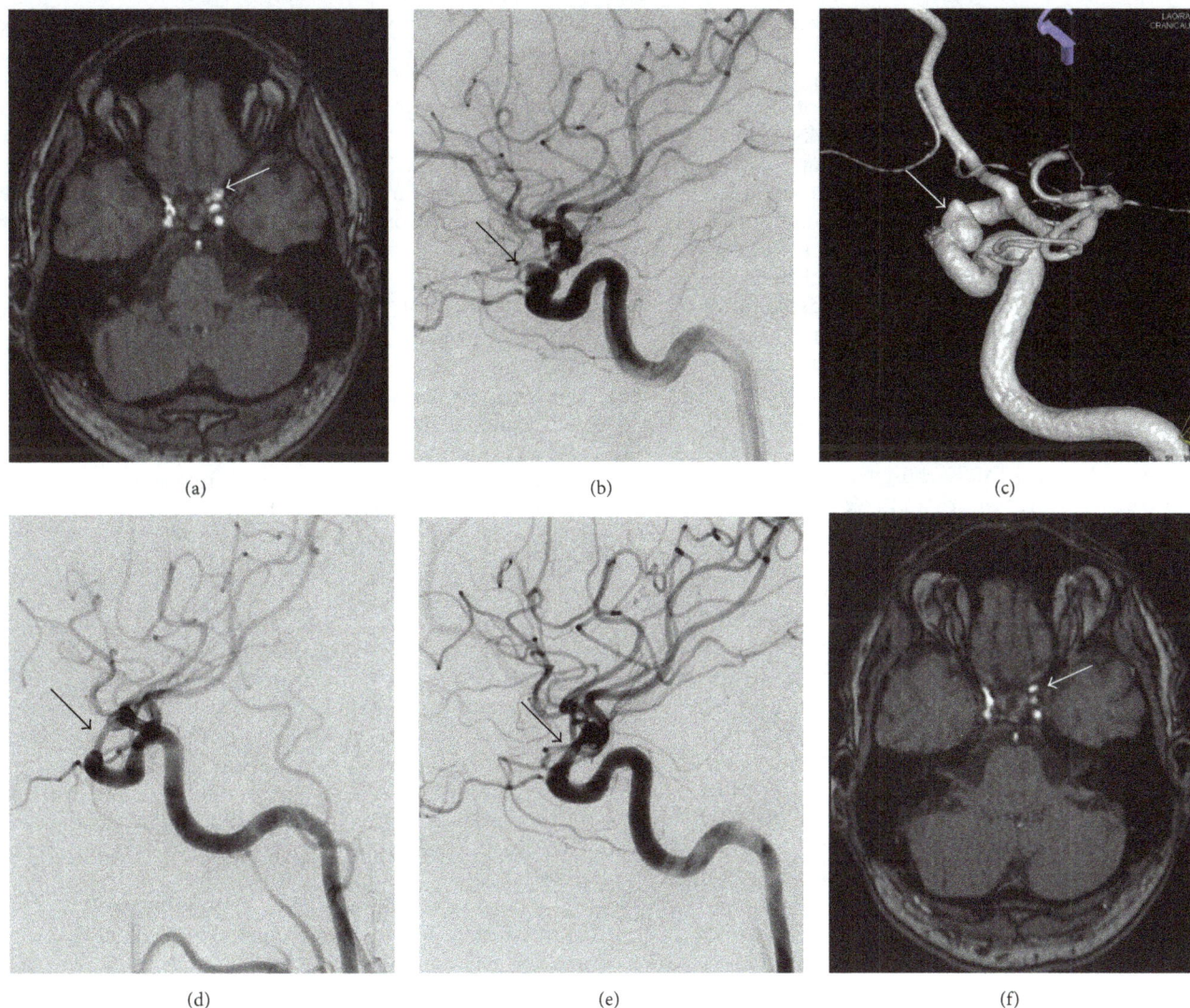

FIGURE 2: Postinterventional stenosis (patient number 25). 44-year-old man with incidental finding of aneurysm in the left carotid artery on MR angiography (a), confirmed by digital subtraction angiography (b, c). After flow diverter treatment, nonsymptomatic stenosis was detected and was stable in 6 months' follow-up (d); stenosis improved at 12 months' follow-up (e) and further noninvasive examinations.

TABLE 1: Clinical data.

Aneurysm location		Aneurysm size (mm)		Clinical symptoms		Configuration	
Anterior circulation	20	<10	15	SAH	7	Wide-necked	19
BA	4	10–20	11	Incidentally	4	Fusiform	7
VA	4	>20	2	Focal symptoms (*cranial nerve palsy*)	17 (*12*)	other	2

This table summarizes location, size, and configuration of aneurysms as well as the clinical symptoms of the patient cohort. BA: basilar artery; SAH: subarachnoid hemorrhage; VA: vertebral artery.

<5 mm, in 43% the diameter was 5–10 mm (12/28 patients), and in 18% the diameter was >10 mm (5/28 patients). The configuration appeared in 19 cases wide-necked (68%) and in 7 cases fusiform (25%). The aneurysms were mainly located in the anterior carotid circulation (71%; 20/28). Most of them were detected in the internal carotid artery (ICA = 19; 68%) and one was detected in the medial cerebral artery (MCA = 1;

4%). Four aneurysms were located in the basilar artery (14%) and four in one of the vertebral arteries (14%).

2.2. Endovascular Treatment and Stent Data.
All procedures were performed under general anaesthesia. All cases were discussed in an interdisciplinary conference. The indication was established in more complex, formerly untreated aneurysms

(especially wide-neck, giant, and fusiform) or pretreated reperfused ones.

For the endovascular treatment of aneurysms by flow diversion we used two different high profile stents. For 23/28 patients we chose the SILK flow diverter (SFD, Balt Extrusion, Montmorency, France). We implanted two SFDs in a telescoping way in 2 patients (25 SFDs were placed in 23 patients). The SFD is a flexible, self-expanding device specifically designed to produce a hemodynamic flow diversion and to reconstruct laminar flow in the parent artery. The device is a braided mesh cylinder with flared ends, composed of 48 nickel-titanium (nitinol) alloy and platinum microfilaments of approximately 35 μm. It is designed to provide 35% to 55% metal coverage of the target vessel's inner surface with a pore size of 110 to 250 μm at nominal diameter [9].

In 5/28 cases the Pipeline Embolization Device (PED, Covidien, Mansfield, Massachusetts) was chosen for the reconstruction of the vessel wall. We placed 9 PEDs in 5 patients; four of them got 2 PEDs. The PED is a composite braided mesh tube of 48 strands with 75% cobalt chromium and 25% platinum. The diameter of the single wire is 30 μm. At the nominal diameter, the pore size is 0.02–0.05 mm^2 and the radial force is about 2.0 mN/mm (3.0 mm vessel diameter), which is similar to a SFD. The braided wires are loose on both ends. The PED is preinstalled on a stainless steel wire and is attached distal to a capture coil. A radiopaque 15 mm platinum tip extends beyond the end of the PED [4].

The diameter of the high profile FD employed ranged in size within 2.5–5.5 mm and in length within 15–50 mm.

In 7 procedures side branches of the aneurysm-sustaining artery were covered by the device (3 in the basilar artery).

In 23 cases (82%), implantation of the FD was placed as the first treatment. The remaining 5 cases received the implantation of a FD as a retreatment after clipping of another aneurysm (n = 2; 7%), another case after clipping and stent-supported coiling of the same aneurysm (n = 1; 4%), and again another case after stent-supported coiling of the same aneurysm (n = 1, 4%). In one woman a FD was implanted in another center. Four of those patients, who were pretreated, had previous SAH. Therefore we implanted FD as the first treatment in the parent artery of ruptured aneurysms in 3 cases.

2.3. Drug Management. All patients received dual antiplatelet therapy (aspirin 100 mg/d and clopidogrel 75 mg/d) from 2 to 28 days before procedure (mean: 12.9 days). One woman received prasugrel instead of clopidogrel because of previous implantation of a drug-eluting stent in a coronary artery. In this case we did not change medication. If the period to procedure was less than 3 days, a loading dose of 500 mg aspirin and 300 mg clopidogrel was applied. Responder status for aspirin and clopidogrel was detected before treatment (8% nonresponder aspirin; 16% nonresponder clopidogrel). For this purpose the assay for the quantitative in vitro determination of platelet function triggered by TRAP (thrombin receptor activating peptide) was used. Cut-off level for aspirin nonresponder was TRAP test > 60 U and aspirin > 70 U and for clopidogrel nonresponder was TRAP test > 60 U and clopidogrel > 45 U. To prevent the peri-interventional

formation of a thrombus, heparin was provided controlled by antiplatelet clotting time (ACT). The therapeutic protocol after treatment in the case of normal responders was as follows: dual antiplatelet therapy for three months (aspirin 100 mg/d and clopidogrel 75 mg/d); after three months clopidogrel was stopped while aspirin 100 mg/d was continued as a life-long regime. In patients who did not sufficiently respond to aspirin or clopidogrel, we applied double-dose and repeated check of response in the course.

2.4. Follow-Up Schedule. In the course of the observation period, 26/28 patients underwent DSA at least once (most of them 3 months after treatment). One patient moved abroad and was therefore lost to follow-up by DSA. Another patient with multiple myeloma got MR imaging instead of DSA to prevent kidney dysfunction. A third patient was lost to follow-up 6 months after the procedure due to intracerebral bleeding (ICB) with lethal effect during a second FD session. Computed Tomography Angiography (CTA; n = 22), Magnetic Resonance Imaging (MRI; n = 2), or Digital Subtraction Angiography (DSA; n = 4) was performed in all patients during their hospital stay within three days after treatment. Follow-up was carried out by DSA, CTA, or MRI on 6 weeks, 3 months, 6 months, 1 year, 2 years, and 3 years. Angiographic outcome of treated aneurysms was assessed using a simplified type of the O'Kelly-Marotta grading scale (OKM), which classifies aneurysm based on angiographic filling and stasis of contrast material exclusively in the arterial phase in a four-level scale (A-D) as follows: A—complete (>95%); B—incomplete (5–95%); C—neck remnant (<5%), or D—no filling (0%) [10]. The clinical treatment effect was rated on a four-level scale (1—improvement, 2—delayed improvement, 3—no improvement, and 4—fatal outcome) and was not applicable (n.a.) in asymptomatic patients with incidental aneurysm.

3. Results

3.1. Technical Findings in Stent Deployment and Additional Appliance. The FD could be placed in a proper position across the parent artery of the aneurysm in 19/28 patients. Stent size was changed in one case to ensure complete unfolding. Due to suboptimal opening in a circumscribed part of the FD, in 6 patients additional balloon-dilatation was performed in an attempt to gain better results. In one of these patients (broad-based aneurysm arising from a fenestration located at the confluence of both vertebral arteries), additional stenting was performed to achieve better aneurysm occlusion. In 3 patients, a second FD, placed in a telescopic way during the on-going session, was necessary for sufficient haemodynamic exclusion of the aneurysm sack.

During two procedures, thrombotic material accumulated at the inner surface of the stent. In both cases abciximab (Reopro®, Janssen Biologics, Netherlands) was applied locally with resolution of the thrombotic material, followed by a continuous infusion of a maintenance dose for 12 h.

3.2. Postprocedural Neurological Events. During the early postprocedural period, 4/28 (14%) patients had neurological deficits related to the procedure. One patient (patient number 6) with a complex proximal basilar artery aneurysm and peri-interventional thrombotic clots requiring application of abciximab developed dysarthria and paresis of the right arm. MR imaging two days following the procedure demonstrated ischemic lesions on both sides of the cerebellum and within the thalamus and splenium of the left side. One patient (patient number 26) who presented initially with a ruptured aneurysm remained intubated because of recurrent nasopharyngeal bleeding under combined heparin and antiplatelet therapy. At the time of transfer to another center, neurological symptoms including ptosis and anisocoria were still present as a result of the SAH. In another case (patient number 14), aphasia occurred after intervention during the hospital stay with complete resolution of the symptoms at discharge. In correlation to this symptom, CTA showed a circumscribed intraparenchymal bleeding of 15 mm diameter in the dorsal temporal lobe of the left hemisphere with treated ICA aneurysm on the right side. Patient number 3 showed transient psychotic symptoms including agitation and loss of time orientation. No early or delayed aneurysm rupture occurred.

A complete recovery of headache related to the aneurysm was observed in one patient within the postprocedural hospital stay; an improvement was observed in further 6 patients with previous restriction of cranial nerve function. In those 6 patients a regression of ptosis, diplopic images, hemianopsia, and an improvement of vision were observed. The symptoms have been preexisting for 9 days to 6 months till the deployment of a FD.

3.3. Radiological Follow-Up and Aneurysm Occlusion.

Due to the flow diverting effect of the high profile stent and thus the reduction of the blood flow into the aneurysm, we witnessed initiating thrombosis in 2/28 patients (7%) already at the end of procedure. In another 9 patients (32%) a delayed inflow and contrast material stagnation inside the aneurysm lumen was observed periprocedurally. Brain imaging by MRA and/or CTA performed within 2-3 days after deployment of a FD showed complete aneurysm occlusion in 4 of 28 cases (14%). One of those had been treated with additional coil packing at the same session and another one a second FD.

After discharge, during a follow-up range from 6 weeks to 3 years, control-imaging studies were available for 27/28 patients (after 6 months 26/28) at different time intervals. 3 months after procedure we observed complete aneurysm occlusion in 16 of 27 patients (59%). Six months after stent implantation, 63% (17/27) of the aneurysms were eliminated, a proportion that increased to 73% (19/26) after 1 year and 77% (20/26) two years after intervention.

When we applied the OKM, we evaluated the occlusion rate only of those patients who underwent DSA because the grading scale is based on recognizable angiographic characteristics [10]. During the course of the observation period, 26 of 28 patients got DSA imaging. The distribution of the different OKM degrees is shown in Table 2.

77% (20/26) achieved best results according to OKM grade D (no filling). In 14 of those 20 cases (70%) we observed best results with no contrast material filling of the aneurysm 3

TABLE 2: Best results according to O'Kelly-Marotta grading scale.

	Frequency	%
A	1	4
B	1	4
C	4	15
D	20	77
Total amount	26	100

This table shows the follow-up results of digital subtraction angiography (DSA) in 26 patients (in 2 patients only CTA or MRI was performed). OKM: A total filling, B subtotal filling, C entry remnant, and D no filling.

TABLE 3: Point in time (months) of OKM grade D (no filling).

Months	Frequency	Cumulative %
3	14	70
6	2	80
12	2	90
24	2	100
Total amount	20	100

Point in time (months) of the 20 patients who were rated as OKM grade D (no aneurysm filling).

months after FD deployment, 90% after 1 year and 100% after 2 years (see Table 3).

Most of the patients (22/26) underwent control imaging by DSA till 3 months after procedure. At this time, besides 14 patients with grade D, 6 of 22 patients (27%) had grade C (entry remnant) and 2 patients (9%) had grade B (subtotal filling). None of them had grade A (total filling). During follow-up we did not detect any aneurysm recurrence or progress in aneurysm filling.

A vessel originating from the aneurysm or the base of the aneurysm was evident in 18% (5/28 patients). Three (patients numbers 9, 20, and 22) achieved OKM grade D within the 3 months' follow-up, one patient (patient number 19) achieved OKM grade B after 3 months, and one patient (patient number 2) achieved OKM grade D after 2 years. However, due to the small number, no statistically significant results of this subgroup can be stated.

In 4 of 6 patients who did not achieve grade D (except one who have not achieved best result until 2 years after FD deployment), proximal and/or distal stent overlapping ≥5 mm was not guaranteed sufficiently.

3.4. Neurological Results and Complications during Follow-Up.

In addition, the clinical-neurological outcome following stent implantation was evaluated. 8/17 patients (47%) with former focal symptoms or cranial nerve palsy were rated as clinically improved (level 1). None of them had to be retreated and no recurrence was seen. We ranked 5/17 patients (29%) among category 2 (delayed improvement); in three cases (18%) no regression of former focal symptoms was seen (treatment effect level 3). In one of those cases (patient number 12) even worsening visual impairment was observed. The period between the appearances of the first symptoms until treatment was 6 months. Concerning another patient

(patient number 21) the damage of the abducens nerve by prolonged compression preceded the intervention for 1.5 years. In this patient no recovery was observed. The third patient (patient number 15) with level 3 presented with a giant aneurysm (max. diameter 22 mm) with a strong jet-like flow. We decided to implant two FDs in a telescoped way to ensure the reconstruction of the parent artery. This patient was lost to follow-up. That is why time lacked to improve. Consequently we had to rank this patient in level 3. In one patient (patient number 19) an ICB in the contralateral hemisphere occurred shortly after the second FD session with lethal effect (treatment effect level 4).

The most frequent complication during follow-up (4/27; 15%) was in-stent stenosis (ISS, see Figure 2). The majority of the stenoses (3 of 4) had no hemodynamic or clinical relevance and showed a regression in the degree of stenosis during follow-up. In only one case of ISS (patient number 7), additional percutaneous transluminal angioplasty (PTA) was performed (balloon-dilatation 5 months after FD placement and stenting 7 months after FD placement) due to high grade of stenosis. Being initial clopidogrel nonresponder, this patient took clopidogrel 150 mg/d for 1.5 years. After reperfusion of the aneurysm, clopidogrel was reduced. Two years after treatment the aneurysm occluded and clopidogrel was stopped. In the remaining 3 patients with ISS no PTA was needed but we continued clopidogrel therapy with a higher dose (150 mg/d). The 3 remaining stenosis cases fortunately achieved OKM grade D 3 months after FD placement and had no subsequent reperfusion. During follow-up we observed vascular obliteration in 2 patients (7%). In one case the anterior inferior cerebellar artery (AICA) occluded which originated from the aneurysm basis with complete leptomeningeal collateralisation after one year (patient number 22). In the other case a segmental obliteration of the left vertebral artery (VA) on a level with the parent artery of the aneurysm occurred (patient number 28). In both cases the patients did not show any clinical-neurological abnormalities. A second FD was placed in one of two patients (patient numbers 14 and 17) who developed an endoleak 3 to 9 months after treatment. OKM grade D could be reached 6 months after former FD deployment. No delayed SAH was observed during follow-up. Complications during follow-up are summarized in Table 4.

A supplementary table providing all patients' clinical symptoms, aneurysm size, and location as well as treatment effects is provided (see supplementary materials).

4. Discussion

The primary goals of aneurysm treatment should be a complete occlusion of the aneurysm sack to prevent delayed SAH or recurrence of the aneurysm lumen as well as recovery from neurologic symptoms. However, it is hard to define the optimal management, especially dealing with incidental finding on an imaging study undertaken for another purpose. The dilemma arises whether the risk associated with preventive surgical or endovascular treatment is outweighed by the risk of death or disability from rupture of the untreated aneurysm. Korja et al. [11] report that the lifelong risk of an unruptured

TABLE 4: Complications during follow-up.

	Frequency	%
None	18	67
Endoleak	2	7
Stenosis	4	15
Vascular obliteration	2	7
ICB	1	4
Total amount	27	100

This table summarizes complications during follow-up. There was no need for subsequent intervention except one in-stent stenosis and one endoleak. One patient with intracerebral bleeding (ICB) during the second FD session died.

intracranial aneurysm rupture depends strongly on the risk factors, also other than the size and location (e.g., cigarette smoking, sex, and systolic blood pressure), and these should be taken into account when making treatment decisions. Another study details that the rupture risk of growing unruptured cerebral aneurysms is 5% in 5 years. They identified additional risk factors like lobulated configuration, multiple aneurysms, and growth [12].

The International Subarachnoid Aneurysm Trial (ISAT) and other recently published data confirm and reinforce their preliminary findings that rebleeding was more likely after endovascular coiling than after neurosurgical clipping, but the risk was small and the probability of disability-free survival was significantly greater in the endovascular group than in the neurosurgical group at 10 years [13, 14].

To improve occlusion rate and to overcome the faintness of coil compaction, aneurysm recurrence, and rebleeding after coiling, a paradigm shift in interventions from an endosaccular to an endoluminal reconstruction was promoted by the design of the FD. The aneurysm itself does no longer have to be catheterized. Comparison of flow diversion and coiling of large unruptured aneurysms shows a significantly higher proportion of aneurysms treated with PED with complete obliteration and fewer necessities of retreatment compared with coiled aneurysms [15].

Meanwhile, the FD asserts itself not only in the treatment of large saccular aneurysms but also in wide-necked and fusiform ones or aneurysms that have a branch incorporated into the sac. The latter, flow through the FD, is maintained into the branch originating from the sac while occlusion of the aneurysm is still possible [2]. Our results do not deviate from this mechanism, except one occlusion of the AICA in a patient showing preexisting extreme atherosclerosis and without clinical relevance in the follow-up. Referring to this, another survey, dealing with SFD implantation in the basilar artery, distinguishes between occlusion of a side branch shortly after FD implantation by narrowing the orifice mechanically or blocking the orifice by tiny thrombi formed on the surface of the FD and late infarcts caused by neointimal overgrowth and progressive narrowing of the perforator's orifice [9]. The mechanism that keeps the side branches and perforators open might be the blood downstream, following the pressure gradient to the low-pressure tissue. The fact that the supplied area acts as a consumer might contribute to the maintenance of sufficient perfusion. Both cases of vessel occlusion in our series (AICA and segment of VA) appeared in patients with extreme atherosclerotic transformation, which has to be considered when making treatment decisions.

In our series, the aneurysmal occlusion rate turns out to be 59% after 3 months, increasing to 77% due to implantation of a second FD or deviation of the antiplatelet regime. Subtotal occlusion was obtained in further 15%. Summing up, 92% of the patients achieved best or good results concerning occlusion rate. It seems to be controversial that a small neck remnant at follow-up is often accepted as adequate treatment after conventional aneurysm coiling, whereas slight filling of an aneurysm treated with a FD may be enough to perpetuate continued mass effect, progressive aneurysm growth, and in some cases spontaneous rupture [10]. According to the OKM grading scale 77% achieved grade D, 70% of them already 3 months after procedure and 80% after 6 months. These results go along with data from a meta-analysis where complete occlusion rate was 76% (95% CI, 70%–81%) at 6 months [1]. The rate and time of complete occlusion were not correlated with the aneurysm size as in other retrospective studies [4, 16–18].

Analysing the characteristics of aneurysm thrombosis, we found out that broad stent overlapping of the aneurysm orifice (≥5 mm proximal and distal) is an important predictor of early aneurysm occlusion. In 4 of 6 patients who did not achieve grade D (except one who has not achieved best result until 2 years after FD deployment), proximal and/or distal stent overlapping ≥5 mm was not guaranteed sufficiently. This kind of device deformation was also described in a clinical case report supplemented by in vitro studies [19]. Estrade et al. [19] tried to identify the causes and effects of device deformation. The main finding of this report is that, upon deployment of oversized FDs, landing zones of insufficient length may lead to device deformation with terminal stenosis. Even though the stenosis may not be flow limiting, the inadequate apposition of the device to the wall of the parent vessel may cause thromboembolic complications. Implanting an oversized FD sometimes cannot be avoided because of diameter alteration between proximal and distal parent artery of the aneurysm. The highest coverage (and therefore least porosity) is achieved at full expansion of the device. Particularly the transitional zone between the constrained part and the fully opened part shows reduced coverage when the oversized device opens to its nominal size within the aneurysm [19, 20]. A residual more turbulent inflow into the aneurysm sac may result that can explain failures and recurrences [19]. More recent generation of ED devices with higher radial forces and tapered design may further improve occlusion rates by allowing correct stent sizing despite diverging parent vessel diameters. Consequently the selection of the adequate length and diameter of the device to guarantee a proper stent adhesion to the vessel wall remains important. As shown in haemodynamic analysis of aneurysm occlusion by flow diversion in rabbits, imperfect deployments can have a substantial impact on the occlusion time and outcome of flow diverting procedures [18].

It is important to mention that 2 of the 6 patients who did not achieve best results in aneurysm occlusion had a situation with 2 branching vessels jailed, which might be conducive to delayed aneurysm exclusion from blood flow. The presence of incorporated vessels has already been reported causing delayed occlusion at 6 months' follow-up and 1 year' follow-up, but not at 2+ years in a recent published study of Chiu et al. [16], which is in concordance with our experience. 2/5 patients in this subgroup did not achieve OKM grade D within 3 months.

The therapeutic effect of the endovascular treatment by flow diversion became most obvious by looking at the most common aneurysm related symptom, the cranial nerve palsy (12/28 patients; 43%). It becomes clear that the patients with visual loss, perimetric restriction, or palsy of the inner or outer ocular muscles achieved better results when treated by FD within 3 months after principal appearance of the symptoms. The time of their total or partial recovery ranged from 3 days to 9 months after procedure. Progressive aneurysm thrombosis and adjacent oedema after treatment might even cause initial worsening of neurological symptoms. Particularly pulsation of the aneurysm wall and adjacent oedema after treatment are responsible for the cranial nerve palsy [21]. If time range between first symptoms and FD implantation exceeds 3 months, the patients have a very restricted chance of recovery so that impairment of the inner or outer ocular muscles or a perimetric or visual restriction remains. Long period till treatment can be an indicator for recovery failure, because of gradually occurring partial calcification of the aneurysm wall and thus less potential of significant reduction in size and simultaneous reduction in mass effect and pulsation leading to cranial nerve decompression. The FD actually should surpass coiling in this feature. That is why treatment should be as prompt as possible after occurrence of first symptoms.

As no ischemic events or aneurysm rupture during follow-up occurred among the patients we treated, we cannot confirm the declaration that SFD is more likely to cause these delayed device-related complications than PED [22]. But, aside from the lower number of patients we treated with PED, we experienced the ISS to be the most frequent complication (4/27 patients; 15%). All of the patients who developed ISS were clinically asymptomatic, except one patient with an unspecific symptom like headache. In asymptomatic patients the angiographic finding was managed medically and with serial follow-up imaging. Additional PTA was performed in only one case. None of the patients with ISS underwent additional balloon-dilatation during their first FD session, which repels the idea that parent artery injury could be a trigger for neointimal proliferation. Analysing the data, we found neither any other correlation between the developments of ISS and other potentially relating factors, such as cardiovascular risk factors, nor lack of response to antiplatelet therapy. Despite the fact that the ingrowth of tissue over the stented segment very likely promotes the durability of blood flow redirection and aneurysm occlusion, occasionally the stenosis may result in neurological symptoms that require retreatment to restore flow. Although the majority of patients with ISS are asymptomatic, the induction of a symptomatic intracranial stenosis in this previously asymptomatic patient population represents a considerable issue [23].

Furthermore, it seems to be challenging to find a balance between aneurysm occlusion and prevention of ISS by varying in dose and period of antiplatelet therapy while facing the additional problem with therapy of nonresponder. A recently published study found a wide variability in the initial patient response to the standard 75 mg daily clopidogrel dose. They suggest that an "acceptable" 60–240 P2Y12 reaction units (PRU) range would not lead to increased thromboembolic or hemorrhagic complications in a larger patient population, but further studies are needed to ensure this statement [24].

The antiplatelet medication and additional anticoagulation during procedure might be responsible for the fatal outcome of an ICB on the contralateral hemisphere of the target aneurysm during a subsequently performed FD procedure in one of our patients (4%). This result equals the rate of Brinjikji's et al. [1] meta-analysis regarding procedure-related mortality of 4% (95% CI, 3%–6%) and is comparable with their ICB rate of 3% (95% CI, 2%–4%), with 3% experiencing early ICB and 2% experiencing late ICB. Aneurysm size and location were not significantly associated with ICB rate. The indication for a second FD in our patient was provided with persistent perfusion of the aneurysm despite termination of dual antiplatelet therapy and proceeding deprivation of vision. The complication became noticeable after delayed awakening and was confirmed by CT. Other cases of ICB are reported. Unlike our case report, all haemorrhages were anatomically remote from the treated aneurysm, but the hematomas were situated in the ipsilateral cerebral hemisphere. The occurrence of ICB seems to be more frequent than delayed aneurysm rupture (1% in the RADAR survey [25]). Therefore ICB has recently emerged as a threatening complication of intracranial aneurysm treatment with FDs. While the mechanism and related factors of ICB during FD procedure remain poorly understood, several considerations could be proposed to explain the occurrence of delayed ipsilateral ICB after flow diversion procedure. Haemodynamic alteration from flow diverter placement, haemorrhagic transformation of ischemic stroke, dual antiplatelet therapy, and cardiovascular risk factors are presumed mechanisms [26].

5. Conclusion

In conclusion, endovascular reconstruction using a FD represents an effective and safe treatment in those aneurysms that are not suitable for conventional interventional or surgical treatment. In giant, wide-necked, and fusiform aneurysms, the occlusion rate is encouraging and in our series no recurrence or delayed SAH occurred. Nevertheless, we found a noteworthy incidence of in-stent stenosis (ISS, 4/27 patients; 15%), but fortunately among those the incidence of symptomatic ISS or the necessity of retreatment is very low (1/4). Another complication that comes along with increased thrombogenicity is the occlusion of the parent artery, especially in very atherosclerotic vessels with clinical relevance depending on the degree of collateralisation. The heterogeneity of the response [25] to clopidogrel could

explain the ISS on one hand and the haemorrhagic events on the other and has to be considered strictly.

However, the complexity of the described issues underlines the necessity of an interdisciplinary consensus concerning treatment in this cohort.

Conflict of Interests

The authors declare that there is no conflict of interests regarding the publication of this paper.

References

[1] W. Brinjikji, M. H. Murad, G. Lanzino, H. J. Cloft, and D. F. Kallmes, "Endovascular treatment of intracranial aneurysms with flow diverters: a meta-analysis," *Stroke*, vol. 44, no. 2, pp. 442–447, 2013.

[2] I. Saatci, K. Yavuz, C. Ozer, S. Geyik, and H. S. Cekirge, "Treatment of intracranial aneurysms using the pipeline flow-diverter embolization device: a single-center experience with long-term follow-up results," *American Journal of Neuroradiology*, vol. 33, no. 8, pp. 1436–1446, 2012.

[3] G. K. C. Wong, M. C. L. Kwan, R. Y. T. Ng, S. C. H. Yu, and W. S. Poon, "Flow diverters for treatment of intracranial aneurysms: current status and ongoing clinical trials," *Journal of Clinical Neuroscience*, vol. 18, no. 6, pp. 737–740, 2011.

[4] S. Fischer, Z. Vajda, M. Aguilar Perez et al., "Pipeline embolization device (PED) for neurovascular reconstruction: initial experience in the treatment of 101 intracranial aneurysms and dissections," *Neuroradiology*, vol. 54, no. 4, pp. 369–382, 2012.

[5] M. M. Y. Tse, B. Yan, R. J. Dowling, and P. J. Mitchell, "Current status of pipeline embolization device in the treatment of intracranial aneurysms: a review," *World Neurosurgery*, vol. 80, no. 6, pp. 829–835, 2013.

[6] L. Pierot and A. K. Wakhloo, "Endovascular treatment of intracranial aneurysms: current status," *Stroke*, vol. 44, no. 7, pp. 2046–2054, 2013.

[7] A Randomized Trial Comparing Flow Diversion and Best-standard Treatment—The FIAT Trial, March 2015, https://clinicaltrials.gov/ct2/show/study/NCT01349582.

[8] "LARGE Aneurysm Randomized Trial: Flow Diversion Versus Traditional Endovascular Coiling Therapy," 2015, https://clinicaltrials.gov/ct2/show/NCT01762137?term=LARGE&rank=2.

[9] Z. Kulcsár, U. Ernemann, S. G. Wetzel et al., "High-profile flow diverter (silk) implantation in the basilar artery: efficacy in the treatment of aneurysms and the role of the perforators," *Stroke*, vol. 41, no. 8, pp. 1690–1696, 2010.

[10] C. J. O'Kelly, T. Krings, D. Fiorella, and T. R. Marotta, "A novel grading scale for the angiographic assessment of intracranial aneurysms treated using flow diverting stents," *Interventional Neuroradiology*, vol. 16, no. 2, pp. 133–137, 2010.

[11] M. Korja, H. Lehto, and S. Juvela, "Lifelong rupture risk of intracranial aneurysms depends on risk factors: a prospective Finnish cohort study," *Stroke*, vol. 45, no. 7, pp. 1958–1963, 2014.

[12] T. Inoue, H. Shimizu, M. Fujimura, A. Saito, and T. Tominaga, "Annual rupture risk of growing unruptured cerebral aneurysms detected by magnetic resonance angiography: clinical article," *Journal of Neurosurgery*, vol. 117, no. 1, pp. 20–25, 2012.

[13] A. J. Molyneux, R. S. Kerr, L.-M. Yu et al., "International subarachnoid aneurysm trial (ISAT) of neurosurgical clipping

versus endovascular coiling in 2143 patients with ruptured intracranial aneurysms: a randomised comparison of effects on survival, dependency, seizures, rebleeding, subgroups, and aneurysm occlusion," *The Lancet*, vol. 366, no. 9488, pp. 809–817, 2005.

[14] A. J. Molyneux, J. Birks, A. Clarke, M. Sneade, and R. S. C. Kerr, "The durability of endovascular coiling versus neurosurgical clipping of ruptured cerebral aneurysms: 18 year follow-up of the UK cohort of the International Subarachnoid Aneurysm Trial (ISAT)," *The Lancet*, vol. 385, no. 9969, pp. 691–697, 2015.

[15] N. Chalouhi, S. Tjoumakaris, R. M. Starke et al., "Comparison of flow diversion and coiling in large unruptured intracranial saccular aneurysms," *Stroke*, vol. 44, no. 8, pp. 2150–2154, 2013.

[16] A. H. Chiu, A. K. Cheung, J. D. Wenderoth et al., "Long-term follow-up results following elective treatment of unruptured intracranial aneurysms with the pipeline embolization device," *American Journal of Neuroradiology*, vol. 36, no. 9, pp. 1728–1734, 2015.

[17] M. Leonardi, L. Cirillo, F. Toni et al., "Treatment of intracranial aneurysms using flow-diverting silk stents (BALT): a single centre experience," *Interventional Neuroradiology*, vol. 17, no. 3, pp. 306–315, 2011.

[18] B. Chung, F. Mut, R. Kadirvel, R. Lingineni, D. F. Kallmes, and J. R. Cebral, "Hemodynamic analysis of fast and slow aneurysm occlusions by flow diversion in rabbits," *Journal of NeuroInterventional Surgery*, vol. 7, no. 12, pp. 931–935, 2015.

[19] L. Estrade, A. Makoyeva, T. E. Darsaut et al., "In vitro reproduction of device deformation leading to thrombotic complications and failure of flow diversion," *Interventional Neuroradiology*, vol. 19, no. 4, pp. 432–437, 2013.

[20] Pipeline Embolization of Cerebral Aneurysma, http://neuroangio.org/neurointerventional-techniques/pipeline-embolization-of-cerebral-aneurysms/.

[21] S. Patel, K. M. Fargen, K. Peters, P. Krall, H. Samy, and B. L. Hoh, "Return of visual function after bilateral visual loss following flow diversion embolization of a giant ophthalmic aneurysm due to both reduction in mass effect and reduction in aneurysm pulsation," *Journal of Neurointerventional Surgery*, vol. 7, no. 1, article e1, 2015.

[22] S. B. Murthy, S. Shah, A. Shastri, C. P. Venkatasubba Rao, E. M. Bershad, and J. I. Suarez, "The SILK flow diverter in the treatment of intracranial aneurysms," *Journal of Clinical Neuroscience*, vol. 21, no. 2, pp. 203–206, 2014.

[23] D. Fiorella, F. C. Albuquerque, H. Woo, P. A. Rasmussen, T. J. Masaryk, and C. G. McDougall, "Neuroform in-stent stenosis: incidence, natural history, and treatment strategies," *Neurosurgery*, vol. 59, no. 1, pp. 34–42, 2006.

[24] J. E. D. Almandoz, Y. Kadkhodayan, B. M. Crandall, J. M. Scholz, J. L. Fease, and D. E. Tubman, "Variability in initial response to standard clopidogrel therapy, delayed conversion to clopidogrel hyper-response, and associated thromboembolic and hemorrhagic complications in patients undergoing endovascular treatment of unruptured cerebral aneurysms," *Journal of NeuroInterventional Surgery*, vol. 6, no. 10, pp. 767–773, 2014.

[25] The ESMINT Retrospective Analysis of Delayed Aneurysm Ruptures after Flow Diversion (RADAR) Study, 2012, http://www.ejmint.org/original-article/1244000088.

[26] C. Tomas, A. Benaissa, D. Herbreteau, K. Kadziolka, and L. Pierot, "Delayed ipsilateral parenchymal hemorrhage following treatment of intracranial aneurysms with flow diverter," *Neuroradiology*, vol. 56, no. 2, pp. 155–161, 2014.

23

Preoperative Quantitative MR Tractography Compared with Visual Tract Evaluation in Patients with Neuropathologically Confirmed Gliomas Grades II and III

Anna F. Delgado,[1,2] Markus Nilsson,[3] Francesco Latini,[4]
Johanna Mårtensson,[1] Maria Zetterling,[4] Shala G. Berntsson,[5]
Irina Alafuzoff,[6] Jimmy Lätt,[7] and Elna-Marie Larsson[1]

[1] *Department of Surgical Sciences, Radiology, Uppsala University, 75105 Uppsala, Sweden*
[2] *Department of Neuroradiology, Karolinska University Hospital, Department of Clinical Neuroscience,
Karolinska Institute, 17177 Stockholm, Sweden*
[3] *Bioimaging Center, Lund University, 22100 Lund, Sweden*
[4] *Department of Neuroscience, Neurosurgery, Uppsala University, 75105 Uppsala, Sweden*
[5] *Department of Neuroscience, Neurology, Uppsala University, 75105 Uppsala, Sweden*
[6] *Section of Pathology, Uppsala University Hospital and Department of Immunology, Genetics and Pathology,
Uppsala University, 75105 Uppsala, Sweden*
[7] *MR Department, Centre for Medical Imaging and Physiology, Lund University Hospital, 22185 Lund, Sweden*

Correspondence should be addressed to Anna F. Delgado; anna.falk-delgado@karolinska.se

Academic Editor: Paul Sijens

Background and Purpose. Low-grade gliomas show infiltrative growth in white matter tracts. Diffusion tensor tractography can noninvasively assess white matter tracts. The aim was to preoperatively assess tumor growth in white matter tracts using quantitative MR tractography (3T). The hypothesis was that suspected infiltrated tracts would have altered diffusional properties in infiltrated tract segments compared to noninfiltrated tracts. *Materials and Methods.* Forty-eight patients with suspected low-grade glioma were included after written informed consent and underwent preoperative diffusion tensor imaging in this prospective review-board approved study. Major white matter tracts in both hemispheres were tracked, segmented, and visually assessed for tumor involvement in thirty-four patients with gliomas grade II or III (astrocytomas or oligodendrogliomas) on postoperative neuropathological evaluation. Relative fractional anisotropy (rFA) and mean diffusivity (rMD) in tract segments were calculated and compared with visual evaluation and neuropathological diagnosis. *Results.* Tract segment infiltration on visual evaluation was associated with a lower rFA and high rMD in a majority of evaluated tract segments (89% and 78%, resp.). Grade II and grade III gliomas had similar infiltrating behavior. *Conclusion.* Quantitative MR tractography corresponds to visual evaluation of suspected tract infiltration. It may be useful for an objective preoperative evaluation of tract segment involvement.

1. Introduction

Gliomas comprise approximately 30% of all CNS tumors and 80% of all malignant brain tumors [1]. In adults, these tumors consist mainly of astrocytomas grades II–IV and oligodendrogliomas grades II-III [2]. In suspected low-grade gliomas, preoperative MRI shows a high signal intensity lesion on T2-FLAIR images, usually without but sometimes with faint/patchy contrast enhancement [3, 4]. Low-grade gliomas are less common than grade IV gliomas, and patients with low-grade gliomas are often younger and have a high quality of life and a longer survival [5]. Survival in patients with glioma increases with the extent of tumor resection at surgery [6, 7]. Total resection of the tumor is hampered by infiltrative growth along white matter tracts [8]. Planning the surgical resection of these tumors is facilitated by knowledge about infiltration of the adjacent tracts. Intraoperative subcortical mapping using direct electrical stimulations under awake surgery is the gold standard to directly assess the functional connectivity of tracts adjacent to the tumor [9]. Retrospective studies have shown increased extent of resection and preserved functions with the help of preoperative physiological MRI, intraoperative neuronavigation, and neurophysiological intraoperative testing [10–12]. Presurgical planning is thus of importance in this group because maximal tumor resection has to be balanced with the preservation of neurological function [13, 14].

Astrocytomas and oligodendrogliomas grade II and grade III have overlapping radiologic features, and on contrast enhanced CT or MRI they can be identified by their lack of typical grade IV features like ring-like contrast enhancement and central necrosis [15, 16]. Gliomas grade II and grade III can be separated on the basis of cytological features, cell density, and mitotic figures on neuropathological assessment. Grade IV gliomas have neuropathological characteristics of irregular vascularization with areas of necrosis [2]. Despite their relatively sharp demarcation on T2-weighted images, low-grade gliomas are known for their infiltrative growth pattern along white matter tracts [17, 18].

Morphological MRI with conventional T1- and T2-weighted images and contrast agent injection provides information about tumor location, the extent of bulk tumor growth, and blood-brain-barrier breakdown and edema, but it does not readily aid in the evaluation of specific white matter tracts. White matter tracts can be displaced, infiltrated, or destroyed by tumor growth as evaluated by brain tumor specimen for histopathological evaluation [19–21]. Preoperative noninvasive assessment of white matter structure and glioma growth by diffusion MRI is a promising tool in the presurgical clinical evaluation.

DTI (diffusion tensor imaging) enables the depiction of anisotropic diffusion, which is dependent on white matter fiber orientation [22]. Diffusion tensor tractography (DTT) shows anisotropic diffusion, measured with DTI as color-coded streamlines [23]. DTT depicts white matter fiber orientation and allows visualization of tumor influence on white matter tracts, beyond that of morphological MRI [24]. MD (mean diffusivity) and FA (fractional anisotropy) can be extracted from DTI. MD describes the mean diffusion in tissues and FA describes the directional diffusion in tissues [25]. MD is low in tissue with high cell density and FA is high in tissues with ordered and orientationally coherent microstructure [25]. Previous studies have shown a correlation between lower FA and white matter destruction by tumor. A study by Wang et al. from 2012 demonstrated reduced FA in white matter invaded by tumor cells in a rat glioma model [19]. Reduced FA has also been correlated with increased cell density in gliomas in humans [26].

Earlier studies have evaluated MD and FA in single regions of interest in gliomas showing differences in diffusion between glioma grades [27, 28]. Retrospective studies have evaluated glioma infiltration in tracts by DTT showing the infiltrative growth pattern in gliomas [29]. Quantitative DTT has been reported to correlate with symptoms in glioma patients [30]. The value of DTT in pre- and perioperative imaging has been studied [11, 12, 31–33]. Although a promising method, DTT has several limitations and clinical implications still need further validation [34].

A well-conducted previous study has evaluated and validated DTT in a cohort of normal individuals [35]. Based on these earlier DTT descriptions, the aim of this study was to compare quantitative analysis of MD and FA in tract segments of the major associative, projection, and commissural bundles with visual tract evaluation in patients with nonnecrotic suspected low-grade gliomas and subsequent confirmed neuropathological diagnosis of glioma grade II or grade III. Taking into account the variation in diffusion along the same tract, we systematically divided each bundle into segments using anatomical landmarks [36–38]. To reduce interindividual differences based on, for example, age and degenerative changes in the white matter between patients we normalized the ipsilateral tract segments to the contralateral tract. The resulting DTT findings were compared with visual tract evaluation and neuropathological tumor diagnosis. The hypothesis was that suspected infiltrated tracts would have altered diffusional properties in infiltrated tract segments compared to noninfiltrated tracts.

2. Materials and Methods

Fifty consecutive patients were asked to participate in this prospective study, approved by the regional ethical review board in Uppsala (2010/015), which was undertaken from May 2010 to February 2014. Two patients declined participation in the study and were not included. All patients ($n =$ 48) gave written informed consent before taking part in the study. Patients eligible for inclusion were those referred to the neurosurgical department with clinical and radiological suspicion of a low-grade glioma. Inclusion criteria were tumors appearing low-grade on morphological MRI with no contrast enhancement or only patchy and faint contrast enhancement [4]. Exclusion criteria were the appearance of high-grade glioma features on morphological MRI with ring-like contrast enhancement and central necrosis. Previously published results from parts of this cohort have evaluated methionine-PET, perfusion, and diffusion characteristics [39, 40]. No study evaluating diffusion tensor tractography in this cohort has been reported. Included patients underwent presurgical radiological imaging, including morphological and physiological MRI with DTI, except for one patient (patient number 3) who had a biopsy 6 months prior to the study MRI. Patients eligible for tractographic evaluation and statistical analysis were those with a neuropathological report following surgery or biopsy of an astrocytoma or oligodendroglioma grade II or III. Exclusion criteria for statistical analysis were the following: no neuropathological diagnosis or diagnosis other than astrocytoma or oligodendroglioma grade II or III on neuropathological assessment.

MRI. MRI was performed on a 3 T scanner (Philips Achieva, Philips Medical Systems, Best, Netherlands) and a 32-channel head coil.

2.1. Morphological MRI. Morphological sequences included axial T2-FLAIR (TR/TE 11,000/125 ms; 90-degree flip angle; 512 × 512 matrix; and 0.45 × 0.45 × 6.00 mm^3 voxel size), axial T1-weighted spin echo sequences (TR/TE 600/10 ms; 70-degree flip angle; 512 × 512 matrix; and 0.45 × 0.45 × 5.00 mm^3 voxel size) before and after intravenous administration of gadobutrol (Gadovist®, Bayer Schering Pharma, Wedding, Berlin, Germany), sagittal T1-weighted 3D turbo field echo (TFE) after contrast agent injection (TR/TE: 8.1/3.7 ms; voxel size 1 × 1 × 1 mm), and sagittal T2-weighted turbo spin echo (SE) (TR/TE = 3,000/80 ms; slice thickness = 4 mm; and slice gap = 0.8 mm). Sequences acquired but not assessed in this study were axial T2-weighted turbo spin echo (SE), coronal T2-FLAIR, and perfusion weighted imaging during contrast agent injection.

2.2. Diffusion MRI. Diffusion MRI was performed with SE EPI sequence with the following scan parameters: TR/TE 6,683 ms/77 ms; 60 slices with a thickness of 2 mm; SENSE = 2; 128 × 128 matrix; FOV 256 × 256 mm; and diffusion encoding in 48 directions, with $b = 1,000 \, \text{s/mm}^2$, for a total scan time of 6 minutes. All postprocessing was performed using in-house developed software, implemented in MATLAB (The Mathworks, Natick, MA, USA). Motion and eddy current distortions were corrected by registering the diffusion-weighted volumes to the volume acquired with $b = 0 \, \text{s/mm}^2$, using ElastiX [41, 42]. In this process, the diffusion-weighted images were smoothed using 3D Gaussian kernel with a full width at half maximum of 2 mm. We used in-house developed software based on linear least-squares fitting with heteroscedasticity correction. Streamline tractography was performed using the Diffusion Toolkit and TrackVis (Ruopeng Wang, Van J. Wedeen, TrackVis.org, Martinos Center for Biomedical Imaging, Massachusetts General Hospital, MA, USA). The whole brain was seeded from two randomly positioned seeds in each voxel using FA threshold of 0.1 and an angular threshold of 45 degrees.

2.3. Tract Segmentation and Evaluation. ROIs (regions of interest) for tracking were delineated in EvalGUI, in-house developed software, based on earlier white matter atlas descriptions [43–45] and previous tractography evaluation of the normal brain [35]. Tracts were subdivided into segments that were defined based on anatomical landmarks, and ROI-delineation is visualized in Supplementary Figures 1 a-i (see Supplementary Material available online at http://dx.doi.org/10.1155/2016/7671854). These ROIs defined the anatomical landmarks. The ROI positions perpendicular to the tracts defined the segments. ROIs for each tract segment were positioned in the ipsilateral hemisphere and in the contralateral hemisphere in all patients; ROIs were

adjusted when tract segment trajectory was altered due to tumor growth. TrackVis was used for visual confirmation of the tract positions (Figures 1(a)–1(i)).

Whole tracts were visually assessed in EvalGUI after selecting ROI positions. Tract segments were visually inspected in 3D using TrackVis. Figure 2 shows an example of the cingulum with associated ROIs and tract segments.

The following tracts were evaluated in all patients: the corticospinal tract, the inferior frontooccipital fasciculus, the retrosplenial and parahippocampal parts of the cingulum [46], the arcuate fasciculus, the inferior longitudinal fasciculus, the uncinate fasciculus, fornix, and the forceps minor of the corpus callosum (Figures 1(a)–1(i)). Segments were numbered 1-2 or 1–3 from caudal to cranial ones, from anterior to posterior ones, or from midline to lateral ones depending on tract course (Figures 1(a)–1(i)). All tract segments were assessed for infiltration or dislocation by the tumor with reference standard for tumor area set as high signal intensity on T2-weighted images by a resident in neuroradiology with 5 years of experience in brain tumor evaluation. A tract segment was visually classified as infiltrated if it coursed through the tumor area defined as high signal intensity on T2-FLAIR weighted images. A tract segment was visually classified as dislocated if it deviated from its expected pathway on FA-color maps and was located outside the increased signal intensity on T2-FLAIR defined as tumor. Tumor location in the left or right hemisphere and lobes was determined on T2-weighted images.

2.4. Neuropathological Evaluation. All histopathological slides were reevaluated by one neuropathologist with extensive clinical experience of glioma diagnosis. The diagnoses followed the 2007 WHO classification of central nervous system tumors. The tumors were classified as either astrocytomas or oligodendrogliomas based on the dominating cell type [2].

2.5. Statistical Analysis. To standardize diffusion measurements, adjust for differences between hemispheres, and decrease interindividual variations between patients, a relative FA (rFA) was calculated for each tract segment by dividing the mean FA in the ipsilateral tract segment by the mean FA in the corresponding contralateral tract segment in each patient. The corresponding calculation was performed for mean MD, yielding relative MD (rMD). The FA and MD in tract segments are the mean values of all voxels in that segment. rFA and rMD were compared between groups based on radiographic features (tumor infiltration, tumor dislocation, and hemisphere location left/right) and neuropathological features (tumor type, tumor grade) with the Mann-Whitney U test. The Wilcoxon matched pairs test was used to evaluate differences in rFA between different segments of a tract partially infiltrated by tumor. The chi-squared test was used to investigate the distributions of visually infiltrating gliomas between grades II and III. The cut-off for significant results was set to a p value of <0.05. Statistical analyses were performed in Statistica version 12 (StatSoft, Dell Software, TX, USA).

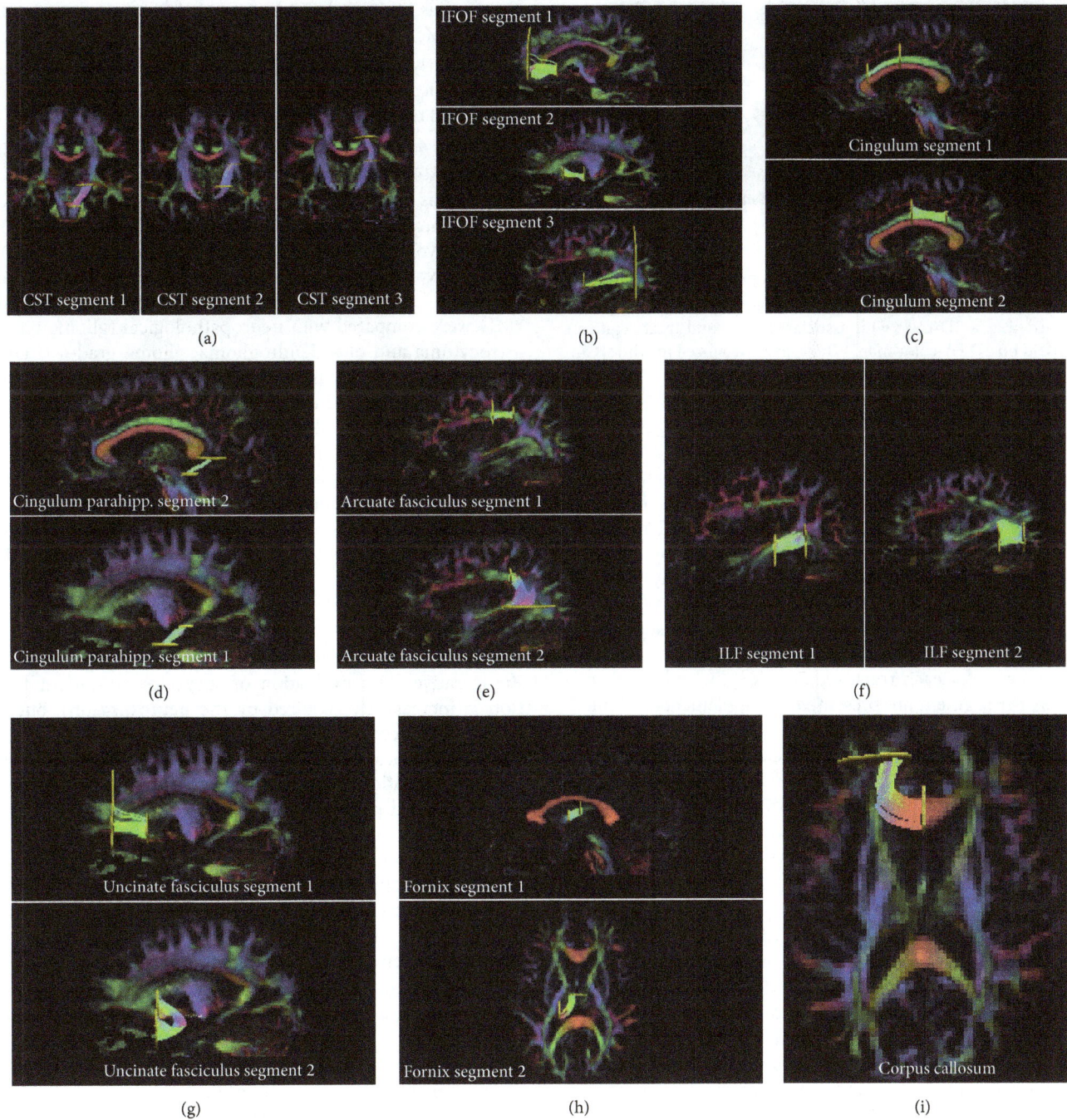

FIGURE 1: 3D-tractography in TrackVis in all tract segments in one patient, in the hemisphere contralateral to the tumor. (a) Corticospinal tract: segments 1–3. (b) Inferior frontooccipital fasciculus: segments 1–3. (c) Cingulum: segments 1 and 2. (d) Parahippocampal cingulum: segments 1 and 2. (e) Arcuate fasciculus: segments 1 and 2. (f) Inferior longitudinal fasciculus: segments 1 and 2. (g) Uncinate fasciculus: segments 1 and 2. (h) Fornix: segments 1 and 2. (i) Corpus callosum: forceps minor.

3. Results

Thirty-four patients had tumors appearing low-grade on morphological MRI without ($n = 24$ patients) or with ($n = 10$ patients) patchy and faint contrast enhancement. Patient age at study entry was 48 ± 15 years (mean $\pm$ SD). The time between MRI and surgery was 3 ± 7 months (mean $\pm$ SD). The study population included 18 males and 16 females. Included patients had undergone presurgical radiological imaging, including morphological and physiological MRI with DTI (except for one patient, patient number 3, who had a biopsy 6 months prior to study MRI). Patients eligible for tracto-graphic evaluation included in the statistical analysis were those with an astrocytoma ($n = 18$) or oligodendroglioma

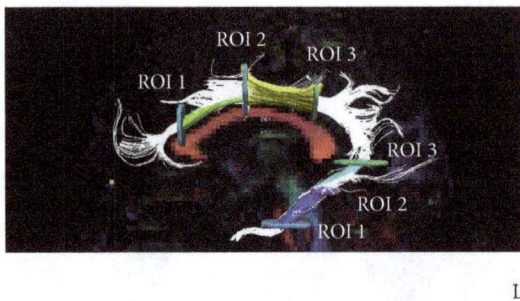

FIGURE 2: Example tract of cingulum with ROIs and tract segments. The cingulum and the parahippocampal part of the cingulum visualized as a 3D-tract with associated ROIs and tract segments overlaid on 2D FA-color map. Whole tract visualized in white. Cingulum: segment 1, green, and segment 2, yellow. Parahippocampal cingulum: segment 1, blue, and segment 2, turquoise.

(n = 16) grade II or III according to postoperative neuropathological reevaluation. Patients with diagnosis other than astrocytoma or oligodendroglioma grade II or III on neuropathological assessment or patients not yet operated on were not included in the analysis. Tractography was successfully performed in 98% of the tract segments (635 tract segments out of 646, with 34 patients × 19 tract segments = 646). Technical details on tract segments regarding number of segments for each tract, segment length, and number of voxels per segment are presented in Supplementary Table 1. All segments except one were longer than 2 cm. A total of 19 segments from nine tracts were evaluated with DTT in each patient (Figures 1(a)–1(i)). The total number of segments in all tracts in each hemisphere was 19, and, out of these, 18 could be analyzed with rFA and rMD. rFA and rMD for segment one of the fornix could not be calculated because of its midline position.

3.1. Infiltration and Dislocation Based on Visual Assessment.
On visual evaluation, 28 of the 34 included patients had at least one infiltrated tract segment (82%). Seventeen of the 34 patients (50%) had at least one dislocated tract segment. Thirteen of these 17 patients (76%) had other tract segments that were infiltrated on visual evaluation. Details concerning tract segment infiltration and dislocation and tumor location are presented in Table 1.

Based on visual and quantitative evaluation, gliomas grade II and gliomas grade III had an equal propensity to infiltrate tract segments (chi-squared test, p = 0.75) and showed similar diffusion alterations (Supplementary Table 2). Figures 3(a)–3(d) show an example of one infiltrated and one dislocated tract in two different patients.

3.2. Relative FA and MD Compared with Visual Assessment and Neuropathological Report (Glioma Type Astrocytoma or Oligodendroglioma, Glioma Grade II or III).
rFA and rMD were calculated for all tract segments and compared between tract segments visually classified as infiltrated and those visually classified as not infiltrated. rFA decreased in all tracts visually classified as infiltrated compared to those not

classified as infiltrated, reaching statistical significance in all but two tract segments (89%, 16/18 segments), Table 2.

Similarly, rMD was higher in 89% of tract segments visually classified as infiltrated, reaching statistical significance in 78% (14/18 tract segments) (Table 3).

Figure 4 shows a box plot of rFA and rMD in tract segment infiltration.

rFA was higher in one dislocated tract segment compared to the contralateral not dislocated tract segment, 6% (1/18). Tumor involvement often included several lobes (Table 1). In the involved lobes, several tract segments were often dislocated or infiltrated (Table 1). Furthermore, rFA and rMD were compared with neuropathological (glioma types astrocytoma and oligodendroglioma, glioma grades II and III) and radiological (visual tract segment dislocation or not, hemisphere location in right or left hemisphere) features. Detailed results from all comparisons are presented in Supplementary Table 2. rFA and rMD in tract segments did not differ significantly between gliomas grade II and gliomas grade III. Significant differences were found between rFA and rMD between astrocytomas (lower FA and higher MD) and oligodendrogliomas in 22% of all evaluated tract segments (4/18).

4. Discussion

Preoperative DTT evaluation of suspected tumor infiltration is increasingly required by the neurosurgeons, but it has not yet become a clinical routine procedure in every neuroradiological center. The method has been validated in normal populations but needs further evaluation in patients with suspected glioma to prove its clinical value [35]. We systematically assessed major associative, projection, and commissural bundles and compared quantitative analysis of tract segments with visual tract evaluation and neuropathological diagnosis in patients with nonnecrotic gliomas grades II and III. We divided the tracts into segments in order to improve the detection of partial tract infiltration.

Previous studies have reported on the usefulness of tractography for preoperative assessment of glioma infiltration along tracts with regard to surgical planning [11, 31]. Retrospective evaluation of gliomas has shown longer survival in patients with noninfiltrative gliomas [21, 47]. No prospective study has to our knowledge evaluated DTT in a cohort of prospectively included suspected low-grade gliomas. Our main finding was that radiological suspicion of glioma infiltration on visual evaluation was confirmed by significantly reduced rFA in 89% (16/18) of the evaluated tract segments. 11% (2/18) had lower rFA but did not reach statistical significance. In segment two of the fornix only two out of 32 patients had visual infiltration making the comparison less likely to show statistical significance. In consistency with earlier reports, dislocated tract segments had no significant alterations of rFA or rMD in 94% compared with not dislocated tract segments, Supplementary Table 2.

Reduced FA in tumor-infiltrated white matter regions is the most studied finding related to DTI tumor evaluation. Supported by DTI experiment in rat glioma models, reduced

TABLE 1: A summary of infiltrated or dislocated tract segments.

Patient number	Glioma type	Glioma grade	Lobe	Displaced tracts	Displaced segments	Infiltrated tracts	Infiltrated segments
1	Astrocytoma	II	Parietal	None	None	AF	AF segments 1 and 2
2	Astrocytoma	III	Frontal lobe, not extending to the motor area	None	None	None	None
3	Astrocytoma	II	Frontoparietotemporal	None	None	ILF IFOF CST CG CG para AF Fornix	ILF segment 2 IFOF segment 3 CST segments 2 and 3 CG segments 1 and 2 CG para segment 2 AF segments 1 and 2 Fornix segment 2
4	Oligodendroglioma	II	Frontal lobe, not extending to the motor area	None	None	UF IFOF CC Fmin	UF segment 1 IFOF segment 1 CC Fmin
5	Astrocytoma	II	Frontal and insular	IFOF AF CST	IFOF segment 2 AF segment 1 CST segments 2 and 3	None	None
6	Astrocytoma	III	Frontal lobe extending to the precentral sulcus	CST	CST segments 2 and 3	AF	AF segments 1 and 2
7	Astrocytoma	III	Temporooccipital	CST	CST segment 2	UF ILF IFOF CG para Fornix	UF segments 1 and 2 ILF segments 1 and 2 IFOF segments 2 and 3 CG para segments 1 and 2 Fornix segment 2
8	Astrocytoma	III	Frontoparietotemporal	ILF IFOF CST	ILF segment 2 IFOF segment 3 CST segments 2 and 3	AF	AF segments 1 and 2
9	Oligodendroglioma	II	Frontal lobe, not extending to the motor area	None	None	UF IFOF CC Fmin CG	UF segments 1 and 2 IFOF segments 1 and 2 CC Fmin CG segments 1 and 2
10	Oligodendroglioma	II	Frontal	CG	CG segments 1 and 2	CST AF	CST segments 2 and 3 AF segment 1
11	Oligodendroglioma	II	Parietal	None	None	None	None
12	Astrocytoma	III	Frontal lobe, not extending to the motor area	None	None	UF IFOF CC Fmin	UF segments 1 and 2 IFOF segment 1 CC Fmin
13	Astrocytoma	II	Frontoparietal	AF	AF segment 1	CST CG	CST segment 3 CG segments 1 and 2
14	Astrocytoma	III	Frontotemporoparietooccipital	ILF IFOF	ILF segments 1 and 2 IFOF segment 3	CST CG CG para AF	CST segment 3 CG segments 2 and 1 CG para segments 1 and 2 AF segment 2

TABLE 1: Continued.

Patient number	Glioma type	Glioma grade	Lobe	Displaced tracts	Displaced segments	Infiltrated tracts	Infiltrated segments
15	Astrocytoma	III	Frontoparietotemporal	None	None	AF	AF segments 1 and 2
16	Astrocytoma	II	Parietotemporooccipital	None	None	IFOF CST AF	IFOF segment 3 CST segment 3 AF segment 2
17	Oligodendroglioma	II	Temporal	CG para	CG para segment 1	UF IFOF	UF segments 1 and 2 IFOF segment 2
18	Oligodendroglioma	II	Frontal lobe, not extending to the motor area	None	None	CC Fmin	CC Fmin
19	Astrocytoma	II	Frontotemporoparietal	None	None	UF ILF IFOF CG para	UF segments 1 and 2 ILF segments 1 and 2 IFOF segments 2 and 3 CG para segments 1 and 2
20	Oligodendroglioma	II	Frontal	AF	AF segment 1	None	None
21	Astrocytoma	II	Frontal	CG	CG segments 1 and 2	None	None
22	Oligodendroglioma	II	Temporoparietal	ILF IFOF	ILF segment 1 IFOF segment 3	None	None
23	Astrocytoma	II	Frontotemporoinsular	CST	CST segments 1 and 2	UF ILF IFOF	UF segments 1 and 2 ILF segment 1 IFOF segments 2 and 3
24	Astrocytoma	II	Temporooccipitoparietal	None	None	ILF IFOF CST ARC	ILF segments 1 and 2 IFOF segment 3 CST segments 2 and 3 FA segments 1 and 2
25	Oligodendroglioma	II	Frontal lobe extending to the precentral sulcus	CG	CG segments 1 and 2	CST ARC	CST segments 2 and 3 AF segment 1
26	Astrocytoma	III	Frontotemporoparietooccipital	CST	CST segments 1 and 2	UF ILF IFOF CG para ARC	UF segments 1 and 2 ILF segments 1 and 2 IFOF segments 1–3 CG para segments 1 and 2 AF segment 2
27	Oligodendroglioma	II	Frontal lobe, not extending to the motor area	CG	CG segment 1	UF CC Fmin	UF segments 1 and 2
28	Oligodendroglioma	II	Frontal lobe extending to the precentral sulcus	CST	CST segments 2 and 3	AF	AF segment 1
29	Oligodendroglioma	II	Frontotemporoinsular	AF CST	AF segments 1 and 2 CST segments 2 and 3	UF ILF IFOF	UF segments 1 and 2 ILF segment 1 IFOF segments 1–3
30	Oligodendroglioma	III	Frontal	None	None	CST	CST segment 3
31	Oligodendroglioma	II	Frontal lobe, not extending to the motor area	None	None	CC Fmin	CC Fmin

TABLE 1: Continued.

Patient number	Glioma type	Glioma grade	Lobe	Displaced tracts	Displaced segments	Infiltrated tracts	Infiltrated segments
32	Oligodendroglioma	III	Frontotemporoinsular	None	None	UF ILF IFOF CC Fmin	UF segments 1 and 2 ILF segment 1 IFOF segments 1–3 CC Fmin
33	Astrocytoma	III	Frontoinsular, not extending to the precentral sulcus	None	None	UF IFOF CC Fmin	UF segment 1 IFOF segments 1 and 2 CC Fmin
34	Oligodendroglioma	III	Frontoinsular, not extending to the precentral sulcus	None	None	UF IFOF CC Fmin	UF segment 1 IFOF segments 1 and 2 CC Fmin

AF = arcuate fasciculus, ILF = inferior longitudinal fasciculus, IFOF = inferior frontooccipital fasciculus, CG = cingulum, CG para = parahippocampal cingulum, UF = uncinate fasciculus, CC Fmin = forceps minor of the corpus callosum, and CST = corticospinal tract.

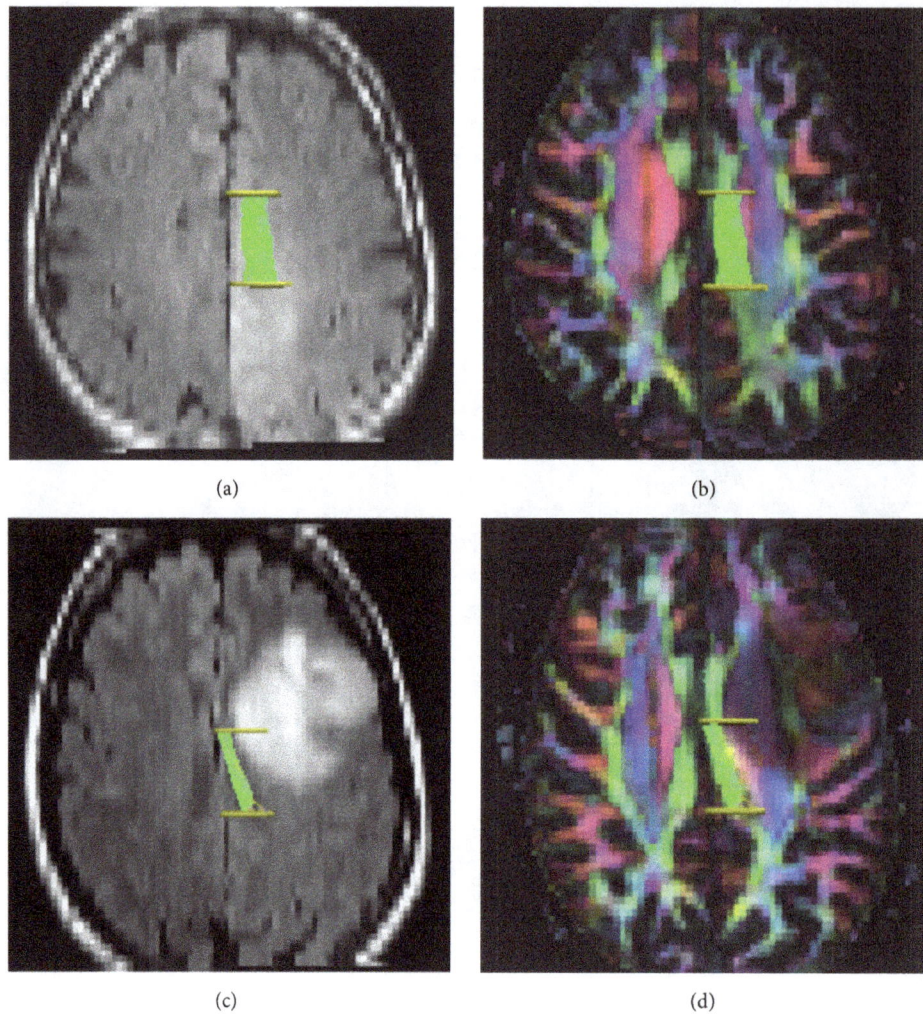

FIGURE 3: Tractography of segment 2 of the cingulum in two different patients (patient number 14 and patient number 25). ((a)-(b)) Patient with an astrocytoma grade III. (a) 3D-tractography of segment 2 of the cingulum overlaid on T2-FLAIR image shows tumor infiltrating the area of the tract segment. ROIs number two and three in yellow. (b) 3D-tractography in the same patient, segment two of the cingulum overlaid on 2D FA-color map. ((c)-(d)) Patient with an oligodendroglioma grade II. (c) 3D-tractography of segment 2 of the cingulum overlaid on T2-FLAIR image shows tumor dislocation of the tract segment. ROIs number two and three in yellow. (d) 3D-tractography in the same patient, segment two of the cingulum overlaid on 2D FA-color map.

rFA in investigated tract segments indicates glioma growth [19]. In general, rFA and rMD in tract segments showed a poor association with glioma grade and type in our study. Gliomas grades II and III had an equal distribution of visual tract segment infiltration, highlighting the intrinsic propensity for infiltrative growth in both tumor grades.

In consistency with earlier reports on glioma infiltration and dislocation of tracts, several patients had infiltration of some tracts combined with dislocation of others [47]. Why gliomas infiltrate some tracts and dislocate others has still to be elucidated. The vulnerability of specific white matter tracts, tumor location, neuropathological glioma characteristics, and progressive disease or tumor volume could all play a role in the processes that influence gliomas growth.

Suspected low-grade gliomas share common imaging criteria: no or patchy and faint contrast enhancement, no extensive mass effect, and no edema. These inclusion criteria, as well as earlier studies showing that low-grade gliomas are mainly confined within the hyperintensity on T2-weighted images, support that our findings of lower rFA and higher rMD in infiltrated segments are related to tumor growth, and not edema. The fact that these tumors (suspected low-grade) do not exhibit surrounding edema makes the changes in diffusion found in visually infiltrated tracts most likely due to bulk tumor infiltration.

The strengths of this study are attributed to the extensive analysis of 19 segments in nine white matter pathways in a prospectively gathered cohort of patients with suspected low-grade gliomas. Segment-wise tractography rather than averaging across a whole tract increases the regional specificity. All patients included in the analysis had a confirmed

TABLE 2: Results from tractography, fractional anisotropy.

Track	Corticospinal tract		p		Corticospinal tract		p		Corticospinal tract		p
DTI scalars	rFA mean (SD)				rFA mean (SD)				rFA mean (SD)		
Segment	Segment 1				Segment 2				Segment 3		
Infiltrated tract segment	n = 8	0.96 (0.03)	0.006135	n = 8	0.93 (0.06)		0.021797	n = 8	0.95 (0.08)		0.138
Not infiltrated tract segment	n = 26	1.01 (0.05)		n = 26	1.00 (0.06)			n = 26	1.01 (0.08)		

Track	Inferior frontooccipital fasciculus		p		Inferior frontooccipital fasciculus		p		Inferior frontooccipital fasciculus		p
DTI scalars	rFA mean (SD)				rFA mean (SD)				rFA mean (SD)		
Segment	Segment 1				Segment 2				Segment 3		
Infiltrated tract segment	n = 14	0.80 (0.14)	0.00029	n = 15	0.74 (0.16)		0.000027	n = 14	0.89 (0.11)		0.000218
Not infiltrated tract segment	n = 19	0.99 (0.07)		n = 19	0.98 (0.08)			n = 19	1.03 (0.06)		

Track	Cingulum		p		Cingulum		p
DTI scalars	rFA mean (SD)				rFA mean (SD)		
Segment	Segment 1				Segment 2		
Infiltrated tract segment	n = 4	0.64 (0.16)	0.004241	n = 4	0.58 (0.22)		0.001471
Not infiltrated tract segment	n = 30	1.02 (0.17)		n = 30	1.03 (0.07)		

Track	Parahippocampal cg		p		Parahippocampal cg		p
DTI scalars	rFA mean (SD)				rFA mean (SD)		
Segment	Segment 1				Segment 2		
Infiltrated tract segment	n = 5	0.61 (0.21)	0.002188	n = 5	0.55 (0.14)		0.000463
Not infiltrated tract segment	n = 29	0.98 (0.10)		n = 29	0.98 (0.11)		

Track	Arcuate fasciculus		p		Arcuate fasciculus		p
DTI scalars	rFA mean (SD)				rFA mean (SD)		
Segment	Segment 1				Segment 2		
Infiltrated tract segment	n = 12	0.76 (0.16)	0.000386	n = 10	0.76 (0.11)		0.000026
Not infiltrated tract segment	n = 22	0.98 (0.06)		n = 21	1.00 (0.07)		

Track	Inferior longitudinal fasciculus		p		Inferior longitudinal fasciculus		p
DTI scalars	rFA mean (SD)				rFA mean (SD)		
Segment	Segment 1				Segment 2		
Infiltrated tract segment	n = 8	0.75 (0.18)	0.000173	n = 8	0.84 (0.09)		0.000173
Not infiltrated tract segment	n = 26	0.99 (0.08)		n = 26	1.00 (0.07)		

Track	Uncinate fasciculus		p		Uncinate fasciculus		p
DTI scalars	rFA mean (SD)				rFA mean (SD)		
Segment	Segment 1				Segment 2		
Infiltrated tract segment	n = 12	0.76 (0.09)	0.000003	n = 12	0.77 (0.18)		0.001058
Not infiltrated tract segment	n = 21	1.01 (0.08)		n = 21	1.00 (0.10)		

TABLE 2: Continued.

Track		Fornix	p		Fornix	p
DTI scalars		FA ratio			rFA mean (SD)	
Segment		1, midline			Segment 2	
Infiltrated tract segment	NA*	NA*	NA*	$n = 2$	0.88 (0.10)	0.056
Not infiltrated tract segment	NA*	NA*	NA*	$n = 30$	1.02 (0.09)	

Track		Callosal body minor forceps	p
DTI scalars		rFA mean (SD)	
Segment		Segment 1	
Infiltrated tract segment	$n = 9$	0.88 (0.12)	**0.00301**
Not infiltrated tract segment	$n = 25$	1.01 (0.05)	

*No ratio due to tract segment in midline.

rFA in infiltrated and not infiltrated tract segment presented as mean and standard deviation with results from Mann-Whitney U tests. $p < 0.05$ was regarded as statistically significant.

rFA = relative fractional anisotropy (ipsilateral mean FA/contralateral mean FA), SD = standard deviation, cg = cingulum, and NA = not available.

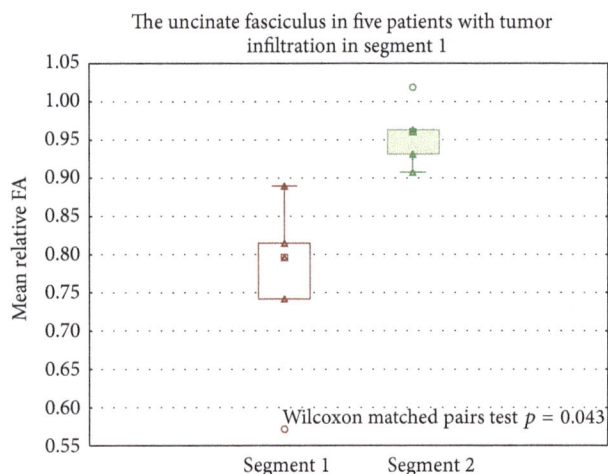

FIGURE 4: Box plot of rFA in tract segments. rFA in segments 1 and 2 in the uncinate fasciculus, in five patients with tumor infiltration in segment 1. Significantly lower rFA in segment 1 compared to segment 2. Wilcoxon matched pairs test, $p = 0.043$. rFA = relative fractional anisotropy.

neuropathological diagnosis of astrocytoma or oligodendroglioma grade II or grade III.

Preoperative knowledge about suspected tumor tract infiltration and tumor tract dislocation can aid surgical preoperative planning and indicates the need for an extended preoperative evaluation including also neurophysiological assessment. It might also aid upon informing the patient about the expected neurological outcome after surgery, which may depend on the extent of tract involvement.

Based on our findings, future studies evaluating measurement of diffusion properties in multiple tract segments may provide new important information about the extent of glioma infiltration. Future applications of this method might also give insight into tract segment infiltration related to different histological subtypes of gliomas.

We acknowledge three major limitations of the present study. First, the limited number of patients included in this study is a disadvantage in a study of heterogeneous tumors with different locations in the brain. Small differences in subgroups can be missed, and our findings need to be interpreted with care and need confirmation in larger cohorts [32]. However, the results on diffusion changes in visually infiltrated tract segments were a consistent finding over different patients and different tracts segments.

Second, infiltrated tracts were visually classified based on T2-FLAIR and FA-color maps; however, this study lacks neuropathological verifications of these findings. To evaluate the visual assessment of tract segment infiltration we compared the results from visual analysis with quantitative data from tract segments. In support of our findings regarding low rFA in infiltrated tract segments, Stadlbauer et al. 2007 showed an association between lower FA values and increasing tumor cell numbers [48].

The third limitation concerns the tractography method. A weakness of the DTT technique is the difficulty of successful tractography in regions with crossing fibers [49, 50]. We strove to minimize this influence by avoiding tracts and segments with known difficulties when deterministic tractography is used. In the segmentation of the tracts, we balanced segment length and tractography quality, and, thus, a majority of investigated tracts (7/9) comprised two segments. This limited the possibility of studying variation in FA and MD along tracts and at different distances from the tumor. Also, FA is affected by both white matter integrity and orientation dispersion and methods to separate the two have been devised recently but require high b-value data [51].

Since intraoperative subcortical mapping using direct electrical stimulations under awake surgery is the gold standard to directly visualize the subcortical connectivity future DTT studies should be compared with intraoperative observation of subcortical tracts [9].

TABLE 3: Results from tractography, mean diffusivity.

Track	Corticospinal tract		p		Corticospinal tract		p		Corticospinal tract		p
DTI scalars	rMD mean (SD)				rMD mean (SD)				rMD mean (SD)		
Segment	Segment 1				Segment 2				Segment 3		
Infiltrated tract segment	n = 8	0.98 (0.05)	0.383	n = 8	1.01 (0.04)		0.761	n = 8	1.08 (0.10)		**0.009935**
Not infiltrated tract segment	n = 26	0.99 (0.04)		n = 26	1.01 (0.04)			n = 26	1.00 (0.04)		
Track	Inferior frontooccipital fasciculus		p		Inferior frontooccipital fasciculus		p		Inferior frontooccipital fasciculus		p
DTI scalars	rMD mean (SD)				rMD mean (SD)				rMD mean (SD)		
Segment	Segment 1				Segment 2				Segment 3		
Infiltrated tract segment	n = 14	1.19 (0.21)	**0.000122**	n = 15	1.20 (0.26)		**0.009287**	n = 14	1.07 (0.09)		**0.018801**
Not infiltrated tract segment	n = 19	1.00 (0.02)		n = 19	1.01 (0.04)			n = 19	0.99 (0.06)		
Track	Cingulum		p		Cingulum		p				
DTI scalars	rMD mean (SD)				rMD mean (SD)						
Segment	Segment 1				Segment 2						
Infiltrated tract segment	n = 4	1.19 (0.15)	**0.002116**	n = 4	1.47 (0.55)		**0.001471**				
Not infiltrated tract segment	n = 30	1.03 (0.04)		n = 30	1.01 (0.04)						
Track	Parahippocampal cg		p		Parahippocampal cg		p				
DTI scalars	rMD mean (SD)				rMD mean (SD)						
Segment	Segment 1				Segment 2						
Infiltrated tract segment	n = 5	1.44 (0.34)	**0.001574**	n = 5	1.37 (0.25)		**0.000793**				
Not infiltrated tract segment	n = 29	1.03 (0.10)		n = 29	1.01 (0.08)						
Track	Arcuate fasciculus		p		Arcuate fasciculus		p				
DTI scalars	rMD mean (SD)				rMD mean (SD)						
Segment	Segment 1				Segment 2						
Infiltrated tract segment	n = 12	1.34 (0.28)	**0.000166**	n = 10	1.22 (0.21)		**0.001226**				
Not infiltrated tract segment	n = 22	1.00 (0.04)		n = 21	1.01 (0.04)						
Track	Inferior longitudinal fasciculus		p		Inferior longitudinal fasciculus		p				
DTI scalars	rMD mean (SD)				rMD mean (SD)						
Segment	Segment 1				Segment 2						
Infiltrated tract segment	n = 8	1.19 (0.15)	**0.000602**	n = 8	1.11 (0.11)		**0.002844**				
Not infiltrated tract segment	n = 26	1.01 (0.04)		n = 26	1.00 (0.06)						
Track	Uncinate fasciculus		p		Uncinate fasciculus		p				
DTI scalars	rMD mean (SD)				rMD mean (SD)						
Segment	Segment 1				Segment 2						
Infiltrated tract segment	n = 12	1.18 (0.15)	**0.000146**	n = 12	1.24 (0.27)		0.15				
Not infiltrated tract segment	n = 21	1.01 (0.03)		n = 21	1.01 (0.04)						

TABLE 3: Continued.

Track		Fornix	p		Fornix	p
DTI scalars		rMD mean (SD)			rMD mean (SD)	
Segment		1, midline			Segment 2	
Infiltrated tract segment	NA*	NA*	NA*	$n = 2$	1.09 (0.02)	0.371
Not infiltrated tract segment	NA*	NA*	NA*	$n = 30$	1.03 (0.19)	

Track		Callosal body minor forceps	p
DTI scalars		rMD mean (SD)	
Segment		Segment 1	
Infiltrated tract segment	$n = 9$	1.13 (0.08)	**0.000209**
Not infiltrated tract segment	$n = 25$	1.01 (0.02)	

*No ratio due to tract segment in midline.
rMD in infiltrated and not infiltrated tract segment presented as mean and standard deviation with results from Mann-Whitney U tests. $p < 0.05$ was regarded as statistically significant.
rMD = relative mean diffusivity (ipsilateral mean diffusivity/contralateral mean diffusivity), SD = standard deviation, cg = cingulum, and NA = not available.

5. Conclusion

Quantitative MR tractography is applicable in patients with nonnecrotic gliomas grades II and III and corresponds to visual evaluation of suspected tract infiltration. It is thus a promising objective tool for the preoperative evaluation of tract segment involvement in these tumors.

Abbreviations

rFA: Relative fractional anisotropy
rMD: Relative mean diffusivity
DTT: Diffusion tensor tractography
DTI: Diffusion tensor imaging
ROI: Region of interest.

Competing Interests

The authors declare that they have no competing interests.

Authors' Contributions

All authors participated in the study design: Johanna Mårtensson, Jimmy Lätt, and Markus Nilsson postprocessed the data; Anna F. Delgado performed the tractography and statistical analyses and drafted the paper. All authors critically revised the paper and approved the final version.

Acknowledgments

Uppsala county council has provided financial support for the study. Grant from Swedish Cancer Society was received.

References

[1] M. L. Goodenberger and R. B. Jenkins, "Genetics of adult glioma," *Cancer Genetics*, vol. 205, no. 12, pp. 613–621, 2012.

[2] D. N. Louis, H. Ohgaki, O. D. Wiestler et al., "The 2007 WHO classification of tumours of the central nervous system," *Acta Neuropathologica*, vol. 114, no. 2, pp. 97–109, 2007.

[3] M. Waqar, S. Hanif, A. R. Brodbelt et al., "Prognostic factors in lobar world health organization grade II astrocytomas," *World Neurosurgery*, vol. 84, no. 1, pp. 154–162, 2015.

[4] J. Pallud, L. Capelle, L. Taillandier et al., "Prognostic significance of imaging contrast enhancement for WHO grade II gliomas," *Neuro-Oncology*, vol. 11, no. 2, pp. 176–182, 2009.

[5] R. Dubrow and A. S. Darefsky, "Demographic variation in incidence of adult glioma by subtype, United States, 1992–2007," *BMC Cancer*, vol. 11, article 325, 2011.

[6] K. Gousias, J. Schramm, and M. Simon, "Extent of resection and survival in supratentorial infiltrative low-grade gliomas: analysis of and adjustment for treatment bias," *Acta Neurochirurgica*, vol. 156, no. 2, pp. 327–337, 2014.

[7] L. Capelle, D. Fontaine, E. Mandonnet et al., "Spontaneous and therapeutic prognostic factors in adult hemispheric World Health Organization Grade II gliomas: a series of 1097 cases," *Journal of Neurosurgery*, vol. 118, no. 6, pp. 1157–1168, 2013.

[8] J. Pallud, P. Varlet, B. Devaux et al., "Diffuse low-grade oligodendrogliomas extend beyond MRI-defined abnormalities," *Neurology*, vol. 74, no. 21, pp. 1724–1731, 2010.

[9] J. Boetto, L. Bertram, G. Moulinié, G. Herbet, S. Moritz-Gasser, and H. Duffau, "Low rate of intraoperative seizures during awake craniotomy in a prospective cohort with 374 supratentorial brain lesions: electrocorticography is not mandatory," *World Neurosurgery*, vol. 84, no. 6, pp. 1838–1844, 2015.

[10] Z. Farshidfar, F. Faeghi, M. Mohseni, A. Seddighi, H. H. Kharrazi, and J. Abdolmohammadi, "Diffusion tensor tractography in the presurgical assessment of cerebral gliomas," *Neuroradiology Journal*, vol. 27, no. 1, pp. 75–84, 2014.

[11] A. Castellano, L. Bello, C. Michelozzi et al., "Role of diffusion tensor magnetic resonance tractography in predicting the extent of resection in glioma surgery," *Neuro-Oncology*, vol. 14, no. 2, pp. 192–202, 2012.

[12] L. Bello, A. Gambini, A. Castellano et al., "Motor and language DTI Fiber Tracking combined with intraoperative subcortical

mapping for surgical removal of gliomas," *NeuroImage*, vol. 39, no. 1, pp. 369–382, 2008.

[13] Y. N. Yordanova, S. Moritz-Gasser, and H. Duffau, "Awake surgery for WHO grade II gliomas within 'noneloquent' areas in the left dominant hemisphere: toward a 'supratotal' resection. Clinical article," *Journal of Neurosurgery*, vol. 115, no. 2, pp. 232–239, 2011.

[14] J. A. Wilden, J. Voorhies, K. M. Mosier, D. P. O'Neill, and A. A. Cohen-Gadol, "Strategies to maximize resection of complex, or high surgical risk, low-grade gliomas," *Neurosurgical Focus*, vol. 34, no. 2, article E5, 2013.

[15] B. L. Dean, B. P. Drayer, C. R. Bird et al., "Gliomas: classification with MR imaging," *Radiology*, vol. 174, no. 2, pp. 411–415, 1990.

[16] M.-L. Schäfer, M. H. Maurer, M. Synowitz et al., "Low-grade (WHO II) and anaplastic (WHO III) gliomas: differences in morphology and MRI signal intensities," *European Radiology*, vol. 23, no. 10, pp. 2846–2853, 2013.

[17] H. J. Scherer, "The forms of growth in gliomas and their practical significance," *Brain*, vol. 63, no. 1, pp. 1–35, 1940.

[18] C. Gerin, J. Pallud, C. Deroulers et al., "Quantitative characterization of the imaging limits of diffuse low-grade oligodendrogliomas," *Neuro-Oncology*, vol. 15, no. 10, pp. 1379–1388, 2013.

[19] S. Wang and J. Zhou, "Diffusion tensor magnetic resonance imaging of rat glioma models: a correlation study of MR imaging and histology," *Journal of Computer Assisted Tomography*, vol. 36, no. 6, pp. 739–744, 2012.

[20] S. J. Price, R. Jena, N. G. Burnet et al., "Improved delineation of glioma margins and regions of infiltration with the use of diffusion tensor imaging: an image-guided biopsy study," *American Journal of Neuroradiology*, vol. 27, no. 9, pp. 1969–1974, 2006.

[21] H. D. Moulding, D. P. Friedman, M. Curtis et al., "Revisiting anaplastic astrocytomas I: an expansive growth pattern is associated with a better prognosis," *Journal of Magnetic Resonance Imaging*, vol. 28, no. 6, pp. 1311–1321, 2008.

[22] D. Le Bihan, J.-F. Mangin, C. Poupon et al., "Diffusion tensor imaging: concepts and applications," *Journal of Magnetic Resonance Imaging*, vol. 13, no. 4, pp. 534–546, 2001.

[23] P. Douek, R. Turner, J. Pekar, N. Patronas, and D. Le Bihan, "MR color mapping of myelin fiber orientation," *Journal of Computer Assisted Tomography*, vol. 15, no. 6, pp. 923–929, 1991.

[24] K. Kallenberg, T. Goldmann, J. Menke et al., "Glioma infiltration of the corpus callosum: early signs detected by DTI," *Journal of Neuro-Oncology*, vol. 112, no. 2, pp. 217–222, 2013.

[25] C. Pierpaoli, P. Jezzard, P. J. Basser, A. Barnett, and G. Di Chiro, "Diffusion tensor MR imaging of the human brain," *Radiology*, vol. 201, no. 3, pp. 637–648, 1996.

[26] T. Beppu, T. Inoue, Y. Shibata et al., "Fractional anisotropy value by diffusion tensor magnetic resonance imaging as a predictor of cell density and proliferation activity of glioblastomas," *Surgical Neurology*, vol. 63, no. 1, pp. 56–61, 2005.

[27] T. Inoue, K. Ogasawara, T. Beppu, A. Ogawa, and H. Kabasawa, "Diffusion tensor imaging for preoperative evaluation of tumor grade in gliomas," *Clinical Neurology and Neurosurgery*, vol. 107, no. 3, pp. 174–180, 2005.

[28] H. Y. Lee, D. G. Na, I.-C. Song et al., "Diffusion-tensor imaging for glioma grading at 3-T magnetic resonance imaging: analysis of fractional anisotropy and mean diffusivity," *Journal of Computer Assisted Tomography*, vol. 32, no. 2, pp. 298–303, 2008.

[29] I.-F. Talos, K. H. Zou, R. Kikinis, and F. A. Jolesz, "Volumetric assessment of tumor infiltration of adjacent white matter based on anatomic MRI and diffusion tensor tractography," *Academic Radiology*, vol. 14, no. 4, pp. 431–436, 2007.

[30] A. Stadlbauer, C. Nimsky, S. Gruber et al., "Changes in fiber integrity, diffusivity, and metabolism of the pyramidal tract adjacent to gliomas: a quantitative diffusion tensor fiber tracking and MR spectroscopic imaging study," *American Journal of Neuroradiology*, vol. 28, no. 3, pp. 462–469, 2007.

[31] G. Bertani, G. Carrabba, F. Raneri et al., "Predictive value of inferior fronto-occipital fasciculus (IFO) DTI-fiber tracking for determining the extent of resection for surgery of frontal and temporal gliomas preoperatively," *Journal of Neurosurgical Sciences*, vol. 56, no. 2, pp. 137–143, 2012.

[32] A. S. Field, A. L. Alexander, Y.-C. Wu, K. M. Hasan, B. Witwer, and B. Badie, "Diffusion tensor eigenvector directional color imaging patterns in the evaluation of cerebral white matter tracts altered by tumor," *Journal of Magnetic Resonance Imaging*, vol. 20, no. 4, pp. 555–562, 2004.

[33] F.-P. Zhu, J.-S. Wu, Y.-Y. Song et al., "Clinical application of motor pathway mapping using diffusion tensor imaging tractography and intraoperative direct subcortical stimulation in cerebral glioma surgery: a prospective cohort study," *Neurosurgery*, vol. 71, no. 6, pp. 1170–1183, 2012.

[34] S. Pujol, W. Wells, C. Pierpaoli et al., "The DTI challenge: toward standardized evaluation of diffusion tensor imaging tractography for neurosurgery," *Journal of Neuroimaging*, vol. 25, no. 6, pp. 875–882, 2015.

[35] S. Wakana, A. Caprihan, M. M. Panzenboeck et al., "Reproducibility of quantitative tractography methods applied to cerebral white matter," *NeuroImage*, vol. 36, no. 3, pp. 630–644, 2007.

[36] A. F. Santillo, J. Mårtensson, O. Lindberg et al., "Diffusion tensor tractography versus volumetric imaging in the diagnosis of behavioral variant frontotemporal dementia," *PLoS ONE*, vol. 8, no. 7, Article ID e66932, 2013.

[37] J. Mårtensson, M. Nilsson, F. Ståhlberg et al., "Spatial analysis of diffusion tensor tractography statistics along the inferior fronto-occipital fasciculus with application in progressive supranuclear palsy," *Magnetic Resonance Materials in Physics, Biology and Medicine*, vol. 26, no. 6, pp. 527–537, 2013.

[38] G. Gerig, S. Gouttard, and I. Corouge, "Analysis of brain white matter via fiber tract modeling," in *Proceedings of the 26th Annual International Conference of the IEEE Engineering in Medicine and Biology Society (IEMBS '04)*, pp. 4421–4424, San Francisco, Calif, USA, September 2004.

[39] S. G. Berntsson, A. Falk, I. Savitcheva et al., "Perfusion and diffusion MRI combined with ^{11}C-methionine PET in the preoperative evaluation of suspected adult low-grade gliomas," *Journal of Neuro-Oncology*, vol. 114, no. 2, pp. 241–249, 2013.

[40] A. Falk, M. Fahlström, E. Rostrup et al., "Discrimination between glioma grades II and III in suspected low-grade gliomas using dynamic contrast-enhanced and dynamic susceptibility contrast perfusion MR imaging: a histogram analysis approach," *Neuroradiology*, vol. 56, no. 12, pp. 1031–1038, 2014.

[41] S. Klein, M. Staring, K. Murphy, M. A. Viergever, and J. P. Pluim, "Elastix: a toolbox for intensity-based medical image registration," *IEEE Transactions on Medical Imaging*, vol. 29, no. 1, pp. 196–205, 2010.

[42] R. Dambe, S. Hähnel, and S. Heiland, "Measuring anisotropic brain diffusion in three and six directions: influence of the off-diagonal tensor elements," *The Neuroradiology Journal*, vol. 20, no. 1, pp. 18–24, 2007.

[43] M. Thiebaut de Schotten, D. H. ffytche, A. Bizzi et al., "Atlasing location, asymmetry and inter-subject variability of white matter tracts in the human brain with MR diffusion tractography," *NeuroImage*, vol. 54, no. 1, pp. 49–59, 2011.

[44] M. Catani and M. Thiebaut de Schotten, "A diffusion tensor imaging tractography atlas for virtual in vivo dissections," *Cortex*, vol. 44, no. 8, pp. 1105–1132, 2008.

[45] M. Catani, D. K. Jones, and D. H. Ffytche, "Perisylvian language networks of the human brain," *Annals of Neurology*, vol. 57, no. 1, pp. 8–16, 2005.

[46] D. K. Jones, K. F. Christiansen, R. J. Chapman, and J. P. Aggleton, "Distinct subdivisions of the cingulum bundle revealed by diffusion MRI fibre tracking: implications for neuropsychological investigations," *Neuropsychologia*, vol. 51, no. 1, pp. 67–78, 2013.

[47] X. Guan, S. Lai, J. Lackey et al., "Revisiting anaplastic astrocytomas II: further characterization of an expansive growth pattern with visually enhanced diffusion tensor imaging," *Journal of Magnetic Resonance Imaging*, vol. 28, no. 6, pp. 1322–1336, 2008.

[48] A. Stadlbauer, C. Nimsky, R. Buslei et al., "Diffusion tensor imaging and optimized fiber tracking in glioma patients: histopathologic evaluation of tumor-invaded white matter structures," *NeuroImage*, vol. 34, no. 3, pp. 949–956, 2007.

[49] R. Seizeur, N. Wiest-Daessle, S. Prima, C. Maumet, J.-C. Ferre, and X. Morandi, "Corticospinal tractography with morphological, functional and diffusion tensor MRI: a comparative study of four deterministic algorithms used in clinical routine," *Surgical and Radiologic Anatomy*, vol. 34, no. 8, pp. 709–719, 2012.

[50] M. L. Mandelli, M. S. Berger, M. Bucci, J. I. Berman, B. Amirbekian, and R. G. Henry, "Quantifying accuracy and precision of diffusion MR tractography of the corticospinal tract in brain tumors: clinical article," *Journal of Neurosurgery*, vol. 121, no. 2, pp. 349–358, 2014.

[51] F. Szczepankiewicz, S. Lasič, D. van Westen et al., "Quantification of microscopic diffusion anisotropy disentangles effects of orientation dispersion from microstructure: applications in healthy volunteers and in brain tumors," *NeuroImage*, vol. 104, pp. 241–252, 2015.

24

Imaging of Hip Pain: From Radiography to Cross-Sectional Imaging Techniques

Fernando Ruiz Santiago,[1] Alicia Santiago Chinchilla,[2]
Afshin Ansari,[3] Luis Guzmán Álvarez,[1] Maria del Mar Castellano García,[1]
Alberto Martínez Martínez,[1] and Juan Tercedor Sánchez[4]

[1]Radiology Department, Hospital of Traumatology, Carretera de Jaen, S/N, 18014 Granada, Spain
[2]Radiology Department, Ciudad Sanitaria Virgen de las Nieves, Avenida de las Fuerzas Armadas 2, 18014 Granada, Spain
[3]Radiology Department, North Tyneside General Hospital, Rake Lane, North Shields NE29 8NH, UK
[4]Orthopedic Department, Hospital of Traumatology, Carretera de Jaen, S/N, 18014 Granada, Spain

Correspondence should be addressed to Fernando Ruiz Santiago; ferusan12@gmail.com

Academic Editor: Andreas H. Mahnken

Hip pain can have multiple causes, including intra-articular, juxta-articular, and referred pain, mainly from spine or sacroiliac joints. In this review, we discuss the causes of intra-articular hip pain from childhood to adulthood and the role of the appropriate imaging techniques according to clinical suspicion and age of the patient. Stress is put on the findings of radiographs, currently considered the first imaging technique, not only in older people with degenerative disease but also in young people without osteoarthritis. In this case plain radiography allows categorization of the hip as normal or dysplastic or with impingement signs, pincer, cam, or a combination of both.

1. Introduction

In the last years, advancements in knowledge of biomechanics and hip joint functional anatomy, as well as improvements in arthroscopy procedures and refinements of imaging techniques, have widened the spectrum of diagnoses causing pain around the hip joint.

Radiologists, as part of the diagnostic team, have to know the appropriate use of different imaging techniques in order to reach an accurate diagnosis without delaying patient management.

2. Causes of Hip Pain

Causes of pain around the hip joint may be intra-articular, extra-articular, or referred pain from neighboring structures, such as sacroiliac joint, spine, symphysis pubis, or the inguinal canal [1].

Intra-articular causes include the following: labral tears, chondromalacia, degenerative changes, intra-articular bone injury, ligamentum teres rupture, arthritis (inflammatory, infectious, etc.), and synovial proliferative disorders.

Extra-articular causes include the following: tendinopathy, bursitis, iliotibial band syndrome, muscle injury, and piriformis syndrome.

This editorial review is going to focus mainly on intra-articular causes of hip pain.

3. Hip Pain Imaging: Need for Clinical Correlation

Imaging of the hip needs to be complementary to the clinical history and physical examination because it is well known that imaging findings do not always correlate with the presence of pain and vice versa.

Clinical tests are adapted to identify the source of pain as intra-articular or extra-articular. The flexion-abduction-external rotation (FABER), internal range of motion with overpressure (IROP), and scour tests show sensitivity values

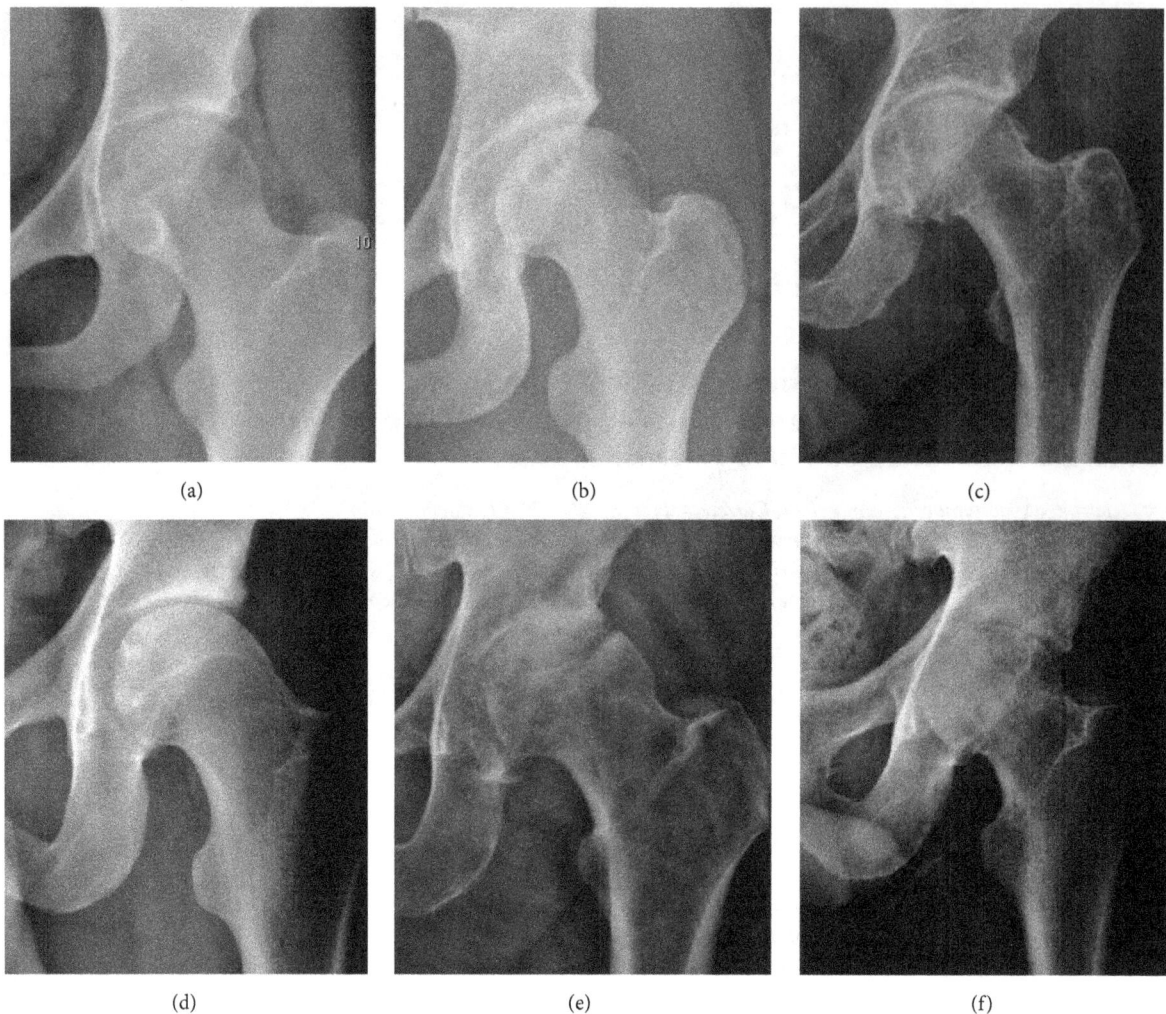

FIGURE 1: Radiography in normal hip (a), hip dysplasia (b), pincer impingement type (c), and cam (d). Hip in osteoarthritis (e) and septic arthritis (f).

in identifying individuals with intra-articular pathology ranging from 0.62 to 0.91 [2].

In the next subheadings, we are going to describe the main indications and role of different imaging modalities (X-ray, magnetic resonance imaging (MRI), computed tomography (CT), ultrasound, and scintigraphy) in studying intra-articular causes of hip pain.

4. X-Ray: A Basic Approach

Radiographs are currently useful not only in older patients in whom osteoarthritis of the hip is suspected but also in younger patients without osteoarthritis, who are being evaluated for femoroacetabular impingement (FAI) or hip dysplasia.

Plain radiography allows us to categorize the hip as normal or dysplastic or with impingement signs (pincer, cam, or a combination of both). Besides these, pathologic processes like osteoarthritis, inflammatory diseases, infection, or tumors can also be identified (Figure 1).

4.1. X-Ray in Pediatric Age. Radiographs of infants should be obtained with the pelvis in neutral position with the lower limbs held in neutral rotation and slight flexion. Reliability of measurements increases if indicators of pelvic alignment are taken into account. Tönnis introduced a quotient of pelvic rotation by dividing the horizontal diameter of the obturator foramen of the right side and that of the left. In neutral rotation the ratio is 1 but is considered to be acceptable when it is between 0.56 and 1.8. The symphysis os-ischium angle of Tönnis evaluates the pelvic position in the sagittal plane. Lines are drawn from the highest point of the ischium to the most prominent point of the symphysis, joining at the inside of the pelvis. The range of normal values is from 90 to 135° and is related to the infant's age [3].

Despite the widespread of ultrasound, pelvis radiographs are still frequently used to diagnose and/or monitor DDH or for assessing other congenital conditions or bone tumors [4]. The Tönnis method is the most widely used radiographic system to classify DDH [5]. It relies on the presence of the femoral head ossification center. Because eccentric position

(a)   (b)

(c)

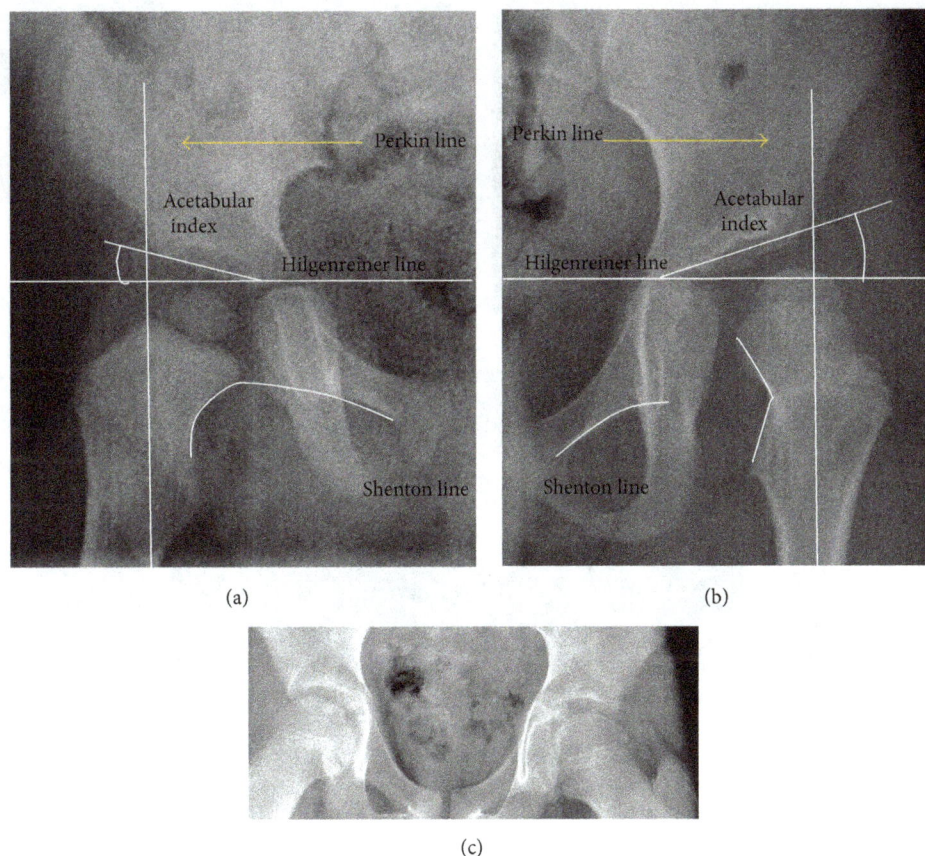

FIGURE 2: Radiological measurements in pediatric normal (a) and dysplastic hip (b). (c) AP view of a patient with left hip effusion secondary to trauma showing widening of the medial joint space.

or delayed appearance of the ossific nucleus is a common finding in DDH, a new radiographic classification system has been developed by the International Hip Dysplasia Institute (IHDI), which uses the mid-point of the proximal femoral metaphysis as a reference landmark [6].

The most useful lines and angles that can be drawn in the pediatric pelvis assessing DDH are shown in Figure 2.

(A) *Hilgenreiner Line*. It is considered a basal line joining the top aspect of the triradiate cartilages. This line is used to measure the acetabular angle and as a reference for Perkin line.

(B) Perkin line is perpendicular to Hilgenreiner line, touching the lateral margin of the acetabulum. This leads to four quadrants and a normal femoral head has to be located in the inferomedial quadrant. We can measure the lateral displacement of the femoral head with regard to the Perkin line by dividing the width of the head that crosses the Perkin line by the diameter of the head. The value for patients under 3 years must be 0 and in older children this ranges from 0 to 22%.

(C) Shenton line is a continuous arc drawn from the inner edge of the femoral neck to the superior margin of the obturator foramen. This should be smooth and undisrupted; otherwise it may indicate a fracture or hip dysplasia.

(D) The acetabular index measures the acetabular roof slope. It is the most useful measure of acetabular dysplasia until 6 years of age. It is formed between Hilgenreiner line and the acetabular roof. In newborns, values of 26°±5° in males and 30°±4° in females are considered normal. Gradually this angle becomes smaller, with a mean value of 18° ± 4° in males and 20° ± 3° in females at 1 year of age [7].

(E) The medial articular joint space is measured between the medial border of the femoral head or neck (when epiphysis is not ossified) and the acetabular platform. Normal values range between 5 and 12 mm. Differences greater than 1.5 mm between the two sides are considered abnormal [8].

Most cases of Legg-Calvé-Perthes disease (LCPD) develop between the ages of 4 and 10 years (Figure 3). Classification of its severity can be assessed by radiographs. Herring or lateral pillar classifications and the patient's age strongly correlate with the outcome [9]. In Group A, which has a better prognosis, there are no loss of height in the lateral third of the femoral head and little density changes; in Group B, there is lucency and lateral height loss of less than 50%; and in Group C, the most severe form, there is more than 50% loss of lateral height. Group B/C is considered when the loss of lateral pillar height is at 50% [10]. Patients who are over the age of 8 years

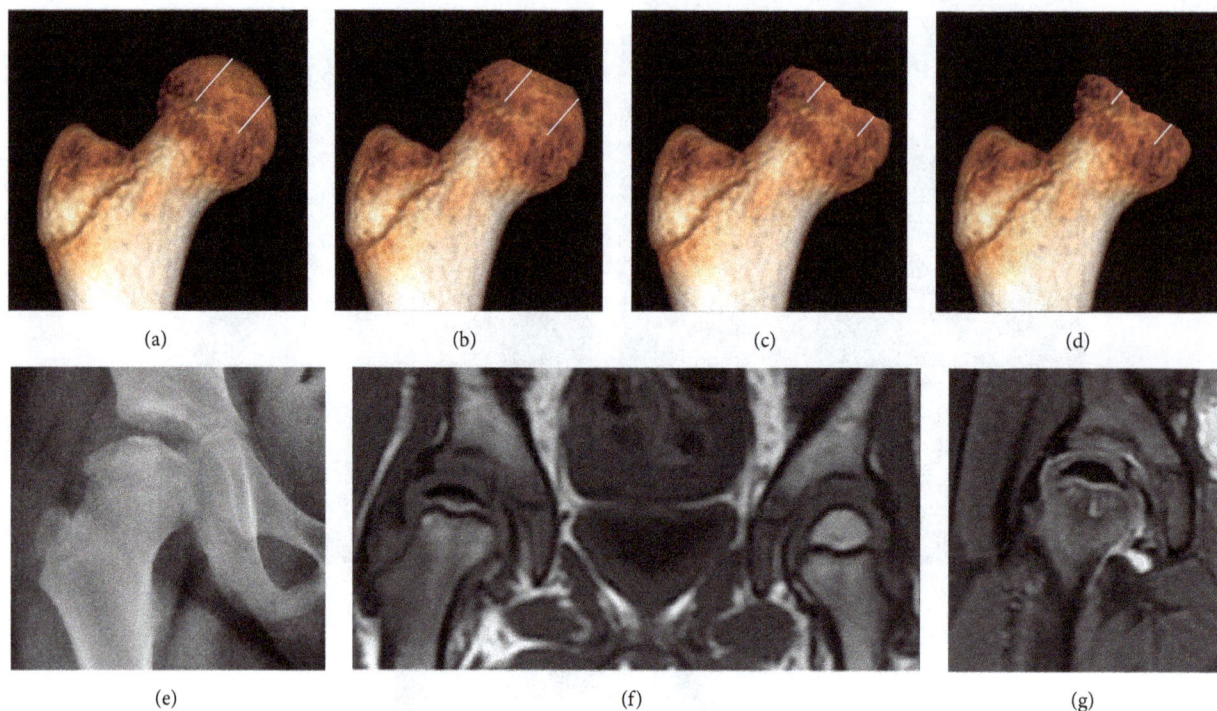

FIGURE 3: Herring lateral pillar classification. Groups A (a), B (b), B/C (c), and C (d). AP radiograph (e), coronal T1 (f), and PD fat sat (g) weighted images showing loss of fat signal of the epiphysis, edema, and cyst formation in femoral metaphysis in a grade C Perthes disease.

at the time of onset and have a hip in the lateral pillar B group or B/C border group have a better outcome with surgical treatment than they do with conservative treatment. Group B hips in children who are less than 8 years at the time of onset have a very favorable outcome unrelated to the treatment, whereas Group C hips in children of all ages usually have poor outcome unrelated to the treatment [11].

Slipped Capital Femoral Epiphyses (SCFE) usually affect 11- to 14-year-old patients (Figure 4). Radiographs may show widening and irregularity of the physis and posterior inferior displacement of the capital femoral epiphysis. On the AP view Klein's line, tangent to the lateral aspect of the femoral neck, does not intersect the femoral head indicating that it is displaced. SCFE may compromise the blood supply to the femoral head and cause avascular necrosis, mainly when there is instability between the fragments [12].

4.2. X-Ray in Adult Age. In the adult hip there are important landmarks to be recognized on plain film radiographs (Figure 5):

(A) Iliopectineal or iliopubic line is formed by the arcuate line of the ilium and the superior border of the superior pubic ramus up to the pubic symphysis. It conforms to the inner margin of the pelvic ring and it is part of the anterior column of the acetabulum.

(B) The ilioischial line of Köhler begins at the medial border of the iliac wing and extends along the medial border of the ischium to end at the ischial tuberosity. It is part of the posterior column of the acetabulum.

(C) *Acetabular Floor.* In normal conditions the floor of the acetabular fossa is lateral to the ilioischial line by 2 mm in men and 1 mm in women. When the acetabular floor overlaps or overpasses the ilioischial line, the diagnosis of coxa profunda can be made. Nevertheless, coxa profunda had been found in 76% of asymptomatic hips, mainly in women. Therefore, this as an isolate criterion is not enough to make the diagnosis of pincer-type impingement [13]. A more severe condition is protrusio acetabuli, diagnosed when the femoral head overlaps or overpasses the ilioischial line (Figure 5).

(D) The teardrop represents a summation of shadows. Its medial aspect corresponds to the inner cortex of the pelvis and the lateral edge with the acetabular notch and the anteroinferior portion of the quadrilateral plate [14]. It is not present at birth but gradually develops due to pressure of the femoral head.

In the adult hip, normal joint space ranges from 3 to 5 mm and must be uniform. Values under 2 mm are consistent with joint space narrowing [15]. The most important measurements are detailed in Figure 6 and Table 1.

Acetabular depth value under 250 characterizes the dysplastic hip [16].

In normal conditions the acetabulum covers 75% of the femoral head. This coverage can be determined by three different measurements: lateral center-edge angle of Wiberg, anterior center-edge angle, and femoral extrusion index. Femoral extrusion index measures the percentage of

TABLE 1: Measurements in adult hip.

Measurement	Measure	Normal value
Acetabular depth ratio	Deepness of acetabulum	>250
Center-edge angle	Coverage of acetabulum	20–40
Tönnis angle	Slope of the sourcil	0–10°
Sharp angle	Acetabular slope	<45°
Crossing ratio	Percentage of acetabular walls crossing	<20%
Alpha angle	Degree of bulging of the femoral head-neck junction	Male > 68° Female > 50°
Femoral head-neck offset	Offset of the femoral head with regard to most prominent aspect of the femora neck	>10 mm
Offset percentage	Femoral head-neck offset related to femoral head diameter	>0.18

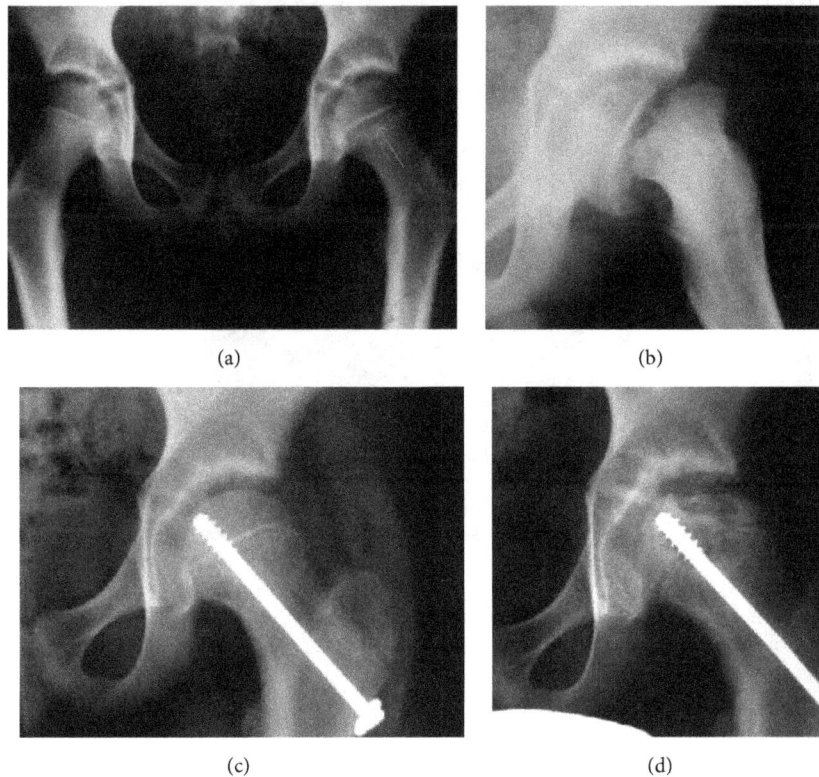

(a) (b)

(c) (d)

FIGURE 4: (a) X-ray of a 10-year-old child with left hip pain. It was considered normal at emergency despite the widening of the left physis (arrow). Two weeks later epiphysiolysis was evident (b). Despite appropriate surgical reduction (c) osteonecrosis developed and femoral head collapsed 1 month later (d).

the femoral head that lies outside of the acetabular roof. This percentage must be inferior to 25% in adults.

Center-edge Wiberg's angle measures the superior-lateral coverage of the femoral head. It is useful in children older than 5 years and in adulthood. For children between 5 and 10 years the minimum normal value is 15°, and in adults it is about 20°, although after 55 years this minimum increases to 24° [17]. Values over 40° indicate overcoverage.

Anterior center-edge Lequesne's angle can be measured in a false profile view of the hip or in a sagittal CT scan. In this case the tangent line touches the anterior rim of the acetabulum. Values under 20° indicate undercoverage of the femoral head [18].

The acetabular slope can also be measured by different methods. The Tönnis angle quantifies the slope of the sourcil (the sclerotic weight-bearing portion of the acetabulum). Values over 10° are considered a risk factor for instability, while values under 0° are considered a risk factor for pincer impingement.

The Sharp angle is a global way to measure the acetabular slope. Angles over 45° are indicative of acetabular dysplasia.

Normal acetabulum is oriented in anteversion. Its value ranges from 15 to 20° in the equatorial plane of the acetabulum and decreases gradually towards the acetabular roof, where normal values range from 0 to 5°. Retroversion of the upper part of the acetabulum has been related with

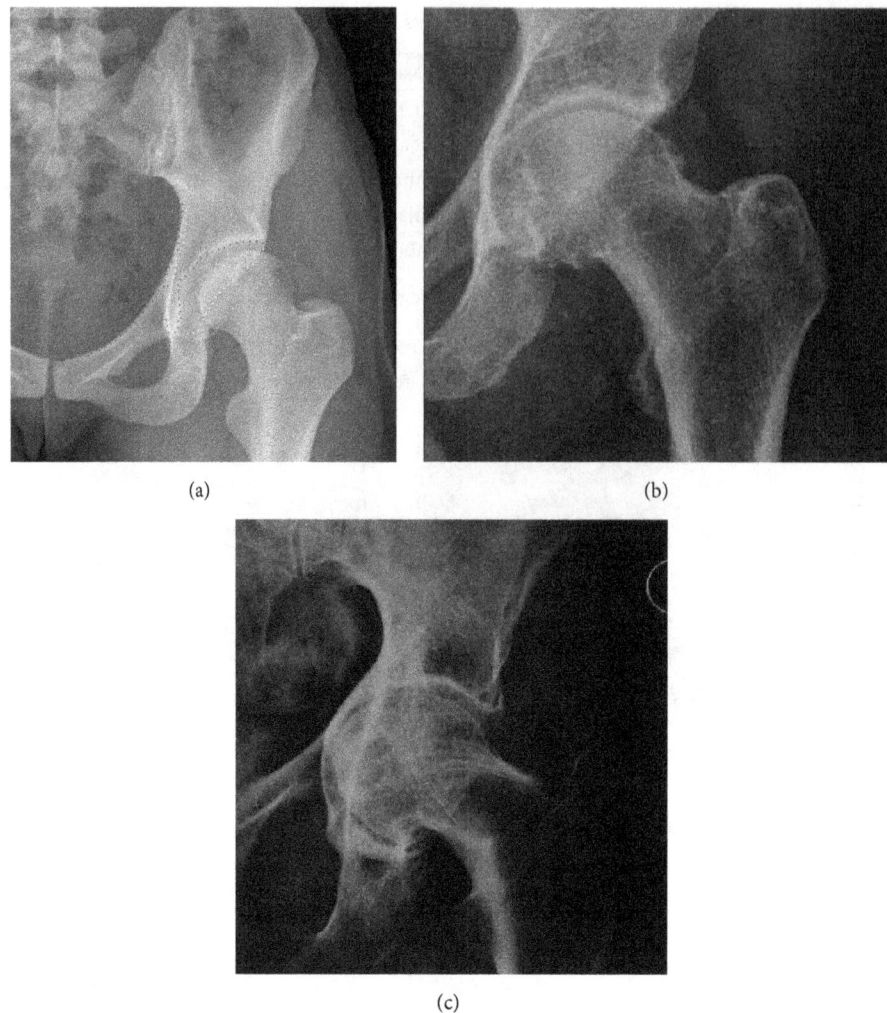

FIGURE 5: (a) Iliopectineal line (red), ilioischial line (yellow), tear drop (blue), acetabular fossa (brown), and anterior (white) and posterior (green) wall of the acetabuli showing mild upper crossover sign. (b) Coxa profunda. (c) Protrusio acetabuli.

pincer type impingement. In radiography the presence of a "crossover sign" is produced when the posterior wall of the acetabulum crosses the anterior wall before reaching the acetabular roof. It is a sign of acetabular retroversion and it has been linked with overcoverage and pincer impingement. Nevertheless, this sign has been described in 6% of the normal population [19]. Therefore, more important than its presence is the percentage of crossing. This ratio is considered significant if it is over 20% [20].

Other signs associated with acetabular retroversion are the sciatic spine and posterior wall signs. The first one is considered positive when the sciatic spine is projected medial to the iliopectineal line in an AP radiography of the spine, indicating that it is not just the acetabulum but the whole hemipelvis that is twisted into retroversion. The second sign is considered positive when the posterior wall edge is medial to the center of the femoral head, indicating deficiency of the posterior wall.

In normal conditions there is a symmetric concave contour at the junction of the anterior and posterior profile of the femoral head and neck. Loss of this concavity or bone bulging may lead to cam type impingement. The degree of this deformity can be measured by the alpha angle. Although it can be measured in the cross-lateral view, the 45° Dunn view is considered more sensitive and the frog leg view more specific in determining pathologic values. Debate about which values are considered normal is still in progress. Based on the Copenhagen Osteoarthritis Study, a recent work defined three ranges of values for the α-angle: pathological ($\geq 83°$ in men and $\geq 57°$ in women), borderline (69° to 82° in men, 51° to 56° in women), and normal ($\leq 68°$ in men and $\leq 50°$ in women) [21].

The offset between the neck and femoral head can also be calculated in the lateral projection of the hip. A value of less than 10 mm is considered pathologic. The percentage is calculated by dividing the distance between the femoral head and the neck lines by the femoral head diameter. If this percentage is under 0.18 there is high probability of cam type impingement [22].

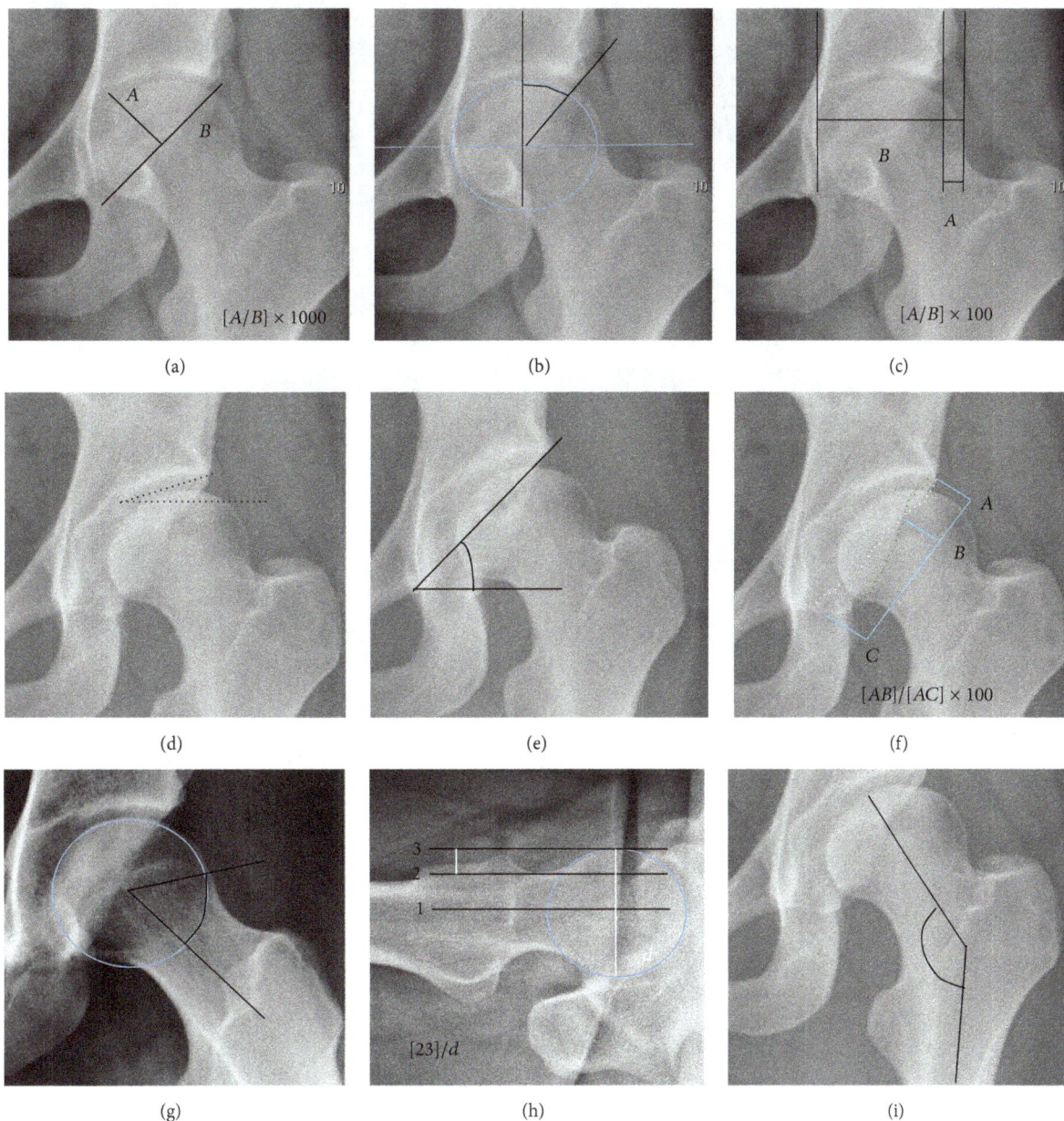

FIGURE 6: (a) Acetabular depth ratio. (b) Center-edge angle of Wiberg. (c) Femoral extrusion index. (d) Tönnis angle. (e) Sharp angle. (f) Crossing ratio. (g) Alpha angle measured in 45° Dunn view. (h) Offset percentage measured in cross-lateral view. (i) Cervical diaphyseal angle.

The angle formed between the femoral neck and femoral diaphysis ranges from 120° to 140°. Coxa valga is diagnosed if the angle is higher and coxa vara if the angle is lower than this normal range.

Although femoral version or torsion can be measured by radiographs, CT overcomes the inconsistencies demonstrated in the measurements made by biplane radiography [23].

In adults, one of the main indications for radiographs is the detection of osteoarthritic changes (Figure 1(e)). Nevertheless, radiographs usually detect advanced osteoarthritis that can be graded according to the Tönnis classifications. The grading system ranges from 0 to 3, where 0 shows no sign of osteoarthritis. Intermediate grade 1 shows mild sclerosis

of the head and acetabulum, slight joint space narrowing, and marginal osteophyte lipping. Grade 2 presents with small cysts in the femoral head or acetabulum, moderate joint space narrowing, and moderate loss of sphericity of the femoral head. Grade 3 is the severest form of osteoarthritis, which manifests as severe narrowing of the joint space, large subchondral cyst with productive bone changes that may lead to deformity of the bone components of the joint [24], while secondary osteoarthritis due to calcium pyrophosphate deposition can be diagnosed when calcification of hyaline cartilage and fibrocartilage is detected [25].

There are other pathological conditions that can affect the hip joint and radiographs help to make the appropriate diagnosis. Acute bacterial septic arthritis can be diagnosed by

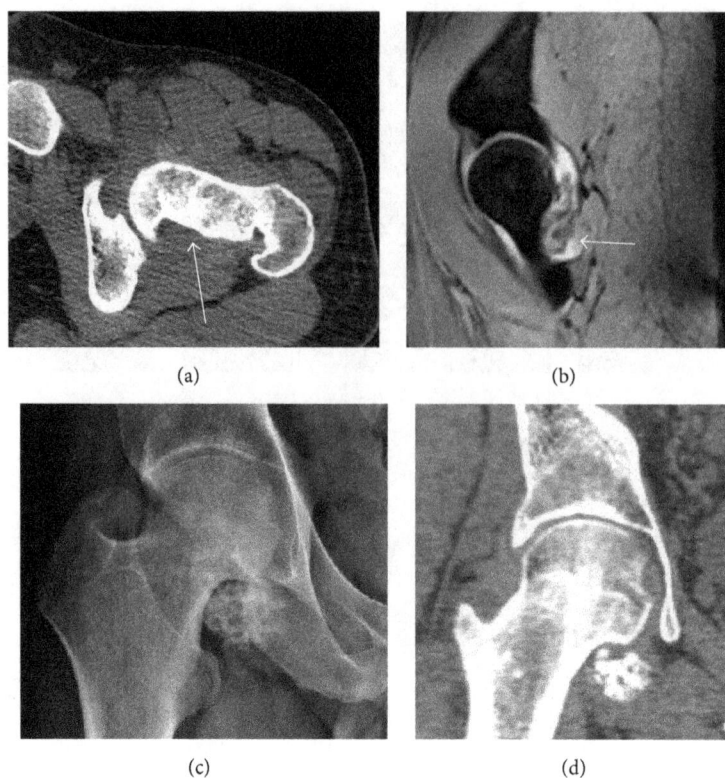

FIGURE 7: (a) Axial CT image of pigmented villonodular synovitis eroding the posterior cortex of the femoral neck. (b) Sagittal T2* gradient echo image showing a posterior soft tissue mass with hypointense areas secondary to hemosiderin deposition. (c) X-ray film and computed tomography (d) in synovial chondromatosis.

radiographs when a fast regional osteoporosis and destructive monoarticular process develops (Figure 1(f)). In case of tuberculous or brucella arthritis it is manifested as a slow progressive process, and diagnosis may be delayed [26].

Synovial chondromatosis can be confidently diagnosed by X-ray when calcified cartilaginous chondromas are seen. However, other synovial proliferative processes, such as pigmented villonodular synovitis, require MRI for accurate diagnosis, although noncalcified synovitis can be suspected in radiographs by indirect signs, such as soft tissue swelling and/or erosions in the femoral head, femoral neck, or acetabulum (Figure 7) [27].

Radiological signs of transient osteoporosis of the hip include localized osteoporosis of the femoral head and neck (Figure 8). Nevertheless, final diagnosis has to be made with MRI to differentiate it from avascular necrosis and from insufficiency or stress fractures of the femoral head or neck. In case of AVN, radiographs can only demonstrate delayed or advanced signs. Staging according to Ficat classification ranges between normal appearance (stage I), slight increased density in the femoral head (stage II), subchondral collapse of the femoral head with or without "crescent" sign (stage III), and advanced collapse with secondary osteoarthritis (stage IV) [28]. In the case of stress or insufficiency fractures X-ray sensitivity has been proven to be much lower than MRI, which is currently the gold standard [29].

5. Magnetic Resonance

Many pathological conditions of the hip are detected early by MRI due to its high soft tissue resolution and sensitivity. Its accuracy in studying acute hip pain in children has proved to be superior to ultrasound and plan film radiography. However, MRI accessibility and the need of sedation relegate its use to selected cases in which diagnosis is not clear with less demanding techniques. These include differentiating transient synovitis from a septic arthritis or osteomyelitis [30], diagnosis of inflammatory joint disease or bone tumors, and early detection and follow-up of Perthes disease.

MRI findings correlate with prognosis in LCPD. These include extent and distribution of epiphyseal necrosis, subchondral ossified nucleus fracture, involvement of the lateral pillar, and disturbance of physeal growth, including presence of transphyseal neovascularity or bridging [31].

Recent studies have been focused on the role of diffusion weighted MRI because it does not need contrast medium administration. ADC ratio of the femoral metaphysis was positively correlated with the Herring classification. ADC ratio superior to 1.63 indicates bad prognosis with 89% sensitivity and 58% specificity [32].

In adult patients, MRI is currently playing a definite role in the assessment of osteoarthritis. Although traditionally belonging to the arena of radiographs, the role of MRI has

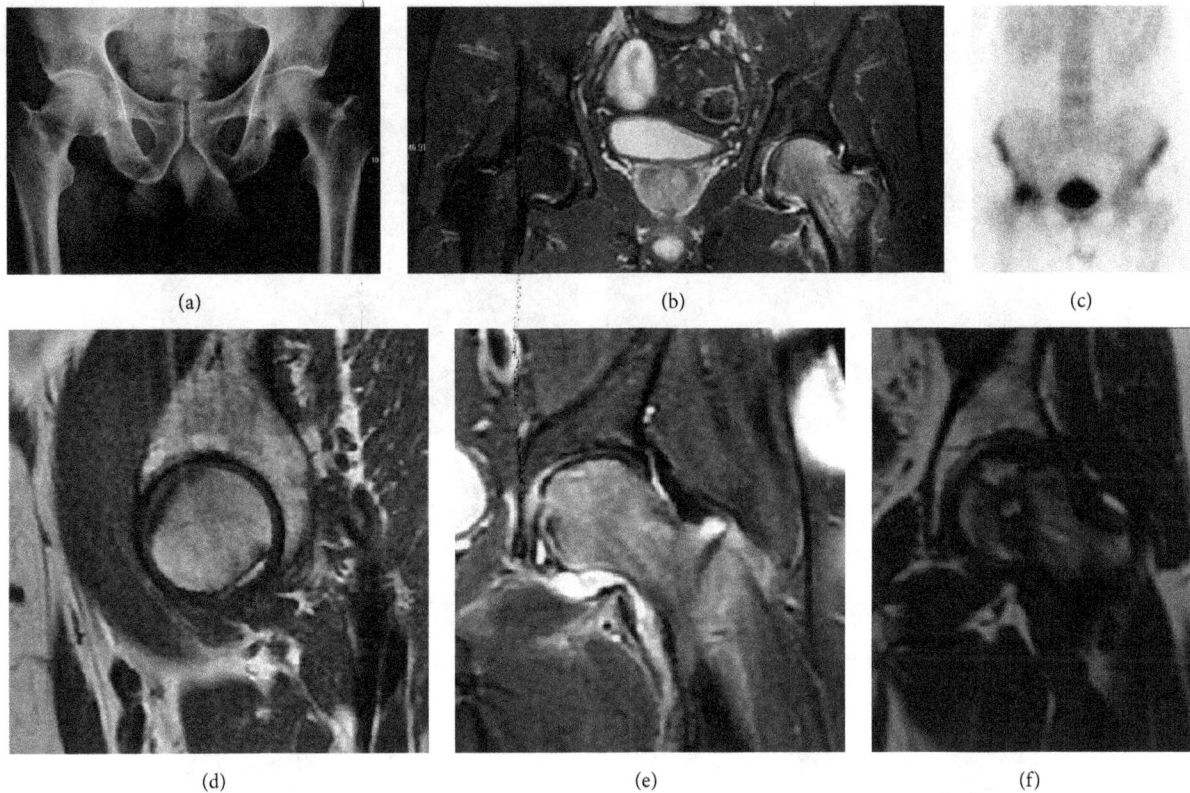

(a) (b) (c)

(d) (e) (f)

FIGURE 8: (a) X-ray of a patient with transient osteoporosis of the left hip showing osteoporosis. (b) Coronal stir imaging showing diffuse edema. Scintigraphy (c), sagittal T1 (d), and coronal PD fat sat (e) of a patient with a subchondral fracture of the femoral head with convex shape to the articular surface. Coronal T1 (f) of a patient with avascular necrosis of the femoral head.

been stressed after the term femoral acetabular impingement was coined in 2003 [33]. Growing interest has been focused in accurate diagnosis of the acetabular and femoral morphological abnormalities that may lead to early osteoarthritis.

MR imaging is considered paramount to these objectives, mainly when surgery is considered, due to the ability of MRI to portray the whole section of the femoral neck surface, as well as to image the labrum and articular cartilage.

Diagnosis of impingement can only be achieved if, besides imaging findings, there are also clinical symptoms and positive impingement maneuvers [34].

Most of the angles and measurements described in the plain radiograph section can be accurately reproduced on MRI. In addition, the superiority of MRI resolution with intra-articular contrast allows detection of labral and chondral abnormalities that may influence the choice of medical, percutaneous, or surgical management (Figure 9).

MR arthrography has proven superior in accuracy when compared to native MR imaging. It is considered the best technique to assess the labrum. Knowledge of the normal variable morphology of the labrum helps to differentiate tears from normal variants. A triangular shape is most commonly seen in 66% of asymptomatic volunteers, but round, flattened, and absent labra can also be found in asymptomatic populations [35]. MR arthrography has demonstrated sensitivity over 90% and specificity close to 100% in detecting labral

tears. Loose bodies are demonstrated as filling defects surrounded by the hyperintense gadolinium [36, 37].

Association between labral tears and chondral damage has been demonstrated. This underscores the interaction between cartilage and labrum damage in the progression of osteoarthritis [38]. Chondral damage to the posteroinferior part of the acetabulum as a contrecoup lesion occurs in approximately one-third of pincer cases secondary to persistent abutment on the anterior part of the joint leading to a slight posteroinferior subluxation. This is considered a bad prognosis sign [39].

MR arthrography can also demonstrate ligamentum teres rupture or capsular laxity, which are debated causes of microinstability of the hip [40]. Elongation of the capsule or injury to the iliofemoral ligament or labrum may be secondary to microtrauma in athletes [41]. MR can demonstrate abnormalities in these cases, such as increased joint volume or a ligamentum teres tear (Figure 9).

Intra-articular osseous causes of pain include several conditions: avascular necrosis (AVN), transient osteoporosis of the hip (TOH), tumors, and stress or insufficiency fractures. All these entities may present with a pattern of bone marrow edema characterized by decreased signal intensity on T1 weighted images and increased signal intensity on fluid sensitive sequences, such as fat saturated T2-weighted or STIR images. When there is no evidence of a focal lesion

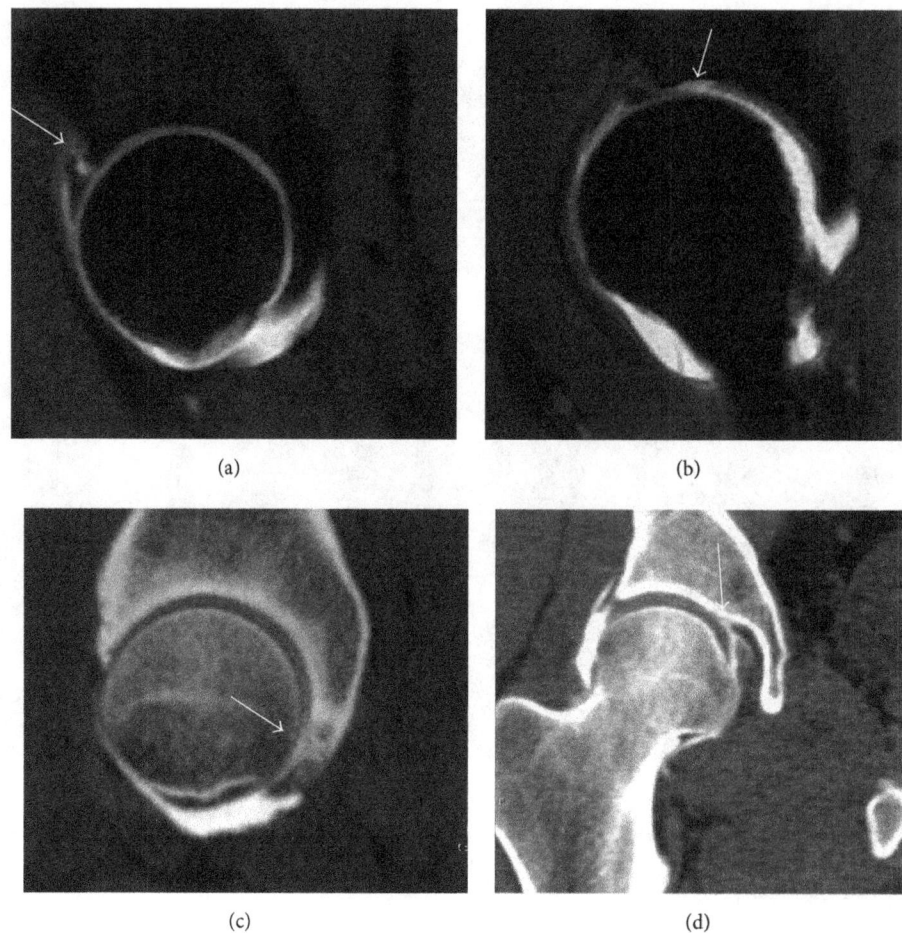

(a)

(b)

(c)

(d)

FIGURE 9: Sagittal T1 weighted images showing anterosuperior labral tear (a) and chondral lesion (b). Sagittal CT-arthrography showing posteroinferior chondral injury (c) and coronal CT-arthrography (d) showing ligamentum teres tear.

associated with the edema pattern, TOH is suspected [42]. When a band of low intensity is seen inside the edematous area, the shape and length of this band become important. It is generally convex to the articular surface in the case of subchondral stress or insufficiency fractures, whereas it is concave, circumscribing all of the necrotic segment, in cases of AVN. When doubts do persist, gadolinium-enhanced MRI tends to show that the proximal portion beyond the band is enhanced in fractures but is not in AVN [43].

MRI has been shown to have 100% sensitivity and specificity in prospective studies of occult hip fractures. These fractures were diagnosed by bone marrow edema and a low signal fracture line, mainly on T1 or T2 weighted images [44] (Figure 10).

In synovial proliferative disorders, MRI demonstrates synovial hypertrophy. In the case of PVNS, characteristic foci of low signal intensity related to hemosiderin deposition are better seen on gradient echo T2* images [45] (Figure 7). In the case of synovial osteochondromatosis, the synovial hypertrophy is accompanied by intermediate signal cartilaginous loose bodies and/or low signal calcified loose bodies [46].

6. Computed Tomography

Due to radiation concerns, CT has been relegated after MRI in the study of intra-articular causes of hip pain. The only exception where CT is considered superior to MRI is in bone tumors, because of its ability in characterizing matrix calcifications, and in depicting the anatomy of acute traumatic fractures. Typical matrix calcifications include the following: (a) osteoid mineralization, like a dense cloud, (b) chondroid calcification, reproducing a punctate popcorn pattern, or (c) fibrous calcification, ground glass-like appearance. There are also tumors that typically do not show matrix calcification. CT is also used for accurate localization of the nidus in osteoid osteomas and this must be differentiated from Brodie's abscess or a stress fracture [47]. The current standard treatment of osteoid osteoma is percutaneous radiofrequency ablation and this is usually performed under CT guidance [48].

Quite often, CT is widely available unlike MRI, especially in the acute setting. CT is performed in this setting when doubt about the existence of a fracture persists following plain radiograph. Modern multidetector computed tomography

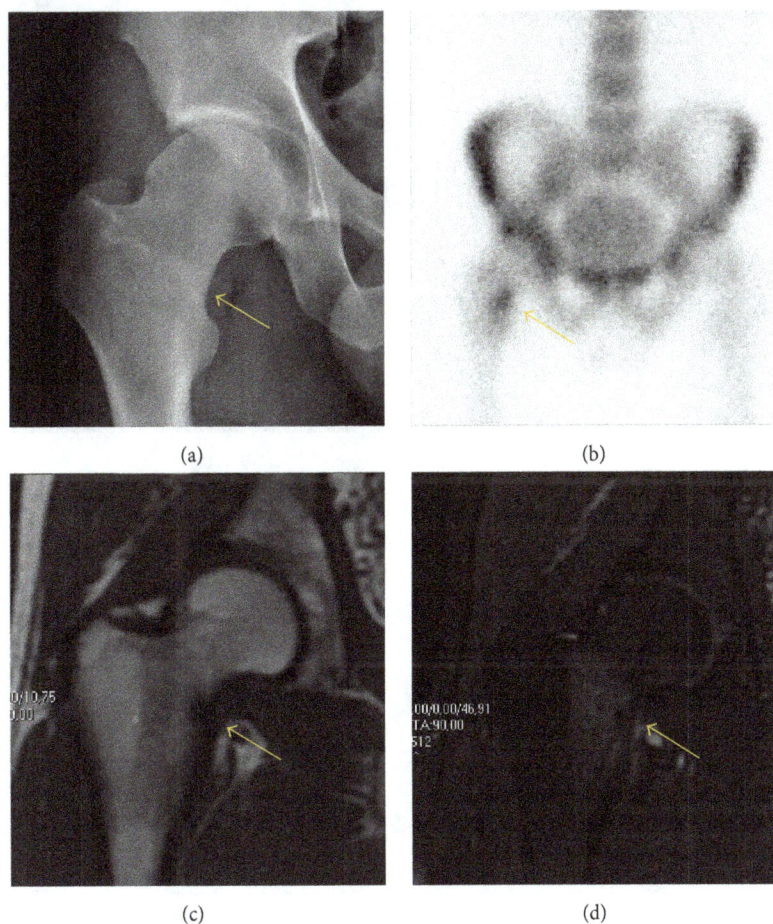

(a)   (b)

(c)   (d)

FIGURE 10: Stress femoral neck fracture in a young athlete barely visible in X-ray film as a sclerotic line (arrow) (a). Tc 99 scintigraphy shows a band of uptake (b), while T1 (c) and DP fat saturated (d) weighted MR images showed the fracture line and a pattern of edema.

(MDCT) shows results comparable with MRI for detecting occult fractures [49].

Due to the submillimeter resolution of MDCT arthrography, many authors consider this technique complementary to MR arthrography. It may even have superior sensitivity in detecting cartilage pathology, but lesser detecting labral tears [50, 51].

CT can also be used to obtain accurate measurement of the femoral version and torsion. The femoral version is measured by an angle formed between a line through the femoral head-neck axis and another horizontal line drawn between both ischial tuberosities. Normal values range between 5 and 25°. Retroversion is considered abnormal.

Femoral torsion is the angle between a line along the femoral head and neck axis and a second line that is touching the posterior border of both femoral condyles. The normal value at birth is approximately 32° and decreases gradually with age. In adults, the normal value ranges from 10° to 20° [52].

7. Ultrasound

Ultrasound is the first-choice technique for diagnosis of newborns hip dysplasia. In experienced hands with appropriate technology, ultrasound can also be useful during the first year of life [53]. Some European healthcare systems encourage universal ultrasound screening in neonates between the sixth and eighth weeks. Although it shows higher initial costs caused, it leads to significant reduction in the total number and overall costs of dysplastic hips undergoing operative and nonoperative treatment [54, 55].

Ultrasound allows categorizing pediatric hips, according to Graf's criteria, in four main types: normal, immature, and dysplastic (subluxed and dislocated) [56]. This classification is based on measurements of the acetabular inclination angle (alpha), cartilage roof angle (beta), and infant age [57]. The femoral head coverage can also be determined by dividing the length of the femoral head covered by the acetabular fossa and the diameter of the femoral head. Its lower normal limits are 47% for boys and 44% for girls [58] (Figure 11).

In a recent study, including newborns with high clinical suspicion for DDH [59] (Ortolani/Barlow test, asymmetry in abduction of 20° or greater, breech presentation, leg-length discrepancy, and first-degree relative treated for DDH), hip sonography led to a change in clinical diagnosis in 52% of hips and to a change in management plan in 32% of hips. It obviated further follow-up in 23%, strengthening its role as an important technique reassuring the clinical diagnosis [60].

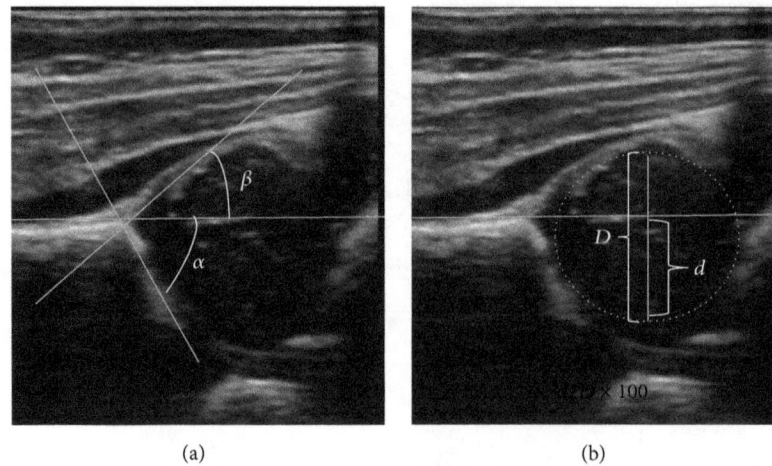

(a)   (b)

FIGURE 11: (a) Useful ultrasound measures in neonatal hip sonography, alpha and beta angles. (b) Measurement of femoral head coverage.

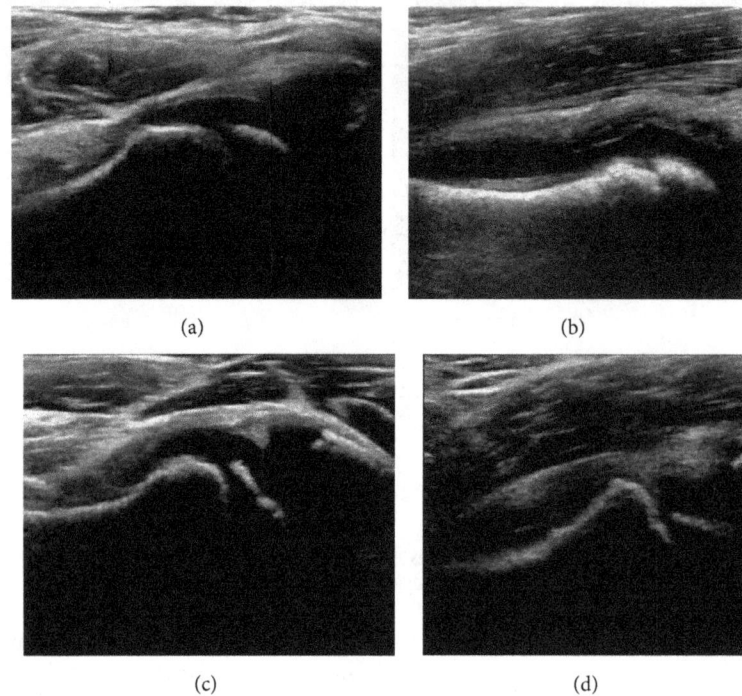

(a)   (b)

(c)   (d)

FIGURE 12: (a) Normal ultrasound appearance of the femoral head-neck junction. (b) Joint effusion in transient synovitis of the hip. (c) Flattening of the femoral head in a patient with Perthes disease. (d) Step in the femoral head-neck junction in a patient with SCFE.

During childhood, ultrasound is a quick method to assess hip pain and quite often may be used to avoid use of irradiating techniques, such as radiography or CT. Ultrasound allows evaluation of joint effusion, synovial thickening and neovascularity, the bone/cartilage contour, and the femoral head-neck alignment. Although sonography is extremely sensitive in detecting increased synovial fluid, it is nonspecific and cannot be used with accuracy to determine the type of fluid. Transient synovitis of the hip, despite being the most frequent cause of pain in children between 3 and 10 years, remains a diagnosis of exclusion. It usually shows

anechoic fluid, but echogenic fluid can also be found [61]. The effusion is considered pathologic when it is measured at >2 mm in thickness [62]. The differential diagnosis is wide, including osteomyelitis, septic arthritis, primary or metastatic lesions, LCPD, and SCFE [63]. Discrimination from septic arthritis is challenging, often requiring joint aspiration. In septic arthritis, US is able to demonstrate a hip joint effusion, synovial thickening, and cartilage damage, although the appearances are nonspecific [64].

A step between the head and the physis can be detected in children with SCFE, while abnormalities in the femoral head contour may suggest the presence of LCPD. In both cases, radiographs are mandatory to confirm diagnosis and severity [65] (Figure 12).

In adults, the most common application for US is to detect tendon or muscle injuries, effusion or synovitis within the hip joint or its adjacent bursae [66]. Joint effusions may be due to many intra-articular processes and this may need another imaging technique to achieve a specific diagnosis.

8. Nuclear Medicine

Bone scanning in patients with hip pain can be complementary to other imaging studies, mainly in indeterminate bone lesions to clarify whether it is an active lesion with abnormal radiotracer accumulation. Nevertheless, MRI has replaced scintigraphy in the diagnosis of most of these conditions. An example is stress or insufficiency fractures: increased uptake is usually present in around 80% of fractures within 24 h, and 95% of fractures reveal activity by 72 h following trauma [67], showing an overall sensitivity of 93% and specificity of 95% [68]. MRI is superior to bone scans in terms of sensitivity (99%-100%) and specificity (100%) [69, 70]. Moreover, a bone scan does not provide detailed anatomical location of the fracture, and further imaging is usually required [71].

Conflict of Interests

The authors declare that there is no conflict of interests regarding the publication of this paper.

References

[1] L. M. Tibor and J. K. Sekiya, "Differential diagnosis of pain around the hip joint," *Arthroscopy*, vol. 24, no. 12, pp. 1407–1421, 2008.

[2] E. Maslowski, W. Sullivan, J. F. Harwood et al., "The diagnostic validity of hip provocation maneuvers to detect intra-articular hip pathology," *PM & R*, vol. 2, no. 3, pp. 174–181, 2010.

[3] D. Tönnis, "Normal values of the hip joint for the evaluation of X-rays in children and adults," *Clinical Orthopaedics and Related Research*, vol. 119, pp. 39–47, 1976.

[4] H. Omeroğlu, A. Kaya, and B. Güçlü, "Evidence-based current concepts in the radiological diagnosis and follow-up of developmental dysplasia of the hip," *Acta Orthopaedica et Traumatologica Turcica*, vol. 41, supplement 1, pp. 14–18, 2007.

[5] D. Tönnis, *Congenital Dysplasia and Dislocation of the Hip in Children and Adults*, Springer, Berlin, Germany, 1987.

[6] U. Narayanan, K. Mulpuri, W. N. Sankar, N. M. P. Clarke, H. Hosalkar, and C. T. Price, "Reliability of a new radiographic classification for developmental dysplasia of the hip," *Journal of Pediatric Orthopaedics*, vol. 35, no. 5, pp. 478–484, 2015.

[7] J. R. Dwek, C. B. Chung, and D. J. Sartoris, "Developmental dysplasia of the hip," in *Diagnosis of Bone and Joint Disorders*, D. Resnick, Ed., pp. 4355–4381, Saunders, Philadelphia, Pa, USA, 4th edition, 2002.

[8] E. J. Eyring, D. R. Bjornson, and C. A. Peterson, "Early diagnostic and prognostic signs in Legg-Calvé-Perthes disease," *American Journal of Roentgenology*, vol. 93, pp. 382–387, 1965.

[9] C. Gigante, P. Frizziero, and S. Turra, "Prognostic value of Catterall and Herring classification in Legg-Calvé-Perthes disease: follow-up to skeletal maturity of 32 patients," *Journal of Pediatric Orthopaedics*, vol. 22, no. 3, pp. 345–349, 2002.

[10] J. A. Herring, H. T. Hui, and R. Browne, "Legg-Calvé-Perthes disease. Part I: classification of radiographs with use of the modified lateral pillar and stulberg classifications," *The Journal of Bone & Joint Surgery*, vol. 86, no. 10, pp. 2103–2120, 2004.

[11] J. A. Herring, T. K. Hui, and R. Browne, "Legg-Calvé-Perthes disease. Part II: prospective multicenter study of the effect of treatment on outcome," *The Journal of Bone & Joint Surgery—American Volume*, vol. 86, no. 10, pp. 2121–2134, 2004.

[12] R. T. Loder, "Correlation of radiographic changes with disease severity and demographic variables in children with stable slipped capital femoral epiphysis," *Journal of Pediatric Orthopaedics*, vol. 28, no. 3, pp. 284–290, 2008.

[13] J. J. Nepple, C. L. Lehmann, J. R. Ross, P. L. Schoenecker, and J. C. Clohisy, "Coxa profunda is not a useful radiographic parameter for diagnosing pincer-type femoroacetabular impingement," *The Journal of Bone & Joint Surgery*, vol. 95, no. 5, pp. 417–423, 2013.

[14] V. B. Vare Jr., "The anatomy of the pelvic tear figure," *The Journal of Bone & Joint Surgery—American Volume*, vol. 34, no. 1, pp. 167–169, 1952.

[15] A. Troelsen, L. Rømer, S. Kring, B. Elmengaard, and K. Søballe, "Assessment of hip dysplasia and osteoarthritis: variability of different methods," *Acta Radiologica*, vol. 51, no. 2, pp. 187–193, 2010.

[16] D. R. Pedersen, C. A. Lamb, L. A. Dolan, H. M. Ralston, S. L. Weinstein, and J. A. Morcuende, "Radiographic measurements in developmental dysplasia of the hip: reliability and validity of a digitizing program," *Journal of Pediatric Orthopaedics*, vol. 24, no. 2, pp. 156–160, 2004.

[17] A. Ozcelik, H. Omeroglu, U. Inan, and S. Seber, "Center-edge angle values in normal hips of children and adults in Turkish population," *Journal of Arthroplasty Arthroscopic Surgery*, vol. 12, pp. 115–119, 2001.

[18] L. B. Laborie, T. G. Lehmann, I. Ø. Engesæter, L. B. Engesæter, and K. Rosendahl, "Is a positive femoroacetabular impingement test a common finding in healthy young adults?" *Clinical Orthopaedics and Related Research*, vol. 471, no. 7, pp. 2267–2277, 2013.

[19] M. Ezoe, M. Naito, and T. Inoue, "The prevalence of acetabular retroversion among various disorders of the hip," *The Journal of Bone & Joint Surgery—American Volume*, vol. 88, no. 2, pp. 372–379, 2006.

[20] C. Diaz-Ledezma, T. Novack, O. Marin-Peña, and J. Parvizi, "The relevance of the radiological signs of acetabular retroversion among patients with femoroacetabular impingement," *Bone and Joint Journal B*, vol. 95, no. 7, pp. 893–899, 2013.

[21] K. K. Gosvig, S. Jacobsen, S. Sonne-Holm, and P. Gebuhr, "The prevalence of cam-type deformity of the hip joint: a survey of 4151 subjects of the Copenhagen Osteoarthritis study," *Acta Radiologica*, vol. 49, no. 4, pp. 436–441, 2008.

[22] H. Eijer, M. Leunig, M. N. Mahomed, and R. Ganz, "Crosstable lateral radiograph for screening of anterior femoral head–neck offset in patients with femoro-acetabular impingement," *Hip International*, vol. 11, pp. 37–41, 2001.

[23] T. Y. Kuo, J. G. Skedros, and R. D. Bloebaum, "Measurement of femoral anteversion by biplane radiography and computed tomography imaging: comparison with an anatomic reference," *Investigative Radiology*, vol. 38, no. 4, pp. 221–229, 2003.

[24] J. C. Clohisy, J. C. Carlisle, P. E. Beaulé et al., "A systematic approach to the plain radiographic evaluation of the young adult hip," *The Journal of Bone & Joint Surgery—American Volume*, vol. 90, supplement 4, pp. 47–66, 2008.

[25] H. K. Ea and F. Lioté, "Calcium pyrophosphate dihydrate and basic calcium phosphate crystalinduced arthropathies: update on pathogenesis, clinical features, and therapy," *Current Rheumatology Reports*, vol. 6, no. 3, pp. 221–227, 2004.

[26] A. Pourbagher, M. A. Pourbagher, L. Savas et al., "Epidemiologic, clinical, and imaging findings in brucellosis patients with osteoarticular involvement," *American Journal of Roentgenology*, vol. 187, no. 4, pp. 873–880, 2006.

[27] M. A. Bhimani, J. F. Wenz, and F. J. Frassica, "Pigmented villonodular synovitis: keys to early diagnosis," *Clinical Orthopaedics and Related Research*, vol. 386, pp. 197–202, 2001.

[28] R. P. Ficat, "Idiopathic bone necrosis of the femoral head. Early diagnosis and treatment," *The Journal of Bone & Joint Surgery—British Volume*, vol. 67, no. 1, pp. 3–9, 1985.

[29] R. Chana, A. Noorani, N. Ashwood, U. Chatterji, J. Healy, and P. Baird, "The role of MRI in the diagnosis of proximal femoral fractures in the elderly," *Injury*, vol. 37, no. 2, pp. 185–189, 2006.

[30] W. J. Yang, S. A. Im, G.-Y. Lim et al., "MR imaging of transient synovitis: differentiation from septic arthritis," *Pediatric Radiology*, vol. 36, no. 11, pp. 1154–1158, 2006.

[31] J. R. Dillman and R. J. Hernandez, "MRI of Legg-Calvé-Perthes disease," *American Journal of Roentgenology*, vol. 193, no. 5, pp. 1394–1407, 2009.

[32] C. Baunin, D. Sanmartin-Viron, F. Accadbled et al., "Prognosis value of early diffusion MRI in Legg Perthes Calvé disease," *Orthopaedics and Traumatology: Surgery & Research*, vol. 100, no. 3, pp. 317–321, 2014.

[33] R. Ganz, J. Parvizi, M. Beck, M. Leunig, H. Nötzli, and K. A. Siebenrock, "Femoroacetabular impingement: a cause for osteoarthritis of the hip," *Clinical Orthopaedics and Related Research*, vol. 417, pp. 112–120, 2003.

[34] M. Lequesne and L. Bellaïche, "Anterior femoroacetabular impingement: an update," *Joint Bone Spine*, vol. 79, no. 3, pp. 249–255, 2012.

[35] F. E. Lecouvet, B. C. Vande Berg, J. Malghem et al., "MR imaging of the acetabular labrum: variations in 200 asymptomatic hips," *American Journal of Roentgenology*, vol. 167, no. 4, pp. 1025–1028, 1996.

[36] G. A. Toomayan, W. R. Holman, N. M. Major, S. M. Kozlowicz, and T. P. Vail, "Sensitivity of MR arthrography in the evaluation of acetabular labral tears," *American Journal of Roentgenology*, vol. 186, no. 2, pp. 449–453, 2006.

[37] B. A. Freedman, B. K. Potter, P. A. Dinauer, J. R. Giuliani, T. R. Kuklo, and K. P. Murphy, "Prognostic value of magnetic resonance arthrography for Czerny stage II and III acetabular labral tears," *Arthroscopy*, vol. 22, no. 7, pp. 742–747, 2006.

[38] J. C. McCarthy, P. C. Noble, M. R. Schuck, J. Wright, and J. Lee, "The Otto E. Aufranc Award: the role of labral lesions to development of early degenerative hip disease," *Clinical Orthopaedics and Related Research*, vol. 393, pp. 25–37, 2001.

[39] M. Tannast, K. A. Siebenrock, and S. E. Anderson, "Femoroacetabular impingement: radiographic diagnosis—what the radiologist should know," *American Journal of Roentgenology*, vol. 188, no. 6, pp. 1540–1552, 2007.

[40] L. Cerezal, A. Kassarjian, A. Canga et al., "Anatomy, biomechanics, imaging, and management of ligamentum teres injuries," *RadioGraphics*, vol. 30, no. 6, pp. 1637–1651, 2010.

[41] B. Shu and M. R. Safran, "Hip instability: anatomic and clinical considerations of traumatic and atraumatic instability," *Clinics in Sports Medicine*, vol. 30, no. 2, pp. 349–367, 2011.

[42] F. Ruiz-Santiago, F. C. Pérez, and J. M. T. Fernández, "Clinical and radiological follow-up until its resolution of a case of subchondral fracture of the femoral head," *European Journal of Radiology Extra*, vol. 61, no. 3, pp. 105–108, 2007.

[43] S. Ikemura, T. Yamamoto, G. Motomura, Y. Nakashima, T. Mawatari, and Y. Iwamoto, "MRI evaluation of collapsed femoral heads in patients 60 years old or older: differentiation of subchondral insufficiency fracture from osteonecrosis of the femoral head," *American Journal of Roentgenology*, vol. 195, no. 1, pp. W63–W68, 2010.

[44] P. D. Evans, C. Wilson, and K. Lyons, "Comparison of MRI with bone scanning for suspected hip fracture in elderly patients," *The Journal of Bone & Joint Surgery*, vol. 76, no. 1, pp. 158–159, 1994.

[45] C. Fang and J. Teh, "Imaging of the hip," *Imaging*, vol. 15, no. 4, pp. 205–216, 2003.

[46] S. H. Kim, S. J. Hong, J. S. Park et al., "Idiopathic synovial osteochondromatosis of the hip: radiographic and MR appearances in 15 patients," *Korean Journal of Radiology*, vol. 3, no. 4, pp. 254–259, 2002.

[47] J. W. Chai, S. H. Hong, J.-Y. Choi et al., "Radiologic diagnosis of osteoid osteoma: from simple to challenging findings," *RadioGraphics*, vol. 30, no. 3, pp. 737–749, 2010.

[48] F. Ruiz Santiago, M. del Mar Castellano García, L. Guzmán Álvarez, J. L. Martínez Montes, M. Ruiz García, and J. M. Tristán Fernández, "Percutaneous treatment of bone tumors by radiofrequency thermal ablation," *European Journal of Radiology*, vol. 77, no. 1, pp. 156–163, 2011.

[49] S. K. Gill, J. Smith, R. Fox, and T. J. S. Chesser, "Investigation of occult hip fractures: the use of CT and MRI," *The Scientific World Journal*, vol. 2013, Article ID 830319, 4 pages, 2013.

[50] T. Nishii, H. Tanaka, K. Nakanishi, N. Sugano, H. Miki, and H. Yoshikawa, "Fat-suppressed 3D spoiled gradient-echo MRI and MDCT arthrography of articular cartilage in patients with hip dysplasia," *American Journal of Roentgenology*, vol. 185, no. 2, pp. 379–385, 2005.

[51] E. Perdikakis, T. Karachalios, P. Katonis, and A. Karantanas, "Comparison of MR-arthrography and MDCT-arthrography for detection of labral and articular cartilage hip pathology," *Skeletal Radiology*, vol. 40, no. 11, pp. 1441–1447, 2011.

[52] M. A. Westcott, M. C. Dynes, E. M. Remer, J. S. Donaldson, and L. S. Dias, "Congenital and acquired orthopedic abnormalities in patients with myelomeningocele," *RadioGraphics*, vol. 12, no. 6, pp. 1155–1173, 1992.

[53] R. M. Schwend, P. Schoenecker, B. S. Richards, J. M. Flynn, and M. Vitale, "Screening the newborn for developmental dysplasia of the hip. Now what do we do?" *Journal of Pediatric Orthopaedics*, vol. 27, no. 6, pp. 607–610, 2007.

[54] M. Thaler, R. Biedermann, J. Lair, M. Krismer, and F. Landauer, "Cost-effectiveness of universal ultrasound screening compared with clinical examination alone in the diagnosis and treatment of neonatal hip dysplasia in Austria," *The Journal of Bone & Joint Surgery—British Volume*, vol. 93, no. 8, pp. 1126–1130, 2011.

[55] A. Gray, D. Elbourne, C. Dezateux, A. King, A. Quinn, and F. Gardner, "Economic evaluation of ultrasonography in the diagnosis and management of developmental hip dysplasia in the United Kingdom and Ireland," *The Journal of Bone & Joint Surgery—American Volume*, vol. 87, no. 11, pp. 2472–2479, 2005.

[56] R. Graf, "Classification of hip joint dysplasia by means of sonography," *Archives of Orthopaedic and Traumatic Surgery*, vol. 102, no. 4, pp. 248–255, 1984.

[57] R. Graf, "Hip sonography: 20 years' experience and results," *HIP International*, vol. 17, supplement 5, pp. S8–S14, 2007.

[58] T. Terjesen, T. Bredland, and V. Berg, "Ultrasound for hip assessment in the newborn," *The Journal of Bone & Joint Surgery*, vol. 71, no. 5, pp. 767–773, 1989.

[59] A. Roposch, L. Q. Liu, F. Hefti, N. M. P. Clarke, and J. H. Wedge, "Standardized diagnostic criteria for developmental dysplasia of the hip in early infancy," *Clinical Orthopaedics and Related Research*, vol. 469, no. 12, pp. 3451–3461, 2011.

[60] E. Ashby and A. Roposch, "Diagnostic yield of sonography in infants with suspected hip dysplasia: diagnostic thinking efficiency and therapeutic efficiency," *American Journal of Roentgenology*, vol. 204, no. 1, pp. 177–181, 2015.

[61] G. J. Marchal, M. T. van Holsbeeck, M. Raes et al., "Transient synovitis of the hip in children: role of US," *Radiology*, vol. 162, no. 3, pp. 825–828, 1987.

[62] W. K. Rohrschneider, G. Fuchs, and J. Tröger, "Ultrasonographic evaluation of the anterior recess in the normal hip: a prospective study on 166 asymptomatic children," *Pediatric Radiology*, vol. 26, no. 9, pp. 629–634, 1996.

[63] S. U. Fischer and T. F. Beattie, "The limping child: epidemiology, assessment, and outcome," *The Journal of Bone & Joint Surgery—British Volume*, vol. 81, no. 6, pp. 1029–1034, 1999.

[64] M. M. Zamzam, "The role of ultrasound in differentiating septic arthritis from transient synovitis of the hip in children," *Journal of Pediatric Orthopaedics—Part B*, vol. 15, no. 6, pp. 418–422, 2006.

[65] C. E. Konstantoulakis, D. V. Petratos, M. Kokkinakis, E. Morakis, and J. N. Anastasopoulos, "Initial diagnostic approach of the irritable hip in childhood: is ultrasound really useful?" *Acta Orthopaedica Belgica*, vol. 77, no. 5, pp. 603–608, 2011.

[66] C. Martinoli, I. Garello, A. Marchetti et al., "Hip ultrasound," *European Journal of Radiology*, vol. 81, no. 12, pp. 3824–3831, 2012.

[67] P. Matin, "The appearance of bone scans following fractures, including immediate and long-term studies," *Journal of Nuclear Medicine*, vol. 20, no. 12, pp. 1227–1231, 1979.

[68] L. E. Holder, C. Schwarz, P. G. Wernicke, and R. H. Michael, "Radionuclide bone imaging in the early detection of fractures of the proximal femur (hip): multifactorial analysis," *Radiology*, vol. 174, no. 2, pp. 509–515, 1990.

[69] M. C. Cabarrus, A. Ambekar, Y. Lu, and T. M. Link, "MRI and CT of insufficiency fractures of the pelvis and the proximal femur," *American Journal of Roentgenology*, vol. 191, no. 4, pp. 995–1001, 2008.

[70] S. J. Rubin, J. D. Marquardt, R. H. Gottlieb, S. P. Meyers, S. M. S. Totterman, and R. E. O'Mara, "Magnetic resonance imaging: a cost-effective alternative to bone scintigraphy in the evaluation of patients with suspected hip fractures," *Skeletal Radiology*, vol. 27, no. 4, pp. 199–204, 1998.

[71] O. Lubovsky, M. Liebergall, Y. Mattan, Y. Weil, and R. Mosheiff, "Early diagnosis of occult hip fractures: MRI versus CT scan," *Injury*, vol. 36, no. 6, pp. 788–792, 2005.

25

The Disruption of Geniculocalcarine Tract in Occipital Neoplasm: A Diffusion Tensor Imaging Study

Yan Zhang,[1] Sihai Wan,[2] Ge Wen,[3] and Xuelin Zhang[3]

[1]Zhongshan Ophthalmic Center, State Key Laboratory of Ophthalmology, Sun Yat-sen University, Guangzhou, Guangdong 510060, China
[2]Department of Radiology, Lu Shan Sanatorium, Nanjing Military Region, Jiujiang, Jiangxi 332000, China
[3]Department of Radiology, Nanfang Hospital, Southern Medical University, Guangzhou, Guangdong 510515, China

Correspondence should be addressed to Xuelin Zhang; 13828470864@126.com

Academic Editor: Andreas H. Mahnken

Aim. Investigate the disruption of geniculocalcarine tract (GCT) in different occipital neoplasm by diffusion tensor imaging (DTI). *Methods.* Thirty-two subjects (44.1 ± 3.6 years) who had single occipital neoplasm (9 gliomas, 6 meningiomas, and 17 metastatic tumors) with ipsilateral GCT involved and thirty healthy subjects (39.2 ± 3.3 years) underwent conventional sequences scanning and diffusion tensor imaging by a 1.5T MR scanner. The diffusion-sensitive gradient direction is 13. Compare the fractional anisotropy (FA) and mean diffusivity (MD) values of healthy GCT with the corresponding values of GCT in peritumoral edema area. Perform diffusion tensor tractography (DTT) on GCT by the line propagation technique in all subjects. *Results.* The FA values of GCT in peritumoral edema area decreased ($P = 0.001$) while the MD values increased ($P = 0.002$) when compared with healthy subjects. There was no difference in the FA values across tumor types ($P = 0.114$) while the MD values of GCT in the metastatic tumor group were higher than the other groups ($P = 0.001$). GCTs were infiltrated in all the 9 gliomas cases, with displacement in 2 cases and disruption in 7 cases. GCTs were displaced in 6 meningiomas cases. GCTs were displaced in all the 7 metastatic cases, with disruption in 7 cases. *Conclusions.* DTI represents valid markers for evaluating GCT's disruption in occipital neoplasm. The disruption of GCT varies according to the properties of neoplasm.

1. Introduction

The eloquent white matter tracts can be delineated by diffusion tensor imaging (DTI) in patients with intracranial neoplasm. On the one hand, the exact relative position between the neoplasm and white matter tracts can be investigated and prompted for dysfunction [1–4]. For instance, motor disability with neoplasm related to the corticospinal tract has been investigated. DTT could visualize the exact location of tumors relevant to eloquent tracts and was found to be beneficial in the neurosurgical planning and postoperative assessment [5, 6]. On the other hand, diffusion indices may prompt neoplasm's histopathology type, tumor fraction, and axonal disruption of fiber tracts since their changes provide information for the underlying microanatomic changes or pathological changes [7–11].

Geniculocalcarine tract (GCT) is a fiber tract that originates from lateral geniculate body (LGB), passes through the sublenticular internal capsule and lenticular nucleus, along the lateral sagittal plane besides the occipital horn, and shapes like a convex lamina, and finally terminates in the calcarine fissure of occipital lobe. It conducts nervous impulse from LGB to the primary visual cortex in occipital lobe. Investigating the disruption of GCT in different occipital neoplasm may assist in identifying conditions occult to structural imaging and provide relational information that is critical to clinical decision making [12–15]. For instance, Salmela et al. used optic nerve tractography to aid in surgical planning for pediatric suprasellar tumors [15]. However, GCT involved in occipital neoplasm has not been delineated well in general.

TABLE 1: The parameters of each acquisition sequence in MRI scanning.

Acquisition sequences	TR/TE (ms)	Matrix size	FOV (cm)	NEX	Slice thickness/interslice separation (mm)	Acquisition time (min:sec)
T_1-FLAIR	2500/11.9	320×256	24×18	2	5/1.5	3:28
T_2WI	4900/99.3	320×224	24×18	2	5/1.5	1:42
T_2-FLAIR	8500/128	320×192	24×24	1	5/1.5	2:24
DTI SE-EPI	6000/60.1	128×128	24×24	2	3/0	6:52

In this research, we investigated GCTs in different occipital neoplasm by DTI and assumed that diffusion indices were valid markers in evaluating GCTs' disruption. We compared fractional anisotropy (FA) and mean diffusivity (MD) values of healthy GCTs with corresponding values of GCTs in peritumoral edema area and performed DTT on GCTs in all subjects.

2. Materials and Methods

2.1. Standard Protocol Approvals and Patient Consent. The research protocol was approved by the ethics committees for clinical research. All of the procedures involving the participants were conducted following the Declaration of Helsinki and institutional guidelines in compliance with the stated regulations. Written informed consent was obtained from all of the participants.

2.2. Subjects. The study group consisted of 32 subjects (17 males and 15 females; age: 44.1 ± 3.6 years, range: 35–61) who had single occipital neoplasm with ipsilateral GCT involved. These cases included 9 gliomas (World Health Organization grade II, 2 cases; grades III and IV, 7 cases), 6 meningiomas, and 17 metastatic tumors (lung cancer, 14 cases; breast cancer, 2 cases; gastric cancer, 1 case). All cases were certified by pathological examinations of surgical specimens. 14 subjects had homonymous hemianopia in the half visual field contralateral to the neoplasm.

For the control group, 30 healthy volunteers (15 males and 15 females; age: 39.2 ± 3.3 years, range: 20–63) were recruited from the outpatients.

Inclusion criteria consisted of (1) being right handed, (2) in the study group, each subject having a single occipital neoplasm with ipsilateral GCT involved in conventional MR scanning, (3) in the control group, no occupied lesion or abnormal findings in conventional MR scanning, (4) no history of neurological diseases including cerebrovascular disease, neurodegenerative disease, and trauma in both groups, and (5) no drug, alcohol, or addictive substance abuse.

2.3. Data Acquisition. MRIs were performed using a 1.5-Tesla scanner (Signa Twin, GE, USA) with an 8-channel head-phased array coil. The baseline scan was in the axial plane. Head movement was limited by vacuum fixation cushions.

All the subjects underwent conventional sequences scanning, including T_1-fluid attenuated inversion recovery (FLAIR), T_2WI, and T_2-FLAIR. Consecutive slices were acquired in all sequences. DTI was performed in a spin echo-echo planar imaging (SE-EPI) diffusion tensor sequence in the axial plane right after the conventional sequences scanning ($b = 0/1000 \, \text{s/mm}^2$; diffusion-sensitive gradient direction = 13; voxel size = $0.9 \, \text{mm} \times 0.9 \, \text{mm} \times 0.9 \, \text{mm}$). The acquisition parameters of each sequence were listed in Table 1.

2.4. Data Analysis. The neoplasm of each subject was defined in the occipital horn planes of T_1WI and T_2WI images.

DTI datasets were processed using Volume One 1.72 (GE Healthcare, USA) and Diffusion Tensor Visualizer 1.72 software (Tokyo University, Tokyo, Japan). In the control group, region of interest (ROI) of GCT was drawn on the axial directionally encoded color (DEC) image in the occipital horn plane (Figure 1(a)). To investigate the diffusion indices of GCT in peritumoral edema area, select the most edematous area adjacent to neoplasm as the ROI in the study group (Figures 2(b), 3(b), and 4(b), circles). Obtain the FA and MD values of each ROI. Repeat the measurement by the same reader in three continuous slices, three ROIs each slice. Obtain the mean value of all the measurements as the final result of FA and MD values of each ROI.

Perform DTT on GCT by the line propagation techniques. The lateral geniculate body (LGB), which is located at the posterior lateral of thalamus, was taken as the seed point and the occipital lobe as the termination in the cross plane of DEC image. The termination of tractography was as follows: FA < 0.15, step < 160, and So < 120. Repeat the measurement by two readers with similar experience in DTI [16].

Witwer et al. [17] categorized the disruption of white matter (WM) tracts as edematous, displaced, and infiltrated in the following rules: (1) displaced: the WM tracts had abnormal pattern and location but normal FA values; (2) disrupted: the WM tracts disappeared in images with significant decrease in FA values; (3) infiltrated: the FA values decreased when compared with normal WM tracts. The WM tracts had abnormal pattern and location but they still can be identified by tractography.

2.5. Statistical Analysis. Two-sample t-test was used to compare the FA and MD values of GCT between the study group and the control group. One-way ANOVA was used to compare the FA and MD values of GCT in peritumoral edema area across tumor types. LSD t-test was used to compare the

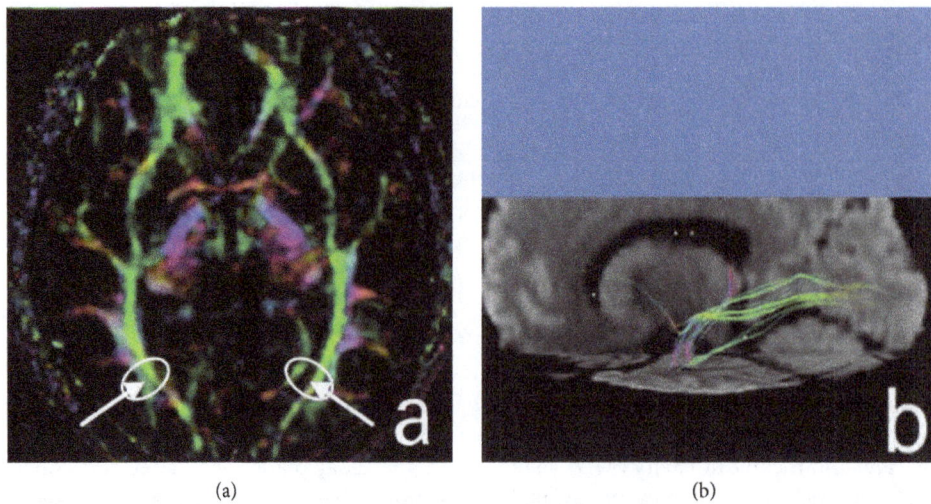

(a)   (b)

FIGURE 1: The GCT fibers ((a), white arrows) appear completely as green fiber tracts besides the paracele in healthy volunteers. It is a fiber tract from LGB and terminates in the calcarine fissure of occipital lobe (b).

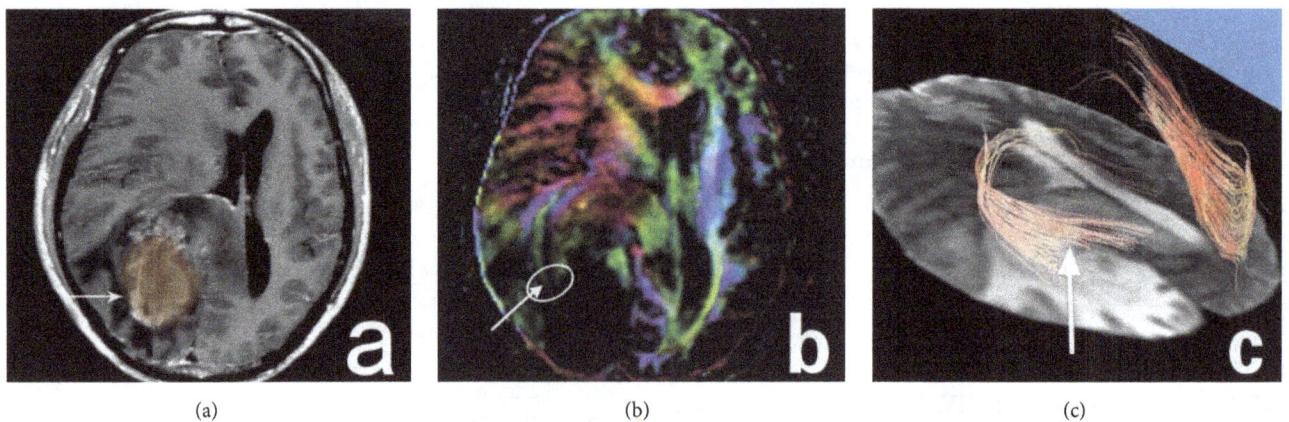

(a)   (b)   (c)

FIGURE 2: The contrast T_1WI image of right occipital lobe gliomas in a 55-year-old man ((a), arrow). The FA value of the right GCT decreases significantly and it can not be identified in the DEC map ((b), arrow). DTT map shows disruption and infiltration of the right GCT fibers ((c), arrow).

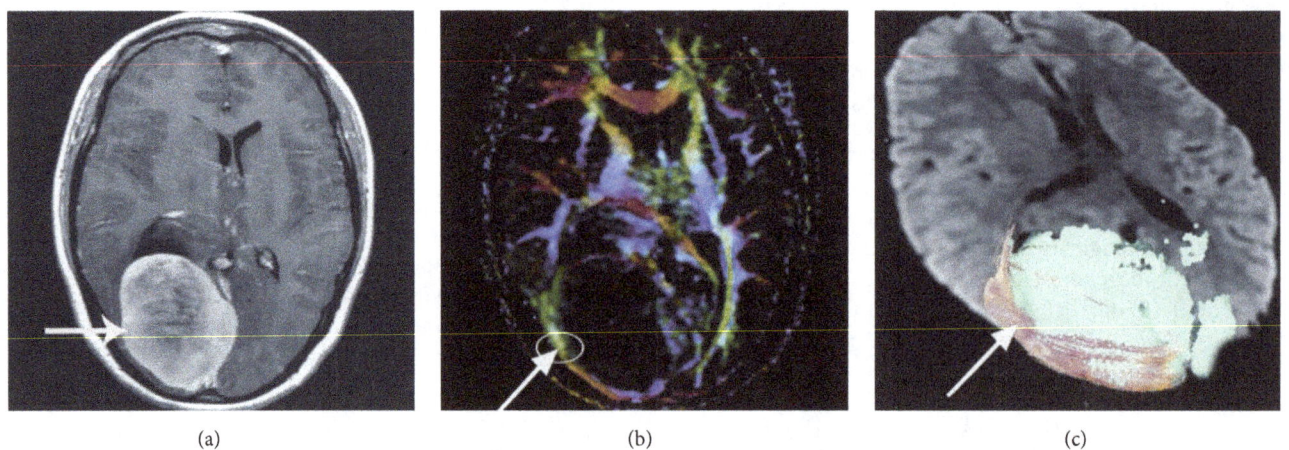

(a)   (b)   (c)

FIGURE 3: The contrast T_1WI image of right occipital lobe meningioma in a 42-year-old woman ((a), arrow). The FA value of right GCT decreases mildly ((b), arrow). DTT map shows the right GCT fibers are displaced ((c), arrow).

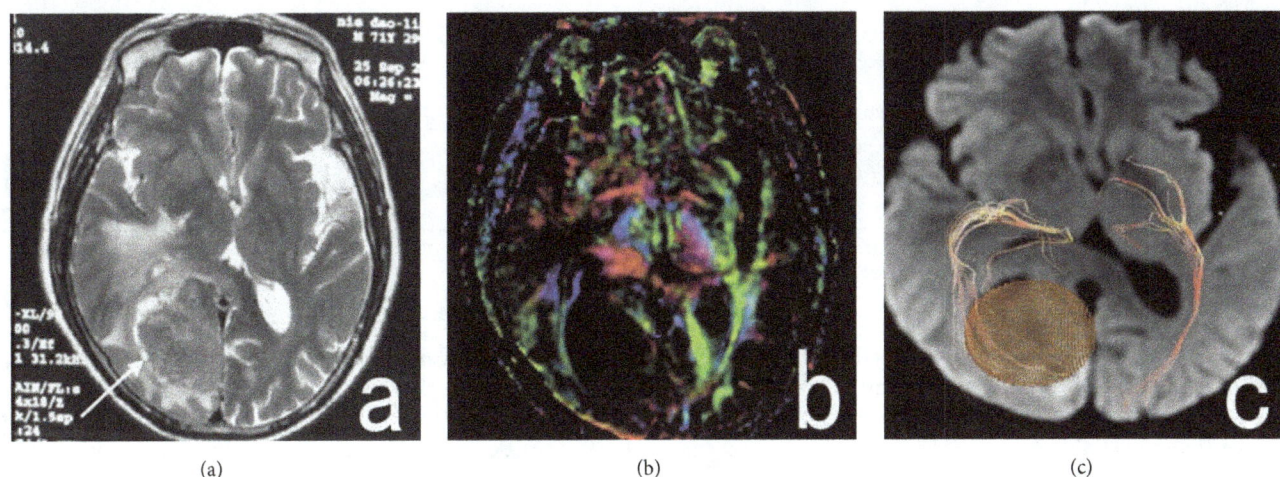

(a)   (b)   (c)

FIGURE 4: The T_2WI image of right occipital lobe metastases in a 71-year-old man ((a), arrow). The FA value of right GCT decreases ((b), arrow). DTT map shows the right GCT fibers ((c), arrow) are disrupted by the metastasis (brown mass).

FA and MD values of GCT between each two types of neoplasm. Kappa-test was used to test the consistency of different readers in categorizing GCT's deformation. $P < 0.05$ was used to determine statistical significance. All analyses were performed by the Statistical Package for the Social Sciences software, Version 13.0 (SPSS, Chicago, Illinois, USA).

3. Results

The FA values of GCT in peritumoral edema area decreased ($P = 0.001$) while the MD values increased when compared with the control group ($P = 0.002$). The MD values of peritumoral edema area in the metastatic tumor group were higher than the other two groups ($P = 0.001$) while the FA values had no difference ($P = 0.114$) (Table 2).

The GCTs in healthy subjects were green fiber tracts besides the paracele triangular on DEC images (Figure 1).

GCT deformation differentiates in various types of neoplasm, which presents as round lesions in T_1WI and T_2WI images (Figures 2(a), 3(a), and 4(a), arrows). The two readers had consistency in categorizing GCTs deformation ($K = 0.784$). The GCTs in gliomas group were all infiltrated (9 cases). The GCTs in grade II gliomas were displaced (2 in 9 cases). But the GCTs in grades III and IV gliomas were disrupted (7 in 9 cases) (Figure 2(c)). The GCTs in meningiomas were compressed and shifted without disruption (Figure 3(c)). DTT images showed that GCT in metastases all had displacement (17 cases), and some companied with disruption (7 in 17 cases) (Figure 4(c)).

4. Discussion

The FA values of GCT in peritumoral edema area decreased while the MD values increased when compared with the control group. FA value stands for the anisotropy of water molecules in each voxel. Decreased FA value may be due to the disorganization of axons and disruption of myelin sheath and the increase in extracellular water content [18].

In peritumoral edema area, the ordered axonal arrangements and the integrity of myelin sheath are damaged. The diffusion resistance decreases with the disintegration of these restrictive barriers. The water molecules lose their directivity parallel to the fiber tract and present in a chaotic state. The extracellular space and the water content of tissues increase in peritumoral edema area, which induce MD value to increase [19].

The FA values of GCT in peritumoral edema area had no difference across tumor types in our study (Table 2). Provenzale et al. made the same conclusion from their investigation. They found that the difference in FA decrease in peritumoral hyperintense regions was not significant between glioma and meningiomas [20]. Lu et al. also found that the peritumoral FA value did not differ significantly between high grade gliomas and metastatic tumors [21]. However, peritumoral fiber tracts alterations in gliomas were more complex as described so far since there were competing findings [20–22]. Investigating and categorizing peritumoral fiber tract alterations with FA values may not be credible enough to make a conclusion. Not only tumoral infiltration but also increase of water content in mesenchyme caused by the damage of blood brain barrier and blood-vessel osmotic increase can be found in the peritumoral hyperintensive regions of high grade gliomas. Using multimodel neuroimaging tools may provide more complementary information and understanding of it [22].

The MD values of GCT in peritumoral edema area in metastatic tumor group were higher than the other two groups (Table 2). This was in accordance with Lu et al.'s study that the peritumoral MD of metastatic lesions measured significantly greater than that of gliomas [21]. MD values increase with the water content of tissue and suggest vasogenic edema. The extracellular space also increases in the presence of elevated MD values. Some researchers considered that increased MD values suggest the infiltration of malignant cell, which destructed the ultrastructure in extracellular matrix and caused the movements of water molecules to be

TABLE 2: FA and MD of GCT in the study group and the control group ($\times 10^{-3}$ mm^2/s).

| | Control group | Study group | | | | | | | | P |
		(1) Gliomas	(2) Meningiomas	(3) Metastases	Total	P(1, 2, 3)	P(1-2)	P(1-3)	P(2-3)	
N	30	9	6	17	32					
FA	0.505 ± 0.028	0.205 ± 0.061	0.197 ± 0.028	0.171 ± 0.285	0.192 ± 0.125	0.114	0.978	0.306	0.245	0.001
MD	0.735 ± 0.047	1.379 ± 0.186	1.335 ± 0.202	1.695 ± 0.270	1.467 ± 0.218	0.001	0.964	0.003	0.015	0.002

P is the value of comparison between the study group and the control group.
P(1, 2, 3) is the value of comparison across tumor types.

less restricted [23]. But most of researchers thought that a reliable differentiation between infiltration and vasogenic edema is not yet possible on the basis of DTI parameters [24, 25]. For instance, Tropine et al. determined that the FA and MD can not differentiate between accompanying edema and tumor cell infiltration of WM beyond the tumor edge in gliomas [26]. Kinoshita et al. also concluded that diffusion tensor-based tumor infiltration index cannot discriminate vasogenic edema from tumor-infiltrated edema from investigation with meningioma and glioma [27].

In our study, the disruption of GCT varied in different neoplasm. The pattern and location of displaced GCTs change but the fiber integrity keeps normal, which means the axons are not destructed. Displaced GCTs are mostly seen in meningioma. As the most frequent intracalvarium benign tumor is located outside the brain, meningioma shifts and compresses the brain but does not destroy WM tracts [28]. The function of GCT in subject with meningioma may recover when the lesion has been removed. Many metastatic tumors also cause the displacement of GCT when they are far away from it. Yet displacement always companies with disruption when the GCTs are in close relationship with metastatic tumors [29].

The FA values of disrupted GCT decreased significantly. This suggests a reduction in axonal density and arrangement of the GCT so its prognosis is pessimistic. The movement of water molecule along the fiber of GCT is constrained by the axon sheath [26, 29, 30]. The destruction of axons will cause water molecules to lose their directivity parallel to the fiber tract and present in a chaotic state, which leads to significant decrease of FA. WM tract disruption always develops in high grade (grades III and IV) gliomas and metastatic tumors. GCTs in high grade gliomas and metastatic tumors were disrupted with adjacent white matter infiltrated in our study.

Infiltration is a deformation between displacement and disruption. The infiltrated GCT has abnormal pattern and location with decreased FA values but still can be identified in FA images. This suggests that the axonal destructions are less serious than the disrupted ones. Infiltrated GCTs all developed in gliomas in our study. This may be because gliomas originate from myelin sheath gliocytes without specific boundary from normal nervous tissue. GCT is gradually destructed by malignant tumor cells in high grade gliomas.

Though the FA and MD in peritumoral edema area can not supply certain information for the involved tracts, they supply a direction to investigate tracts' alterations and potentially predictions of patients' prognosis [31, 32]. As a noninvasive technique to evaluate the WM integrity and fiber connectivity in vivo, DTI can assist neurosurgeons in identifying conditions occult to structural imaging and provide relational information that is critical to neurosurgery decision making [33]. Even if the classification of WM tracts' disruption in neoplasm lacks unified standard and seems to be oversimplified, DTT still acts as the most visual method for presenting function damage and estimating possible outcome from stereoscopic images of target WM tracts so far.

5. Conclusion

In this study, we investigated the disruption of GCT in different occipital neoplasm by DTI. The disruption of GCT varies according to the properties of neoplasm and can be categorized as disrupted, displaced, and infiltrated. DTI indices represent valid markers for GCT disruption in occipital lobe neoplasm.

Abbreviations

DTI: Diffusion tensor imaging
DTT: Diffusion tensor tractography
GCT: Geniculocalcarine tract
FA: Fractional anisotropy
MD: Mean diffusivity
FLAIR: Fluid attenuated inversion recovery
SE-EPI: Spin echo-echo planar imaging
DEC: Directionally encoded color
ROI: Regions of interest
LGB: Lateral geniculate body
WM: White matter.

Competing Interests

There are no competing interests.

Acknowledgments

This work was supported by Natural Science Foundation of Guangdong Province (no. 2015A030313076) and Fundamental Research Funds of the State Key Laboratory of Ophthalmology.

References

[1] A. Stadlbauer, C. Nimsky, R. Buslei et al., "Diffusion tensor imaging and optimized fiber tracking in glioma patients: histopathologic evaluation of tumor-invaded white matter structures," NeuroImage, vol. 34, no. 3, pp. 949–956, 2007.

[2] R. Kleiser, P. Staempfli, A. Valavanis, P. Boesiger, and S. Kollias, "Impact of fMRI-guided advanced DTI fiber tracking techniques on their clinical applications in patients with brain tumors," *Neuroradiology*, vol. 52, no. 1, pp. 37–46, 2010.

[3] I.-F. Talos, K. H. Zou, R. Kikinis, and F. A. Jolesz, "Volumetric assessment of tumor infiltration of adjacent white matter based on anatomic MRI and diffusion tensor tractography," *Academic Radiology*, vol. 14, no. 4, pp. 431–436, 2007.

[4] I. S. Khayal, S. R. Vandenberg, K. J. Smith et al., "MRI apparent diffusion coefficient reflects histopathologic subtype, axonal disruption, and tumor fraction in diffuse-type grade II gliomas," *Neuro-Oncology*, vol. 13, no. 11, pp. 1192–1201, 2011.

[5] S. Y. Chun, K. C. Li, Y. Xuan, M. J. Xun, and W. Qin, "Diffusion tensor tractography in patients with cerebral tumors: a helpful technique for neurosurgical planning and postoperative assessment," *European Journal of Radiology*, vol. 56, no. 2, pp. 197–204, 2005.

[6] J. Rademacher, U. Bürgel, S. Geyer et al., "Variability and asymmetry in the human precentral motor system: a cytoarchitectonic and myeloarchitectonic brain mapping study," *Brain*, vol. 124, no. 11, pp. 2232–2258, 2001.

[7] T. Beppu, T. Inoue, Y. Shibata et al., "Measurement of fractional anisotropy using diffusion tensor MRI in supratentorial astrocytic tumors," *Journal of Neuro-Oncology*, vol. 63, no. 2, pp. 109–116, 2003.

[8] S. Sinha, M. E. Bastin, I. R. Whittle, and J. M. Wardlaw, "Diffusion tensor MR imaging of high-grade cerebral gliomas," *American Journal of Neuroradiology*, vol. 23, no. 4, pp. 520–527, 2002.

[9] S. Wang, S. Kim, S. Chawla et al., "Differentiation between glioblastomas, solitary brain metastases, and primary cerebral lymphomas using diffusion tensor and dynamic susceptibility contrast-enhanced MR imaging," *American Journal of Neuroradiology*, vol. 32, no. 3, pp. 507–514, 2011.

[10] C.-H. Toh, M. Castillo, A. M.-C. Wong et al., "Primary cerebral lymphoma and glioblastoma multiforme: differences in diffusion characteristics evaluated with diffusion tensor imaging," *American Journal of Neuroradiology*, vol. 29, no. 3, pp. 471–475, 2008.

[11] V. A. Coenen, K. K. Huber, T. Krings, J. Weidemann, J. M. Gilsbach, and V. Rohde, "Diffusion-weighted imaging-guided resection of intracerebral lesions involving the optic radiation," *Neurosurgical Review*, vol. 28, no. 3, pp. 188–195, 2005.

[12] T. J. D. Byrnes, T. R. Barrick, B. A. Bell, and C. A. Clark, "Diffusion tensor imaging discriminates between glioblastoma and cerebral metastases in vivo," *NMR in Biomedicine*, vol. 24, no. 1, pp. 54–60, 2011.

[13] S. Chanraud, N. Zahr, E. V. Sullivan, and A. Pfefferbaum, "MR diffusion tensor imaging: a window into white matter integrity of the working brain," *Neuropsychology Review*, vol. 20, no. 2, pp. 209–225, 2010.

[14] N. R. Miller, "Diffusion tensor imaging of the visual sensory pathway: are we there yet?" *American Journal of Ophthalmology*, vol. 140, no. 5, pp. 896–897, 2005.

[15] M. B. Salmela, K. A. Cauley, T. Andrews, J. V. Gonyea, I. Tarasiewicz, and C. G. Filippi, "Magnetic resonance diffusion tensor imaging of the optic nerves to guide treatment of pediatric suprasellar tumors," *Pediatric Neurosurgery*, vol. 45, no. 6, pp. 467–471, 2010.

[16] J.-D. Tournier, S. Mori, and A. Leemans, "Diffusion tensor imaging and beyond," *Magnetic Resonance in Medicine*, vol. 65, no. 6, pp. 1532–1556, 2011.

[17] B. P. Witwer, R. Moftakhar, K. M. Hasan et al., "Diffusion-tensor imaging of white matter tracts in patients with cerebral neoplasm," *Journal of Neurosurgery*, vol. 97, no. 3, pp. 568–575, 2002.

[18] A. M. Ulug, D. F. Moore, A. S. Bojko, and R. D. Zimmerman, "Clinical use of diffusion-tensor imaging for diseases causing neuronal and axonal damage," *American Journal of Neuroradiology*, vol. 20, no. 6, pp. 1044–1048, 1999.

[19] Y. Zhang, S. Wan, and X. Zhang, "Geniculocalcarine tract disintegration after ischemic stroke: a diffusion tensor imaging study," *American Journal of Neuroradiology*, vol. 34, no. 10, pp. 1890–1894, 2013.

[20] J. M. Provenzale, P. McGraw, P. Mhatre, A. C. Guo, and D. Delong, "Peritumoral brain regions in gliomas and meningiomas: investigation with isotropic diffusion-weighted MR imaging and diffusion-tensor MR imaging," *Radiology*, vol. 232, no. 2, pp. 451–460, 2004.

[21] S. Lu, D. Ahn, G. Johnson, and S. Cha, "Peritumoral diffusion tensor imaging of high-grade gliomas and metastatic brain tumors," *American Journal of Neuroradiology*, vol. 24, no. 5, pp. 937–941, 2003.

[22] A. Stadlbauer, T. Hammen, P. Grummich et al., "Classification of peritumoral fiber tract alterations in gliomas using metabolic and structural neuroimaging," *Journal of Nuclear Medicine*, vol. 52, no. 8, pp. 1227–1234, 2011.

[23] K.-I. Morita, H. Matsuzawa, Y. Fujii, R. Tanaka, I. L. Kwee, and T. Nakada, "Diffusion tensor analysis of peritumoral edema using lambda chart analysis indicative of the heterogeneity of the microstructure within edema," *Journal of Neurosurgery*, vol. 102, no. 2, pp. 336–341, 2005.

[24] D. van Westen, J. Lätt, E. Englund, S. Brockstedt, and E.-M. Larsson, "Tumor extension in high-grade gliomas assessed with diffusion magnetic resonance imaging: values and lesion-to-brain ratios of apparent diffusion coefficient and fractional anisotropy," *Acta Radiologica*, vol. 47, no. 3, pp. 311–319, 2006.

[25] A. Server, B. Kulle, J. Mæhlen et al., "Quantitative apparent diffusion coefficients in the characterization of brain tumors and associated peritumoral edema," *Acta Radiologica*, vol. 50, no. 6, pp. 682–689, 2009.

[26] A. Tropine, G. Vucurevic, P. Delani et al., "Contribution of diffusion tensor imaging to delineation of gliomas and glioblastomas," *Journal of Magnetic Resonance Imaging*, vol. 20, no. 6, pp. 905–912, 2004.

[27] M. Kinoshita, T. Goto, Y. Okita et al., "Diffusion tensor-based tumor infiltration index cannot discriminate vasogenic edema from tumor-infiltrated edema," *Journal of Neuro-Oncology*, vol. 96, no. 3, pp. 409–415, 2010.

[28] G. X. Zhun, "Intracranial tumor," in *Practice of Internal Medicine*, J. Z. Chen, L. T. Liao, B. H. Yang, X. H. Weng, G. W. Lin, and Z. X. Pan, Eds., pp. 2683–2688, People's Medical Publishing House, Beijing, China, 12th edition, 2005.

[29] S.-K. Song, S.-W. Sun, M. J. Ramsbottom, C. Chang, J. Russell, and A. H. Cross, "Dysmyelination revealed through MRI as increased radial (but unchanged axial) diffusion of water," *NeuroImage*, vol. 17, no. 3, pp. 1429–1436, 2002.

[30] P. J. Basser, S. Pajevic, C. Pierpaoli, J. Duda, and A. Aldroubi, "In vivo fiber tractography using DT-MRI data," *Magnetic Resonance in Medicine*, vol. 44, no. 4, pp. 625–632, 2000.

[31] M. L. White, Y. Zhang, F. Yu, and S. A. Jaffar Kazmi, "Diffusion tensor MR imaging of cerebral gliomas: evaluating fractional anisotropy characteristics," *American Journal of Neuroradiology*, vol. 32, no. 2, pp. 374–381, 2011.

[32] S. Lu, D. Ahn, G. Johnson, M. Law, D. Zagzag, and R. I. Gross-man, "Diffusion-tensor MR imaging of intracranial neoplasia and associated peritumoral edema: Introduction of the tumor infiltration index," *Radiology*, vol. 232, no. 1, pp. 221–228, 2004.

[33] O. Ciccarelli, A. T. Toosy, G. J. M. Parker et al., "Diffusion tractography based group mapping of major white-matter pathways in the human brain," *NeuroImage*, vol. 19, no. 4, pp. 1545–1555, 2003.

Permissions

List of Contributors

Ujwala Shivarama Shetty
A J Institute of Dental Science and Hospital, Mangalore, Karnataka, India

Krishna N. Burde, Venkatesh G. Naikmasur and Atul P. Sattur
SDM College of Dental Science and Hospital, Dharwad, Karnataka, India

William D. Kerridge
Department of Radiology and Imaging Sciences, Indiana University School of Medicine, Indianapolis, IN 46202, USA

Oleksandr N. Kryvenko
Departments of Pathology and Urology, University of Miami Miller School of Medicine, Miami, FL 33136, USA

Afua Thompson
Department of Radiology, Meharry Medical College, Nashville, TN 37208, USA

Biren A. Shah
Department of Radiology, Henry Ford Hospital, Detroit, MI 48202, USA

Yasir Jamil Khattak, Rana Hamid Shoaib, Raza Sayani, Tanveer-ul Haq and Muhammad Awais
Department of Radiology, Aga Khan University Hospital, Karachi, Pakistan

Tariq Alam
Department of Radiology, French Medical Institute for Children, Aliabad, Kabul, Afghanistan

Daisuke Tsurumaru, Kiyohisa Hiraka, Masahiro Komori and Hiroshi Honda
Department of Clinical Radiology, Graduate School of Medical Sciences, Kyushu University, 3-1-1 Maidashi, Higashi-ku, Fukuoka City 812-8582, Japan

Yoshiyuki Shioyama
Department of Heavy Particle Therapy and Radiation Oncology, Graduate School of Medical Sciences, Kyushu University, 3-1-1 Maidashi, Higashi-ku, Fukuoka City 812-8582, Japan

Masaru Morita
3Department of Surgery and Sciences, Graduate School of Medical Sciences, Kyushu University, 3-1-1 Maidashi, Higashi-ku, Fukuoka City 812-8582, Japan

Muhammad Ali, Tanveer Ul Haq, Basit Salam, Madiha Beg, Raza Sayani and Muhammad Azeemuddin
Radiology Department, Aga Khan University Hospital, Stadium Road

Pankaj Gupta, Anindita Sinha, Kushaljit Singh Sodhi, Anupam Lal, Uma Debi and Niranjan Khandelwal
Department of Radiodiagnosis and Imaging, Post Graduate Institute of Medical Education and Research (PGIMER), Chandigarh 160012, India

Babu R. Thapa
Pediatric Gastroenterology, Post Graduate Institute of Medical Education and Research (PGIMER), Chandigarh 160012, India

Thorsten Jentzsch, James Geiger, Stefan M. Zimmermann, Ksenija Slankamenac and Clément M. L. Werner
Division of Trauma Surgery, Department of Surgery, University Hospital Zürich, Rämistrasse 100, 8091 Zürich, Switzerland

Thi Dan Linh Nguyen-Kim
Institute of Diagnostic and Interventional Radiology, University Hospital Zürich, Rämistrasse 100, 8091 Zürich, Switzerland

J. Gossner
Department of Clinical Radiology, G̈ottingen-Weende Hospital, An der Lutter 24, 37074 Göttingen, Germany

R. Nau
Department of Geriatric Medicine, G̈ottingen-Weende Hospital, An der Lutter 24, 37074 Göttingen, Germany

Sunita Dhanda
Department of Diagnostic Imaging, National University Hospital, Level 2, Main Building, 5 Lower Kent Ridge Road, Singapore 119074
Tata Memorial Hospital, Dr. E. Borges Marg, Parel, Mumbai, Maharashtra 400012, India

Subhash Ramani and Meenkashi Thakur
Tata Memorial Hospital, Dr. E. Borges Marg, Parel, Mumbai, Maharashtra 400012, India

Catherine Maldjian, Vineet Khanna and Richard Adam
Department of Radiology, University of Pittsburgh, Pittsburgh, PA 15213-2582, USA

James Bradley
Department of Orthopedic Surgery, UPMC, Pittsburgh, PA 15213-2582, USA

Nieves Gómez León and Beatriz Bandrés
Department of Radiology, Research Institute La Princesa, La Princesa University Hospital, C/Diego de León 62, 28006Madrid, Spain

Sofía Escalona and Daniel Callejo
Health Technology Assessment Unit, Lain Entralgo Agency, C/Gran Vía 27, 28013 Madrid, Spain

Cristobal Belda
National School of Health, Sinesio Delgado 4, 28029 Madrid, Spain

Juan Antonio Blasco
Health Technology Assessment Unit, Lain Entralgo Agency, C/Gran V´ıa 27, 28013 Madrid, Spain
Institute for Health and Consumer Protection, Joint Research Centre, European Commission, Via E. Fermi 2749, 21027 Ispra, Italy

Pedro A. Gómez Damián
GE Global Research, 85748 Garching bei München, Germany
Medical Engineering, Tecnológico de Monterrey, 64849 Monterrey, NL, Mexico
Medical Engineering, Technische Universität München, 85748 Garching bei München, Germany

Jonathan I. Sperl, Floriann Wiesinger, Rolf F. Schulte and Marion I. Menzel
GE Global Research, 85748 Garching bei München, Germany

Martin A. Janich
GE Global Research, 85748 Garching bei München, Germany
Nuclear Medicine, Technische Universität München, 81675 Munich, Germany
Chemistry, Technische Universität München, 85748 Garching bei München, Germany

Oleksandr Khegai
GE Global Research, 85748 Garching bei München, Germany
Chemistry, Technische Universität München, 85748 Garching bei München, Germany

Steffen J. Glaser
Chemistry, Technische Universität München, 85748 Garching bei München, Germany

Axel Haase
Medical Engineering, Technische Universität München, 85748 Garching bei München, Germany

Markus Schwaiger
Nuclear Medicine, Technische Universität München, 81675 Munich, Germany

Elahe Pirayesh, Mahasti Amoui and Maryam Khorrami
Department of Nuclear Medicine, Shohada-e-Tajrish Medical Center, Shahid Beheshti University of Medical Sciences, Tehran, Iran

Shahram Akhlaghpoor
Department of Interventional Radiology, Noor Medical Imaging Center, Tehran, Iran

Shahnaz Tolooee, Hossain Poor Beigi and Shahab Sheibani
Department of Nuclear Sciences, Iranian Atomic Energy Organization, Tehran, Iran

Majid Assadi
The Persian Gulf Nuclear Medicine Research Center, Bushehr University of Medical Sciences, Bushehr, Iran

Morteza Sanei Taheri, Mohammad Ali Karimi, Hamidreza Haghighatkhah and Ramin Pourghorban
Department of Radiology, Shohada-e-Tajrish Hospital, Shahid Beheshti University of Medical Sciences, Tehran, Iran

Mohammad Samadian
Department of Neurosurgery, Loghman Hakim Hospital, Shahid Beheshti University of Medical Sciences, Tehran, Iran

Hosein Delavar Kasmaei
Department of Neurology, Shohada-e-Tajrish Hospital, Shahid Beheshti University of Medical Sciences, Tehran, Iran

Manabu Watanabe, Takashi Ikehara, Michio Kogame, Mie Shinohara, Masao Shinohara, Koji Ishii, Yoshinori Igarashi and Yasukiyo Sumino
Division of Gastroenterology and Hepatology, Department of Internal Medicine, Toho University Medical Center, Omori Hospital, 6-11-1 Omorinishi, Ota-ku, Tokyo 143-8541, Japan

Hiroyuki Makino
Division of Gastroenterology and Hepatology, Department of Internal Medicine, Saiseikai Yokohamashi Tobu Hospital, 3-6-1 Shimosueyoshi, Tsurumi-ku, Yokohama-shi, Kanagawa 230-0012, Japan

Kazue Shiozawa
Division of Gastroenterology and Hepatology, Department of Internal Medicine, Toho University Medical Center, Omori Hospital, 6-11-1 Omorinishi, Ota-ku, Tokyo 143-8541, Japan
Division of Gastroenterology and Hepatology, Department of Internal Medicine, Saiseikai Yokohamashi Tobu Hospital, 3-6-1 Shimosueyoshi, Tsurumi-ku, Yokohama-shi, Kanagawa 230- 0012, Japan

João Palas, António P. Matos and Miguel Ramalho
Radiology Department, Hospital Garcia de Orta, 2801-951 Almada, Portugal

Boniface Moifo
Department of Radiology and Radiation Oncology, Faculty of Medicine and Biomedical Sciences, The University of Yaoundé, Yaoundé, Cameroon
Radiology Department, YaoundéI Gynaecology, Obstetrics and Pediatrics Hospital (YGOPH), YaoundéI, Cameroon

Ulrich Tene, Justine Tchemtchoua Youta and Joseph Gonsu Fotsin
Department of Radiology and Radiation Oncology, Faculty of Medicine and Biomedical Sciences, The University of Yaoundé, Yaoundé, Cameroon

Jean Roger Moulion Tapouh
Department of Radiology and Radiation Oncology, Faculty of Medicine and Biomedical Sciences, The University of Yaoundé, Yaoundé, Cameroon
Radiology Department, Yaoundé University Teaching Hospital Yaoundé, Cameroon

Odette Samba Ngano
Department of Radiation Oncology, Yaoundé General Hospital, Yaoundé, Cameroon

Augustin Simo
National Radiation Protection Agency (NRPA), Yaoundé, Cameroon

Shamar J. Young and Tina S. Sanghvi
Department of Radiology, University of Minnesota, 420 Delaware St SE, Minneapolis, MN 55455, USA

Ronald G. Quisling and Sharatchandra Bidari
Department of Diagnostic Radiology, University of Florida, 1600 SW Archer Rd, Gainesville, FL 32610, USA

Sharon Chen
Department of Medical Imaging and Radiological Sciences, Kaohsiung Medical University, Kaohsiung 807, Taiwan

Yu-Chang Tyan
Department of Medical Imaging and Radiological Sciences, Kaohsiung Medical University, Kaohsiung 807, Taiwan
Center for Infectious Disease and Cancer Research, Kaohsiung Medical University, Kaohsiung 807, Taiwan
Graduate Institute of Medicine, College of Medicine, Kaohsiung Medical University, Kaohsiung 807, Taiwan
Institute of Medical Science and Technology, National Sun Yat-sen University, Kaohsiung, Taiwan

Jui-Jen Lai and Chin-Ching Chang
Department of Medical Imaging, Kaohsiung Medical University Hospital, Kaohsiung 807, Taiwan

Lucie Sukupova
Department of the Director, Institute for Clinical and Experimental Medicine, Videnska 1958/9, 140 21 Prague 4, Czech Republic

Ondrej Hlavacek and Daniel Vedlich
Radiodiagnostic and Interventional Radiology Department, Institute for Clinical and Experimental Medicine, Videnska 1958/9, 140 21 Prague 4, Czech Republic

Emma Olsson, Ronnie Wirestam and Emelie Lind
Department of Medical Radiation Physics, Lund University, Skåne University Hospital Lund, 22185 Lund, Sweden

Anna-Katharina Breu, Till-Karsten Hauser, Ulrike Ernemann and Achim Seeger
Department of Diagnostic and Interventional Neuroradiology, Eberhard Karls University, Hoppe-Seyler-Street 3, 72076 Tübingen, Germany

Florian H. Ebner
Department of Neurosurgery, Eberhard Karls University, Hoppe-Seyler-Street 3, 72076 Tübingen, Germany

Felix Bischof
Department of Neurology, Eberhard Karls University, Hoppe-Seyler-Street 3, 72076 Tübingen, Germany

Johanna Mårtensson and Elna-Marie Larsson
Department of Surgical Sciences, Radiology, Uppsala University, 75105 Uppsala, Sweden

Anna F. Delgado
Department of Surgical Sciences, Radiology, Uppsala University, 75105 Uppsala, Sweden
Department of Neuroradiology, Karolinska University Hospital, Department of Clinical Neuroscience, Karolinska Institute, 17177 Stockholm, Sweden

Markus Nilsson
Bioimaging Center, Lund University, 22100 Lund, Sweden

Francesco Latini and Maria Zetterling
Department of Neuroscience, Neurosurgery, Uppsala University, 75105 Uppsala, Sweden

Shala G. Berntsson
Department of Neuroscience, Neurology, Uppsala University, 75105 Uppsala, Sweden

Irina Alafuzoff
Section of Pathology, Uppsala University Hospital and Department of Immunology, Genetics and Pathology, Uppsala University, 75105 Uppsala, Sweden

Jimmy Lätt
MR Department, Centre for Medical Imaging and Physiology, Lund University Hospital, 22185 Lund, Sweden

Fernando Ruiz Santiago, Luis Guzmán Álvarez, Maria del Mar Castellano García and Alberto Martínez Martínez
Radiology Department, Hospital of Traumatology, Carretera de Jaen, S/N, 18014 Granada, Spain

Alicia Santiago Chinchilla
Radiology Department, Ciudad Sanitaria Virgen de las Nieves, Avenida de las Fuerzas Armadas 2, 18014 Granada, Spain

Afshin Ansari
Radiology Department, North Tyneside General Hospital, Rake Lane, North Shields NE29 8NH, UK

Juan Tercedor Sánchez
Orthopedic Department, Hospital of Traumatology, Carretera de Jaen, S/N, 18014 Granada, Spain

Yan Zhang
Zhongshan Ophthalmic Center, State Key Laboratory of Ophthalmology, Sun Yat-sen University, Guangzhou, Guangdong 510060, China

Sihai Wan
Department of Radiology, Lu Shan Sanatorium, Nanjing Military Region, Jiujiang, Jiangxi 332000, China

Ge Wen and Xuelin Zhang
Department of Radiology, Nanfang Hospital, Southern Medical University, Guangzhou, Guangdong 510515, China

Index

www.ingramcontent.com/pod-product-compliance
Lightning Source LLC
Chambersburg PA
CBHW080514200326
41458CB00012B/4207